NEURODEGENERATIVE DISEASES

Edited by **Uday Kishore**

Neurodegenerative Diseases
http://dx.doi.org/10.5772/45957
Edited by Uday Kishore

Contributors

Alexander Gow, Ferihan Cetin, George E. Barreto, Ricardo Cabezas, Marco Fidel Ávila, Janneth Gonzalez, Ramon El-Bachá, Ludis Morales, Daniel Torrente, Juan Andres Orellana, Masahiro Kawahara, Tomohiro Chiba, Zhang, Luca Lovrecic, Stavros J Baloyannis, Cenk Suphioglu, Justin Read, Yang, Ivana Delalle, Manuel J Rojas, Camilo Orozco Sanabria, Francisco Olea, Christian Lefebvre D'Hellencourt, Avinash Parimisetty, Rana Awada, Antonio Ibarra, Humberto Mestre, Daniel Zajarias-Fainsod, Yael Cohen-Minian, Eyer, Eva Babusikova, Marisol Herrera-Rivero, Yusuf Tutar, Aykut Ozgur, Lutfi Tutar, Weili Xu, Anna Marseglia, Camilla Ferrari, Hui-Xin Wang, Iuliana Nicola-Antoniu, Analava Mitra, Faraz Farooq, Martin Holcik, Alex MacKenzie, Uday Kishore

Published by InTech

Janeza Trdine 9, 51000 Rijeka, Croatia

Publishing Process Manager Iva Simcic
Technical Editor InTech DTP team
Cover InTech Design team

Additional hard copies can be obtained from orders@intechopen.com

Neurodegenerative Diseases, Edited by Uday Kishore
p. cm.
ISBN 978-953-51-1088-0

For EU product safety concerns:
IN TECH d.o.o., Prolaz Marije Krucifikse Kozulić 3, 51000 Rijeka, Croatia,
info@intechopen.com or visit our website at intechopen.com.

Meet the editor

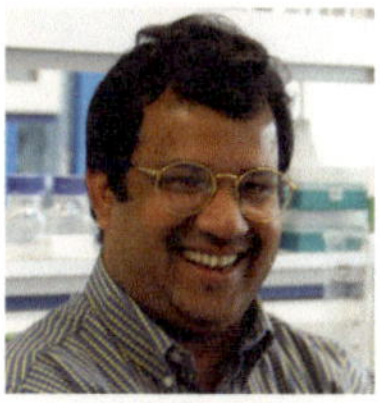

Dr. Uday Kishore is the Director of the Centre for Infection, Immunity and Disease Mechanisms, Brunel University, London. He earned his MSc and PhD from the University of Delhi, India, followed by post-doctoral training at the Salk Institute, California, USA and University of Oxford, UK (MRC Immunochemistry Unit and Weatherall Institute of Molecular Medicine, John Radcliffe Hospital). He has been a recipient of fellowships awarded by NASA, Wellcome Trust, Humboldt Foundation and Medical Research Council. Dr Kishore has authored over 80 peer-reviewed research papers, edited two books, and is currently writing a text book on host pathogen interaction. In addition to innate immunity, complement system and host-pathogen interaction, Dr Kishore's research interests include dissecting role of complement system in neuroinflammation and neurodegeneration.

Contents

Preface

It is my pleasure to present to you this book that I edited with great interest and anticipation. My own research interests include examining the role of complement proteins in neuroinflammation and neurodegeneration using the models of Alzheimer's disease as well as British and Danish familial dementia. However, through my own studies and during the course of editing this book, it became evident that one needs to have a holistic view about the pathophysiology of various neurodegenerative diseases. These are multi-factorial and complex disease processes that require a range of multi-disciplinary approaches from various angles and directions in order to achieve diagnostic and therapeutic outcomes. This book is a small but significant step in highlighting the complexities of issues relevant for basic and translational research in the area of neuroinflammation and neurodegeneration.

The book has three major sections addressing disease mechanisms and therapeutic interventions in Alzheimer's disease, followed by generic mechanisms in other forms of the neurodegenerative diseases. The book ends with its last miscellaneous section that is a small conglomeration of chapters on Spinal Muscular Atrophy, Acute Ischemic Stroke, and Cognitive dysfunction syndrome. I sincerely hope that this book is an exciting point of reference for many clinical and non-clinical neuroscientists.

I am ever so indebted to all the authors who have contributed various chapters for this book. I am also grateful to Daria Nahtigal and Iva Simcic of the InTech Europe for inviting me to edit this book. I would like to thank Dr Annapurna Nayak, Dr Patrick Waters, Dr Marco Bonifati, Dr Abhishek Shastri and Dr Janez Ferluga for stimulating discussions during the course of editing this book. Many thanks are also due to Prof Bob Sim, Prof Nick Willcox and Prof Angela Vincent for priming me into the field of neuroimmunology.

Dr Uday Kishore
Director
Centre for Infection, Immunity and Disease Mechanisms
Brunel University
London, UK

Section 1

Disease Mechanisms in Alzheimer's Disease

Chapter 1

Alzheimer's Disease: A Clinical Perspective

Weili Xu, Anna Marseglia, Camilla Ferrari and Hui-Xin Wang

Additional information is available at the end of the chapter

http://dx.doi.org/10.5772/54539

1. Introduction

Dementia is defined as a clinical syndrome characterized by progressive deterioration in multiple cognitive domains that are severe enough to interfere with daily functioning, including social and professional functioning. Alzheimer disease (AD) is the most common form of dementia often diagnosed in people over 65 years old, even though the early-onset AD can occur much earlier since 40 years of age. AD is a multifactorial disorder in which the causes and the progression are still not well-understood. Aging is the most common non-modifiable cause of dementia in the elderly, but it accounts only for approximately half of all cause. Research identified other potential causes among the interaction between modifiable environmental factors, such as vascular disease and genetic susceptibility. The recent genetic discoveries have shown that mutation of the β-amyloid precursor protein on chromosome 21, and the mutations of presenilin 1 and presenilin 2 on chromosome 14 and 1, were associated with increased susceptibility of AD. Finally, the presence of the ε4 allele of Apolipoprotein E (APOE) is considered as a risk factor for late-onset of AD. The Diagnostic and Statistical Manual on Mental Disorders, fourth edition text revised (DSM-IV-TR), defines dementia as an acquired disease characterized by decline in memory and at least one other cognitive function such as attention, visuo-spatial skills, language, or executive functions. Beside the cognition, the disease affects the emotional abilities and interferes significantly with work and daily-life activities. Dementia can be defined as either possible, or probable based on the recent published diagnostic criteria [1]. Since 1980s, numerous community-based prospective studies of aging and health have been implemented in the world; many of which have focused on dementia and its main subtypes of AD and vascular dementia (VaD). In this Chapter, we review the literature of clinical and epidemiological research in the dementias by focusing on most recent studies.

AD is an age-related phenomenon and is the most common cause of dementia, but increasing evidence from population-based neuropathological and neuroimaging studies shows that mixed brain pathology (neurodegenerative and vascular) account for a large number of dementia cases, especially in very old people [2]. According to the World Alzheimer Report, there were 35.6 million people living with dementia worldwide in 2010, a number that will increase to 65.7 million by 2030 and 115.4 million by 2050 unless effective means of reducing disease incidence are introduced. The total estimated worldwide costs of dementia were US $604 billion in 2010, including the costs of informal care, direct costs of social care, and the direct costs of medical care [3]. Increasing age is a well-established risk factor for dementia and AD. Both prevalence and incidence of AD increases exponentially with advancing age, and 70% of all dementia cases occur in people aged 75+ years [4]. Notwithstanding, despite the incidence rate of AD increases almost exponentially until 85 years of age, it remains uncertain whether the incidence continues to increase even at more advances ages or reaches a plateau [5]. In Europe, the age-adjusted prevalence is 6.4% for dementia in general, and 4.4% for AD among people 65 years and older [6]. In the US, has been estimated that the 9.7% of people aged 70+ years has AD [7]. More than 25 million people in the world are affected by dementia; most of them suffer from AD, with about 5 million new cases every year [8, 9]. The estimated global annual incidence is around 7.5 per 1000 people [8]. The incident rate increases from approximately one per 1000 person-year in people aged 60-64 to more than 70 per 1000 person-year in 90+ years-old. In Europe, the pooled incidence rate of AD in people aged 65 years and older was 19.4 per 1000 person-year. The incidence rates of AD across different regions are quite similar in the younger-old, but greater variations have been seen among the older ages, but this is probably because of differences in methodology such as study designs and case ascertainment [5]. In conclusion, the worldwide population aging explains the epidemic proportions for dementia making the disease an important issue for the public health.

2. Pathogenesis and mechanisms of AD

Alzheimer's disease has not a single cause but is the results of the interaction of multiple mechanisms that can be grouped into aging, genetic influence, vascular pathology, inflammation and environmental influence such as toxic exposure. However, currently, the precise pathogenesis of AD is not known. One of the most important pathologic features characterising AD is the brain atrophy which results by loss of neurons, synapses and dendritic arborization in the cerebral cortex and subcortical regions. Cerebral atrophy is associated with the presence of neurofibrillary tangles and amyloid plaques, two hallmarks over-expressed in AD brain [10]. Neurofibrillary tangles are insoluble aggregates of hyperphoshorylated microtubule-associated tau protein that become accumulate inside the cells themselves. Changes in tau protein lead to the disintegration of the brain microtubules, the main neuron's transport system [11]. Amyloid plaques are dense and insoluble extracellular deposits of β-amyloid peptide (Aβ). Aβ derived from APP protheolisis. This transmembrane protein is divided into smaller fragments by three different enzymes: α, β, and γ–secretases. The

http://dx.doi.org/10.5772/54539

cleavage of APP by β, and γ–secretases creates Aβ42 peptide, while the cleavage by α-secretase produce Aβ40. Aβ42 peptide aggregates more readily than Aβ 40, and the ratio of these two isoforms influence the formation of the senile plaques [12]. Genetic studies [13] have identified mutations in APP and presenilin 1 and 2 (components of the γ-secretase) that cause rare, dominantly inherited familial AD. These findings strongly supported the amyloid hypothesis [14], which posits that β-amyloid peptides play a pivotal role in AD pathogenesis. The amyloid cascade hypothesis suggests that deposition of Aβ triggers neuronal dysfunction and death in the brain. In the original hypothesis, this neuronal dysfunction and death was thought to be a toxic effect of the total amyloid load.

As knowledge of pathological changes in Alzheimer's disease increased, research identified Aβ oligomers as the principle players of the toxic effect [10]. Changes in tau phosphorylation status and consequent neurofibrillary tangles formation are also triggered by toxic concentrations of Aβ [14]. All the factors mentioned above (aging, genes, inflammation, and vascular pathology) can increase the production of Aβ. Despite genetic and cell biological evidence support the amyloid hypothesis [15], which is also the target of the new immunotherapies for AD, it is becoming clear that AD etiology is complex and that Aβ alone is unable to account for all the aspects of the disease. Others amyloid- independent hypothesis have been proposed [16]. The inflammatory hypothesis is based on the presence of activated microglia in AD brain. These cells, which have been shown to cluster around senile plaques, produce massive amounts of oxygen radicals and inflammatory mediators that are toxic to brain cells ultimately destroying them [17]. There is general agreement that the overproduction of free radicals generated from oxidative stress has a major role in neurodegeneration [18] and, as a reactive process, it may be involved in cell cycle regulation contributing to cell death [19]. In brain, a variety of stressants can induce oxidative stress as cerebral hypoperfusion, inflammation, aging, hypoxia, cigarette smoking, excess alcohol, or cardiovascular disease. There is also a vascular hypothesis that suggests that cerebral hypoperfusion in the presence of vascular risk factors can further lower cerebral blood flow to a critical level that threatens neuronal survival [20, 21]. Many other mechanisms have been suggested and can be involved in AD neurodegeneration, anyhow none hypothesis alone can explain the pathogenesis of AD [22].

3. Risk factors

The aetiology of dementia and AD has been extensively studied trying to find efficacious prevention and treatment strategies. As said, dementia is a multifactorial disorder caused by complex interaction between environmental and genetic factors. It has been estimated that 1-5% of AD cases are due to genetic mutations, while the most part are ascribable to modifiable environmental factors and their interaction with genetic susceptibility [10]. Age is the most powerful determinant of dementia, suggesting that aging-related biological process may be involved in the pathogenesis of AD [23]. In actuality, the association between age and AD is mediated by the cumulative effect of other risk and protective factors over the lifespan. The major risk and protective factors for AD can be summarized basing on the different etiological hypotheses including genetic susceptibility hypothesis, vascular pathway hypothesis, psychosocial hypothesis, nutrition and dietary hypothesis, and others (e.g., toxic or inflammatory factors). While the role of genetic, vascular and psychosocial factors in the AD onset is supported by strong to moderate epidemiological, neuroimaging and neuropathological researches, the evidences for the other factors are controversial and insufficient [5]. Following age, the presence of Apolipoprotein E ε4 allele (APOE ε4) is the most established genetic risk factor for developing late-onset AD. There are three forms of APOE alleles, ε2, ε3, and ε4, APOE ε4 increased the risk of AD by three times in heterozygote and more in homozygote, while ε2 decreases the risk [24, 25]. APOE allele ε4 is a susceptibility gene, being neither necessary nor sufficient for the development of AD.

In the last decade many others AD susceptibility genes have been identified, highlighting the importance of a genetic susceptibility for AD development [26]. Over the last decade, great attention has been paid to figure out which AD-related factors may be modified to decrease the risk of AD. Two groups of modifiable factors for late-life dementias have been identified as "vascular risk factors" that have been strongly associated with an increased risk of dementia; and the "psychosocial factors" that may contribute to the delay of dementia onset. Strong epidemiological evidences suggested that cardiovascular risk factors and vascular disease are associated with an increased risk of symptomatic AD [27].Thus, studies revealed age-dependents associations with AD for several aging-related conditions. The most important cardiovascular risk factors for subsequent AD include cigarette smoking [28, 29], heavy alcohol consumption [30], midlife high blood pressure [31], atrial fibrillation and heart failure [32], spontaneous cerebral emboli [33], midlife obesity or central adiposity as well as low BMI in late-life [34-36], midlife high cholesterol levels [37], diabetes mellitus and impaired glucose regulation [38-40], neuroinflammation [41, 42], and elevated plasma and total homocysteine levels [43].

Other risk factors for AD may include traumatic brain injury, late-life metabolic syndrome and depression, but their role is not clear and studies with long-term follow-up need to support the risk factors hypothesis [44, 45]. About psychological factors epidemiological research has been accumulating that some psychosocial factors and healthy lifestyle such as the social network and social engagement, weekly-to-daily physical activity, higher educational and socio-economic status and mentally stimulating activity, may postpone the onset of dementia by enhancing cognitive reserve [3, 46-48]. In addition, several studies reported a decreased risk of AD and dementia associated with a diet rich in both high polyunsaturated and fish-related fatty acids, such as the Mediterranean diet [49], and elevated levels of vitamin B_{12} and folate (50). Finally, controversy exists about the role of hormone replacement therapy with estrogens and progestin and subsequent development of AD. Several studies suggest that normal age-related depletion of estrogens in women and testosterone in men may represent potential risk factors for AD's onset [51], suggesting hormone replacement therapy (HRT) as method to reduce risk of late-life AD in postmenopausal women. Nevertheless, the therapeutic effects of HRT is not supported by the Cochrane's review, which found that HRT or estrogens for improving or maintaining cognition was not indicated for women with AD [52].

4. Clinical features

A peculiar feature of AD is the progressive and multi-focal cognitive deterioration characterized by the insidious onset, the absence of focal neurological signs, and memory disorders. It develops slowly and gets worse overtime. Progressing, the disease damages the most areas of the brain, and this is manifested through the gradually deterioration of memory, attention, executive functions, language, praxia, movement and personality. AD should be suspected when any individual, without alterations of awareness, refers generalized episodic memory disturbances with insidious onset that escalate up to interfere with daily living, social and/or occupational activities. In an attempt to help clinicians in recognizing the severity of disease, the Mayo Clinic group proposes three main stages in the natural history of AD, each characterized by distinctive symptoms and duration. The classification has been made based on clinical experience and generalization. It is not intended to be in an inflexible and taxonomic way, but it is important to realize that AD is the neurodegenerative process of the single person, and thus the duration and the type of symptoms may change from one patients to another. Considering that, it is helpful divide the AD progression into following stages: 1) "Early stage" characterized mainly by memory disorders; 2) "Moderate stage" where appears progressive cortical dysfunction (apraxia, aphasia, visuo-spatial disturbance) and disorders of instrumental functions; 3) "Advanced stage" with disorders of the "Control" functions and rise of neuropsychiatric disorders.

People may manifest mild symptoms long time before the clinical diagnosis of AD and often they are underestimated and mistakenly ascribe to either aging or stress. The early detection of symptoms is difficult because of the absence of a definite time of disease onset, so in the clinical practice patients with dementia are often first diagnosed when the disease is advanced to the early stage with the clear manifestation of cognitive and behavioural disorders [53]. The prodromal stage of the disease is known as "Mild cognitive impairment" (MCI) indicating those people likely to be in the earliest stage of dementia, but with so mild symptoms that cannot be formulate a formal diagnosis of dementia. Patients with MCI typically present forgetfulness due to the episodic memory impairment that leads to difficulties of recall and learning new information, but they do not have a clear deficit in daily functioning, being able to live independently with a minimal help [54]. Not all the subjects with MCI develop dementia, but all subjects affected by AD had first presented this mild stage. It is accepted that AD pathogenesis starts decades before clinical manifestation and that subjects decline slowly in cognition for years before meeting the diagnostic criteria for dementia [55, 56]. Longitudinal studies have shown that people with MCI have a high probability to develop dementia within 1-3 years after diagnosis [54]. When the progression of memory impairment and the decline in other cognitive domains (executive function, visuo-spatial, language, behaviour or personality) significantly interfere with the ability to function at work or at usual activities, the criteria for diagnosis of dementia are met [1]. The AD's "Mild stage" can last from 2 to 4 years. The typical scenario includes memory impairment for recent events with relative sparing for remote events (autobiographical memory), prospective memory disorders (remembering to perform a planned action or intention at the appropriate moment), difficulty with problem solving, complex task and sound judgment, difficulty to organize and express thoughts, deficit in the ability to plan and execute actions in a correct sequence (executive function and apraxia), slowing in the ability to switch from one activity to another [54]. In addition, patients in the mild stage may start to present sporadic language disorders mainly characterized by decreased vocabulary and word fluency with a subsequent impoverishment of the speaking and writing [57].

Neurocognitive studies show that the episodic memory impairment is due to a deficit of storage newly acquired information in long-term memory [58] reflecting an early impairment of the "central executive" component of the working memory with relative sparing of the "slave systems". In this stage it is also likely that personality changes appear and the most prominent is apathy with symptoms of diminished interests and concerns and may be associated with depression. Social withdrawal, fluctuating mood, irritability or anxiety are less frequent. In some cases the non-cognitive symptoms may be more prominent than the cognitive impairment complicating the care of patients with AD. Despite that, they are not present in all patients and are not constantly progressive as the cognitive deficits. Decreased attention and motivation to complete task as well as dresses inappropriately are also common. Towards the end of the mild stage, patients may start to be confused especially in unfamiliar place, reflecting the onset of orientation defects. The "Moderate stage" of AD is the longest stage lasting from 2 to 10 years. The cognitive and behavioural symptoms increase in the severity, people get more confused and forgetful and the progressive deterioration interfere with individual independence, with person being unable to perform most common daily living activities and self-care. On cognition, the middle stage is characterized by a progressive cortical dysfunction with prominent language, praxis, visuo-spatial, executive function and abstract reasoning disorders. Progressive deterioration of oral and written communication includes anomias of aphasic lexico-semantic origin that progress into a fluent aphasia, speech planning defects and "empty speech" because of inability to recall vocabulary which leads to semantic paraphasias, progressive loss of reading and writing. Ideational and ideo-motor apraxia is responsible for difficulties in number processing and calculation. Memory impairment worsen may involve also the autobiographical memory.

Disturbance of visuo-perceptual contour processing and spatial processing evolve leading to deficit in recognizing familiar faces (prosopagnosia) and person, geographical and environmental disorientation, difficulty in coping figure, and visual imagery deficits. Patients become less able to succeed the more demanding tasks of daily living, such as manage finances and driving. The personality and behavioural changes worsen. Psychotic behaviour, paranoia, delusions, auditory or visual hallucinations are not unusual in this stage. Common manifestations are labile affect, irritability, wandering, aggression or resistance to caregiver. Sleep disorders including disruption in the sleep/wake cycle, sundowning, and urinary incontinence can develop. Patients lose awareness of their disease process and limitation (anosognosia). In the AD's "Severe stage" (1-3+ years), patients generally lose the ability to communicate coherently, and experience a great decline in physical abilities becoming mostly dependent on caregiver for feeding and hygiene. Language is reduced to single simple phrases or words. Despite the severity of communication problem, people can understand and return emotional signal. On the behavioural level, aggressiveness can be still present, but severe apathy and exhaustion are common symptoms. Neu-

http://dx.doi.org/10.5772/54539

rological disorders (tonic grasping, echolalia, oral grasping, Kluver-Bucy syndrome and bilateral apraxia), and motor abnormalities can develop. Muscle mass and mobility deteriorate until the patient is completely bedridden and not self-sufficient. People with AD typically die from medical complication as bronchitis, pneumonia, or pressure ulcers, and not because of disease itself [59, 60].

5. Alzheimer's disease diagnosis

The 1984 criteria made by the National Institute of Neurologic, Communicative Disorders and Stroke/Alzheimer's disease and Related Disorders Association (NINCDS-ADRDA) work group [61] were based on doctor's clinical judgment about the cause of patient's symptoms, taking into account reports from the patient and family members, and results of cognitive tests and general neurological assessment. These criteria have been quite successful and they have been widely used in clinical trials and clinical research, showing a sensitivity of 81% and specificity of 70% [62]. However, the increasing knowledge of the clinical manifestations and biology of AD determined the need of criteria revision. After 27 years, in 2011 the National Institute on Aging (NIA) and the Alzheimer's Association recommended new diagnostic criteria and guidelines for Alzheimer's disease [1,55,56]. The notable changes of the 2011 criteria are mainly due to the concept that the pathophysiological process of AD begins years, if not decades, before the diagnosis of clinical dementia, and to the incorporation of biomarkers that can indicate the presence or absence of AD pathology. The new criteria propose three different stages of Alzheimer's disease: preclinical AD, MCI due to AD, dementia due to AD. The preclinical stage occurs before symptoms development and indicates cognitive intact subjects with positive biomarkers of AD-related brain changes [55]. Table 1 shows diagnostic criteria of the different stages of preclinical AD phase. The investigation of the presence of this stage is strictly for research purposes only and usually used for individuals with high genetic risk of AD. Individuals with MCI have mild but measurable changes in cognition that are noticeable to the person affected and to family and friends but that do not affect the individual's ability to carry out everyday activities. Not all the subjects with MCI develop dementia, it is estimated that the rate of progression can be 10% per year. It is unclear why some individual progress into dementia and some others not, however it is believed that MCI can be an early stage of dementia. In the new criteria (Table 2) the use of biomarkers is suggested in order to investigate whether subjects have brain changes that put them at higher risk of developing AD. If biomarkers of AD-pathology result positive the diagnosis is MCI due to AD [56].

The new criteria proposed to classify people with AD dementia in the following groups after meet general criteria for dementia [1]: 1) Probable AD dementia, 2) Possible AD dementia, and 3) Probable or Possible AD dementia with evidence of the AD pathophysiological process. Table 3 shows the revised criteria for AD. The first two have been planned to use in a clinical setting and are very much similar to the previous NINCS-ADRDA criteria of possible and probable AD. The third group has been suggested only for research field.

	Aβ (PET or CSF)	Markers of neuronal injury (tau CZ-F, PET-FDG, MRI)	Evidence of subtle cognitive change
Asymptomatic cerebral amyloidosis	Positive	Negative	Negative
Asymptomatic cerebral amyloidosis + neurodegeneration	Positive	Positive	Negative
Amyloidosis+ neuronal injury+ subtle cognitive/ behavioral decline	Positive	Positive	Positive
(Sperling RA et al. 2011) [55]			

Table 1. Pre-clinical Alzheimer´s Disease stages: National Institute on Aging (NIA) and the Alzheimer's Association diagnostic criteria 2011.

MCI- core clinical criteria • Cognitive concern reflecting a change in cognition reported by patient or informant or clinician (i.e., historical or observed evidence of decline over time) • Objective evidence of impairment in one or more cognitive domains, typically including memory (i.e., formal or bedside testing to establish level of cognitive function in multiple domains) • Preservation of independence in functional abilities • Not demented
Examine etiology of MCI consistent with AD pathophysiological process • Rule out vascular, traumatic, medical causes of cognitive decline, where possible • Provide evidence of longitudinal decline in cognition, when feasible • Report history consistent with AD genetic factors, where relevant
MCI due to AD: Intermediate likelihood Clinical criteria + positive Aβ biomarkers and untested neuronal injury biomarkers Clinical criteria + untested Aβ biomarkers and positive neuronal injury biomarkers High likelihood Clinical criteria+ positive Aβ and neuronal injury biomarkers MCI- unlikely due to AD Clinical criteria + negative Aβ and neuronal injury biomarkers
(Albert SA et al. 2011) [56]

Table 2. Mild Cognitive Impairment due to AD: National Institute on Aging (NIA) and the Alzheimer's Association diagnostic criteria 2011.

Probable AD	A. Insidious onset. Symptoms have a gradual onset over months to years, not sudden over hours or days B. Clear-cut history of worsening of cognition by report or observation; and C. The initial and most prominent cognitive deficit are evident on history and examination in one of the following categories a. Amnestic presentation is the most common syndromic presentation of AD dementia. The deficits should include impairment in lerning and recall of recently learned information. There should also be evidence of cognitve dysfunction in at least one other cognitive domain b. Nonamnestic presentations: • Language presentation: The most prominent deficits are in word-finding, but deficits in other cognitive domains should be present • Visuospatial presentation: The most prominent deficits are in spatial cognition, including object agnosia, impaired face recognition, simultagnosia, and alexia. Deficits in other cognitive domains should be present • Executive dysfunction: The most prominent deficits are impaired reasoning, judgment, and problem solving. Deficits in other cognitive domains should be present
Possible AD	Atypical course A. Atypical course meets the core clinical criteria in terms of the cognitive deficits for AD dementia, but either has a sudden onset of cognitive impairment or demonstrates insufficient historical detail or objective cognitive documentation of progressive decline or Etiologically mixed presentation B. Etiologically mixed presentation meets all core clinical criteria for AD dementia but has evidence as the following: a. Concomitant cerebrovascular disease, defined by a history of stroke temporally related to the onset or worsening of cognitive impairment; or the presence of multiple or extensive infarcts or severe white matter hyperintensity burden; or b. Features of Dementia with Lewy bodies other than the dementia itself; or c. Evidence for another neurological diseases or a non-neurological medical comorbidity or medication use that could have a substantial effect on cognition
Probable AD with three levels of evidence of AD pathophysiology	Intermediate Aβ unavailable or indeterminate Neuronal injury positive Intermediate Aβ positive Neuronal injury unavailable or indeterminate High Aβ positive Neuronal injury positive
Possible AD (atypical presentation) with evidence of AD pathophysiology	High but does not rule out second etiology Aβ positive Neuronal injury positive

Dementia-unlikely due to AD	1. Does not meet clinical criteria for AD dementia. 2. a. Regardless of meeting clinical criteria for probable or possible AD dementia, there is sufficient evidence for an alternative diagnosis such as HIV dementia, dementia of Huntington's disease, or others that rarely, if ever, overlap with AD. b. Regardless of meeting clinical criteria for possible AD dementia, both Aβ and neuronal injury biomarkers are negative

(McKhann GM et al. 2011) [1].

Table 3. Dementia due to AD: National Institute on Aging (NIA) and the Alzheimer's Association diagnostic criteria

The diagnostic procedure in clinical setting is usual divided into two phases. Screening is used to formulate the diagnostic hypothesis and is followed by the diagnostic confirmation. During the screening phase, the main point is to collect detailed information on history not only from the patient itself, but also from the people who take care of patients such as familial or other type of caregiver. Information about history includes medical history (presence of severe medical disease that may cause encephalopathy, psychiatric disease, traumatic brain injury or other neurological disease), medications, family history of dementia, and changes in both basic activities of daily living (such as self-feeding, dressing and bathing, ambulation) and instrumental activities of daily living (such as grooming, homework, manage finances, driving, and leisure). To obtain information on activities daily living could be particularly helpful to use standardized evaluation instruments such as Katz ADL scale [63] Lawton-Brody IADL scale [64], and the Bristol Activities of Daily Living Scale [65]. In addition to the history, a systematic assessment of general cognitive functioning is required through instruments designed for this purpose. There are no screening tools that can quickly assess different levels of cognitive impairment. The American Academy of Neurology guidelines suggested to use the Mini-Mental Status Examination [66], and the Memory Impairment Screen (MIS) [67]. In recent times, the Montreal Cognitive Assessment (MoCA) was developed as a tool to screen patients in who has been hypothesized a mild cognitive decline and usually performed in the normal range on the MMSE [68, 69]. Studies have shown that MoCa is sensitive for the mild stages of AD dementia, whereas MMSE is superior for more advanced stages with the functional impairment. A complete summary of neuropsychological tests has been proposed [70].

After the screening, the second phase consists of a neurological examination, a neuropsychological assessment, and a behavioural disease evaluation. A complete general neurological examination has been recommended as well as accurate neuropsychological evaluation in order to test possible differential diagnosis. The presence of Parkinsonism can suggest a Lewy Body's dementia, while asymmetric tendon reflex or other lateralizing signs can suggest a vascular component. Other neurological signs, for example peripheral neuropathy may indicate toxic or metabolic problems. There is no evidence-based data to support the usefulness of specific routine blood tests for evaluation of those with dementia but these are useful in excluding co-morbidities. Most expert opinion advises to screen for vitamin B12, folate, thyroid stimulating hormone, calcium, glucose, complete blood cell count, renal and liver function abnormalities. Serological tests for syphilis, Borrelia and HIV should be considered in individuals at high risk [71]. Structural neuroimaging, computed tomography (CT) or magnetic resonance imaging (MRI) is recommended as level B in the Dementia Guideline [71] at least once in each patient in order to exclude other condition as neoplasms, subdural hematomas. The lumbar puncture is not recommended unless the suspicion of prion disease or viral encephalitis.

6. Biomarkers

A biomarker is any characteristic that is objectively measured and evaluated as an indicator of biologic or pathogenic process and it should also be reliable, non-invasive and simple to perform [72]. Regarding AD, biomarkers included in the new diagnostic criteria are a measurement of the underline pathology and can be divided in markers of amyloid accumulation (CSF Aβ level, PET with amyloid-tracers) and markers of neuronal injury (atrophy of MTL at MRI, tau level in CSF, metabolic PET) [55]. Table 4 shows all the biomarkers.

6.1. Medial temporal lobe atrophy

Bilateral atrophy of medial temporal lobe structures, including hippocampus, has been found in patients with AD (Figure 1). Moreover it has been reported that the brain atrophy detected with neuroimaging reflects the typical pattern of progression of neuropathology, spreading from entorhinal cortex and hippocampus to the association cortices, as describe by Braak and Braak [73, 74]. In a meta-analysis of studies using visual and linear measurements of medial temporal lobe atrophy (MTA) on MRI, the overall sensitivity and specificity for detection of AD compared with controls was estimated to be 85% and 88%, respectively [75]. A yearly decline in hippocampal volume is approximately 2.5 times greater in patients with AD than in normal aged subjects. In clinical practice simple visual rating scales estimating hippocampal atrophy has proven to be useful to support the diagnosis in the first stage of the disease [74]. Although MTL is a biomarker of neurodegeneration and a good surrogate of disease progression, it has low sensitivity and specificity (51-70% and 68-69%, respectively) in identifying prodromal AD stage [76].

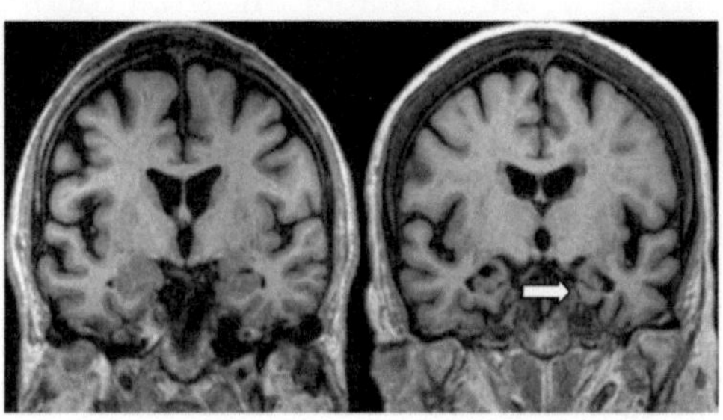

Figure 1. Coronal T1-weighted MRI scans of control (left) and patient with AD (right). The patient with AD shows atrophy of the hippocampus (arrow) [74].

6.2. Metabolic PET

PET with traced glucose (FDG-PET) shows brain metabolism and reflects pattern of neurodegeneration. Metabolic reduction in bilateral temporal- parietal regions and in posterior cingulate is the most commonly described diagnostic criterion for AD [77].This specific pattern significantly predicts decline to AD with an average overall accuracy of 86%, and with sensitivity and specificity about 75-80%. Moreover some studies on pre-symptomatic carriers of genetic mutations for AD revealed FDG-PET hypometabolism many years before the clinical onset of the disease [78,79].

6.3. PET with amyloid-tracers

Interestingly recently has been developed a technique to detect amyloid in vivo using PET. [18F]-FDDNP and [11C] Pittsburgh compound-B (PIB) were the first amyloid PET tracers developed. Both tracers bind with nanomolar affinity to amyloid and enter the brain in amounts sufficient for imaging with PET. Retention of the tracers in neocortical and subcortical brain regions was significantly higher in AD patients than in controls. In subjects with MCI and positive retention the rate of progression to AD is estimated 25% per year [80]. A recent meta-analysis estimated a sensitivity of 93% and specificity of 56.2% [78]. Similarly, genetic at-risk cohorts demonstrate evidence of Aβ accumulation many years before detectable cognitive impairment [79]. This method could be used to follow the therapeutic efficacy of the new AD immunotherapies.

6.4. CSF Aβ and tau

Many reports have demonstrated a decline in CSF Aβ and elevation of total tau, phospho-tau, and tau/Aβ ratio in AD subjects. The reduction of Aβ could be by about 50% in subjects with AD compared with age-matched controls [81] and this phenomenon is thought to result from deposition of Aβ into plaques, leaving less Aβ being available to diffuse into the CSF. CSF total tau reflects the intensity of the neuronal and axonal damage, and it is increased in AD subjects by 2-3 folds compare with controls. However, tau, as a marker of neuronal injury, can be transiently increased after any acute brain injury (such as stroke or trauma) [82]. A comprehensive review [83] reports that Aβ shows a sensitivity and specificity of 86% and 90%, respectively, in differentiating AD from controls. For tau, the sensitivity is 81% and the specificity 90%, and p-tau has a mean sensitivity of 80% when specificity is set at 92%. By use of a combination of concentrations of Aβ42 and t-tau for AD versus controls, high sensitivities (85–94%) and specificities (83–100%) can be reached. The reliability of CSF biomarker has been tested by the comparison with autopsy results, showing high sensitivity and specificity in discriminating AD from both the cognitively normal elderly and from patients with other dementias. These CSF markers have also been shown to predict AD in patients with MCI [84], and to precede symptoms in familial AD [85]. However CSF biomarkers are not related with dementia severity.

Biomarkers, despite their great potential especially in the research field, are not recommended for the routine use in clinical diagnostic setting. Clinical criteria provide very good accu-

http://dx.doi.org/10.5772/54539

racy, there is limited standardization of the biomarkers and the access is limited to university hospitals.

	Specificity	Sensitivity
Biomarkers of Aβ deposition		
CSF Aβ [83]	90%	86%
PET amyloid imaging [78]	56.2%	93.5%
Biomarkers of neuronal injury		
CSF tau [83]	90%	81%
Medial temporal lobe atrophy on MRI [75]	88%	85%
FDG-PET imaging [78]	74%	78.7%

Table 4. Alzheimer´s disease biomarkers: diagnostic accuracy

7. Others biomarkers

7.1. CSF BACE1 and sAPP

APP, amyloid precursor protein, is sequentially cleaved by α-or β-secretase (BACE1), followed by γ-secretase enzyme. The cleavage by BACE1 and γ-secretase generates Aβ peptide, likely to aggregate in plaques, and the N-terminal secreted fragment of APPβ (sAPPβ). In contrast, APP cleavage by α-and γ-secretase generates non-amyloidogenic fragments and secreted fragment of APPα (sAPPα). Thus, CSF BACE1 activity and sAPPβ and sAPPα proteins have been testing to provide information about amyloidogenic vs. nonamyloidogenic processing in the brain. Although some reports have shown higher levels of CSF BACE1 activity in AD compared with healthy controls and higher levels in subjects with MCI who progress to AD, others have not observed these, or have shown a decline of BACE1 activity in AD [86]. It is possible that CSF BACE activity is elevated in incipient AD and subsequently decline with disease progression. Several groups have measured CSF sAPPβ and sAPPα levels from AD and control subjects to understand brain APP metabolism better. Some studies reported higher levels of sAPPβ and a reduction in sAPPα levels in AD, however, these results need further confirmation [86].

7.2. Plasma Aβ

Several studies investigated plasma level of Aβ in AD. One group of researchers reported that in patients with newly acquired Alzheimer's disease, the plasma Aβ levels decline significantly compared with controls or participants with prevalent Alzheimer's disease during an average follow-up period of 3 years [87]. Another study reported that higher baseline plasma Aβ concentrations and greater reductions in plasma Aβ concentrations were associated with cognitive decline in non-demented elderly people over 4 years follow-up [88].

This study indicated that plasma Aβ level is elevated during the pre-symptomatic stage in at-risk individuals, but subsequently start falling with the development of Alzheimer's disease/MCI. Anyhow most groups have not found any significant differences between patients and controls. Wu and colleagues [86] recently tried to measure, through specific antibody, plasma level of BACE1, sAPPβ and sAPPα. They reported significant increase in plasma BACE activity, sAPPβ, and sAPPα in a small sample of AD patients (n=20) compared with age-matched controls (n=30).

7.3. Clinical variants of Alzheimer's disease

The common conception of Alzheimer's disease (AD) is a disorder that initially affects memory function, associated with early pathological changes in medial temporal lobes, and progresses to involve language, visuospatial skills and other cognitive abilities, reflecting progressive involvement of association neocortices [61]. It is recognised, however, that the clinical presentation of AD is variable and in some cases the presenting dominant symptom is not memory [89-91]. Non-amnestic presentations are frequently referred to as "focal" presentations of AD. It is well established that most patients with a progressive disturbance of aspects of visuo-perceptual and spatial abilities, often referred to as posterior cortical atrophy, have underlying AD pathology. In addition, it is now clear that a proportion of patients with progressive aphasia, both fluent and non-fluent type, can have AD as the primary pathology. Recently, cases of corticobasal syndrome (CBS) secondary to AD pathology have also been reported [90]. The existence of a frontal presentation is more controversial. Patients with familial AD secondary to presenilin 1 mutations may have a behavioural onset [92, 93] and there are isolated reports of sporadic AD resembling fronto-temporal dementia (FTD) [91, 94].

7.4. Progressive aphasia

Primary progressive aphasia (PPA) is a clinical syndrome in which cognitive decline is limited to one or more components of the language system. Since Mesulam's first description of the phenomenon [95] clinical, neuropsychological and imaging studies have converged on the existence of three distinct clinical subtypes: semantic dementia (SD), characterized by fluent but empty speech, impaired comprehension and high incidence of dyslexic errors, in association with selective atrophy in anterior temporal regions; non fluent/agrammatic aphasia (PNFA) with phonologically and/or grammatically distorted speech output, preserved single word comprehension, and atrophy focused on the left inferior frontal and insular regions; logopenic variant (LPA), characterized by a slow production rate, long word finding pauses, sparse phonological paraphasias and difficulty with sentence (but not single word) repetition. MRI reveals abnormalities in more posterior brain regions [96]. Pathologically, PNFA and SD are more likely to present an FTD pattern, although in some cases they can be the clinical presentation of atypical AD pathology. In contrast, biochemical, amyloid imaging and post mortem findings in LPA support the idea that the syndrome is a clinical marker of AD pathology [97]. Clinical evolution of that variant leads to mutism and memory impairment.

7.5. Visual variant

Posterior cortical atrophy (PCA) or visual variant of AD is characterized by early impairment of visuo-spatial skills with less prominent memory loss and is associated with atrophy in parieto-occipital and posterior temporal cortices with right predominance [98]. Clinical presentation includes difficulties in reading lines of text, in judging distances, in identifying static objects within the visual field, alexia, and features of Balint's syndrome (simultanagnosia, oculomotor apraxia, optic ataxia, environmental agnosia) and Gerstmann's syndrome (acalculia, agraphia, finger agnosia, left–right disorientation) [99]. Deficits in working memory and limb apraxia have also been noted [100]. By the time PCA has run its course, many patients develop also memory and language deficits. Findings of pathological studies all show that Alzheimer's disease is the most common underlying cause of PCA [101]. Some studies have shown that PCA cases have the greatest density of both plaques and neurofibrillary tangles in visual and visual-association cortices and fewer tangles and senile plaques in the hippocampus and subiculum [101]. CSF biomarkers ($A\beta_,$ tau, and P-tau) show similar pattern in patients with PCA compared with AD subjects, supporting the hypothesis that PCA is associated typically with underlying Alzheimer's disease pathology. However, some cases are attributable to other causes, such as corticobasal degeneration, dementia with Lewy bodies, or prion disease [98].

7.6. Progressive apraxic syndrome

Autopsy proven AD cases can be related to an apraxis clinical syndrome. Patients with these phenotype present progressive loss of use of the limbs which compromises performance on manual tasks such as dressing, handling a knife or a fork and writing. Cognitive assessment reveals apraxia and in less extends deficits in spatial function, with initially preserved memory [102]. The clinical spectrum of that phenotype may also include others symptoms of the corticobasal syndrome (CBS), as asymmetric parkinsonism, ideomotor apraxia and alien limb phenomena. CBS is an unusual clinical manifestation of various neurodegenerative pathologies, AD, FTD, corticobasal degeneration (CBD). The one related to AD presents a temporo-parietal atrophy prevalent on the left side and hypoperfusion of parietal lobe, with less involvement of pre-frontal regions compare with FTD and CBD [103].

7.7. Frontal variant

Sometimes AD patients presents a prevalent impairment of the executive function in the early stages of the disease, but there is also a multidomain deficit [90, 102]. Two reports, [91, 94] have claimed that a behavioural onset of cognitive dysfunction, with disinhibition, apathy and personality change could be also an atypical presentation of AD pathology. Alladi and colleagues [90] after the examination of 28 cases of behavioral variant - FTD found AD pathology in two cases. None of the two patients had amnesia at the onset of the disease, but in both cases diffuse cognitive dysfunction developed early in the course of the disease. Authors concluded that a behavioural variant of AD exists, but in contrast to patients with non-AD pathology, the disease does not appear to remain restricted to the frontal lobes for very long.

8. Treatment and management

Regarding the therapeutic management of a disease generally there are at least three possibilities: (i) prevention strategy, (ii) symptomatic treatment, and (iii) disease modifying therapies. Currently, a long list of factors that can reduce or delay the risk of AD onset has been reported, but so far there is no certain evidence supporting the prevention efficacy in AD. In Europe, there are three ongoing multidomain interventional random clinical trials (RTCs) that focus on the optimal management of vascular risk factors and vascular diseases and include also medical and lifestyle interventions. The results of the RTCs might help in improving strategies of dementia prevention [3]. This indicates the principle type of AD treatment is based on symptomatic drugs. There is no cure for AD, but new types of disease modifying treatments are under investigation. Non-pharmacological interventions have been also recently added in AD patient management.

8.1. Symptomatic treatments: acetylcholinesterase inhibitors

The neuropathology of Alzheimer's disease is characterized by early loss of basal forebrain cholinergic neurons, leading to decreased cholinergic transmission which is involved in many aspects of cognition, including memory and attention. Inhibitors of the acetylcholinesterase enzyme (AChEIs) increase acetylcoline level in brain, which leads to memory improvement. Since the introduction of the first ChEI in 1997, these agents are considered first-line pharmacotherapy for mild to moderate AD stages [71]. Four ChEIs are currently available: tacrine, donepezil, rivastigmine and galantamine. Tacrine (Cognex), the first approved, is not commonly used because of a poor tolerability profile and low oral bioavailability [104]. The Cochrane's Review [105] of placebo controlled trials of ChEIs demonstrated that the treatment determine an improvement of 1.4- to 3.9-point in the ADAS-Cog scale at 6 months and 1 year. In clinical trials, a change of 4 points is considered clinically significant for patients with mild to moderate dementia. In addition to their effects on cognition, these agents also have demonstrated beneficial effects on measures of behavior, activities of daily living (ADLs), and global patient function as reported in a recent meta-analysis [106]. Donepezil (Aricept) was approved in the mid-1990s. The starting dose is 5 mg once daily which can be increased after 4 weeks to 10 mg, if well tolerated. The common side effects are nausea, vomiting, gastritis and diarrhea. The length of the response has been documented up to 52 weeks. When donepezil is discontinued, performance of the subject returns to the same as in the untreated state. Rivastigmine (Exelon) is a pseudo-irreversible inhibitor as it dissociates from the enzyme slowly. Two type of administration are available: oral and transdermal patch. The oral starting dose is 1,5 mg twice daily that can be weekly increase of 1,5 mg until a total amount of 12 mg per day (6 mg twice daily). The transdermal patch last 24 hours and has two dosages: 4,6 mg and 9,5 mg. The target dose, 9,5 mg/24 h, can be reached after 4 weeks if the low dosage is well tolerated. Side effects of oral Rivastigmine are approximately the same as donepezil, while gastrointestinal symptoms are at least three times less prominent with the patch [104]. Rivastigmine is also an inhibitor of butyrylcholinesterase that facilitate cholinergic neurotransmission by slowing the degradation of acetylcholine released by functionally intact cholinergic neurons. The therapy with Galantamine (Remin-

http://dx.doi.org/10.5772/54539

yl) starts with 4 mg twice daily and increases in increments of 4 mg per dose twice a day to a maximum of 12 mg twice daily if tolerated. Currently it is also available in an extended-release formulation that can be taken once daily. Galantamine has some nicotinic receptor activity. All AChEIs can influence cardiac rhytm, but is not common unless a person has an underlying disturbance in cardiac conduction. An electrocardiogram prior to initiating the treatment is recommended. AChEIs may also have an effect on respiratory conditions, such as chronic obstructive pulmonary disease or asthma, or gastrointestinal disease, such as gastric ulcer. The absorption of AChEI is not influenced by food intake. These agents are recommended for the treatment for patient only in the mild and moderate stages [71].

8.2. Memantine

Memantine is an NMDA (N-methyl-D-aspartate) receptor antagonist that reduces glutamatergic excitotoxicity. Based on the glutammatergic hypothesis of AD, Memantine has been claimed to be a disease modifying therapy. Clinical trial with Memantine reports a mild efficacy in maintaning functional level in patients with severe dementia [107]. Memantine is licensed for the treatment of people with moderate-to-severe AD. The starting dose is 5 mg that can be increased of 5 mg every week up to the dose of 20 mg. Side effects are very unusual and include restlessness, hyperexitation and fatigue. There are good evidence of clinical benefit in patients moving into severe stages of AD from a combination therapy with Memantine and an acetylcholinesterase inhibitor [108-110].

8.3. Disease-modifying treatments

Since the role of beta amyloid (Aβ) is considered to be paramount in the development of AD, several research strategies have been undertaken to alter the biochemistry of Aβ in the brain through interference of either the formation or the deposition of Aβ. The amyloid precursor protein can be processed in two different pathways, non-amyloidogenic by α-secretase and amyloidogenic ones by β-secretase followed by γ-secretase [12]. Thus, the inhibition of β or γ-secretase is the target of therapies that aim to reduce the production of Aβ, while new immunotherapeutic strategies promote removal of Aβ from the brain. Drugs that can act as β-secretase inhibitors belong to a group of type 2 diabetes therapies, thiazolidinediones (rosiglitazone and pioglitazone). Despite the promising biological plausibility of these compounds, the results of randomized clinical trials (RCTs) have been disappointing [111-112]. A number of γ-secretase modulators (semagacestat and tarenflurbil) have also failed to provide benefits in the treatment of AD [113,114]. Immunotherapies or "vaccines" are based on both active and passive immunization. Initial approaches based on immunization with Aβ fragments performed extremely well in transgenic mouse models but showed less promise in humans [51]. The most promising of these, AN-1792 (QS-21) resulted in significant Aβ-antibody titers in patients with mild-to-moderate AD in Phase II trials. Postmortem analysis on long-term follow-up also confirmed that the therapy had resulted in a significant reduction in Aβ burden in the brain. However, there was no evidence of any clinical benefit and the trial was halted owing to patients developing aseptic meningoencephalitis, thought to have been induced by cytotoxic T-cell activation. Immunotherapies have since been designed using shorter peptides designed to mimic immunoreactive sections of Aβ, in an effort to avoid severe inflammatory response. There are various immunotherapies taking these approaches. For example, CAD-106, which targets Aβ1–6, resulted in Aβ clearance without collateral immunoreactivity in Phase I trials, and is now in a Phase II RCT. Passive immunotherapy for AD has met with some criticism owing to the challenge of designing an approach that can achieve significant antibody concentrations in the brain. Although some of the data from animal studies do suggest a possible impact on oligomer formation and brain amyloid load. Currently, monoclonal antibody therapies include bapineuzumab (AAB-001) and solanezumab (LY-2062430) that are now in a phase III RCT [115]. The results of these trials are eagerly awaited, but experts' consensus is not anticipating positive outcomes. Despite the facts that vaccines can remove Aβ from the brain, a fundamental debate continues around the clinical benefit of Aβ clearance. Neurofibrillary tangles are another hallmark of AD pathology, however treatments to target tauopathy have received far less attention than amyloid therapies. Very preliminary results in animal models have shown that a tau immunotherapy might be a valuable approach [116].

8.4. Non-pharmacological treatment

In the last ten years there has been a great public interest in possible non-pharmacological therapies to delay disease progression and functional decline. The psychosocial interventions fitted to this goal and they were developed based on the concept of "cognitive reserve". Evidence from meta-analyses and systematic reviews has shown that a higher cognitive reserve is associated with a significantly reduced risk to develop dementia [117]. Generally "cognitive reserve" describes the mind's resistance to damage of the brain. There has been proposed two models to explore the reserve, a passive model called "brain reserve" and an active model knows as "cognitive reserve" [118]. There are several different approaches to neuropsychological and training interventions focusing on cognition with different evidence for efficacy in people with AD. In large part, the psychosocial interventions have shown significant, but modest effect-size when used alone. The American Association for Gertiatric Psychiatry (AAGP) proposed a care/treatment model that combines pharmacological therapies with psychosocial intervention for people with AD [119]. To date, the literature about psychosocial intervention is wide [120-123]. For this reason we decide to illustrate briefly the most important intervention below. The psychosocial interventions can be classified according to the treatment goal and include behaviour, emotion-oriented and stimulation-oriented treatment, and cognitive training [124].

Behaviour-oriented therapy is used to modify dysfunctional behaviour employing behaviour change techniques which increase or decrease the frequency of behaviour through the use of reinforcement, punishment, and extinction following the Experimental Analysis of Behaviour (B.F. Skinner). Behaviour therapy is helpful to reduce typical behaviour's problems such as incontinence and wondering [125-127]. Stimulation-oriented interventions include recreational activities such as creative arts (such as craft, music, dance, andtheatre) and leisure education, art therapy, music therapy, pet therapy, and other formal activities aim to maximize pleasurable activities for the patients. Stimulation improves modestly be-

http://dx.doi.org/10.5772/54539

Drug	Suggested Dosage	Approved indication
Cholinesterase inhibitors		
Donepezil (Aricept)	5 mg once daily, which can be increased to 10 mg/day after 4 weeks	Mild to moderate AD Sever AD in add-on with Memantine
Rivastigmine (Exelon)	Oral: Twice daily starting with 1.5 mg which can be increased up to 6 mg twice daily in 6 weeks Transdermal patch: once daily, 4,6 mg/24 h, or 9,5 mg/24 h.	Mild to moderae AD
Galantamine (Remynil)	Twice daily, beginning with 4 mg and increase after 4 weeks to 8 mg twice daily. A dosage of 12 mg twice daily can also be reached after a medical examination Availabe a new extended-release formulation that can be taken once daily	Mild to moderate AD
NMDA atagonist		
Mematine (Ebixa)	Twice daily beginning with 5 mg increase up to 10 mg twice daily in 4 weeks Available a dosage of 20 mg that can be taken once daily	Moderate to severe AD
Immunotherapies		
Active immunization		Pashe II RCT*
CAD-106		Phase III RCT*
Passive immunization		Phase III RCT*
Bapineuzumab (AAB-001)		
Solanezumab (LY-2062430)		

*RCT= randomize clinical trial

Table 5. Alzheimer's disease pharmacological treatments

haviours and mood, but the main effect is to change the daily-life routine [124]. Emotion-oriented approaches include supportive psychotherapy, reminiscence therapy, validation therapy, sensory integration (snoezelen), and simulated presence therapy (SPT). Supportive psychotherapy has not received formal scientific studies, but can be used to address issue of loss in the early stage of AD and help mildly impaired patients to adapt themselves to a new lifestyle imposed by the disease. Reminiscence therapy remains controversial, individually or in group, on past life events of the patient helped by using external aids such as photographs, household items, music and sound recordings, or other familiar items from the past. The final goal is to improve the psychological well-being, mood, and coping skills of patients with AD [128]. Researches have shown that reminiscence is useful to improve directly emotions in overall mood, thus can improve cognitive functioning [129-132]. Validation therapy [133] is based on the empathic relationship between the patient and the therapist.

Through listening, the therapist examines the reality's perception of the patient in order to create significant emotional and relational contacts. The objectives are to stimulate the patient to take social role, stimulate verbal communication, and encourage social interaction. Validation is intended for patients with severe to moderate dementia. Cognitive training involves guided practice on a set of standard tasks designed to stimulate specific cognitive functions (memory, attention, or problem-solving). The underlying assumption is that practice may improve or maintain functioning in a given domain, generalizing the effects of practice beyond the clinical context to everyday life [121].The aim is to reduce cognitive deficits. The Reality Orientation Therapy (ROT) is a technique widely used in treatment of AD [134-136]. The objective is to stimulate the personal, time, and space orientation in the patient through repeated multimodal stimulation (verbal, visual, and musical), strengthen the basic information with respect to space and time coordinates, and his personal history. The level of stimulation is modulated agree with residual cognitive resource of patient. Other types of cognitive training include skills training and cognitive retraining focusing on cognitive deficits. There has been demonstrated that cognitive training improve cognitive functioning, but effects were transient and often accompanied by negative effects linked to frustration [137]. Finally, the caregivers are also part of the treatment and should be carefully managed overtime.

9. Conclusions

Alzheimer´s disease is a common disorder of aging, and a major cause of dependence and mortality among elderly. Substantial progress has been made over the past few decades in understanding AD. Nevertheless, our knowledge of this disease is still profoundly imperfect, as demonstrated by the failure of all but symptomatic treatments for clinically diagnosed AD. We know that in people aged >85 years, dementia and cognitive impairment are common, reaching a combined prevalence >50% in the oldest old, and that the incidence of dementia continues to rise in the oldest age groups. Thus, screening is essential to identify cognitively normal individuals in midlife or old age who have a high risk of developing MCI and AD, so that interventions, when available, can be administered to stop the development of specific disease-related pathologies. Although the exact pathogenetic mechanism of AD is still unclear, thanks to new technologies, we are now able to detect in vivo subjects with AD-related brain pathological changes. Many studies have provided evidence that AD pathology begins as many as 20 years before symptoms appear. These findings determined a new concept of AD, where the symptom of dementia represents the final part of the "continuum" of AD. Recently, based on the new knowledge about AD, some disease modifying therapies have been developed and their results are eagerly awaited.

Acknowledgements

Research grants were received from the Swedish council for working life and social research, the Swedish Research Council in Medicine and the Swedish Brain Power. This study

http://dx.doi.org/10.5772/54539

was also supported in part by funds from the Loo and Hans Ostermans Foundation and the Foundation for Geriatric Diseases at Karolinska Institutet, the Gamla Tjänarinnor Foundation, Demens fonden and the Bertil Stohnes Foundation.

Author details

Weili Xu[1,2*], Anna Marseglia[2,3], Camilla Ferrari[2,4] and Hui-Xin Wang[2]

*Address all correspondence to: weili.xu@ki.se

1 Department of Epidemiology, Tianjin Medical University, Tianjin, P.R. China

2 Aging Research Center, Karolinska Institutet-Stockholm University, Stockholm, Sweden

3 Institute of Neuroscience - Aging Branch, National Council of Research (CNR), Padua, Italy

4 Department of Neuroscience, University of Florence, Italy

References

[1] McKhann GM, Knopman DS, Chertkow H, Hyman BT, Jack CR, Jr., Kawas CH, et al. The diagnosis of dementia due to Alzheimer's disease: recommendations from the National Institute on Aging-Alzheimer's Association workgroups on diagnostic guidelines for Alzheimer's disease. Alzheimers Dement. 2011;7(3):263-9.

[2] Schneider JA, Arvanitakis Z, Bang W, Bennett DA. Mixed brain pathologies account for most dementia cases in community-dwelling older persons. Neurology. 2007;69(24):2197-204.

[3] Mangialasche F, Kivipelto M, Solomon A, Fratiglioni L. Dementia prevention: current epidemiological evidence and future perspective. Alzheimers Res Ther. 2012;4(1):6.

[4] Fratiglioni L, Launer LJ, Andersen K, Breteler MM, Copeland JR, Dartigues JF, et al. Incidence of dementia and major subtypes in Europe: A collaborative study of population-based cohorts. Neurologic Diseases in the Elderly Research Group. Neurology. 2000;54(11 Suppl 5):S10-5.

[5] Qiu C, Kivipelto M, von Strauss E. Epidemiology of Alzheimer's disease: occurrence, determinants, and strategies toward intervention. Dialogues Clin Neurosci. 2009;11(2):111-28.

[6] Lobo A, Launer LJ, Fratiglioni L, Andersen K, Di Carlo A, Breteler MM, et al. Prevalence of dementia and major subtypes in Europe: A collaborative study of popula-

tion-based cohorts. Neurologic Diseases in the Elderly Research Group. Neurology. 2000;54(11 Suppl 5):S4-9.

[7] Plassman BL, Langa KM, Fisher GG, Heeringa SG, Weir DR, Ofstedal MB, et al. Prevalence of dementia in the United States: the aging, demographics, and memory study. Neuroepidemiology. 2007;29(1-2):125-32.

[8] Ferri CP, Prince M, Brayne C, Brodaty H, Fratiglioni L, Ganguli M, et al. Global prevalence of dementia: a Delphi consensus study. Lancet. 2005;366(9503):2112-7.

[9] Brookmeyer R, Johnson E, Ziegler-Graham K, Arrighi HM. Forecasting the global burden of Alzheimer's disease. Alzheimers Dement. 2007;3(3):186-91.

[10] Ballard C, Gauthier S, Corbett A et al. Alzheimer's disease. Lancet 2011; 377: 1019-1031

[11] Hernandez F, Avila J. Tauopathies. Cell Mol Life Sci. 2007;64(17):2219-33.

[12] Schaeffer EL, Figueiro´ IM, Wagner F, et al. Insights into Alzheimer disease pathogenesis from studies in transgenic animal models. CLINICS 2011;66(S1):45-54

[13] Price DL, Tanzi RE, Borchelt DR, Sisodia SS et al. Alzheimer's disease: genetic studies and transgenic models. Annu Rev Genet.19998; 32:461– 493.

[14] Hardy JA, Higgins GA. Alzheimer's disease: the amyloid cascade hypothesis. Science. 1992;256:184-185

[15] Bettens K, Sleegers K, Van Broeckhoven C. Current status on Alzheimer disease molecular genetics; from past, to present, to future. Hum Mol Genet 2010; 19: R4–R11

[16] Pimplikar SW, Nixon RA, Robakis NK. Et al. Amyloid-independent mechanisms in Alzheimer's disease pathogenesis. J Neurosci. 2010 ;30(45):14946-54

[17] McGeer PL, McGeer EG, Yasojima K et al. Alzheimerndisease and neuroinflammation. J Neural Transm Suppl. 2000; 59: 53-57

[18] Guglielmotto M, Tamagno E, Danni O et al. Oxidative stress and hypoxia contribute to Alzheimer's disease pathogenesis: two sides of the same coin. Scientific World Journal. 2009; 9:781-791.

[19] Yang Y. Mufson EJ, Herrup K et al. Neuronal cell death is preceded by cell cycle events at all stages of Alzheimer's disease. J Neurosci. 2003; 23: 2557-2563.

[20] de la Torre JC. Critically attained threshold of cerebral hypoperfusion: the CATCH hypothesis of Alzheimer's pathogenesis. Neurobiol Aging 2000; 21: 331-342.

[21] de la Torre JC, Mussivand T. Can disturbed brain microcirculation cause Alzheimer's disease? Neurol Res 1993; 15:146-153.

[22] de la Torre JC. Three Postulates to Help Identify the Cause of Alzheimer's Disease. Journal of Alzheimer's Disease. 2011; 24: 657–668

[23] Herrup K. Re-imagining Alzheimer's disease – an age-based hypothesis. J Neurosci. 2010; 30(50):16755-62

[24] Huang Y, Weisgraber HK, Mucke L et al. Apolipoprotein E. Diversity of Cellular Origins, Structural and Biophysical Properties, and Effects in Alzheimer's Disease. J Mol Neurosci 2004; 23(3):189-204

[25] Ahn Jo S, Ahn K, Kim JH, Kang BH, Kim E, Jo I, et al. ApoE-epsilon 4-dependent association of the choline acetyltransferase gene polymorphisms (2384G>A and 1882G>A) with Alzheimer's disease. Clin Chim Acta. 2006;368(1-2):179-82

[26] Cohn-Hokke PE, Elting MW, Pijnenburg YAL, van Swieten JC. Genetics of Dementia: Update and Guidelines for the Clinician. Am J Med Genet Part B. 2012; 159B:628–643

[27] Qiu C. Epidemiological findings of vascular risk factors in Alzheimer's disease: implications for therapeutic and preventive intervention. Expert Rev Neurother. 2011;11(11):1593-607.

[28] Barnes DE, Haight TJ, Mehta KM et al. Secondhand smoke, vascular disease, and dementia incidence: findings from the cardiovascular health cognition study. Am J Epidemiol. 2010; 1: 171 (3): 292-302

[29] Rusanen M, Kivipelto M, Quensenberry CP et al. Heavy smoking in midlife and long-term risk of Alzheimer disease and vascular dementia. Arch Intern Med.2011; 171(4):333-339

[30] Anttila T, Helkala EL, Viitanen M, Kareholt I, Fratiglioni L, Winblad B, et al. Alcohol drinking in middle age and subsequent risk of mild cognitive impairment and dementia in old age: a prospective population based study. BMJ. 2004; 329(7465):539.

[31] Qiu C, Winblad B, Fratiglioni L. The age-dependent relation of blood pressure to cognitive function and dementia. Lancet Neurol. 2005;4(8):487-99.

[32] Qiu C, Winblad B, Marengoni A, Klarin I, Fastbom J, Fratiglioni L. Heart failure and risk of dementia and Alzheimer disease: a population-based cohort study. Arch Intern Med. 2006;166(9):1003-8.

[33] Purandare N, Burns A, Daly KJ, Hardicre J, Morris J, Macfarlane G, et al. Cerebral emboli as a potential cause of Alzheimer's disease and vascular dementia: case-control study. BMJ. 2006; 332(7550):1119-24.

[34] Beydoun MA, Lhotsky A, Wang Y, Dal Forno G, An Y, Metter EJ, et al. Association of adiposity status and changes in early to mid-adulthood with incidence of Alzheimer's disease. Am J Epidemiol. 2008;168(10):1179-89.

[35] Atti AR, Palmer K, Volpato S, Winblad B, De Ronchi D, Fratiglioni L. Late-life body mass index and dementia incidence: nine-year follow-up data from the Kungsholmen Project. J Am Geriatr Soc. 2008; 56(1):111-6.

[36] Hassing LB, Dahl AK, Thorvaldsson V, Berg S, Gatz M, Pedersen NL, et al. Overweight in midlife and risk of dementia: a 40-year follow-up study. Int J Obes (Lond). 2009; 33(8):893-8.

[37] Solomon A, Kivipelto M. Cholesterol-modifying strategies for Alzheimer's disease. Expert Rev Neurother. 2009; 9(5):695-709.

[38] Xu W, Qiu C, Winblad B, Fratiglioni L. The effect of borderline diabetes on the risk of dementia and Alzheimer's disease. Diabetes. 2007; 56(1):211-6.

[39] Lu FP, Lin KP, Kuo HK. Diabetes and the risk of multi-system aging phenotypes: a systematic review and meta-analysis. PLoS One. 2009;4(1):e4144.

[40] Xu W, Caracciolo B, Wang HX, Winblad B, Backman L, Qiu C, et al. Accelerated progression from mild cognitive impairment to dementia in people with diabetes. Diabetes. 2010; 59(11):2928-35.

[41] Tan ZS, Beiser AS, Vasan RS, Roubenoff R, Dinarello CA, Harris TB, et al. Inflammatory markers and the risk of Alzheimer disease: the Framingham Study. Neurology. 2007; 68(22):1902-8.

[42] Sundelof J, Kilander L, Helmersson J, Larsson A, Ronnemaa E, Degerman-Gunnarsson M, et al. Systemic inflammation and the risk of Alzheimer's disease and dementia: a prospective population-based study. J Alzheimers Dis. 2009; 18(1):79-87.

[43] Van Dam F, Van Gool WA. Hyperhomocysteinemia and Alzheimer's disease: A systematic review. Arch Gerontol Geriatr. 2009;48(3):425-30.

[44] Ownby RL, Crocco E, Acevedo A, John V, Loewenstein D. Depression and risk for Alzheimer disease: systematic review, meta-analysis, and metaregression analysis. Arch Gen Psychiatry. 2006; 63(5):530-8.

[45] Raffaitin C, Gin H, Empana JP, Helmer C, Berr C, Tzourio C, et al. Metabolic syndrome and risk for incident Alzheimer's disease or vascular dementia: the Three-City Study. Diabetes Care. 2009; 32(1):169-74.

[46] Rovio S, Kareholt I, Helkala EL, Viitanen M, Winblad B, Tuomilehto J, et al. Leisure-time physical activity at midlife and the risk of dementia and Alzheimer's disease. Lancet Neurol. 2005;4(11):705-11.

[47] Karp A, Andel R, Parker MG, Wang HX, Winblad B, Fratiglioni L. Mentally stimulating activities at work during midlife and dementia risk after age 75: follow-up study from the Kungsholmen Project. Am J Geriatr Psychiatry. 2009;17(3):227-36.

[48] Paillard-Borg S, Fratiglioni L, Winblad B, Wang HX. Leisure activities in late life in relation to dementia risk: principal component analysis. Dement Geriatr Cogn Disord. 2009;28(2):136-44

[49] Scarmeas N, Stern Y, Tang MX, Mayeux R, Luchsinger JA. Mediterranean diet and risk for Alzheimer's disease. Ann Neurol. 2006 Jun;59(6):912-21

[50] Hooshmand B, Solomon A, Kareholt I, Leiviska J, Rusanen M, Ahtiluoto S, et al. Homocysteine and holotranscobalamin and the risk of Alzheimer disease: a longitudinal study. Neurology. 2010; 75(16):1408-14.

[51] Barron AM, Pike CJ. Sex hormones, aging, and Alzheimer's disease. Front Biosci (Elite Ed). 2012; 4:976-97.

[52] Hogervorst E, Yaffe K, Richards M, Huppert FA. Hormone replacement therapy to maintain cognitive function in women with dementia. Cochrane Database Syst Rev. 2009(1):CD003799.

[53] Callahan CM, Hendrie HC, Tierney WM. Documentation and evaluation of cognitive impairment in elderly primary care patients. Ann Intern Med. 1995; 122(6):422-9.

[54] Petersen RC, Doody R, Kurz A, Mohs RC, Morris JC, Rabins PV, et al. Current concepts in mild cognitive impairment. Arch Neurol. 2001;58(12):1985-92.

[55] Sperling RA, Aisen PS, Beckett LA., et al. Toward defining the preclinical stages of Alzheimer's disease: Recommendations from the National Institute on Aging-Alzheimer's Association workgroups on diagnostic guidelines for Alzheimer's disease. Alzheimers Dement. 2011; 7(3): 280–292.

[56] Albert MS, DeKosky ST, Dickson D, et al. The diagnosis of mild cognitive impairment due to Alzheimer's disease: Recommendations from the National Institute on Aging- Alzheimer's Association workgroups on diagnostic guidelines for Alzheimer's disease. Alzheimers Dement. 2011; 7(3): 270–279.

[57] Taler V, Phillips NA. Language performance in Alzheimer's disease and mild cognitive impairment: a comparative review. J Clin Exp Neuropsychol. 2008; 30(5):501-56.

[58] Mohs RC. The clinical syndrome of Alzheimer's disease: aspects particularly relevant to clinical trials. Genes Brain Behav. 2005;4(3):129-33.

[59] The Swedish Council on Technology Assessment in Health Care. Dementia- Etiology and Epidemiology: A Systematic Review. 2008

[60] Vellas B, Hausner L, Frölich L et al. Progression of Alzheimer disease in Europe: Data from the European ICTUS study. Curr Alzheimer Res. 2012 Jun 26

[61] McKhann, G., Drachman, D., Folstein, et al. Clinical diagnosis of Alzheimer's disease: report of the NINCDS-ADRDA Work Group under the auspices of Department of Health and Human Services Task Force on Alzheimer's Disease. Neurology. 1984; 34, 939-944.

[62] Knopman DS, DeKosky ST, Cummings JL, Chuit H, Corey-Bloom J, Relkin N, et al. Practice parameter: diagnosis of dementia (an evidence-based review). Neurology. 2001; 56:1143–53.

[63] Katz S, Ford AB, Moskowitz RW, Jackson BA, Jaffe MW. Studies of Illness in the Aged. The Index of Adl: A Standardized Measure of Biological and Psychosocial Function. JAMA. 1963; 185:914-9.

[64] Lawton MP, Brody EM. Assessment of older people: self-maintaining and instrumental activities of daily living. Gerontologist. 1969; 9(3):179-86.

[65] Bucks RS, Ashworth DL, Wilcock GK, Siegfried K. Assessment of activities of daily living in dementia: development of the Bristol Activities of Daily Living Scale. Age Ageing. 1996; 25(2):113-20.

[66] Folstein MF, Folstein SE, McHugh PR. "Mini-mental state". A practical method for grading the cognitive state of patients for the clinician. J Psychiatr Res. 1975; 12(3): 189-98.

[67] Buschke H, Kuslansky G, Katz M, Stewart WF, Sliwinski MJ, Eckholdt HM, et al. Screening for dementia with the memory impairment screen. Neurology. 1999; 52(2): 231-8.

[68] Price CC, Cunningham H, Coronado N, Freedland A, Cosentino S, Penney DL, et al. Clock drawing in the Montreal Cognitive Assessment: recommendations for dementia assessment. Dement Geriatr Cogn Disord. 2011; 31(3):179-87.

[69] Damian AM, Jacobson SA, Hentz JG, Belden CM, Shill HA, Sabbagh MN, et al. The Montreal Cognitive Assessment and the mini-mental state examination as screening instruments for cognitive impairment: item analyses and threshold scores. Dement Geriatr Cogn Disord. 2011; 31(2):126-31.

[70] Lezack M, Howieson DB, Bigler ED, Tranel D. Neuropsychological assessment. 5th ed. New York: Oxford University press; 2012.

[71] Hort J, O´Brien JT, Gainotti G, Pirttila T, Popescu BO et al. EFNS guidelines for the diagnosis and managment f Azlehimer´s disease. European Journal of Neurology. 2010; 17:1236-1248

[72] Wright CF, Hall A, Matthews FE and Brayne C. biomarkers, dementia and Public Health. Ann. N.Y. Acad. Sci. 2009; 11880:11-19

[73] Braak H, Braak E. Morphological criteria for recognition of Alzheimer´s disease and the distribution pattern of cortical changes related to this disorder. Neurobiol Aging. 1994; 15:355-356

[74] Scheltens P. Imaging in Alzheimer´s disease. Dialogues Clin Neurosci. 2009; 11: 191–199.

[75] Sluimer JD, van der Flier WM, Karas GB, et al. Whole-brain atrophy rate and cognitive decline: longitudinal MR study of memory clinic patients. Radiology. 2008; 248:590-598.

[76] Bruno Dubois B, Feldman HH, Jacova C, DeKosky ST et al. Research criteria for the diagnosis of Alzheimer's disease: revising the NINCDS–ADRDA criteria. Lancet Neurol 2007; 6: 734–46

[77] Coleman RE. Positron emission tomography diagnosis of Alzheimer's disease. Neuroimaging Clin N Am. 2005; 15: 837–46.

[78] Zhang. S, Han D, Tan X et al. Diagnostci accuracy of 18F-FDG and 11C-PIB-PET for predict of short-term conversion to Alzheimer´s disease in subjects with mild cognitive impairment. Int J Clin Pract. 2012; 66 (2): 185-198

[79] Ringman JM, Younkin SG, Pratico D, Seltzer W, Cole GM, Geschwind DH, et al. Biochemical markers in persons with preclinical familial Alzheimer disease. Neurology. 2008; 71:85–92.

[80] Nordberg A, Carter SF, Rinne J, Drzezga A, Brook DJ et al. A European multicentre PET study of fibrillar amyloid in Alzheimer's disease. Eur J Nucl Med Mol Imaging. 2012. Sept 8.

[81] Sunderland, T., Linker, G., Mirza, N., Putnam, K.T., Friedman, D.L.,Kimmel, L.H., Bergeson, J., Manetti, G.J., Zimmermann, M., Tang, B., Bartko, J.J., Cohen, R.M. Decreased beta-amyloid1-42 and increased tau levels in cerebrospinal fluid of patients with Alzheimer disease. JAMA.2003; 289: 2094–2103

[82] Hesse, C., Rosengren, L., Andreasen, N., Davidsson, P., Vanderstichele,H., Vanmechelen, E., Blennow, K. et al. Transient increase in total tau but not phospho-tau in human cerebrospinal fluid after acute stroke.Neurosci. Lett. 2001; 297:187–190.

[83] Blennow K, Zetterberg H and Fagan AM. Fluid Biomarkers in Alzheimer Disease. Cold Spring Harb Perspect Med 2012; 2:a006221

[84] Snider BJ, Fagan AM, Roe C, Shah AR, Grant EA, Xiong C, Morris JC, Holtzman DM. Cerebrospinal fluid biomarkers and rate of cognitive decline in very mild dementia of the Alzheimer type. Arch Neurol. 2009; 66: 638–645.

[85] Moonis M, Swearer JM, Dayaw MP, St George-Hyslop P, Rogaeva E, Kawarai T, et al. Familial Alzheimer disease: decreases in CSF Abeta42 levels precede cognitive decline. Neurology. 2005; 65:323–5.

[86] Wu G, Sankaranarayanan S, Wong J, Tugusheva K et al. Characterization of Plasma b-Secretase (BACE1) Activity and Soluble Amyloid Precursor Proteins as Potential Biomarkers for Alzheimer's Disease . Journal of Neuroscience Research. 2012. Jul 16.

[87] Mayeux R, Honig LS, Tang MX, Manly J, Stern Y, Schupf N, Mehta PD. Plasma Ab40 and Ab42 and Alzheimer's disease: relation to age, mortality, and risk. Neurology 2003; 61:1185–1190.

[88] Pomara N, Willoughby LM, Sidtis JJ, Mehta PD. Selective reductions in plasma Ab1–42 in healthy elderly subjects during longitudinal followup: a preliminary report. Am J Geriatr Psychiatry 2005;13:914–917

[89] Galton CJ, Patterson K, Xuereb JH and Hodges JR. Atypical and typical presentations of Alzheimer's disease: A clinical, neuropsychological, neuroimaging and pathological study of 13 cases. Brain. 2000; 123: 484-498.

[90] Alladi S, Xuereb J, Bak T, et al. Focal cortical presentations of Alzheimer's disease. Brain 2007; 130 (10):2636–2645.

[91] von Gunten A, Bouras C, Kovari E, Giannakopoulos P, Hof PR. Neural substrates of cognitive and behavioral deficits in atypical Alzheimer's disease. Brain Res Rev 2006; 51: 176–211

[92] Portet F, Dauvilliers Y, Campion D, Raux G, Hauw JJ, Lyon-Caen O, et al. Very early onset AD with a de novo mutation in the presenilin 1 gene (Met 233 Leu). Neurology 2003; 61: 1136–7.

[93] Mendez MF, McMurtray A. Frontotemporal dementia-like phenotypes associated with presenilin-1 mutations. Am J Alzheimer's Dis Other Demen 2006; 214: 281–6.

[94] Johnson JK, Head E, Kim R, Starr A, Cotman CW. Clinical and pathological evidence for a frontal variant of Alzheimer disease. Arch Neurol 1999; 56: 1233–9.

[95] Mesulam MM. Slowly progressive aphasia without generalized dementia. Ann Neurol 1982;11:592e8.

[96] Gorno-Tempini ML, Hillis AE, Weintraub S, et al. Classification of primary progressive aphasia and its variants. Neurology 2011; 76:1006e14.

[97] Ahmed S, de Jager CA, Haigh AF, Garrard P et al. Logopenic aphasia in Alzheimer's disease: clinical variant or clinical feature? J Neurol Neurosurg Psychiatry. 2012; 10.1136/jnnp-2012-302798

[98] Renner JA, Burns JM, Hou CE, McKeel DW Jr, Storandt M, Morris JC. Progressive posterior cortical dysfunction: a clinicopathologic series. Neurology 2004; 63: 1175–80.

[99] McMonagle P, Deering F, Berliner Y, Kertesz A. The cognitive profile of posterior cortical atrophy. Neurology 2006; 66: 331–38.

[100] Kas A, de Souza LC, Samri D, et al. Neural correlates of cognitive impairment in posterior cortical atrophy. Brain 2011; 134: 1464–78.

[101] Crutch SJ, Lehmann M, Schott JM, et al. Posterior cortical atrophy. Lancet Neurol. 2012 ; 11(2):170-8. Review

[102] Snowden JS, Stopford CL, Julien CL et al.Cognitive phenotypes in Alzheimer′disease and genetic risk. Cortex. 2007; 43:835-845

http://dx.doi.org/10.5772/54539

[103] Hassan A, Whitwell JL, and Josephs KA. The corticobasal syndrome–Alzheimer's disease conundrum Expert Rev Neurother. 2011; 11(11): 1569–1578.

[104] Sadowsky CH, and Galvin JE. Guidelines for the Management of Cognitive and Behavioral Problems in Dementia J Am Board Fam Med. 2012; 25:350 –366.

[105] Birks J. Cholinesterase inhibitors for Alzheimer's disease. Cochrane Database Syst Rev 2006;(1): CD005593

[106] Trinh NH, Hoblyn J, Mohanty S, Yaffe K. et al. Efficacy of cholinesterase inhibitors in the treatment of neuropsychiatric symptoms and functional impairment in Alzheimer disease: a meta-analysis. JAMA 2003; 289:210–6.

[107] Winblad B and Poritis N. Memantine in severe dementia: results of the 9M-BEST study (benefit and efficacy in severely demented patients during treatment with memantine). Int. J. Geriat. Psychiatry, 1999; 14:135-146

[108] Tariot PN, Farlow MR, Grossberg GT, Graham SM, McDonald S, Gergel I. Memantine treatment in patients with moderate to severe Alzheimer disease already receiving donepezil: a randomized controlled trial. JAMA 2004; 291(3), 317–324.

[109] Atri A, Shaughnessy LW, Locascio JJ, Growdon JH. Long-term course and effectiveness of combination therapy in Alzheimer disease. Alzheimer Dis. Assoc. Disord. 2008; 22(3), 209–221.

[110] Howard R, McShane R, Lindesay J et al. Donepezil and memantine for moderate-to-severe Alzheimer's disease. N. Engl. J. Med. 2012; 366, 893–903.

[111] Landreth G, Jiang Q, Mandrekar S, Heneka M. PPARgamma agonists as therapeutics for the treatment of Alzheimer's disease. Neurotherapeutics . 2008; 5(3), 481–489

[112] Gold M, Alderton C, Zvartau-Hind ME et al. Effects of rosiglitazone as monotherapy in apoE4-stratified subjects with mild-to-moderate Alzheimer's disease. Alzheimers Dement. 2009; 5(4), 86

[113] Henley DB, May PC, Dean RA, Siemers ER. Development of semagacestat (LY450139), a functional gamma-secretase inhibitor, for the treatment of Alzheimer's disease. Expert Opin. Pharmacother. 2009; 10(10): 1657–1664.

[114] Green RC, Schneider LS, Amato DA et al. Effect of tarenflurbil on cognitive decline and activities of daily living in patients with mild Alzheimer disease: a randomized controlled trial. JAMA. 2009; 302(23): 2557–2564.

[115] Anne Corbett1, Jessica Smith1 and Clive Ballard. New and emerging treatments for Alzheimer's disease Expert Rev. Neurother. 2012; 12(5):535–543.

[116] Wilcock DM, Colton CA. Anti-Ab immunotherapy in Alzheimer's disease; relevance of transgenic mouse studies to clinical trials J. Alzheimers Dis. 2008;15(4): 555–569.

[117] Valenzuela MJ, Sachdev P. Brain reserve and dementia: a systematic review. Psychol Med. 2006;36(4):441-54.

[118] Stern Y. What is cognitive reserve? Theory and research application of the reserve concept. J Int Neuropsychol Soc. 2002;8(3):448-60.

[119] Lyketsos CG, Colenda CC, Beck C, Blank K, Doraiswamy MP, Kalunian DA, et al. Position statement of the American Association for Geriatric Psychiatry regarding principles of care for patients with dementia resulting from Alzheimer disease. Am J Geriatr Psychiatry. 2006;14(7):561-72.

[120] De Vreese LP, Neri M, Fioravanti M, Belloi L, Zanetti O. Memory rehabilitation in Alzheimer's disease: a review of progress. Int J Geriatr Psychiatry. 2001; 8:794-809.

[121] Clare L, Woods RT, Moniz Cook ED, Orrell M, Spector A. Cognitive rehabilitation and cognitive training for early-stage Alzheimer's disease and vascular dementia. Cochrane Database Syst Rev. 2003; 4:CD003260.

[122] Wilson BA. Neuropsychological rehabilitation. Annu Rev Clin Psychol. 2008; 4:141-62.

[123] Yamaguchi H, Maki Y, Yamagami T. Overview of non-pharmacological intervention for dementia and principles of brain-activating rehabilitation. Psychogeriatrics. 2010;10(4):206-13.

[124] Rabins PV, Blacker D, Rovner BW, Rummans T, Schneider LS, Tariot PN, et al. American Psychiatric Association practice guideline for the treatment of patients with Alzheimer's disease and other dementias. Second edition. Am J Psychiatry. 2007; 164(12 Suppl):5-56.

[125] Doody RS, Stevens JC, Beck C, Dubinsky RM, Kaye JA, Gwyther L, et al. Practice parameter: management of dementia (an evidence-based review). Report of the Quality Standards Subcommittee of the American Academy of Neurology. Neurology. 2001; 56(9):1154-66.

[126] Hermans DG, Htay UH, McShane R. Non-pharmacological interventions for wandering of people with dementia in the domestic setting. Cochrane Database Syst Rev. 2007(1):CD005994.

[127] Robinson L, Hutchings D, Dickinson HO, Corner L, Beyer F, Finch T, et al. Effectiveness and acceptability of non-pharmacological interventions to reduce wandering in dementia: a systematic review. Int J Geriatr Psychiatry. 2007; 22(1):9-22.

[128] Tadaka E, Kanagawa K. Effects of reminiscence group in elderly people with Alzheimer disease and vascular dementia in a community setting. Geriatrics & Gerontology International 2007; 7(2):167-73.

[129] Bohlmeijer E, Smit F, Cuijpers P. Effects of reminiscence and life review on late-life depression: a meta-analysis. Int J Geriatr Psychiatry. 2003; 18(12):1088-94.

http://dx.doi.org/10.5772/54539

[130] Bohlmeijer E, Valenkamp M, Westerhof G, Smit F, Cuijpers P. Creative reminiscence as an early intervention for depression: results of a pilot project. Aging Ment Health. 2005; 9(4):302-4.

[131] Katsuaki T, Yukiko Y, Yoshio K, Kazuki S, Ayako M, Ryuhei N, et al. Improved cognitive function, mood and brain blood flow in single photon emission computed tomography following individual reminiscence therapy in an elderly patient with Alzheimer's disease. Geriatrics & Gerontology International. 2007; 7(3):305-9.

[132] Afonso R, Bueno B. [Reminiscence with different types of autobiographical memories: Effects on the reduction of depressive symptomatology in old age]. Psicothema. 2010; 22(2):213-20.

[133] Neal M, Briggs M. Validation therapy for dementia. Cochrane Database Syst Rev. 2003; 3:CD001394.

[134] Spector A, Orrell M, Davies S, Woods B. Reality orientation for dementia. Cochrane Database Syst Rev. 2000; 4:CD001119.

[135] Spector A, Orrell M, Davies S, Woods B. WITHDRAWN: Reality orientation for dementia. Cochrane Database Syst Rev. 2000; 3:CD001119.

[136] Savorani G, Chattat R, Capelli E, Vaienti F, Giannini R, Bacci M, et al. Immediate effectiveness of the "new identity" reality orientation therapy (ROT) for people with dementia in a geriatric day hospital. Arch Gerontol Geriatr Suppl. 2004; 9:359-64.

[137] Spector A, Thorgrimsen L, Woods B, Royan L, Davies S, Butterworth M, et al. Efficacy of an evidence-based cognitive stimulation therapy programme for people with dementia: randomised controlled trial. Br J Psychiatry 2003; 183:248-54.

Chapter 2

Late-Onset Alzheimer's Disease: Risk Factors, Clinical Diagnosis and the Search for Biomarkers

Marisol Herrera-Rivero

Additional information is available at the end of the chapter

http://dx.doi.org/10.5772/53775

1. Introduction

Even with the progress that has been made in the past years on our understanding of Alzheimer's disease (AD) we don't seem to be closer to finding a cure than we were before. AD is a complex disorder wherein the pathophysiology is influenced by a great number of environmental and genetic factors, thus making it difficult to uncover the triggering events underlying disease's onset. In this chapter, we will first discuss some common conditions within the general population that have been associated with an increased risk to develop late-onset Alzheimer's disease (LOAD), such as hypertension, type 2 diabetes mellitus and high serum cholesterol and triglycerides levels, and the way they might be contributing to cognitive decline; depression and traumatic brain injuries, amongst others, will also be boarded.

Misdiagnosis is a frequent issue with important repercussions not only for the patient's condition but also for family members. For this reason, in the second part we will review the main basic aspects that should be involved in AD diagnosis, from laboratory tests to neuroimaging technologies, highlighting the importance of seeking a differential diagnosis of dementias in the elderly and the crucial role an accurate diagnosis may play in therapeutic outcomes as well as the implications for quality of life.

Early diagnosis of Alzheimer's may be the best tool we could find, as for now, to improve treatment outcomes by slowing the disease progression rate. This idea has led an important number of scientists around the globe to the search for biomarkers using a wide variety of approaches in the brain, cerebrospinal fluid (CSF) and blood. On this matter, we will briefly comment on our preliminary study using lymphocytes from cognitively healthy people and neuropsychological patients affected not only with LOAD but other types of neuropathologies as well to analyse in blood cells the expression of the main genes directly related to AD in brain cells. This study included 72 subjects in whom the expression of the microtubule-associated protein tau (MAPT), the amyloid precursor protein (APP), nicastrin (NCSTN), a component of the γ-secretase, and β-secretase (beta-site APP cleaving enzyme 1, BACE1) were analysed through 4 groups of cognitively healthy individuals ranging from 25 to 92 years of age and in conditions such as LOAD, vascular dementia (VaD) and Parkinson's disease (PD) in elderly individuals. We also aimed to discover the manner in which the expression of these genes might be affected by conditions associated with increased risk for LOAD such as hypertension and glucose, cholesterol and triglycerides serum levels.

2. Risk factors for AD

A wide variety of factors have been associated with an increased risk to develop LOAD; nevertheless, a number of these associations remain controversial. Age is the main risk factor to develop AD of the sporadic type and is only followed by apolipoprotein E (ApoE) genotype. However, other genetic and environmental conditions have also been proven to influence the risk of developing the disease and the rate of cognitive decline which affects disease progression. Amongst these are found cardiovascular risk factors, type 2 diabetes mellitus, sleep disorders, depression, education, smoking, alcohol, traumatic brain injury (TBI) and several single nucleotide polymorphisms (SNPs) in a growing list of candidate genes.

2.1. Environmental

a. Cardiovascular risk factors.

Within the risk factors for vascular disease hypertension and high cholesterol levels are most importantly associated with LOAD. Various longitudinal studies have shown an association between a diagnosis of hypertension in midlife and the development of AD in late life [1,2]. On this regard, hypertension may cause cerebrovascular disease which would contribute to accelerate AD processes, even when there are reports on a decrease in blood pressure during the disease course probably due to affection of the brain regions implicated in its regulation [3]. Cholesterol and its metabolism is associated with AD by several proposed mechanisms including regulation of beta-amyloid (Aβ) generation by an increase in β-secretase activity, APP membrane localization and cleavage variations by changes in cholesterol rich lipid rafts and ApoE-regulated interactions between cholesterol and Aβ.

b. Type 2 diabetes mellitus.

Diabetes and even high glucose levels in the absence of a diabetes diagnosis are associated with an increased risk to develop AD involving various mechanisms, primarily being changes in the blood brain barrier (BBB) and the transport within cerebral small vessels [4].

c. Traumatic brain injury.

TBI has been associated with an increased risk to develop AD by longitudinal and retrospective studies, suggesting an effect between severity and repetitive episodes of TBI particularly by an increase in amyloid deposition [5, 6].

d. Depression.

It has been subject for debate whether depression might be an early manifestation of AD or a contributing factor for development of the disease. If one thing is sure is that depression contributes to cognitive decline and may by itself cause a condition known as "depressive pseudo-dementia" which can frequently evolve to a true dementia (mainly AD) when not treated, particularly in the elderly [7]. A history of major depressive disorder or susceptibility to depression during an individual's lifetime has therefore been associated with an increased risk to develop LOAD [8].

e. Sleep.

Chronic sleep deprivation and other sleep disorders have a negative effect on cognitive function primarily due to the role sleep plays in memory and learning processes and possibly in synaptic plasticity, although it is also believed there is an increase in Aβ during the waking hours [9]. History of sleep disorders has thus been linked to an increase in the risk to develop LOAD; furthermore, sleep disorders occurring as part of the aging process and those related to coexisting medical conditions contribute to cognitive decline and behavioural problems in AD patients.

f. Education.

People with a lower level of education show an increased risk to develop LOAD. This might be due to the relative lack of constant stimulation of cognitive processes (such as learning and memory) compared to individuals with a higher education degree. In fact, cognitive stimulation therapies are widely used for helping the treatment of people with dementia [10].

g. Diet.

It is well known that diet affects every aspect of an individual's health. A number of medical conditions associated with an increased risk for developing AD have a strong nutritional background as cholesterol, glucose and vitamin B_{12} levels, just to mention a few, importantly influence the risk for dementia [11], particularly in old age.

h. Alcohol and smoking.

It remains unclear whether alcohol and smoking increase the risk for AD as their association has been inconsistent. Although smoking is a strong risk factor for vascular disease, and the association of the latter with AD has been established, the possibility of a neuroprotective effect of nicotine by a smoking-induced increase in nicotinic receptors exists [3]. Similar is the case of alcohol where wine presents protective effects because of its antioxidant contents while associations between other types of alcohol and risk of AD remain controversial.

2.2. Genetic

Medical conditions and lifestyle in midlife, especially when a group of these factors coexist in an individual creating a synergistic effect, can contribute to cellular and molecular alterations ultimately leading to the hallmark pathological processes of AD later in life. Although environmental factors appear to play an important role in the development of LOAD, a number of them may depend on a genetic-influenced predisposition. Genetic variations in candidate genes have been widely investigated for associations with an increased risk of development, age of onset and progression of AD and, while results on several studies are controversial or inconclusive, it remains clear that common genetic variations do associate with LOAD whether in a general or population-specific manner. The AlzGene database holds information on 2973 polymorphisms in 695 genes reported in 1395 studies. We summarize in Table 1 some of the main findings on this field.

Gene	*Chromosome*	*SNP*	*Odds ratio*	*Studies*
APOE	19	e2/3/4	3.68 (4 vs. 3)	37
BIN1	2	rs744373	1.17	21
CLU	8	rs11136000	0.89	33
ABCA7	19	rs3764650	1.23	10
CR1	1	rs3818361	1.15	27
PICALM	11	rs3851179	0.88	27
MS4A6A	11	rs610932	0.90	11
CD33	19	rs3865444	0.89	5
MS4A4E	11	rs670139	1.08	11
CD2AP	6	rs9349407	1.12	5
EPHA1	7	rs11767557	0.89	5
GSTO1	10	rs4925	0.97	7
TOMM40	19	rs8106922	0.66	7
SORL1	11	rs2282649	1.10	23
PVRL2	19	rs6859	1.50	8
NCSTN	1	rs2274185	0.90	5
BDNF	11	270C/T	1.09	20
GAB2	11	rs2373115	0.85	13

Source: Meta-analysis for all studies from AlzGene-field synopsis of genetic association studies in AD (www.alzgene.org)

Table 1. Some widely studied genetic variations associated with an increased risk of AD.

At this point there is a need to highlight that prevention of LOAD may only be achieved by a healthy lifestyle implemented early in life, most importantly by those individuals with a genetic susceptibility.

http://dx.doi.org/10.5772/53775

3. Clinical diagnosis of LOAD

To perform a clinical diagnosis of AD or other dementias may not be challenging when symptoms are from moderate to severe and well differentiated; however, it might be more difficult to achieve an accurate diagnosis in the early stages of the disease, especially in elderly individuals where initial manifestations of AD can be taken as an effect of aging. Early detection of cognitive decline in primary care thus becomes crucial for canalization of the patient to an adequate specialist and a subsequent early accurate diagnosis which allows a better management of disease progression. In the first stages of AD, memory processes are the most affected but since a number of other treatable medical conditions also present with deficiencies in memory performance, a differential diagnosis based on all available tools must always be pursued. Clinical diagnosis of LOAD should include laboratory and neuropsychological tests as well as structural and functional imaging of the brain which, together with the clinical history and interviews with those living closest to the patient, would provide a better idea of the patient's overall condition.

3.1. Initial evaluation

Clinical history and, importantly, interviews with close family members and friends provide valuable information on patient's medical history, lifestyle and disease onset and progression. Several issues may be considered though when evaluating an aged individual: clinical manifestations of psychiatric disorders differ from younger patients; life events, social and financial situations as well as physical status are also relevant aspects to be taken into account.

3.2. Laboratory tests

Running laboratory tests is important to identify secondary causes of dementia and medical conditions common in the aged population. It is advisable to perform a complete blood count, serum electrolytes, glucose, vitamin B12, BUN/creatinine ratio and thyroid and hepatic function panels. Electrocardiography (ECG), electroencephalography (EEG) and thorax x-rays can also be included. Increase in total tau protein (t-tau) and decrease in $A\beta_{42}$ in CSF are found in AD.

3.3. Neuropsychological evaluation

Neuropsychological evaluation is fundamental for dementia diagnosis providing evidence of cognitive dysfunction and specific patterns helping to uncover the cause. AD diagnosis is based on NINCDS-ADRDA (National Institute of Neurological and Communicative Disorders and the Alzheimer's Disease and Related Disorders Association) criteria and is classified as definitive (clinical diagnosis with histological confirmation), probable (typical clinical features without histological confirmation) or possible (atypical clinical features, no apparent alternative diagnosis and no histological confirmation). Diagnosis of probable AD can only be made when objective evidence of significant memory deterioration exists by neuropsychological evaluation together with at least one other biological feature such as abnormal CSF biomarkers and specific positron emission tomography (PET) patterns. Patients are evaluated using structured/semi-structured interviews and neuropsychological batteries with a variety of available tests to explore different aspects of cognition and behaviour. It may be advisable to apply a quick neuropsychological test to patients with apparent cognitive decline at primary care level; this would facilitate a proper canalization and management of the patient. Initial evaluations of general cognitive status can be performed using the popular Mini-Mental State Examination (MMSE) which is quick and easy to apply and provides information on global cognitive efficiency and dementia severity, although is not recommended for a definitive diagnosis.

The issue of neuropsychiatric syndromes should also be addressed during dementia evaluation as their presence is associated with a rapid deterioration of cognition. It is important to notice that AD and cerebrovascular disease frequently coexist and the latter strongly determines presence and severity of clinical symptoms; thus, taking into account vascular risk factors and focal neurological signs as well as Hachinski Ischemic Scale results, combined with neuroimaging, serve as powerful tools to uncover a mixed dementia, especially in elderly individuals.

The most prominent feature of AD is a decline in cognitive function initially characterized by deficient memory for recent events, unusually repetitive omissions and difficulty to learn new information. The Free and Cued Selective Reminding Test (FCSRT) is a useful tool to explore these initial deficiencies in suspected AD patients. Temporo-spatial disorientation appears in early stages of the disease and progresses towards intermediate stages, where the patient can be disoriented in familiar places and aphasia appears with a decrease in verbal comprehension and nominal difficulty. To evaluate the fluency and coherence of language simple and complex orders and naming tests are used.

Confident neuropsychological markers of AD in early stages are deficiencies in episodic memory. Neuropsychological evaluation of AD patients also finds a loss of autonomy with disease progression from higher level to basic daily activities, for which daily living activities tests are applied. Instrumental functions such as language, praxis and visuospatial skills start being affected in intermediate stages of AD. Visuospatial dysfunction is a common feature in this stage of disease and can be evaluated by drawing and copying tests. In moderate to severe stages, difficulty to use objects and dressing apraxia can be observed as well as visual agnosia and a visual processing dysfunction recognized by facial and object recognition tests. Working memory and attention are usually affected by the time of diagnosis.

Deficiency in activities of daily living due to cognitive decline is essential diagnostic criteria for dementia and has great impact on quality of life. Neuropsychological tests to evaluate this feature allow differentiation of dementia from mild cognitive impairment (MCI). These tests measure basic (e.g. dressing, hygiene, feeding) and instrumental (e.g. cooking, cleaning, money management) activities. Activities of the Daily Living (ADL) and Instrumental Activities of the Daily Living (IADL) are widely used scales and provide the advantage of being easily applicable in primary care.

http://dx.doi.org/10.5772/53775

Non-cognitive, psychiatric and behavioural alterations common to dementia such as apathy, aggression, depression, psychosis and sleep disorders vary according to disease severity and may fluctuate; they can also present as initial manifestations of dementia. It is believed that neuropsychiatric alterations may even serve as clinical indicators of MCI conversion to AD. Scales for mood and behaviour not only evaluate the presence/absence of symptoms but their frequency, severity and impact; they can be applied to family and caregivers. The Neuropsychiatric Inventory can evaluate up to 10 behavioural alterations and is considered a standard tool, although a number of different batteries are available for this purpose. In Table 2 we provide a list of neuropsychological tests and batteries available to evaluate different aspects of cognitive and non-cognitive alterations.

General cognitive function	Cognitive Assessment System (CAS)
	Dementia Rating Scale—2 (DRS-2)
	Kaplan Baycrest Neurocognitive Assessment (KBNA)
	Kaufman Brief Intelligence Test (K-BIT)
	Mini-Mental State Examination (MMSE)
	National Adult Reading Test (NART)
	Neuropsychological Assessment Battery (NAB)
	Raven's Progressive Matrices (RPM)
	Repeatable Battery for the Assessment of Neuropsychological Status (RBANS)
	Stanford-Binet Intelligence Scales—5th edition (SB5)
	The Test of Nonverbal Intelligence—3 (TONI-3)
	The Speed and Capacity of Language Processing Test (SCOLP)
	Wechsler Abbreviated Scale of Intelligence (WASI)
	Wechsler Adult Intelligence Scale—III (WAIS-III)
	Woodcock-Johnson III Tests of Cognitive Abilities (WJ III COG)
Executive function	Behavioural Assessment of the Dysexecutive Syndrome (BADS)
	CANTAB
	Category Test (CT)
	Cognitive Estimation Test (CET)
	Delis-Kaplan Executive Function System (D-KEFS)
	Design Fluency Test
	Five Point Test
	Hayling and Brixton Tests
	Ruff Figural Fluency Test (RFFT)
	Self-Ordered Pointing Test (SOPT)
	Stroop Test
	Verbal Fluency
	Wisconsin Card Sorting Test (WCST)
Attention	Brief Test of Attention (BTA)
	Colour Trails Test (CTT)
	Comprehensive Trail Making Test (CTMT)
	Conners' Continuous Performance Test II (CPT-II)

	Integrated Visual and Auditory Continuous Performance Test (IVA + Plus) Paced Auditory Serial Addition Test (PASAT) Ruff 2 & 7 Selective Attention Test (2 & 7 Test) Symbol Digit Modalities Test (SDMT), Test of Everyday Attention (TEA) Test of Variables of Attention (T.O.V.A.) Trail Making Test (TMT)
Memory	Autobiographical Memory Interview (AMI) Benton Visual Retention Test (BVRT-5) Brief Visuospatial Memory Test—Revised (BVMT-R) Brown-Peterson Task Buschke Selective Reminding Test (SRT) California Verbal Learning Test-II (CVLT-II) Doors and People Test (DPT) Hopkins Verbal Learning Test—Revised (HVLT-R) Recognition Memory Test (RMT) Rey-Osterrieth Auditory Verbal Learning Test (RAVLT) Rey Complex Figure Test (ROCF) Rivermead Behavioural Memory Test—2th edition (RBMT-II) Ruff-Light Trail Learning Test (RULIT) Sentence Repetition Test Wechsler Memory Scale—3th edition (WMS-III) Wide Range Assessment of Memory and Learning—2th edition (WRAML2)
Language	Boston Diagnostic Aphasia Examination—3th edition (BDAE-3) Boston Naming Test—2 (BNT-2) Dichotic listening – Words Expressive One-Word Picture Vocabulary Test—3th edition (EOWPVT3) Expressive Vocabulary Test (EVT) Multilingual Aphasia Examination (MAE) Peabody Picture Vocabulary Test—3th edition (PPVT-III) Token Test (TT)
Visual perception	Balloons Test Bells Cancellation Test Clock Drawing Test (CDT) Facial Recognition Test (FRT) Hooper Visual Organization Test (VOT) Judgement of Line Orientation (JLO) Visual Object and Space Perception Battery (VOSP)
Somatosensory and olfactory function, body orientation	Finger localization Right-Left Orientation (RLO) Rivermead Assessment of Somatosensory Performance (RASP) Smell Identification Test (SIT) Tactual Performance Test (TPT)

Motor function	Finger Tapping Test (FTT) Grip Strength Grooved Pegboard Purdue Pegboard Test
Mood, personality and adaptive functions	Beck Depression Inventory—2th edition (BDI-II) Behaviour Rating Inventory of Executive Function (BRIEF) Geriatric Depression Scale (GDS) Instrumental Activities of Daily Living (IADL) Minnesota Multiphasic Personality Inventory-2 (MMPI-2) Personality Assessment Inventory (PAI) Scales of Independent Behaviour—Revised (SIB-R) Trauma Symptom Inventory (TSI)
Activities of the daily living	Activities of the Daily Living (ADL) Instrumental Activities of the Daily Living (IADL) Disability Assessment for Dementia Scale Alzheimer Disease Cooperative Study ADL Scale Functional Activities Questionnaire Progressive Deterioration Scale

Source: Strauss E, Sherman EMS, Spreen O. A compendium of neuropsychological tests: administration, norms, and commentary, 3rd ed. New York: Oxford University Press; 2006.

Table 2. Tests and batteries for neuropsychological evaluation.

3.4. Neuroimaging

Imaging of the brain can reflect anatomical and physiological changes related to specific pathological processes. Structural neuroimaging technologies such as computed tomography (CT) and magnetic resonance imaging (MRI) provide relevant information on brain structures and help to exclude treatable conditions while functional neuroimaging including single photon emission computed tomography (SPECT), PET and functional magnetic resonance imaging (fMRI) informs about brain activity status. CT and MRI on AD evaluation are used to exclude neurosurgical lesions (tumors, subdural hematomas), search for evidence of cerebro-vascular lesions (stroke, white matter lesions) and identify medial temporal lobe atrophy. The overlap of whole-brain atrophy in AD with normal aging and other dementias is considerable and therefore lacks diagnostic value in clinical practice. Absolute values of glucose metabolism in the hippocampus are normal in early stages of AD but decrease progressively during disease course as detected by PET. Hypometabolism in the associative parietal cortex, external temporal area, precuneus, posterior cingulate cortex and dorsolateral frontal cortex can be found in patients with clear dementia symptoms.

AD is characterized by changes in neurotransmission correlating with cognitive decline, particularly acetylcholine. A few PET tracers to measure acetylcholinesterase (AChE) and ligands to muscarinic and nicotinic receptors have been developed on the basis of the role of the cholinergic system in cognition and AD. AChE activity can be measured by its radioactively tagged analogues N-[^{11}C]-methyl-piperidine-4-yl-propionate (^{11}C-PMP) and N-[^{11}C]-methyl-piperidine-4-yl-acetate (^{11}C-MP4A); nicotinic receptors can be measured by ^{11}C-nicotine. A decrease in ^{11}C-nicotine correlates with cognition measured by MMSE [12]. Visualization of amyloid plaques started some 15 years ago initially using Aβ monoclonal antibodies and peptidic fragments and later small radioactively tagged Congo red, chrysamine G and thioflavin analogues for PET and SPECT. ^{18}F tagging may present some advantages for clinical applications compared to ^{11}C. Studies have shown there is less correlation between cognitive decline and the amount of amyloid plaques in the AD brain than between cognitive decline and the amount of neurofibrillary tangles and/or neurotransmitter activity as amyloid deposits are observed in up to 30% of cognitively healthy aged individuals [13]. An increase in microglial activation has also been reported in AD patients using neuroimaging technologies [14].

3.5. Differential diagnosis

Even when AD is the most common dementing syndrome in the elderly, one shall not forget that AD can share symptoms with other disorders. Medical, neurological and psychiatric conditions to which memory loss, depression, disorientation and other symptoms can be attributed must be also investigated for a differential diagnosis of dementia. When performing a diagnosis, it is important to be aware of features found during the patient evaluation providing doubt for the AD diagnosis and bear in mind that the more accurate the diagnosis is, the better the disease can be managed. AD diagnosis can be questioned when the conditions presented in Table 3 exist.

Feature	Possible cause
Early alterations of behaviour: inappropriate social behaviour/feeding alterations	Fronto-temporal dementia (FTD)
Early extrapyramidal signs Early visual hallucinations Early visuospatial and attention deterioration Behavioural disturbances during REM sleep Fluctuation of symptoms	Dementia with Lewy Bodies (DLB)
Vascular lesions in neuroimaging Sudden onset of symptoms Focal neurological signs	Vascular dementia (VaD)
Early language alterations: -Hesitant, forced speech, agrammatism -Progressive loss of knowledge about words and objects-Progressive decline of speech with anomia	Non-fluent progressive aphasia Semantic dementia Logopenic progressive aphasia
Onset with high order visuospatial dysfunction/Balint syndrome: ocular apraxia, optic ataxia, simultagnosia	Progressive posterior cortical atrophy

Table 3. Evaluation findings suggesting a diagnosis different from AD.

http://dx.doi.org/10.5772/53775

4. The search for AD biomarkers

Biomarkers for LOAD could help predict and diagnose the disease as well as follow its progression, evaluate treatments and find new therapeutic targets. Neuroimaging technologies, genomics, transcriptomics and proteomics approaches are being extensively used globally to search for novel biomarkers for AD capable of detecting changes in the brain and peripheral tissues occurring early in the disease. Nevertheless, the finding of biomarkers with good sensitivity and specificity for AD, and furthermore, their validation, is challenging, reason why different combinations of biomarkers, cognitive markers and risk factors may represent a more suitable tool to pursue diagnostic sensitivity and specificity for LOAD.

4.1. Brain biomarkers

Markers of AD pathology have been extensively investigated in the brain of these patients; unfortunately, the task has been challenging due to overlap of a number of these findings with other brain disorders and even with normal ageing, as is the case of whole-brain atrophy. Although some findings might still represent specific biomarkers for AD as shown by a recent study where a decrease in grey matter diffusion values observed mainly in the posterior cingulate gyrus and precuneus area has been suggested as a potential new biomarker for AD in early stages [15].

However, abnormalities in brain imaging (structural and functional), cognitive markers (neuropsychological scores) and molecules (mRNA, proteins) measured in specific brain regions affected by AD are currently demonstrating a better potential to identify AD and differentiate it from other disorders in a number of different combinations. Recent studies on the Alzheimer's Disease Neuroimaging Initiative (ADNI) subjects have shown correlations between temporal lobe atrophy measured by serial MRI scans with CSF p-tau and tau/Aβ_{42} ratio as well as with cognitive markers which apparently may also be able to predict MCI-AD conversion. Hippocampal volume loss showed to correlate with ApoE4 genotype. PET imaging using ^{18}F-fludeoxyglucose (FDG) showed correlations with Aβ_{42}, but using ^{11}C-labelled Pittsburgh compound B (^{11}C-PIB) to specifically bind fibrillar Aβ plaques showed correlations not only with Aβ_{42} but t-tau and p-tau$_{181}$ [16]. However, recently, a comparative study suggested ADNI subjects appear to have a more aggressive pathology than population-based samples, as observed by the rates of decline in hippocampal volume measured by MRI, which may raise concerns about ADNI subjects not being representative of the general population [17]. In any case, we must remember all findings should be validated in different cohorts and here may be the point where reproducibility cannot be achieved, reason why this has become a very active field in AD research.

4.2. Peripheral biomarkers

The search for easily available biomarkers for AD has lead scientists in the past years to investigate a number of molecules in CSF and blood components. From a variety of these studies several molecules were proposed as potential blood biomarkers for the disease (Table 4), although some results remained controversial. Until now, the best biomarker validated for

AD diagnosis is the CSF tau/Aβ_{42} ratio. Other biomarkers in CSF have been investigated though and, recently, protein markers of DNA damage have shown potential as biomarkers for AD and other dementias [18].

Markers involved in APP and Aβ metabolisms	
	Aβ peptides (total Aβ, Aβ_{40} and Aβ_{42})
	Brain-plasma Aβ flux
	Aβ autoantibodies
	APP platelet isoforms
	BACE1 activity
Markers related to cholesterol metabolism and vascular disease	
	Cholesterol
	24S-hydroxycholesterol
	ApoE
	Lp(a)
	Homocysteine
Markers of oxidation	
	Antioxidant levels (carotene, lycopene, vitamins A, C and E, urate, bilirubin)
	Lipid peroxidation (F_2-isoprostanes, 4-hydroxynonenal)
Markers of inflammation	
	C reactive protein
	IL-1β
	TNF-α
	IL-6 and its receptor
	α1-antichymotrypsin
Other proposed markers	
	Total tau (t-tau) and phosphorilated tau (p-tau)
	p97
	GSK3
	MAO-B
	Phospholipase-A2
	α2-macroglobulin
	Complement factor H (CFH)
	Desmosterol

Table 4. Proposed blood biomarkers for AD.

In recent years, the approach for biomarker discovery has changed, now focusing on pattern recognition and combinations of different markers to identify panels capable of differentiating AD from healthy control subjects and, in some cases, from other brain disorders. As the work on this field has been so extensive we will limit ourselves now to briefly mention some of the recent biomarker findings reported principally in blood plasma (Table 5), where protein profiles have been extensively analysed in AD, MCI and control subjects using a wide range of technologies. We shall not forget serum and blood cells are also a potential source of pathologic alterations reflecting disease.

Sample	Cohort	Panel	Change	Ref.
Plasma	AD and controls from the Australian Imaging Biomarker and Lifestyle study (AIBL)	cortisol, pancreatic polypeptide, insulin like growth factor binding protein 2, β2 microglobulin, vascular cell adhesion molecule 1, carcinoembryonic antigen, matrix metalloprotein 2, CD40, macrophage inflammatory protein 1α, superoxide dismutase, and homocysteine	Increase	[19]
		apolipoprotein E, epidermal growth factor receptor, hemoglobin, calcium, zinc, interleukin 17, and albumin	Decrease	
Plasma	MCI, AD and controls from ADNI	eotaxin 3, pancreatic polypeptide, N-terminal protein B-type brain natriuretic peptide, tenascin C	Increase	[20]
		IgM and ApoE	Decrease	
Peripheral blood mononuclear cells (PBMCs)	LOAD and controls	fatty acid amide hydrolase (FAAH) gene expression, protein levels and activity	Increase	[21]
Plasma	MCI-AD converters and controls from ADNI	α2-macroglobulin, angiotensinogen, apolipoprotein A-II (ApoA-II), ApoE, betacellulin (BTC), Fas ligand (FasL), heparin-binding EGF-like growth factor (HB-EGF), macrophage inflammatory protein-1α (MIP-1α), peptide YY (PYY), m glutamic oxaloacetic transaminase (SGOT), transthyretin (TTR)	Signature	[22]
Plasma	AD and controls	ANG-2, CCL5, CCL7, CCL15, CCL18, CXCL8, EGF, G-CSF, GDNF, ICAM-1, IGFBP-6, IL-1α, IL-3, IL-11, M-CSF, PDGF-BB, TNF-α, TRAIL-R4	Signature	[23]
Plasma	AD and controls AD and other dementias	EGF, PDG-BB and MIP-1δ TRAIL-R4	Not stated	[24]
Serum	AD and controls	miR-137, -181c, -9, -29a/b	Down-regulated	[25]
Plasma	MCI, AD and control from AddNeuroMed	complement components C3 and C3a, complement factor-I, γ-fibrinogen and alpha-1-microglobulin	Associate with whole-brain volume	[26]

Table 5. Recent findings on blood biomarkers for AD.

4.2.1. Expression of MAPT, APP, NCSTN and BACE1 in lymphocytes

Neurofibrillary tangles and amyloid plaques are hallmarks in the AD brain involving the microtubule-associated protein tau (MAPT) and Aβ peptides generated from the amyloid precursor protein (APP) by sequential cleavage of the β- and γ-secretases, nicastrin (NCSTN) being a major component of the latter. These molecules have been widely investigated in the brain; nevertheless, little is known about their expression in peripheral cells. The established role of inflammation in the AD pathology lead us to question how these major genes express in peripheral lymphocytes and, furthermore, whether their expression may correlate with common medical conditions in the elderly that have been identified as risk factors for LOAD.

a. Samples

To address this question, we collected blood samples from a total of 72 subjects, including 48 healthy individuals divided into 4 groups by age (25 to 92 years of age), 12 clinically diagnosed AD patients and 12 patients suffering from other brain disorders (vascular dementia-VaD-, Parkinson's disease-PD-, traumatic brain injury-TBI-, cerebrovascular events-CVE-, psychotic disorder) as a comparative group named NP (Table 6). All patients had been previously diagnosed by appropriate professionals in the private practice and healthy subjects volunteered, making this a small population-based cohort with exploratory purposes. For all subjects, blood pressure was measured and history was briefly collected; for all patients, interviews with family members were also performed. All patients are participants in our neuro-rehabilitation program [27] and samples were collected at the time of enrolment.

Group	*n*	*Mean age*	*Diagnosis*
I	12	30	
II	12	44	Cognitively healthy
III	12	58	
IV	12	80	
AD	12	80	LOAD
NP	12	78	PD, MCI, VaD, CVE, TBI, psychotic disorder/ schizophrenia

Table 6. Basic characteristics of the study groups.

b. Methodology

After collection, serum was separated from whole blood to quantify total cholesterol, glucose and triglycerides. Lymphocytes were isolated from EDTA whole blood using Lymphoprep (Nycomed Pharma). After washing the pellet, total RNA was extracted from lymphocytes by the TRIzol method (Invitrogen). Endpoint RT-PCR was selected to semiquantify MAPT, APP, NCSTN and the β-secretase BACE1 expression levels because of our strong interest in the use of the most easily available technologies for small research and clinical laboratories. Glyceraldehyde-3-phosphate-dehydrogenase (GAPDH) was the housekeeping gene of choice.

c. Data analysis

Gene expression values were compared between study groups using Student's *t* and Mann-Whitney's *U* tests. Associations between gene expression levels and between expression with raw values of the analysed risk factor conditions were investigated using Spearman's correlation coefficients. Differences were considered significant at $p<0.05$.

d. Main findings

As the full report of this exploratory study is currently under review for publication, we will limit ourselves here to share only the most relevant of our results. From the four genes analysed, we were not able to detect NCSTN in any AD subjects, therefore showing significant differences between the AD group and all the others, but particularly differing from the group of other brain disorders which showed the highest expression levels for this study (Figure 1). We also investigated the prevalence of commonly elevated variables increasing the risk for AD: blood pressure (taken as systolic/diastolic pressure and pulse), glucose, total cholesterol and triglycerides. High serum triglycerides and cholesterol prevailed in the whole study population whereas the AD group showed no greater prevalence of any of these conditions. Correlation analyses associated NCSTN expression in lymphocytes with that observed for APP and BACE1, as well as with serum total cholesterol levels in the whole study population but, when separated by groups, NCSTN expression only correlated with cholesterol levels in the group NP.

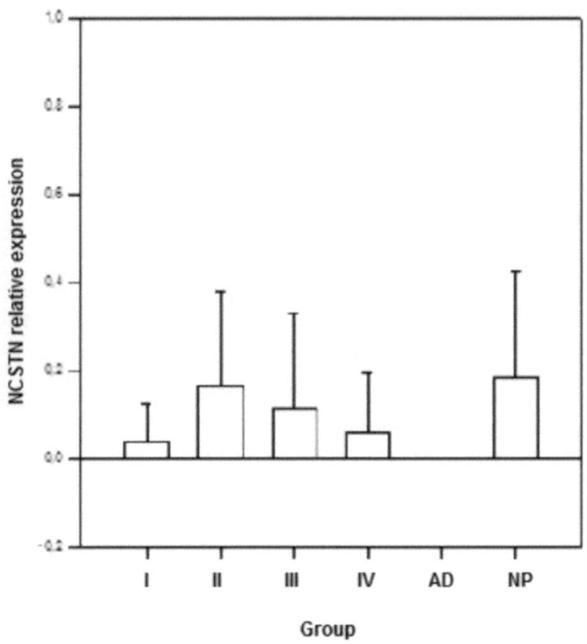

Figure 1. NCSTN relative expression in lymphocytes.

5. Conclusions

Late-onset Alzheimer's disease (LOAD) is the most common dementia in the aged population and therefore great efforts to discover the factors conferring an increased risk for this disease and biomarkers able to help in its diagnosis and prognosis are made worldwide. These intensively active fields of research have produced huge amounts of information, some of which have been controversial but also a good volume showing real potential and waiting to seek further replication and validation. However, while research on biomarkers for AD struggles with the challenge of sensibility, specificity and reproducibility in different cohorts, it is of major importance to assure the best possible performance when clinically diagnosing a patient with LOAD. Clinical diagnosis of dementias may be a bit of a long process which requires some expertise and must include specific laboratory and neuropsychological tests as well as imaging of the brain and family interviews. An accurate diagnosis has implications on therapeutic approaches, disease progression and costs, quality of life of patients, family and caregivers and other important aspects for disease management.

We previously reported the establishment of a neuro-rehabilitation program for AD and other neuropsychological disorders in our locality [27] and made brief mention of a biomarker study for which now we reported results on this occasion. Our major interest resides in using the most easily and widely available technologies for biomarker discovery and therapeutic approaches which could be directed to the general population around the globe in a cost effective manner. Even when our work is in the very first stages of this research, we seek to continue our studies in larger cohorts, including more variables and using better technologies.

Acknowledgements

The author would like to thank to Gonzalo E. Aranda-Abreu, PhD, leading researcher of the original work commented herein, and María E. Hernández Aguilar, PhD, both from the Center of Cerebral Investigations, Universidad Veracruzana. Also thanks to Consejo Nacional de Ciencia y Tecnología (CONACyT, Mexico) for the doctoral scholarship number 223277 in biomedical sciences granted to M.H.R., and the nursing home Emperatríz de las Américas.

Author details

Marisol Herrera-Rivero

Doctorate in Biomedical Sciences, Centre of Biomedical Investigations, Universidad Veracruzana, Xalapa, Veracruz, Mexico

References

[1] Shah NS, Vidal JS, Masaki K, Petrovitch H, Ross GW, Tilley C et al. Midlife blood pressure, plasma beta-amyloid, and the risk for Alzheimer disease. *Hypertension* 2012; 59: 780-86. doi: 10.1161/hypertensionaha.111.178962

[2] Yang YH, Roe CM, Morris JC. Relationship between late-life hypertension, blood pressure, and Alzheimer's disease. *An J Alzheimers Dis Other Demen* 2011; 26(6): 457-62. doi: 10.1177/1533317511421779

[3] Rodríguez-Valdés R, Álvarez-Amador A, Aguilar-Fabré L. Vascular factors and Alzheimer's disease (in Spanish). *Rev Mex Neuroci* 2006; 7(3): 225-230. http://www.medigraphic.com/pdfs/revmexneu/rmn-2006/rmn063h.pdf

[4] Kalaria RN. Cerebral vessels in aging and Alzheimer's disease. *Pharmacol Ther* 1996; 72(3): 193-214. tp://dx.doi.org/10.1016/S0163-7258(96)00116-7

[5] Jellinger KA, Paulus W, Wrocklage C, Litvan I. Traumatic brain injury as a risk factor for Alzheimer's disease: comparison of two retrospective autopsy cohorts with evaluation of ApoE genotype. *MNC Neurol* 2001; 1:3. doi: 10.1186/1471-2377-1-3

[6] Uryu K, Laurer H, McIntosh T, Praticò D, Martínez D, Leight S et al. Repetitive mild brain trauma accelerates Abeta deposition, lipid peroxidation, and cognitive impairment in a transgenic mouse model of Alzheimer amyloidosis. *J Neurosci* 2002; 22(2): 446-54. http://www.jneurosci.org/content/22/2/446.long

[7] Sáez-Fonseca JA, Lee L, Walker Z. Long-term outcome of depressive pseudodementia in the elderly. *J Affect Disord* 2007; 101(1-3): 123-9. doi: 10.1016/j.jad.2006.11.004

[8] Barnes DE, Yaffe K, Byers AL, McCormick M, Schaefer C, Whitmer RA. Midlife vs late-life depressive symptoms and risk of dementia: differential effects for Alzheimer disease and vascular dementia. *Arch Gen Psychiatry* 2012; 69(5): 493-8. doi: 10.1001/archgenpsychiatry.2011.1481

[9] Kang JE, Lim MM, Bateman RJ, Lee JJ, Smyth LP, Cirrito JR et al. Amyloid-beta dynamics are regulated by orexin and the sleep-wake cycle. *Science* 2009; 326(5955): 1005-7. doi: 10.1126/science.1180962

[10] Liberati G, Raffone A, Olivetti Belardinelli M. Cognitive reserve and its implications for rehabilitation and Alzheimer's disease. *Cogn Process* 2012; 13(1): 1-12. doi: 10.1007/s10339-011-0410-3

[11] Lanyau Domínguez Y. The diet in Alzheimer's disease (in Spanish). *Revista Cubana de Salud Pública* 2009; 35(4): 55-64. http://redalyc.uaemex.mx/redalyc/pdf/214/21418848007.pdf

[12] Nordberg A, Lundqvist H, Hartvig P, Lilja A, Langstrom B. Kinetic analysis of regional (S)(-)11C-nicotine binding in normal and Alzheimer brains. In vivo assessments using positron emission tomography. *Alzh Dis Assoc Disord* 1995; 9(1):21-7.

[13] Villemagne VL, Pike KE, Darby D, Maruff P, Savage G, Ng S et al. Abeta deposition in older non-demented individuals with cognitive decline are indicative of preclinical Alzheimer's disease. *Neuropsychologia* 2008; 46(6):1688-97. http://dx.doi.org/10.1016/j.neuropsychologia.2008.02.008

[14] Cagnin A, Brooks DJ, Kennedy AM, Gunn RN, Myers R, Turkheimer FE et al. In vivo measurement of activated microglia in dementia. *Lancet* 2001; 358(9280):461–7. doi: 10.1016/S0140-6736(01)05625-2

[15] Jacobs HI, van Boxtel MP, Gronenschild EH, Uylings HB, Jolles J, Verhey FR. *Alzheimers Dement* 2012. doi: 10.1016/j.jalz.2011.11.004

[16] Trojanowski JQ, Trojanowski JQ, Vandeerstichele H, Korecka M, Clark CM, Aisen PS et al. Update on the biomarker core of the Alzheimer's Disease Neuroimaging Initiative subjects. *Alzheimers Dement* 2010; 6(3): 230-8. doi: 10.1016/j.jalz.2010.03.008

[17] Whitwell JL, Wiste HJ, Weigand SD, Rocca WA, Knopman DS, Roberts RO et al. Comparison of imaging biomarkers in the Alzheimer Disease Neuroimaging Initiative and the Mayo Clinic Study of Aging. *Arch Neurol* 2012; 69(5): 614-44. doi: 10.1001/archneurol.2011.3029

[18] Watabe-Rudolph M, Song Z, Lausser L, Schnack C, Begus-Nahrmann Y, Scheithauer MO et al. Chitinase enzyme activity in CSF is a powerful biomarker of Alzheimer disease. *Neurology* 2012; 78(8): 569-77. doi: 10.1212/WNL.0b013e318247caa1

[19] Doecke JD, Laws SM, Faux NG, Wilson W, Burnham SC, Lam CP et al. Blood-based protein biomarkers for diagnosis of Alzheimer Disease. *Arch Neurol* 2012. doi: 10.1001/archneurol.2012.1282

[20] Soares HD, Potter WZ, Pickering E, Kuhn M, Immermann FW, Shera DM et al. Plasma biomarkers associated with the Apolipoprotein E genotype and Alzheimer disease. *Arch Neurol* 2012. doi: 10.1001/archneurol.2012.1070

[21] D'Addario C, Di Francesco A, Arosio B, Gussago C, Dell'osso B, Bari M et al. Epigenetic regulation of fatty acid amide hydrolase in Alzheimer disease. *PLoS One* 2012; 7(6): e39186. doi: 10.1371/journal.pone.0039186

[22] Johnstone D, Milward EA, Berretta R, Moscato P. Multivariate protein signatures of pre-clinical Alzheimer's disease in the Alzheimer's disease neuroimaging initiative (ADNI) plasma proteome dataset. *PLoS One* 2012; 7(4): e34341. doi: 10.1371/journal.pone.0034341

[23] Ray S, Britschgi M, Herbert C, Takeda-Uchimura Y, Boxer A, Blennow K et al. Classification and prediction of clinical Alzheimer's diagnosis based on plasma signaling proteins. Nat Med 2007; 13(11): 1359-62. doi: 10.1038/nm1653

[24] Björkqvist M, Ohlsson M, Minthon L, Hansson O. Evaluation of a previously suggested plasma biomarker panel to identify Alzheimer's disease. *PLoS One* 2012; 7(1): e29868. doi: 10.1371/journal.pone.0029868

[25] Geekiyanage H, Jicha GA, Nelson PT, Chan C. Blood serum miRNA: non-invasive biomarkers for Alzheimer's disease. *Exp Neurol* 2012; 235(2): 491-6. doi: 10.1016/j.expneurol.2011.11.026

[26] Thambisetty M, Simmons A, Hye A, Campbell J, Westman E, Zhang Y et al. Plasma biomarkers of brain atrophy in Alzheimer's disease. *PLoS One* 2011; 6(12): e28527. doi: 10.1371/journal.pone.0028527

[27] Herrera-Rivero M, Aranda-Abreu GE. Therapeutics of Alzheimer's Disease. In: *Advanced Understanding of Neurodegenerative Diseases,* Raymond Chuen-Chung Chang (Ed.), 2011. ISBN: 978-953-307-529-7, InTech. Available from: http://www.intechopen.com/books/advanced-understanding-of-neurodegenerative-diseases/therapeutics-of-alzheimer-s-disease

Chapter 3

Role of Protein Aggregation in Neurodegenerative Diseases

Yusuf Tutar, Aykut Özgür and Lütfi Tutar

Additional information is available at the end of the chapter

http://dx.doi.org/10.5772/54487

1. Introduction

Proteins and peptides are essential complex macromolecules of organisms and participate in actually every process within cells. Three dimensional structures of proteins play a critical role for biological functions. Therefore, they must be properly folded for performing these functions. Three dimensional structures are determined by composition of amino acid sequence. In addition to hydrophobic forces, covalent and weak interactions direct the formation of native protein conformation [1].

Proteins can be exposed to internal and external forces such as protein-protein interactions, various stresses, mutations etc. Since these forces alternates protein conformation, the biological activity of the protein decreases. However, newly synthesized proteins may not fold correctly, or properly folded proteins cannot spontaneously fold. In this case, proteins have a strong tendency to aggregate [1-3]. Especially, heat shock proteins (chaperones) play a key role in correcting protein folding and prevention of protein aggregation [1, 4, 5].

Protein aggregates has toxic effects when accumulated over a certain amount in the cell. The accumulation of abnormal proteins leads to progressive loss of structure and/or function of neurons, including the death of neurons. Many diseases associate with protein aggregation such as prion, Alzheimer's (AD), Parkinson's (PD), and Huntington's diseases (HD). Thus, dysmnesia, mental retardation, and also cancer are seen in these diseases. Many of the neurodegenerative disorders likely occur due to environmental and genetic factors. Especially, probability of AD and PD occurrence rise with increasing age. Briefly, neurodegenerative diseases have similar pathogenesis and cellular mechanisms [6-10].

Nowadays, mechanisms of protein aggregations and generation of neurodegenerative diseases with misfolded proteins are not clear at the molecular level. Thus, protein aggregation is a bone to pick for biotechnology and pharmaceutical industries. The aim of this chapter is to bring a perspective to the role of misfolded proteins in neurodegenerative diseases in terms of molecular and cellular basis.

2. Overview of protein aggregation

Formation of neurodegenerative diseases has not been elucidated for many years. To date, a variety of mechanisms have been suggested for explaining protein misfolding and protein aggregation, however we cannot understand the mechanism clearly at the molecular and cellular basis.

Functional proteins must pass a quality control process in terms of folding to perform catalysis, cellular transport, signal transmission and regulation. However, variety of structural and environmental factors influence this process negatively [1-3]. In this section, we will focus on aggregation behavior of proteins and these factors.

2.1. Factors affecting protein aggregation in neurodegenerative diseases

2.1.1. Protein structures

The first critical factor is protein structure. Especially, primary and secondary structures of a protein are two of the most important factors for physical and chemical features.

Encoded information in amino acid sequence of a protein determines the three dimensional structure. Position and number of different characteristic amino acid residues in primary structure may lead to an increase or a decrease in aggregation behavior. Number of hydrophobic amino acids in proteins is proportional to tendency of aggregation [2].

Secondary structures of proteins involve in protein misfolding as well as stability. Proteins often fold locally into stable structures that include α-helix and β-sheet. Generally, some β-sheet-rich proteins (such as scrapie infected prion protein) associate with pathological states. During protein aggregation, the secondary structure is converted from α-helix to β-sheet. Thus, protein gets strictness and wide surface area [1, 11, 12].

2.1.2. Mutations

Mutations play determinative role in protein aggregation and they may dramatically alter solubility, stability, and aggregation tendency of proteins [13].

Thermally stable proteins may change its stability even with a point mutation in its structure. For example, a human lysozyme I56T and D67H mutants greatly decreases the lysozyme stability and as a result the lysozyme aggregates easily upon heating. Further aggregation cause amyloid fibrils and these fibrils are deposited in tissues and are associated with neurodegenerative diseases [2].

Recently, scientists have been suggested a new protein for understanding of ALS (amyotrophic lateral sclerosis), AD, cystic fibrosis (CF) and frontotemporal lobar degeneration (FTLD) mechanisms. The transactive response DNA binding protein 43 (TDP-43) is expressed by all mammalian tissues, conformational changes in this protein cause aggregation and loss of function. TDP-43 has been shown to bind to DNA and mRNA and participate in regulation of transcription and translation. TDP-43 has a glycine rich C-terminal tail and mutation occurs from this region. Consequently, TDP-43 is converted to aggregated form which is accumulated in tissues [14].

2.1.3. *Post-translational modifications*

After a protein is synthesized, the posttranslational modifications (PTM) of amino acids may increase the diversity of proteins by additional functional groups (acetate, phosphate, various proteins etc.) and structural changes [15]. In particular, phosphorylation plays a significant role in neurodegenerative diseases. It is also known that, occurrence of AD is associated with tauopathy due to aggregation of the tau protein. In brain, tau protein is found in neurons and it can be phosphorylated with kinase enzymes. Thus, aberrant tau aggregates are formed and they can be accumulated in neurons, thereby their toxic effects are caused neuronal loss and synaptic alteration [16, 17].

Glycosylation is an important PTM for protein stability and aggregation potential. Human prion protein has two potential *N*-glycosylation sites (Asn181 and Asn197). However, in prion pathology, conversion of PrP^{c} to PrP^{Sc} occurs easily if the PrP^{c} is glycosylated. In AD patients, hyperglycosylated tau protein is found in brains [18, 19].

Hyperphosphorylation and hyperglycosylation are seemed to be required for protein aggregation and misfolding in neurodegenerative diseases. Moreover, the other PTMs such as glycation, nitration, truncation, polyamination etc. involve in protein misfolding diseases [17].

2.1.4. *Oxidative stress*

Oxidative stress leads to protein oxidation which is a biomarker for many neurodegenerative diseases. In particular, free radicals and ROS (reactive oxygen species) cause protein oxidation. A variety of oxidants can be occurred in normal aerobic metabolism [20]. Also, lack of antioxidants, excess of oxygen and lipid and metal ions can generate free radicals.

The oxidation of proteins extremely depends on their amino acid compositions. Generally; lysine, histidine, arginine, methionine, cysteine, phenylalanine, tryptophan, threonine, glutamic acid, and proline residues incline oxidation. Some proteins have metal binding regions on its own structure. Metal ions such as copper, zinc, and iron, are capable of redox reactions and electrons are transferred from ions to oxidizing compounds. Therefore, toxic free radicals are formed and proteins can be converted into aggregation forms or proteins can be aggregated by conformational changes [20, 22].

2.1.5. Protein concentration

Protein concentration is an important parameter in protein aggregation. High protein concentration can increase the likelihood of aggregation. Protein-protein interactions and intermolecular interactions (especially interactions among hydrophobic amino acids) may generate abnormal protein structures. Some misfolded protein aggregates can be constituted neurodegenerative diseases above a certain concentration. Moreover, proteins are refolded at low concentrations spontaneously. For example, lysozyme and immunoglobulin G refold itself at low protein concentration however, refolding yield decreases with increasing protein concentration. Therefore, the optimum spontaneous protein concentration range is accepted as 10-50 μg/ml. [2, 23].

2.1.6. pH

Environmental pH is to be critical for protein aggregation due to changes in net charge on protein. Protonation state of ionizable sites of protein and positive net charge are increased in acidic conditions. Especially, organization of salt bridges is changed in parallel with composed new secondary structures [2,20]. In prion diseases, acidic pH facilitates generation of PrP^{Sc}. At low pH, PrP^{c} gains β-sheet structures and shows aggregation tendency [24]. According to the Finl (2006), α-Syn incubated at different temperature and pH values, and the best formation conditions were determined as pH 7.4 and 37°C [25]. α-Syn can be lost its native structures and PD is accelerated in these conditions.

3. Neurodegenerative diseases

In the world, millions of elder people suffer from neurodegenerative diseases and diagnosis and treatment of these diseases costs millions of dollars per year. Unfortunately, the mechanisms of these diseases are still unclear and we don't have effective treatment methods. Neurodegenerative diseases are identified as protein misfolding diseases, proteopathies and protein conformational disorders. All diseases (prion, AD, PD, and HD) show typical symptoms: loss and deterioration of neurons and synaptic alterations.

Protein misfolding leads to protein aggregation and accumulation of these aggregates is implicated as the main reason of neurodegenerative diseases. In brain, some native proteins (prion, tau, β-amyloid, α-synuclein, and huntington) undergo conformational changes via genetic and environmental factors. Therefore, secondary structures of protein convert from α-helix/random coil to β-sheet (Table 1.). Consequently, neurotoxic misfolded protein aggregates are deposited in central nervous systems and brain damage and neurodegenerative diseases are formed. In this section, we will analyse the most important four neurodegenerative diseases; prion diseases, AD, PD, and HD, on the basis of protein aggregation and its molecular and cellular mechanisms [6, 8-10].

http://dx.doi.org/10.5772/54487

Neurodegenerative Diseases	Respective Proteins	Mechanism	Conformation in Aggregates	Inclusion
Prion Diseases	Prion	Protein aggregation	β-sheet	Spongiosis
Alzheimer's Diseases	Tau β-amyloid	Protein aggregation	β-sheet	Neurofibrillary Tangles Senile Plaques
Parkinson's Diseases	α-Synuclein	Protein aggregation	β-sheet	Lewy Bodies
Huntington's Diseases	Huntington	Protein aggregation	β-sheet	Huntington Inclusion

Table 1. Properties of neurodegenerative diseases.

3.1. Prion diseases

The group of prion diseases, including Creutzfeldt-Jakob (CJD), fatal familial insomnia (FFI), Kuru, Gerstmann-Sträussler-Scheinker syndrome (GSS) are seen in humans, and in similar fashion scrapie, bovine spongiform encephalopathy (mad cow disease), chronic wasting diseases (CWD), transmissible mink encephalopathy (TME), feline spongiform encephalopathy (FSE) diseases are observed in animals. All of these diseases give similar neurological symptoms such as dysmnesia, depression, sense disturbances, and psychosis [26].

3.1.1. Structure of PrP^c and PrP^{Sc}

In 1982, prion term coined by Stanley Prusiner and co-workers from "proteinaceous infectious particle". Prion protein is found in two different forms: a cellular form of prion protein (PrP^c) and scrapie isoform of prion protein (PrP^{Sc}). Properly folded form is denoted as PrP^c while misfolded form is denoted as PrP^{Sc} [27].

The PrP^c is an α-helix-rich glycoprotein that is approximately 250 amino acids in length. It is encoded by the *prion protein gene (Prpn)* which is located on chromosome 20. PrP^c is commonly found on neuronal cell membrane by a glycosyl phosphatidylinositol (GPI), however it is also expressed on other cells such as leukocytes and dendritic cells. PrP^c has been assumed a variety of functions including cell adhesion, intracellular signaling, copper metabolism, and protective antioxidant activity [8, 12, 28].

PrP^c is highly conserved protein among mammals during evolution (Fig.1.). When we examine the primary structure of the protein, PrP^c consist of a signal peptide (1-22), five octapeptide repeats (PHGGGWGQ) (51-91), a highly conserved hydrophobic domain (106-126), and a GPI (glyco-sylphosphatidylinositol) anchor. Furthermore, PrP^c contains two N-linked glycosylation sites (^{181}Asn-Ile-Thr and ^{197}Asn-Phe-Thr). Thus, they get dynamic and flexible properties and the glycan covers prevent intermolecular and intramolecular interactions. His96 and His111 are found in metal binding domains of PrP^c and they compose coordination sites with metal ions (Cu^{+2}, Zn^{+2}, Mn^{+2}, Ni^{+2}). A disulfide bond between Cys179 and Cys214 play a significant role for proper folding of PrP^c [9, 18-20, 24, 27].

```
Rabbit    --MAHLGYWMLLLFVATWSDVGLCKKRPKPGGGWNTGGSRYPGQSSPGGN
Bovine    MVKSHIGSWILVLFVAMWSDVGLCKKRPKPGGGWNTGGSRYPGQGSPGGN
Human     --MANLGCWMLVLFVATWSDLGLCKKRPKPGG-WNTGGSRYPGQGSPGGN
Mouse     --MANLGYWLLALFVTMWTDVGLCKKRPKPGG-WNTGGSRYPGQGSPGGN

Rabbit    RYPPQGGGGWGQPHGGGWGQPHGGGWGQPHGGGWGQPHGGGWGQ------
Bovine    RYPPQGGGGWGQPHGGGWGQPHGGGWGQPHGGGWGQPHGGGWGQPHGGGG
Human     RYPPQGGGGWGQPHGGGWGQPHGGGWGQPHGGGWGQPHGGGWGQ------
Mouse     RYPPQGG-TWGQPHGGGWGQPHGGSWGQPHGGSWGQPHGGGWGQ------

Rabbit    --GGGTHNQWGKPSKPKTSMKHVAGAAAAGAVVGGLGGYMLGSAMSRPLI
Bovine    WGQGGTHGQWNKPSKPKTNMKHVAGAAAAGAVVGGLGGYMLGSAMSRPLI
Human     --GGGTHSQWNKPSKPKTNMKHMAGAAAAGAVVGGLGGYMLGSAMSRPII
Mouse     --GGGTHNQWNKPSKPKTNLKHVAGAAAAGAVVGGLGGYMLGSAMSRPMI

Rabbit    HFGNDYEDRYYRENMYRYPNQVYYRPVDQYSNQNSFVHDCVNITVKQHTV
Bovine    HFGSDYEDRYYRENMHRYPNQVYYRPVDQYSNQNNFVHDCVNITVKEHTV
Human     HFGSDYEDRYYRENMHRYPNQVYYRPMDEYSNQNNFVHDCVNITIKQHTV
Mouse     HFGNDWEDRYYRENMYRYPNQVYYRPVDQYSNQNNFVHDCVNITIKQHTV

Rabbit    TTTTKGENFTETDIKIMERVVEQMCITQYQQESQAAYQ--RAAGVLLFSS
Bovine    TTTTKGENFTETDIKMMERVVEQMCITQYQRESQAYYQ--RGASVILFSS
Human     TTTTKGENFTETDVKMMERVVEQMCITQYERESQAYYQ--RGSSMVLFSS
Mouse     TTTTKGENFTETDVKMMERVVEQMCVTQYQKESQAYYDGRRSSSTVLFSS

Rabbit    PPVILLISFLIFLIVG
Bovine    PPVILLISFLIFLIVG
Human     PPVILLISFLIFLIVG
Mouse     PPVILLISFLIFLIVG
```

Figure 1. Multiple protein sequence alignment of prion proteins. Full length amino acid sequences of rabbit (NP_001075490.1), bovine (GenBank: CAA39368.1), human (UniProtKB/Swiss-Prot: P04156.1), and mouse (NP_035300.1) were aligned using the program Clustal W. PHGGGWGQ repeats are shaded in red. Metal binding sites, His96, and His111 are shaded in blue. Glycosylation sites, ^{181}NIT and ^{197}NFT, are shaded in pink. Finally, Cys179 and Cys214 (disulfide bond sites) are shaded in black.

PrP^{Sc} can be defined as an infectious isoform of PrP^{c} and causes fatal prion diseases. PrP^{Sc} is formed by misfolding of PrP^{c} with a lost in α-helical content. PrP^{Sc} has same amino acid sequence with PrP^{c}, but their secondary, tertiary, and quarternary structures are different. Approximately, PrP^{c} includes 3% β-structure and 47% α-helix structure, but nonetheless PrP^{Sc} is composed of 43% β-structure and 30% α-helix structure [24, 29]. It becomes non-soluble and resists to proteolytic degradation with conformational changes, whereas PrP^{c} is soluble and protease sensitive. This insoluble protein accumulates in brain and causes a variety of prion diseases in human and animals.

3.1.2. Molecular pathology of Prion diseases

Previous studies suggested a variety of mechanisms for explaining prion pathology. Oxidative stress and lipid peroxidation are the major factors in prion diseases [20, 30]. In central nervous systems, a variety of oxidative stresses including high level of oxygen and lipid, metal ions, and inadequate antioxidants produce free radicals. In PrP^{Sc} infected mice, superoxide anion (O_2^-) is extremely increased in brain. Therefore, high levels of heme oxygenase-1 and malondialdehyde are observed as oxidative stress markers in brain. Cytochrome c oxidase is a large transmembrane protein in mitochondria and it shows antioxidant activity in mitochondria [12, 31]. The level of lipid peroxidation is increased while Cytochrome c oxidase activities are reduced in scrapie infected animal models. Phospholipase D catalyzes the hydrolysis of phosphatidylcholine to generate choline and phosphatidic acid, and its expression level is induced by H_2O_2 [12]. According to the studies, activity of phospholipase D is increased in the brains of scrapie infected animals. As a result, PrP^c transforms into PrP^{Sc} because of the formation of these free radicals.

As we discussed the effect of metal ions on protein misfolding in section 2.1.4, the metal ions also play key roles in prion formation. Cu^{2+}ions play a critical role in prion diseases. PrP^c has five conserved octapeptide repeats (PHGGGWGQ) which have an affinity for Cu^{2+} ions. In contrast, affinity of other metal ions (Mg^{2+}, Mn^{2+}, Ni^{2+} etc.) is weak or nonexistent. The binding of Cu^{2+} provides formation of protease resistant form: PrP^{Sc}. It is also suggested that, PrP^c protects cells from harmful redox activities. Especially, in copper-rich environment, PrP^c acts as a "copper buffer" that means it inhibits toxic effects of Cu^{2+} ions for central nervous system and helps maintaining neurons in high level of cupper ions. Thus, redox damage of PrP^c has been involved in prion diseases. In brief, copper can convert the cellular prion protein into a protease-resistant species with conformational changes [31-35].

Glycosylation is a stability-enhancing post translational modification in proteins. PrP^c contains two potential glycosylation sites which are Asn181 and Asn197 in human PrP^c [36]. Generally, binding of carbohydrates can protect protein surface from proteases and undesired protein-protein interactions. Moreover, N-glycosylated prion protein is anchored to the lipid membranes via GPI [18, 19].

Interaction of PrP^c with membrane lipid layers play a significant role in conversion of PrP^c to PrP^{Sc}. PrP^c is localized in cholesterol and sphingomyelin rich area on cell surface (known as lipid raft). PrP^c is bound to lipid membranes through its GPI anchor. While leaving PrP^c from the membranes by catalysis of phosphatidylinositol phospholipase C (PIPLC), PrP^{Sc} show resistance to PIPLC. When binding of PrP^c to the lipid membranes, PrP^c is degraded or converted into PrP^{Sc} form [37-40].

3.2. Alzheimer's diseases

Alzheimer's disease (AD) is the most frequent type of neurodegenerative disorder in the world. AD is composed of accumulation of aberrant folded tau protein and beta-amyloid protein ($A\beta$ protein) in brain. In 1906, AD was first described by psychiatrist and pathologist Dr. Alois Alzheimer and then the disease was named with his surname [8-10].

To date, there are no effective treatment methods for AD, but some nuclear medicine applications (MRI and PET) are applied in diagnosis of AD. Dramatically, symptoms of AD rise with increasing age and the first sign is memory lapse. Cellular and molecular mechanisms of AD are not well understood yet. Researchers have been reported that AD is associated with genetic and environmental factors and life-style.

3.2.1. Structure of Tau gene and proteins

A microtubule associated protein, Tau, is a biggest component of AD. In 1975, tau proteins were first discovered by Marc Kirschner in Princeton University. Tau was derived from "**t**ubulin **a**ssociated **u**nit" as a term. It is highly expressed in brain, but other organs such as lung, hearth, and kidney have trace amounts. Many animals (bovine, goat, monkey, goldfish etc.) also have tau proteins [41].

The human *tau gene* is located on chromosome 17q21 and contains 16 exons. Among these exons of the tau gene, exon 2, 3, and 10 are alternatively spliced and these exons allow six combinations (2-3-10-; 2+3-10-; 2+3+10-; 2-3-10+; 2+3-10+; 2+3+10+). Thus, human brain contains six isoforms of tau proteins which range from 352 to 441 amino acids length and approximate molecular weights are between 60 and 70 kDa (Fig. 2.) [16, 17].

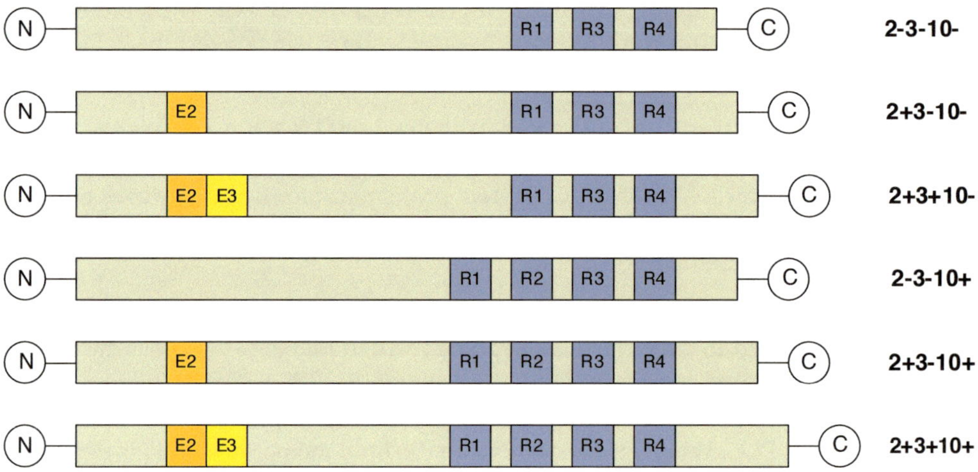

Figure 2. Schematic representation of six human tau isoforms. R1, R2, R3, and R4 (blue boxes) indicate repeat regions. E2 and E3 (orange and yellow box) indicate Exon 2 and Exon 3 respectively (Redrawn from Buee et al., 2000).

Tau protein has four main regions in its primary structures. Acidic region is located in the N-terminal part and it is encoded by exon 2 and exon 3. Prolin-rich region located in the middle of the protein, is encoded by exon 7 and exon 9 and contains several PXXP motifs which can interact with tyrosine kinase. Prolin-rich region works together with acidic region, therefore these two regions are called projection domain which interacts with neural plasma membrane and cytoskeletal elements [16, 17, 41-43].

Tau protein has three to four highly conserved repeats in the C-terminal part for binding to microtubules. Therefore, these repetitive regions are called microtubule binding domains (MBDs) which is encoded by exons 9-12. ^{275}VQJINK^{280} and ^{306}VQJVYK^{311}are conserved hexapeptides which are located at the beginning of the second and third MBDs. These peptides involve in the generation of β-sheet structure during tauopathy [44].

3.2.2. *Aggregation of Tau protein*

Microtubules are major proteins of the cytoskeleton. They have hollow and cylindrical structure and participate in intracellular transport, protection cell structure, and continuity of cell viability. The main function of the tau protein is to stabilize microtubules with binding to microtubules and to other proteins [16, 41]. To perform these functions, tau proteins must be phosphorylated at normal level. However, if tau protein hyperphosphorylate, its biological activity can be lost. Moreover, hyperphosphorylation causes conformational changes and aggregation of tau proteins. Other post-translational modifications such as glycosylation, glycation, polyamination, and nitration may play essential roles in AD [17].

The longest isoform of tau protein (441 amino acids) has seventy nine Ser or Thr phosphorylation sites which are mainly found on prolin-rich regions. Also, Ser^{262}, Ser^{293}, Ser^{324}, and Ser^{356} are located in KXGS motif of R1, R2, R3, and R4 domains. Many of kinases and phosphatases (glycogen synthase kinase-3β (GSK3β), mitogen activated protein kinase (MAPK), tau tubulin kinase 1-2 (TTBK1/2), cyclin dependent kinase 5 (CDK5), microtubule affinity regulating kinase (MARK), and stress activated protein kinase (SAP) are affected in tau phosphorylation [17, 45, 46].

Frontotemporal dementia with parkinsonism-17 (FTDP-17) is a progressive neurodegenerative disease which is caused by mutations in the tau gene. The tau gene is mutated in familial FTDP-17 and this mutation accelerates formation of neurofibrillary tangles (NFTs) in the brain. Furthermore, hyperphosphorylation is promoted by this mutation [47,49].

Excess of NFTs and senile plaques (SPs) are important markers in AD. NFTs are aggregates of hyperphosphorylated tau protein that are most commonly known as a primary marker of AD [50]. NFTs are originated from abnormally hyperphosphorylated tau protein. Normally, tau is a microtubule binding protein that stabilizes and assembles microtubules. However, in AD, tau protein undergoes biochemical changes because it twists into pairs of helical filaments and they twist into tangles. Also, tau is generally located in axons, but in tauopathy, it is located in dendrites. Thus, neuron's transport system may be disintegrated and microtubule cannot function correctly [16, 50].

3.2.3. *Structure of Aβ protein and gene*

Aβ is a relatively small peptide of 4 to 4.4 kDa that is the major component of amyloid deposits. Intracellular Aβ protein is widely found in neurons and it is associated with inflammatory and antioxidant activity, regulation of cholesterol transport, and activation of kinase enzyme. However, Aβ is one of the best known components in formation of neurodegenerative diseases including AD.

Aβ is approximately composed of 36-43 amino acids and it originates from amyloid precursor protein (APP). In human, *APP gene* is encoded on chromosome 21 and contains at least 18 exons. APP is a glycoprotein of 695-770 amino acids which has three main regions: an extracellular N-terminal region, a hydrophobic transmembrane region, and cytoplasmic C-terminal region. Mutations in APP gene cause familial susceptibility to AD. Furthermore, mutations in other three genes, including apoE, PS1, and PS2 are associated with AD and increased production of Aβ protein and amyloidogenicity. In contrast, a coding mutation (A673T) in APP gene shows protective effects for AD [51-53].

APP can be cleaved into fragments by α, β, and γ secretases and Aβ protein is formed by the action of the β and γ secretases. Aβ protein contains two important regions which play a major role in the formation insoluble amyloid fibrils. C-terminal regions (residues 32 to 42) and internal hydrophobic regions (residues 16 to 23) may enhance increasing β-sheet conformation and Aβ protein misfolding [53].

3.2.4. Aggregation mechanisms of Aβ protein

In normal brain, Aβ proteins contain mixture of β-sheet and random coil structures. However, a number of β-sheet structures are increased at high protein concentration. Aβ protein constitutes SPs which are important markers in AD. The formation of SPs is a problem of protein folding because of misfolded and aggregated form of Aβ accumulates and shows toxicity in brain [54].

Genetically, three genes: *APP, PS1,* and, *PS2* are associated with AD. More than 50 different mutations in the APP gene can cause AD. The most frequent APP mutation is a single mutation in the APP at position 717. As a result of this single mutation, a valine residue is replaced by an isoleucine, or phenylalanine, or glycine. *APP* mutations lead to an increased amount of the Aβ proteins which are deposited in neuritic plaques [50, 54].

3.3. Parkinson's diseases

Parkinson's disease (PD) is neurodegenerative movement disorder of the central nervous systems. In 1817, Dr. James Parkinson published *"An Essay on the Shaking Palsy"* in which he first described paralysis agitans and then this disorder was entitled as a Parkinson's disease by Dr. Jean Martin Charcot. The occurrence of an illness is characterized by accumulation of misfolded α-synuclein protein in brain. Generally; anxiety, tremor, rigidity, depression, bradykinesia, and postural abnormalities are the most common symptoms in Parkinson's disease. Also, α-Syn related neurodegenerative diseases are known as "Synucleinopathies" [55].

3.3.1. Structure of α-synuclein

Natively unfolded α-syncline (α-Syn) is a 14 kDa and highly conserved protein that localize different regions of the brain. The name of protein was preferred as "α-synuclein" because of it shows **syn**aptic and **nuc**lear localization. α-Syn regulates dopamine neurotransmission by modulation of vesicular dopamine storage. It interacts with tubulin and can function like tau protein. Also, α-Syn shows a molecular chaperon activity in folding of SNARE (soluble N-ethylmaleimide-sensitive-factor attachment protein receptor) proteins [56].

Natively, α-Syn is an unfolded protein, but obtains its conformation with biological interactions. In cytoplasm, α-Syn is a soluble and in an unfolded state, but it can be found in α-helical conformation for binding to lipid membranes. Also, α-Syn can be in the form of β-sheet for composing Lewy bodies as explained below [56-58].

α-Syn is encoded with *SNCA gene* which is located on chromosome 4q21. Human α-Syn has 140 amino acids and three main domains: **(i)** an amphipathic N-terminal region (residues 1-60), **(ii)** a central hydrophobic region (residues 61-95) and **(iii)** a highly acidic C-terminal region (residues 96-140) (Fig. 3.). Amphipathic N-terminal region contains imperfect six hexamer motif repeats (KTKEGV) which involve in binding of micelles and liposomes.

```
1   MDVFMKGLSKAKEGVVAAAEKTKQGVAEAAGKTKEGVLYVGSKTKEGVVHGVATVAEKTK
61  EQVTNVGGAVVTGVTAVAQKTVEGAGSIAAATGFVKKDQLGKNEEGAPQEGILEDMPVDP
121 DNEAYEMPSEEGYQDYEPEA
```

Figure 3. Primary structure of human α-Syn (Gen Bank: AAL15443.1). Imperfect KTKEGV repeats are colored in blue. Acidic residues are colored in red. Phosphorylation sites (Ser87 and Ser129) are colored in yellow.

Central hydrophobic region contains non-amyloid beta component (NAC) sequences from residue 61 to 95. This region is highly hydrophobic, and it can promote formation of β-sheet structure. The less conserved C-terminal region consists of a large number of acidic amino acids and several prolines [56-60].

3.3.2. Structures of Lewy bodies

At present, biological role and pathogenic processes of Lewy bodies are still unclear. As far as we know, Lewy bodies are aberrant protein aggregates and their deposits cause PD. Lewy bodies are localized not only in PD brains, but also in other neurodegenerative disorders such as AD brains. According to the electron microscopy images, Lewy bodies are 8-30 μm which are consisted of approximately 10 nm amyloidogenic fibrils such as fibrillary α-Syn and neurofilaments. Lewy bodies contain a variety of proteins including α-Syn, neurofilaments, ubiquitinated proteins, and heat shock proteins (Hsp70 and Hsp90). Oxidative stress, mitochondrial dysfunction, inflammation, ubiquitin proteasome system, pH, protein concentration, and high temperature may be affected negatively by Lewy bodies. Therefore, these factors induce misfolding and aggregation of proteins in the Lewy bodies [57, 61].

3.3.3. Mechanisms of α-Syn misfolding and aggregation

α-Syn plays crucial role in PD because α-Syn is a major fibrillary component for Lewy bodies. There are many adjuvant and disincentive factors available in α-Synfibrillogenesis. Two mutations, A53T and A30P, in the α-Syn gene and overexpression of wild type α-Syn are increased misfolding processes and aggregation. Also, accumulation of abnormal form of α-Syn can inhibit proteasomal functions [9, 61, 62].

It is known that, α-Syn is natively unfolded as well as predominantly non-phosphorylated *in vivo*. In PD brains, α-Syn is found to be phosphorylated at Ser87 and Ser129 in aggregates. These serine residues are phosphorylated with casein kinase 1 (CK1) and casein kinase 2 (CK2). Several studies reported that accumulation of phosphorylated α-Syn was observed in animal models of synucleinopathies. Therefore, this post translational modification has a pathological role in fibrillation of α-Syn [63, 64].

As known, oxidative stress is one of the major factors in many diseases as well as the formation of PD [9, 20]. As a result of oxidation, formed free radicals react rapidly with proteins thus, misfolding and aggregation are generated inside the cells. Among twenty amino acids, methionine and cysteine are capable of being easily oxidized. α-Syn doesn't have cysteine residues, but high content of methionine residues oxidize to methionine sulfoxide. Thus, due to methionine content of α-Syn, the protein is readily aggregates at oxidation conditions. On the other hand, α-Syn phosphorylation can be increased with oxidative stresses as well [65].

3.4. Huntington's diseases

Huntington's disease (HD) is a genetic neurodegenerative disorder and the disease is caused by autosomal dominant inheritance. In 1872, HD was first described as a genetic disease by Dr. George Huntington. Involuntary muscle contractions, movement, and mental disorders are progressed in HD. The disease is inherited as an autosomal dominant and effects brain and nervous systems. Huntington protein undergoes conformational changes with mutation and it shows aggregation tendency [66].

3.4.1. Structure of Huntington protein and genes

Huntington (Htt) is a large size protein of 350 kDa that is generally composed of 3144 amino acids. Normal protein is highly expressed in peripheral tissues and brain, and it is involved in endocytosis, cytosketal functions, vesicle trafficking, cellular signal transduction, and membrane recycling. In brains, Htt protein leads to cell damage and toxicity through deposition of misfolded aggregate form of Htt protein [8, 9].

The gene for HD is located on the tip of chromosome 4, and is called the *IT-15 gene*. This part of DNA contains cytosine-adenine-guanine (CAG) repeats which are called trinucleotide repeats. Number of trinucleotide repeats is determined as risk of HD development. The CAG repeats are translated into polyglutamine (polyQ) residues which are located in the N-terminal region [66-68].

Htt proteins interact with a variety of peptides including huntington associated protein 1 (HAP1), huntington interacting protein 1 and 2 (HIP1 and HIP2) and huntington yeast partners A, B, and C (HYPA, HYPB, and HYPC). These peptides are functioned in cell signaling, transport, and transcription processes [67, 69].

3.4.2. Mechanisms of Huntington misfolding and aggregation

In HD, the neuropathology is characterized with accumulation of Htt protein aggregates. HD is caused by a number of CAG repeats in the gene. To date, many theories have been suggested in HD, but functions of CAG repeats and mechanisms of HD cannot be understood yet. However, common opinion is long CAG repeats (polyQ) are the most important promoter for toxicity of Htt protein aggregates. The polyQ region starts at residue 18 and the number of glutamine residues are the most important marker in HD. Surprisingly, 40 or more CAG repeats are always generated neuropathy, while 35 or fewer CAG repeats are never generated neuropathy. However, in childhood, CAG repeats from 27 to 35 can develop neuropathy [66, 70-72].

In 1994, Max Perutz put forward a "**polar zipper**" hypothesis about HD pathology. In this model, many polar glutamine residues can generate anti parallel β-sheet structures with hydrogen bonds. Therefore, aggregation tendency of Htt protein is increased and this state lead to cell death [73-75]. Furthermore, aggregation of Htt protein induces oxidative stress, mitochondria dysfunction, lipid peroxidation etc.

4. Prevention of neurodegenerative diseases and molecular chaperones

Until this section, neurodegenerative diseases have been discussed on the basis of protein aggregation and misfolding. In healthy organisms, a variety of mechanisms work efficiently for prevention of preteopathies. Molecular chaperones are known to be critical for protein folding processes and neurodegenerative diseases. Heat shock proteins (Hsps) are well-known molecular chaperons in living organisms [1, 76-78].

4.1. The Hsp chaperons

Hsps are highly conserved proteins among living organisms. Hsps are an important class of molecular chaperons and they are located in different parts of the cells such as endoplasmic reticulum, cytosol, and mitochondria. Mainly, Hsps are related with formation of proper protein conformation, and also prevention protein aggregation, misfolding, and oligomerization. Proteins can be exposed a number of cellular and environmental factors including high temperature, inflammation, growth factors, oxidative stress etc. which can cause misfolding and protein aggregation. Overexpression of Hsps has been observed under these stress conditions. Several studies have focused on the neuroprotective role of Hsps. Therefore, the expression levels of Hsps are decreased and misfolded protein accumulation can be occurred in brain [1, 76-78].

Generally, Hsps are divided into six groups on the basis of molecular mass. In this section; Hsp40, Hsp60, Hsp70, Hsp90, Hsp100, and small Hsp (sHsp) have been examined and characterized for association with neurodegenerative diseases and protein folding processes [1].

Hsp70 is a highly conserved protein in all living organisms. It makes complex with unfolded or partially denatured proteins. Hsp70 has two functional domains: ATPase domain and substrate binding domain (SBD). The operation of these domains is controlled with hydrolysis of ATP. ATPase domain binds to ATP and hydrolyzes it to ADP. This energy drives the protein folding function of the Hsp70. Similarly, Hsp70 binding to misfolded peptides, increases the ATP hydrolysis. Also, Hsp70 interacts with Hsp40 and Hsp90 to perform protein folding process. Hsp70 serves a neuroprotective role in all of neurodegenerative diseases [79-81]. Auluck and co-workers indicated that, expression of Hsp70 reduced α-Syn aggregation, accumulation, and toxicity in PD animal models [82]. In HD models, Hsp70 shows protective assignment in polyglutamine-induced toxicity [83]. Also, Hsp70 is involved in the folding and functional maintenance of tau protein. In prion diseases, Hsp70 binds aggregate form of prion proteins and it mediates their degradation by the proteasome [81].

Hsp40 is expressed in variety of organisms in different isoforms. It associates with unfolded polypeptides and prevents protein aggregation. Hsp40 can be found in a cell in three different types. All types of Hsp40 contain highly conserved J domain which interacts with Hsp70 ATPase domain. Thus, ATPase activity of Hsp70 is regulated by this interaction. Hsp40 transmits substrate towards Hsp70 SBD domain with an appropriate conformation. Thus, Hsp70 help substrate peptide in its hydrophobic SBD region and assists the peptide to come to a state of proper three-dimensional structure [1, 84]. Hsp40 is extensively found in neurodegenerated brains due to it is association with Hsp70 as a co-chaperon [83].

Hsp100 participates in counteraction of protein aggregation with Hsp70 and Hsp40. This hexameric 100 kDa protein has substrate and ATP binding regions. Large protein aggregates are broken by Hsp100 and formed small aggregates are carried forward by Hsp70-Hsp40 complex. In yeast, overexpression of Hsp100 leads to disassemble of large prion aggregates and generate the small prion seeds for new rounds of prion propagation [1, 83].

Hsp90 is a highly expressed cellular molecular chaperon and also stabilizes certain proteins and aids protein degradation. Hsp90 is a dimeric protein which has a highly conserved N-terminal domain and a C-terminal domain. Hsp90 is one of the main cytosolic molecular chaperons which is activated with Hsp40 and Hsp70 [1, 85]. Uryu and co-workers demonstrated that expression of Hsp90 is increased in transgenic mouse model of PD. Inhibition of Hsp90 lead to generation of tauopathies because of protein hyperphosphorylation and abnormal neuronal activity can be increased in AD [86].

Hsp60 is a heptameric 60 kDa protein which is located particularly in mitochondria. Hsp60 works with Hsp70 coordinately for protein folding. Furthermore, it plays key roles in mitochondrial protein transport, replication and transmission of mitochondrial DNA, and apoptosis. For actin and tubulin, Hsp60 is a specific chaperon which is decreased in AD. In AD effected neurons, aggregated and misfolded tau protein is increased in contrast with expression of Hsp60 is decreased [1, 83].

sHsp has a molecular mass between 12 and 30 kDa [87]. As a molecular chaperone, sHsp are located at different compartments in the cell and they can protect protein structures and activities. Also, overexpression of sHsp have reported in many studies [87-90]. In HD, the expression level of Hsp27 is increased and it prevents polyglutamine induced toxicity in neurons. Furthermore, Hsp27 reduces α-syn-induced toxicity in PD patient brain [82, 88]. The other sHsps including Hsp10, Hsp12, Hsp20, Hsp26 are associated with protein folding diseases [89].

5. Conclusion

More than 600 diseases such as Alzheimer's disease, Huntington's disease, prion diseases, Parkinson's disease, multiple sclerosis (MS), amyotrophic lateral sclerosis (ALS) and others

http://dx.doi.org/10.5772/54487

are characterized by progressive nervous system dysfunction. In the world, millions of people are affected from these diseases. For example, five million people suffer from Alzheimer's disease, one million people from Parkinson's disease and 30.000 people from Huntington's diseases in USA. US government spends approximately 50-100 billions of dollars for diagnosis and therapies [91]. Today, we are using effective methods (PET, MRI, SPECT etc.) for diagnosis of neurodegenerative diseases, but we cannot treat the diseases easily as we diagnose them.

All of neurodegenerative diseases are related with protein misfolding and aggregation. Different native proteins lead to formation of diseases, but practically same factors involve in these diseases. Structurally, β-sheet conformation plays a key role in neuropathies. Furthermore, oxidative stress, pH, mutations, post translational modifications etc. lead to protein folding diseases.

New innovations in biochemical and medicinal fields lead to development of a number of mechanisms for protein aggregation and neurodegenerative diseases. Moreover, a variety of analytical techniques such as IR (infrared spectroscopy), NMR (nuclear magnetic resonance), CD (circular dichroism), calorimeters, and electron microscopy have been used for detection of aggregation process. Nevertheless, we cannot identified cellular mechanisms of protein misfolding and related diseases clearly yet. In the future, scientists will concentrate on design of practical and fast methods for detection of protein aggregation in cells.

Acknowledgements

This work was funded through a seed grant from the Turkish National Academy of Sciences (TUBA GEBIP 2008-29 for YT).

Author details

Yusuf Tutar[1,2,3], Aykut Özgür[4*] and Lütfi Tutar[5]

1 Cumhuriyet University, Faculty of Pharmacy, Department of Biochemistry, Turkey

2 Cumhuriyet University, Faculty of Medicine, Department of Biophysics, Turkey

3 Cumhuriyet University, Faculty of Medicine, CUTFAM Research Center, Sivas, Turkey

4 Gaziosmanpasa University, Faculty of Natural Sciences and Engineering, Department of Bioengineering, Tokat, Turkey

5 Kahramanmaraş Sütçü İmam University, Faculty of Science and Letters, Department of Biology, Kahramanmaraş, Turkey

References

[1] Tutar L, Tutar Y. Heat shock proteins: An overview. Current Pharmaceutical Biotechnology 2010; 11(2):216-222.

[2] Wang W. Protein aggregation and its inhibition biopharmaceutics. International Journal of Pharmaceutics 2005; 289: 1-30.

[3] Stefani M. Protein misfolding and aggregation: new examples in medicine and biology of the dark side of the protein world. BiochimiaetBiophysicaActa 2004; 1739: 5-25.

[4] Chaudhuri TK, Paul S. Protein-misfoldingdiseases and chaperone-based therapeutic approaches. FEBS Journal 2006; 1331-1349.

[5] Adachi H, Katsuno M, Waza M, Minamiyama M, Tanaka F, Sobue G. Heat shock protins in neurodegenerative diseases: Pathogenic roles and therapeutic implications. International Journal of Hyperthermia 2009; 25(8): 647-654.

[6] Soto C, Estrada, LD. Protein misfolding and neurodegeneration. Arch Neurol2008; 65(2): 184-189.

[7] Lee SJ, Lim HS, Masliah E, Lee HJ. Protein aggregate spreading in neurodegenerative diseases: Problems and perspectives. Neuroscience Research 2011; 70: 339-348.

[8] Shastry BS. Neurodegenerative disorders of protein aggregation. Neurochemistry International 2003; 43: 1-7.

[9] Trzesniewska K, Brzyska M, Elbaum D. Neurodegenerative aspects of protein aggregation. ActaNeurobiolExp 2004; 64: 41-52.

[10] Ross CA, Poirier MA. Protein aggregation and neurodegenerative diseases. Nature Medicine 2004; DOI: 10.1038/nm1066.

[11] Philo JS, Arakawa T. Mechanisms of protein aggregation. Current Pharmaceutical Biotechnology 2009; 10: 348-351.

[12] Hur K, Kim JI, Choi SI, Choi EK, Carp RI, Kim YS. The pathogenic mechanisms of prion protein. Mechanisms of Ageing and Development 2002; 123: 1637-1647.

[13] Lee C, Y MH. Protein folding and diseases. Journal of Biochemistry and Molecular Biology 2005; 38(3): 275-280.

[14] Wilson AC, Dugger BN, Dickson DW, Wang DS. TDP-43 in aging and Alzheimer's disease – a review. Int J ClinExpPathol 2011;4(2):147-155.

[15] Karve TM, Cheema AK. Small changes huge impact: The role of protein posttranslational modifications in cellular homeostasis and disease. Journal of Amino Acids 2011; DOI:10.4061/2011/207691

[16] Buee L, Bussiere T, Buee-Scherrer V, Delacourte A, Hof PR. Tau protein isoforms, phosphorylation and role in neurodegenerative disorders. Brain Research Reviews 2000; 33: 95-130.

[17] Martin L, Latypova X, Terro F. Post-translational modifications of tau protein: Implications for Alzheimer's disease. Neurochemistry International 2011; 58: 458-471.

[18] Rudd PM, Merry AH, Wormald MR, Dwek RA. Glycosylation and prion protein. Current Opinion in Structural Biology 2002; 12: 578-586.

[19] Rudd PM, Wormald MR, Wing DR, Prusiner SB, Dwek RA. Prion glycoprotein: Structure, dynamics, and roles for the sugar. Biochemistry 2001; 40(13): 3759-3766.

[20] Guest WC, Plotkin SS, Cashman NR. Toward a mechanisms of prion misfolding and structural models of PrP^{Sc}: Current knowledge and future directions. Journal of Toxicology and Environmental Health, Part A 2011; 74: 154-160.

[21] Pogocki D. Alzheimer's β-amyloid peptide as a source of neurotoxic free radicals: the role of structural effects. ActaNeurobiolExp 2003; 63: 131-145.

[22] Moulton PV, Yang W. Air pollution, oxidative stress, and Alzheimer's Disease. Journal of Environmental and Public Health 2012; DOI:10.1155/2012/472751.

[23] Treuheit MJ, Kosky AA, Brems DN. Inverse relationship of protein concentration and aggregation. Pharmaceutical Research 2002; 19(4): 511-516.

[24] DeMArco ML, Daggett V. Local environmental effects on the structure of the prion protein. C R Biologies 2005; 328: 847-862.

[25] Finl AL. The aggregation and fibrillation of α-synuclein. AccChem Res 2006; 39: 628-634.

[26] Wadsworth JDF, Collinge J. Update on human prion diseases. BiochimiaetBiophysicaActa 2007; 1772: 598-609.

[27] Mehrpour M, Codogno P. Prion protein: From physiology to cancer biology. Cancer Letters 2010; 290: 1-23.

[28] Hu W, Kieseier B, Frohman E, Eagar TN, Rosenberg RN, Hartung HP, Stüve O. Prion protein: Physiological functions and role in neurological disorders. Journal of Neurological Sciences 2008; 264: 1-8.

[29] Cohen FE. Protein misfolding and prion diseases. Journal of Molecular Biology 1999; 293: 131-320.

[30] Milhavet O, McMahon HEM, Rachidi W, Nishida N, Katamine S, Mange A, Arlotto M, Casanova D, Riondel J, Favier A, Lehmann S. Prion infection impairs the cellular response to oxidative stress. PNAS 2000; 97(25): 13937-13942.

[31] Westergard L, Christensen HM, Harris DA. The cellular prion protein (PrP^C): Its physiological function and role in disease. BiochimicaetBiophysicaActa 2007; 1772: 629-644.

[32] Garnett AP, Viles JH. Copper Binding to the octarepeats of the prion protein. Journal of Biological Chemistry 2003; 278(9): 6795-6802.

[33] MilhauserGL. Copper binding in the prion protein. AccChem Res 2004; 37(2): 79-85.

[34] Viles JH, Cohen FD, Prusiner SB, Goodin DB, Wright PE, Dyson HJ. Copper binding to the prion protein: Structural implications of four identical cooperative binding sites. ProcNatlAcadSci 1999; 96: 2042-2047.

[35] Calabrese MF, Miranker AD. Metal binding sheds light on mechanisms of amyloid assembly. Prion 2009; 3(1): 1-4.

[36] Daggett V. Structure-function aspects of prion proteins. Current Opinion in Biotechnology 1998; 9: 359-365.

[37] Taylor DR, Hooper NM. The prion protein and lipid rafts. Molecular Membrane Biology 2006; 23(1) 89-99.

[38] Wang F, Yang F, Hu Y, Wang X, Wang X, Jin C, Ma J. Lipid interaction converts prion protein to a PrP^{Sc}-like proteinase K-resistant conformation under physiological conditions. Biochemistry 2007; 46: 7045-7053.

[39] Critchley P, Kazlauskaite J, Eason R, Pinheiro TJT. Binding of prion proteins to lipid membranes. Biochemical and Biophysical Research Communications 2004; 313: 559-567.

[40] Rushworth JV, Hooper NM. Lipid Rafts: Linking Alzheimer's amyloid-β production, aggregation, and toxicity at neuronal membranes. International Journal of Alzheimer's Disease 2011; DOI:10.4061/2011/603052.

[41] Kolarova M, Garcia-Sierra F, Bartos A, Ricny J, Ripova D. Structure and pathology of tau protein in Alzheimer Disease. International Journal of Alzheimer's Disease 2012; DOI:10.1155/2012/731526.

[42] Bulic B, Pickharth M, Mandelkow EM, Mandelkow E. Tau protein and tau aggregation inhibitors. Neuropharmacy 2010; 59: 276-289.

[43] Li L, Bergen MV, Mandelkow EM, Mandelkow E. Structure, Stability, and Aggregation of paired helical filaments from tau protein and FTDP-17 mutants probed by tryptophan scanning mutagenesis. Journal of Biological Chemistry 2002; 277(44): 41390-41400.

[44] Bergen MV, Friedhoff P, Biernat J, Heberle J, Maldelkox EM, Maldelkow E. Assembly of t protein into Alzheimer paired helicalfilaments depends on a local sequence motif ($^{306}VQIVYK^{311}$) forming β structure. Biochemistry 2000; 97(10): 5129-5134.

[45] Avila J. Tau phosphorylation and aggregation in Alzheimer's diseases pathology. FEBS Letters 2006; 580: 2922-2927.

[46] Du JT, Li YM, Ma QF, Qiang W, Zhao YF, Abe H, Kanazawa K, Qin XR, Aoyagi R, Ishizuka Y, Nemoto T, Nakanishi H. Synthesis and conformational properties of phosphopeptides related to the human tau protein. Regulatory Peptides 2005; 130: 48-56.

[47] Connell JW, Gibb GM, Betts JC, Blacstock WP, Gallo JM, Lovestone S, Hutton M, Anderton BH. E¡ects of FTDP-17 mutations on the in vitro phosphorylation of tau by-glycogen synthase kinase 3β identified by mass spectrometry demonstrate certain mutations exert long-range conformational changes. FEBS Letters 2001; 493: 40-44.

[48] Bunker JM, Kamath K, Wilson L, Jordan MA, Feinstein SC. FTDP-17 Mutations compromise the abilityoftautoregulatemicrotubuledynamicsincells. JBC Papers 2006; DOI: 10.1074/jbc.M509420200.

[49] Goedert M. Tau protein and neurodegeneration. Seminars in Cell&Developmental Biology 2004; 15: 45-49.

[50] Dimakopoulos AC. Protein aggregation in Alzheimer's diseases and other neuropathological disorders. Current Alzheimer Research 2005; 2: 19-28.

[51] Baumketner A, Bernstein SL, Wyttenbach T, Lazo ND, Teplow DB, Bowers MT, Shea JE. Structure of the 21-30 fragment of amyloid β-protein. Protein Science 2006; 15: 1239-1247.

[52] Crescenzi O, Tomaselli S, Guerrini R, Salvadori S, D'Ursi AM, Temussi PA, Picone D. Solution structure of the Alzheimer amyloid β-peptide (1-42) in an apolar microenvironment. Eur J Biochem 2002; 269: 5642-5648.

[53] Estrada LD, Soto C. Disrupting β-amyloid aggregation for Alzheimer diseases treatment. Current Topics in Medicinal Chemistry 2007; 7: 115-126.

[54] Li M, Chen L, Lee DHS, Yu LC, Zhang Y. The role of intracellular amyloid β in Alzheimer's diseases. Progress in Neurobiology 2007; 83: 131-139.

[55] Dauer W, Przedborski S. Parkinson's diseases: Mechanisms and Models. Neuron 2003; 39: 889-909.

[56] Ma QL, Chan P, Yoshii M, Ueda K. α-Synuclein aggregation and neurodegenerative diseases. Journal of Alzheimer's Diseases 2003; 5: 139-148.

[57] McNaught KSP, Olanow CW. Protein aggregation in the pathogenesis of familial and sporadic Parkinson's diseases. Neurobiology of Aging 2006; 27: 530-545.

[58] Valtierra S. α-Synuclein phosphorylation and nitration in Parkinson's disease. Eukaryon 2008; 4: 90-94.

[59] Khandelwal PJ, Dumanis SB, Feng LR, Maguire-Zeiss K, Rebeck GW, Lashuel HA, Moussa CEH. Parkinson-related parkin reduces α-Synuclein phosphorylation in a gene transfer model. Molecular Neurodegeneration 2010; 5(47): 1-13.

[60] Mizuna Y, Hattori N, Mori H. Genetics of Parkinson's diseases. Biomed &Pharmacother 1999; 53: 109-116.

[61] Licker V, Kövari E, Hochstrasser DF, Burkhard PR. Proteomics in human Parkinson's diseases research. Journal of Proteomics 2009; 73: 10-29.

[62] Gitler AD, Chesi A, Geddie ML, Strathearn KE, Hamamichi S, Hill KJ, Caldwell GA, Cooper AA, Rochet JC, Lindquist S. α-Synuclein is part of a diverse and highly conserved interaction network that includes PARK9 and manganese toxicity. Nature Genetics 2009; 41(3): 308-315.

[63] Carla M, Tome L, Tyson T, Rey NL, Grathwohl S, Britscgi M, Brundin P. Inflammati on and α-Synuclein 's prion-like behavior in Parkinson's disease—Is there a link? MolNeurobiol 2012; DOI 10.1007/s12035-012-8267-8.

[64] Kim EJ, Sung JY, Lee HJ, Rhim Y, Hasegawa M, Iwatsubo T, Min DS, Kim J, Paik SR, Chung, KC. Dyrk1A phosphorylates α-synuclein and enhances intracellular inclusion formation. The Journal of Biological Chemistry 2006; 281(44): 33250-33257.

[65] Uverski VN, Yamin G, Souillac PO, Goers J, Glaser CB, Fink AL. Methionine oxidation inhibits fibrillation of human alphasynuclein in vitro. FEBS Letters 2002; 517: 239-244.

[66] Ross RAC. Huntington 's disease: A clinical review. Journal of Rare Diseases 2010; 5(40): 1-8.

[67] Gusella JF, MacDonald ME. Huntington: A single bait hooks many species. Current Opinion in Neurobiology 1998; 8: 425-430.

[68] Ramaswamy S, Shannon KM, Kordower JH. Huntington 's disease: Pathological mechanisms and therapeutic strategies. Cell Transplantation 2007; 16: 1-100.

[69] Margolis RL, Rudnicki DD, Holmes SE. Huntington's disease like-2: Review and update. ActaNeurol Taiwan 2005; 14: 1-8.

[70] Walker FO. Huntington's diseases. Lancet 2007; 369: 218-228.

[71] Perez De-La Cruz V, Santamaria A. Integrative hypothesis for Huntington's disease: A brief review of experimental evidence. Physiol Res 2007; 56: 513-526.

[72] Gudesblatt M, Tarsy D. Huntington's diseases: A clinical review. Neurobiology Reviews 2011.

[73] Perutz M. Polar zippers: Their role in human disease. Protein Science 1994; 3: 1629-1637.

[74] Hoffner G, Djan P. Transglutamine and diseases of the central nervous system. Frontiers in Bioscience 2005; 10: 3078-3092.

[75] Newcomer ME. Trading places. Nature 2001; 8(4): 282-284.

[76] Bukau B, Weissman J, Horwich A. Molecular chaperons and protein quality control. Cell 2006; 125: 443-451.

[77] Mayer MP. Gymnastics of molecular chaperones. Cell 2010; DOI:10.1016/j.molcel.2010.07.012

[78] Dou F, Netzer WJ, Takashima A, Xu H. Heat shock proteins reduce aggregation and facilitate degradation of tau protein. International Congress Series 2003; 1252: 383-393.

[79] Fan CY, Lee S, Douglas MC. Mechanisms for regulation of Hsp70 function by Hsp40. Cell Stress & Chaperones 2003; 8(4): 309-316.

[80] Mapa K, Sikor M, Kudryavtsev V, Waegemann K, Kalinin S, Seidel CAM, Neupert W, Lamb DC, Mokranjac D. The conformational dynamics of the mitochondrial Hsp70 chaperone. Cell 2010; 38: 89-100.

[81] Turturici G, Sconzo G, Geraci F. Hsp70 and its molecular role in nervous system diseases. Biochemistry Research International 2011; DOI: 10.1155/2011/618127.

[82] Luo GR, Chen S, Le WD. Are heat shock proteins therapeutic target for Parkinson's diseases? International Journal of Biological Sciences 2007; 3(1): 20-26.

[83] Söti C, Csermely P. Chaperons and aging: Role in neurodegeneration and in other civilization diseases. Neurochemistry International 2002; 41: 383-389.

[84] Li J, Bingdon SHA. Structure-based mutagenesis studies of the peptide substrate binding fragment of type I heat-shock protein 40. Biochem J 2005; 386: 453-460.

[85] Faou P, Hoogenraad NJ, Tom34: A cytosolic cochaperone of the Hsp90/Hsp70 protein complex involved in mitochondrial protein import. BiochimiaetBiophysicaActa 2012; 1823: 348-357.

[86] Luo W, Sun W, Taldone T, Rodina A, Chiosis G. Heat shock protein 90 in neurodegenerative diseases. Molecular Neurodegeneratin 2010; 5(24): 1-8.

[87] Sun Y, MacRae TH. The small heat shock proteins and their role in human diseases. FEBS Journal 2005; 272: 2613-2627.

[88] Outeiro TF, Klucken J, Strathearn KE, Liu F, Nguyen P, Rochet JC, Hyman BT, McLean PJ. Small heat shock proteins protect against α-synuclein-induced toxicity and aggregation. Biochemical and Biophysical Research Communications 2006; 351: 631-638.

[89] Wilhelmus MMM, Boelens WC, Otte-Höller I, Kamps B, De Wall RMW, VErbeek MM. Small heat shock proteins inhibit amyloid-β protein aggregation and cerebrovascular amyloid-β protein toxicity. Brain Research 2006; 1089: 67-78.

[90] Jiao W, Li P, Zhang J, Zhang H, Chang Z. Small heat-shock proteins function in the insoluble protein complex. Biochemical and Biophysical Research Communications 2005; 335: 227-231.

[91] http://www.neurodiscovery.harvard.edu/challenge/challenge_2.html

Chapter 4

Role of Oxidative Stress in Aβ Animal Model of Alzheimer's Disease: Vicious Circle of Apoptosis, Nitric Oxide and Age

Ferihan Cetin

Additional information is available at the end of the chapter

http://dx.doi.org/10.5772/54718

1. Introduction

The aging process is believed to be closely related to increased oxidative stress. Reactive intermediates of oxidative stress affect the cellular redox status and induce apoptosis [1]. Oxidative stress due to the loss of balance between ROS production and antioxidant defenses affects all the vital organs, resulting in aging [1,2]. Oxidative damage, mitochondrial dysfunction and inflammation underlies many common aging-related neurodegenerative diseases, including AD [2,3]. The major pathological hallmark of AD is the accumulation of Aβ peptides in the brain [4]. Oxidative insults that induce neuronal apoptosis, including agents that induce membrane lipid peroxidation, also have been shown to activate caspases [5]. Increased lipid peroxidation was consistently observed in some animal models of Alzheimer amyloidosis [4, 6]. It has been shown that a single Aβ administration into the rat hippocampus could induce increase of NOS activity and NO level [6]. Nitric oxide is a multifunctional molecule that acts as messenger/modulator in synaptogenesis and potential neurotoxin and is synthesized by three isozymes of Nitric oxide synthase (NOS) [7]. Oxidative stress reflects a situation in which ROS is continuously produced and exceeds the capacity of endogenous antioxidant defense systems. Several studies have suggested that oxidative stress plays a key role in Aβ-mediated neuronal cytotoxicity by triggering or facilitating neurodegeneration through a wide range of molecular events that eventually lead to neuronal cell loss. Aβ significantly increases production and enhances membrane lipid peroxidation, leading to neuronal apoptosis [8,9]. Because multiple factors are involved in the pathogenesis of the AD, it is difficult to find an ideal in vivo model. It is important to determine Aβ 1-42 injection effects especially in hippocampus, temporal and parietal cortex, because a definite atrophy reveals in these regions in the late stage of sporadic AD. The fact that revealing changes with age are the accumulation of ROS and the onset of apoptosis cascade, these interfering subjects have been investigated intensely nearly for two decades. β-amyloid itself is a source of free radicals. One possible mechanism for initiating apoptosis could be the generation of free radicals by the peptide leading to lipid peroxidation and oxidative stress [9,10]. Many recent studies have confirmed the toxicity of peroxynitrite to neurons and the involvement of nitric oxide in neurologic pathologies [10,11]. Other suspects include the superoxide radical hydrogen peroxide, which is implicated in amyloid neurotoxicity, and peroxynitrite, which can be formed by combining superoxide and nitric oxide [9].

Nitric oxide is a multifunctional molecule that acts as messenger/modulator in synaptogenesis and potential neurotoxin and is synthesized by three isozymes of NOS. Entorhinal cortex neurons are highly vulnerable to neurodegeneration in AD express low levels of NOS and the inducible form of NOS is upregulated in AD [14]. They found a significant decrease in the number of cells expressing detectable levels of nNOS mRNA in the white matter underlying the frontal cortex and in the dentate gyrus and CA subfields of the hippocampus in AD. Furthermore, there was also a significant decrease in the number of NADPHd-positive cells in the dentate gyrus and CA subfields of the hippocampus in AD [15].

It has been suggested that the upregulation of nNOS and subsequent NO release in certain classes of cortical interneurons may be one of the earliest events signaling the apoptosis of cortical projection neurons in lesion models [16]. Conflicts may arise from varying emphasis on different cortical areas among these investigators and the complex anatomy of cortical nitrinergic neurons that comprise at least three distinct cell populations, that is, large subcortical whiter matter neurons, large nNOS (+) interneurons, and smaller nNOS (+) interneurons that are often missed because of low levels of nNOS/NADPHd expression [16]. Not only neurons but also activated microglia are capable of releasing neurotoxic molecules, such as proinflammatory cytokines and toxic oxygen and nitrogen species [17]. The relationship between mitochondrial damage, glutathione status/GSH dependent enzymes, oxidative stress, and neuronal dysfunction has been demonstrated by the effects of excessive production of H_2O_2 within mitochondria, which leads to depletion of mitochondrial GSH. Besides, measurements of the activity time course of antioxidant enzymes are important when comparing the alterations induced by Aβ with those found in AD patients [18]. Glutathione is known to protect cells against apoptosis, which is consistent with the suggestion of involvement of $ONOO^-$ mediated cellular events in neuronal apoptosis [2,17].The current literature contains contradictory results about the dual role (neuroprotector/neurotoxic) that NO may play in the aging CNS [19]. It is mostly believed that NO has neurotoxic effects on neurons [20,21]. It is now known that, in aging and Alzheimer brain, nNOS-expressing hippocampal neurons are more vulnerable to oxidative stress [14]. Aβ (25–35) activated nNOS in the cerebral cortex and hippocampus without effect on iNOS activity [6]. Since Aβ neurotoxicity is believed to be mediated by NO and the potential toxic effects of NO depend on the intracellular source of the molecule (i.e. isoform-specific) [7].

http://dx.doi.org/10.5772/54718

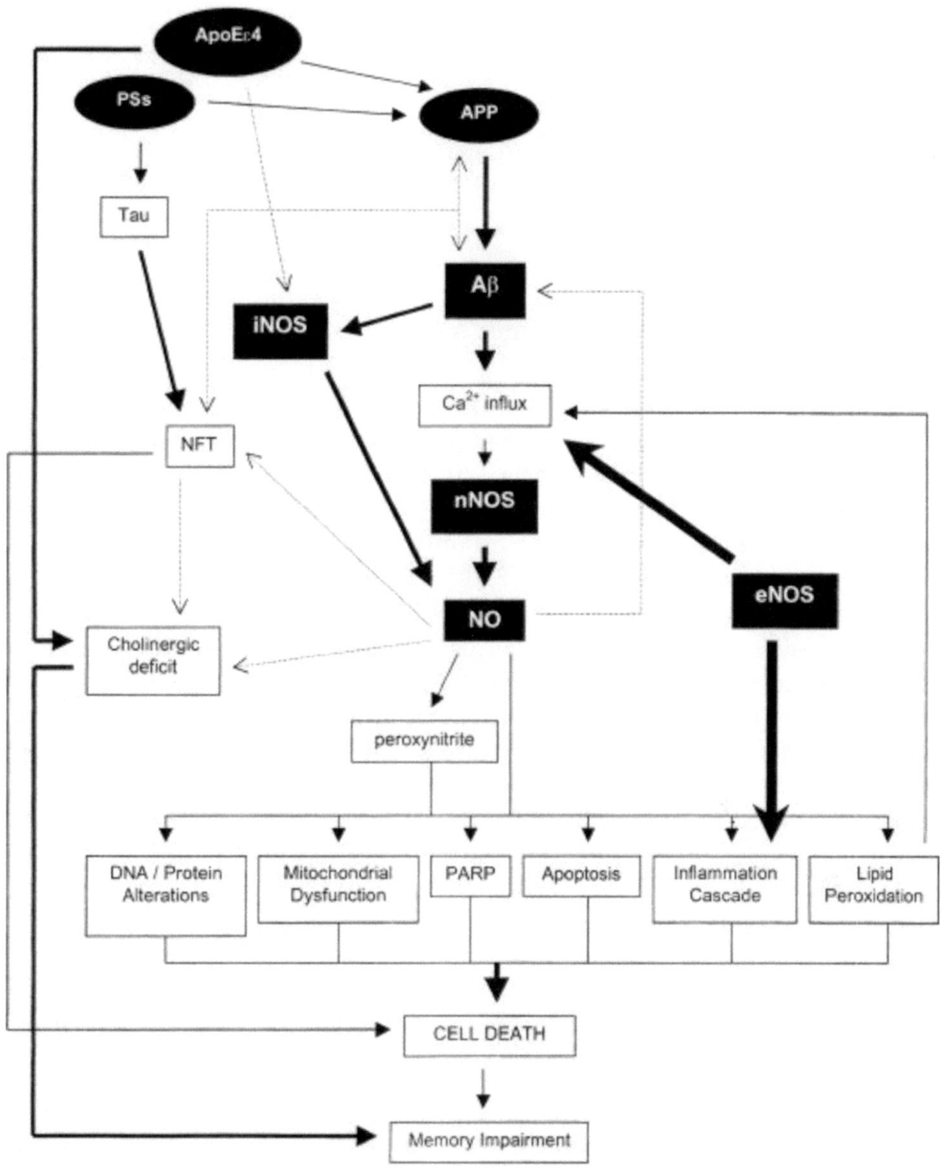

Figure 1. Nitric oxide (NO) neurotoxicity and neuroprotectivity in relation to Alzheimer's disease (AD). Mutations of presenilins (PSs) and amyloid precursor protein (APP) are associated with increased production of Aβ. Neurofibrillary tangles (NFT) formation is the result of tau hyperphosphorylation, which leads to cell death secondary to cellular trafficking disruption. PSs have also been implicated in the process of tau hyperphosphorylation. Apolipoprotein E e4 (ApoE e4) genotype is considered a risk factor for AD. It appears to affect Aβ production and a correlation between ApoE e4 and cholinergic deficit has been established. Cholinergic deficit is one of the most significant findings in AD, and is implicated in memory impairments observed in this disease. Increased production of Aβ induces NO production either by disrupting Ca homeostasis and subsequent increased in intracellular Ca (nNOS and eNOS-mediated NO release) or by interactions with glial cells (iNOS-mediated NO release). NO is a free radical and can produce peroxynitrite. These reactive oxygen species induce a variety of neurotoxic mechanisms, including DNA/ protein alterations, mito-

chondrial dysfunction, poly ADP-ribose polymerase (PARP) overactivation, apoptosis, neuro-inflammation, and lipid peroxidation (which jeopardize cellular membrane integrity, which leads to further Ca influx and NO release). These mechanisms are likely to be involved in cell death and memory impairments observed in AD. Several potential relationships may exist between various AD markers (dashed arrows). ApoE e4 may induce iNOS-mediated NO production. NFT formation may influence Aβ accumulation and vice versa, and that APP metabolism may play a role in tau phosphorylation and subsequent NFT formation. NO, by activating a variety of signalling molecules, may induce Aβ and NFT formation. In ischemia, eNOS-mediated NO production appears to be neuroprotective by decreasing Ca influx and neuro-inflammation (thickened arrows). This NOS isoform may have a similar role in neurodegenerative diseases such as AD. [Law A., Gauthier S., Quiron R., Say NO to Alzheimer's disease: putative links between nitric oxide and dementia of the Alzheimer's type. 2001, ref 7]

2. β-amyloid peptide in Alzheimer's disease

In 1911, Alois Alzheimer described a neuropsychiatric disorder affecting the elderly, which is widely known today as Alzheimer's disease (AD). Early studies of patients afflicted with this disease demonstrated, via silver staining, the presence of lesions in the brain cortex. Those lesions corresponded to neurofibrillary tangles (NFTs), which are histopathologic structures localized within the neuronal cells. The majority of cases of AD correspond to the sporadic form of this disorder. Approximately 5–10% of patients present an autosomal mode of transmission and account for cases called familial Alzheimer's disease (FAD). The role of amyloid deposits in brain as a triggering factor for Alzheimer's disease has obtained increasing scientific support since Glenner's discovery in 1984. The amyloid precursor protein (APP) belongs to a type 1 transmembrane family of glycoproteins that is ubiquitously expressed in several types of cells. The N-terminal moiety of APP is projected toward the extracellular domain or can be localized in the lumen of intracellular vesicles, such as those of the endoplasmic reticulum, Golgi apparatus, and intracellular endosomes. On the other hand, the APP C-terminal region lies in the cytoplasmic domain. APP is sensitive to proteolysis by a set of proteases called α, β, γ secretases. Secretases are responsible for the production of Aβ(1–40) peptide or the Aβ(1–42) variant with a significantly higher capacity to self-aggregate.[22]

3. Aβ animal models

A critical question that must be addressed in examining any animal model of a human disease is how well the animal model mimics the mechanisms and ultimate pathology observed in the human disease. [23] Clearly, there are differences between the present rat model and human AD. First, whereas in a study gliosis and pathology are observed over a time course of 30 d, in human AD the time course is on the order of decades. Second, the amyloid load per unit of brain area is generally higher and the amyloid distribution more extensive in the human AD brain than in their rat model. However, a key difficulty in addressing the mechanisms of pathology in human AD is that one rarely looks at human brain tissue at the initiation of the disease but rather examines the AD brain at the end stage of the disease, long after the initial mechanisms of pathology occur. In behalf of these discrepancies intracerebral or intracerebroventricular Aβ injections or infusions are used to mimic AD.[23,24]

Thus, the results strongly suggest that injection of fibrillar Aβ activates both microglia and astrocytes. Although both microglia and astrocytes show a dramatic upregulation of iNOS expression in response to injection of fAβ, there are marked spatial and morphological differences in the microglia and astrocyte responses to fAβ. Whereas microglia surround and phagocytize fAβ, astrocytes show no evidence of Aβ phagocytosis but rather form a virtual wall between microglia containing fAβ and the surrounding neurons.[23] The fAβ induces neuronal loss and a significant increase in iNOS expression by microglia and astrocytes *in vivo*, suggesting that it is the release of bioactive molecules like nitric oxide by microglia and astrocytes, rather than direct contact between Aβ fibrils and neurons, that mediates Aβ neurotoxicity in AD.[23]

4. Aβ and oxidative stress

In recent years, considerable data have accrued indicating that the brain in AD is under increased oxidative stress and this may have a role in the pathogenesis of neuron degeneration and death in this disorder. The direct evidence supporting increased oxidative stress in AD is: (1) increased brain Fe, Al, and Hg in AD, capable of stimulating free radical generation; (2) increased lipid peroxidation and decreased polyunsaturated fatty acids in the AD brain, and increased 4-hydroxynonenal, an aldehyde product of lipid peroxidation in AD ventricular fluid; (3) increased protein and DNA oxidation in the AD brain; (4) diminished energy metabolism and decreased cytochrome c oxidase in the brain in AD; (5) advanced glycation end products (AGE), malondialdehyde, carbonyls, peroxynitrite, heme oxygenase-1 and SOD-1 in neurofibrillary tangles and AGE, heme oxygenase-1, SOD-1 in senile plaques; and (6) amyloid beta peptide is capable of generating free radicals. [25]

Oxidative insults emanating from within the cell can threaten homeostasis if they are not appropriately resolved. Mitochondria actively and continuously generate ROS during respiration, favoring a situation of mitochondrial oxidative stress. The electron transport chain is an essential mechanism for generation of cellular energy and is localized to the mitochondrial inner membrane. Autooxidation of reduced respiratory chain components cause the production of free radical intermediates, O_2 and H_2O_2, which in the presence of iron can produce hydroxyl radical (•OH). There are two specific sites where electrons may leak out of the chain to partially reduce oxygen. One is the NADH dehydrogenase and the other is at the ubiquinone cytochrome b intersection. These oxygen species are dealt with by superoxide dismutases (SOD), enzymes that are considered to be the first line of defense against oxygen toxicity, and exist in two forms in mammalian tissues: copper, zinc (Cu, Zn SOD), and manganese (Mn SOD) metalloproteins. Although mitochondria are notorious for ROS production, they are not the only sites of intracellular oxidative stress. In the cytosol, the arachadonic acid cascade, yielding prostaglandins, and leukotrienes may generate ROS when the released lipid is metabolized, and some cytochrome P-450 isozymes are notorious O_2^{-2} producers. Several possibilities have been proposed for the mechanisms of NO^--mediated cytotoxicity. [26] First, formation of iron-nitrosyl complexes with critical FeScontaining enzymes (e.g., aconitase), may cause an impairment of mitochondrial function and energy depletion. Second, NO^- may directly damage chromatin by deamination and cross-linking of DNA, which increases mutagenesis. Third, generation of peroxynitrite by a reaction between NO^- and superoxide (O_2^{-2}) may play a significant role in the cytotoxic process. Fourth, NO^- may inactivate several antioxidant enzymes, including catalase, glutathione peroxidase, and superoxide dismutases. Also, NO^- has been reported to induce apoptosis by increasing ceramide generation through caspase-3 activation, induction of mitochondrial permeabilittransition, and activation of the Fas system. The mechanism of action of many exogenous agents involves redox cycling whereby an electron is accepted to form a free radical and it is then transferred to oxygen. [26]

Although NO has many important and beneficial physiologic functions, it also can play a role in neurodegenerative disease pathology. In these diseases, NO is produced in excess by iNOS induction owing to the proinflammatory response, which is a common feature of neurodegenerative disorders. Moreover, NO is much more harmful under pathologic conditions that involve the production of reactive oxygen species (ROS), such as superoxide anion and the formation of peroxynitrite. Two important properties of NO that may contribute to its pathologic functions are its ability to modify proteins through nitrosylation and nitrotyrosination and its ability to react with oxygen to form RNS. [27]

In mature neurons, when cytosolic nNOS is the primary producer of NO, Ca^{2+} entry through overactive NMDA channels stimulates nNOS; thus, NO can then enter the mitochondria, directly inhibiting complex IV (cytochrome c oxidase) of the respiratory chain, which leads to a block of ATP production and eventual cell death due to energetic failure. [27]

Furthermore, NO has been shown to activate both the constitutive and inducible isoforms of cyclooxygenase, which are upregulated in brain cells under proinflammatory conditions. During the catalytic cycle of cyclooxygenase, the release of free radicals and the formation of prostaglandins occur, two events closely related to the development of neuroinflammation. [27]

Hsp90 is another protein associated with AD that undergoes nitrosylation. S-Nitrosylation of Hsp90 abolishes ATPase activity that is necessary for its chaperone function; thus, inactivation of Hsp90 may allow accumulation of tau and Aβ aggregates in the AD brain. It is generally recognized that mitochondria continuously undergo two opposing processes, fission and fusion. The disruption of this dynamic equilibrium may herald cell injury or death and may contribute to developmental and neurodegenerative disorders. Nitric oxide produced in response to β-amyloid protein has been shown to trigger mitochondrial fission, synaptic loss, and neuronal damage, in part through S-nitrosylation of dynamin-related protein. [27]

Many studies showed amyloid-beta interaction with different receptors in the cellular membrane of the vasculature, neurons, oligodendrocytes, and glial cells where it is transported from cell surface into endosomal and lysosomal compartments. The aberrant signalling of these receptors in AD triggered an abnormal accumulation of amyloid-beta into cytosol-inducing cellular stress underlies to neuronal dysfunction and dementia. It is described that these receptors can be megalin, also known as low-density lipoprotein related protein-2 (LRP2), LRP-1, or RAGE (receptors for advanced glycation end products). The interaction of these receptors with amyloid-beta in neurons, microglia, and vascular cells accelerates and amplifies deleterious effects on neuronal and synaptic functions. [28] These findings are further in line with the recently proposed hypothesis of an intracellular amyloid-beta toxicity cascade which suggests that the toxic amyloid-beta species intervening in molecular and biochemical abnormalities may be intracellular soluble aggregates instead of extracellular, insoluble plaques. There are many studies proposing that megalin- and/or RAGE-dependent signalling are involved in the regulation of amyloid-beta clearance and probably may contribute to amyloid pathology and cognitive dysfunction observed in the AD patients and AD mouse model. [28]

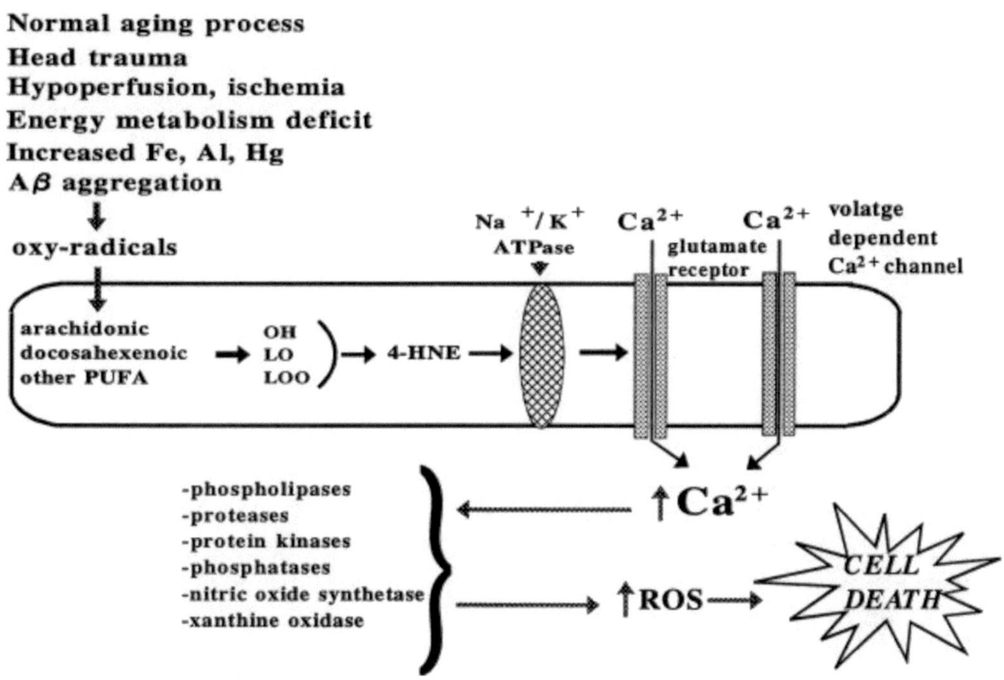

Figure 2. Mechanism of potential neuron death in AD. Anumber of conditions may cause free radical generation that can lead to peroxidation of membrane polyunsaturated fatty acids. This leads to formation of other oxygen radicals and generates aldehydes such as 4-hydroxynonenal (HNE). 4-HNE is capable of altering membrane ATPases leading to increased intracellular calcium, which initiates a cascade of events leading to further free radical generation and neuron death. [Markesbery W.R, 1997, ref 25]

5. Interrelation between amyloid-beta and mitochondria

One of the most interesting events in AD is that mitochondrial oxidative stress occurs early in AD progression, before the onset of Aβ pathology. Mitochondria are the major source of ROS, and, in fact, mitochondrial dysfunction as well as hypometabolism has long been implicated in the onset of the familial and sporadic forms of AD. mtDNA defects have also been linked to an increased incidence of AD. Energy deficiency and mitochondrial dysfunction have been recognized as a prominent, early event in AD. Mitochondrial abnormalities have been found both in neurons and astrocytes, suggesting that both neurons and astrocytes might be damaged by free radicals in the AD brain. Superoxide radicals might be produced in mitochondrial electron transport chain complexes I and III and in components of the Krebs cycle, including αketoglutarate dehydrogenas. In addition, superoxide radicals might be generated in the outer mitochondrial membrane. H_2O_2 and superoxide radicals, released from the mitochondrial matrix and from the inner and outer mitochondrial membranes, might be carried to the cytoplasm and, ultimately, might lead to the oxidation of cytoplasmic proteins. [28]

Both APP and Aβ are present in mitochondrial membrane and interact with mitochondrial proteins, block mitochondrial import channels, impair mitochondrial transport, disrupt the electron transfer chain, increase ROS levels, and cause mitochondrial damage. [28]

APP and amyloid-beta may block mitochondrial translocation of nuclear-encoded proteins, such as components of the electron transport chain, impairing mitochondrial function. Intra-mitochondrial amyloid-beta is able to perturb mitochondrial function in several ways by directly influencing extracellular transport chain complex activities, impairing mitochondrial dynamics, or disturbing calcium storage, thus increasing apoptotic pathways. Moreover, amyloid-beta interacts with mitochondrial matrix components inducing an improper mitochondrial complex function leads to a decreased mitochondrial membrane potential of the organelle and impairing ATP formation. [28]

It is well documented that mtDNA changes are responsible for aging phenotypes.

It has been hypothesized that ongoing oxidative damage to mtDNA may be the underlying mechanism for cellular senescence. Since mtDNA repair mechanisms are limited and because mtDNA is situated in close proximity to the site of ROS production, mtDNA is more vulnerable to oxidative damage than nuclear DNA. With age, oxidation of mtDNA increases compared to nuclear DNA leading to an age dependent accumulation of mtDNA mutations. The effects of these mutations may lead to opening of the mitochondrial permeability transition pore and subsequent neuronal death. Increased ROS levels act at multiple levels to impair mitochondrial function: they induce mtDNA mutations that consequently negatively influence mitochondrial function, enhance amyloid-beta production by guiding APP cleavage pathway toward the amyloidogenesis, increase lipid peroxidation, activate mitophagy, leading to a reduced mitochondrial number, and augment tau hyperphosphorylation and NFT formation impairing organelle trafficking and neuronal function which leads to apoptosis. [28] In addition to its well-known role in glycolysis, GAPDH contributes to nuclear signaling in apoptosis. SNitrosylation of GAPDH terminates its enzymatic activity and allows binding of GAPDH to Siah1, an E3 ubiquitin ligase. Siah1 has a nuclear localization signal and carries GAPDH to the nucleus. GAPDH stabilizes Siah1 in the nucleus and allows degradation of nuclear proteins through ubiquitination. [27]

Protein-disulfide isomerase (PDI) is an endoplasmic reticulum (ER)-associated chaperone protein that prevents neurotoxicity caused by ER stress and protein misfolding and can also function as an NO receptor or donor, depending on the cellular context. PDI is nitrosylated both in AD and PD. Both PD and AD patient postmortem brains exhibit increased levels of nitrosylated PDI as compared with those of healthy controls. PDI nitrosylation prevents PDI-mediated ER stress reduction and allows protein misfolding. [27]

Microglial activation is a key feature in Alzheimer's disease and is considered to contribute to progressive neuronal injury by release of neurotoxic products. Mononuclear phagocytes, such as microglial cells, are crucial components of the innate immune system. Cellular activation in response to pathogen-associated molecular patterns on microorganisms is mediated through interaction with innate immune receptors on the surfaces of mononuclear phagocytes, e.g., Toll-like receptors (TLRs) and the lipopolysaccharide receptor CD14. Lipopolysaccharide (LPS), a component of the cell wall of gram-negative bacteria, was first identified as the TLR ligand. The innate immune receptor Toll-like-receptor 4 (TLR4), localized on the surface of microglia, is a first-line host defense receptor against invading microorganisms. It has been shown that a spontaneous loss-of-function mutation in the *Tlr4* gene strongly inhibits microglial and monocytic activation by aggregated Alzheimer amyloid peptide resulting in a significantly lower release of the inflammatory products IL-6, TNFα and nitric oxide. Treatment of primary murine neuronal cells with supernatant of amyloid peptide-stimulated microglia demonstrates that Tlr4 contributes to amyloid peptide-induced microglial neurotoxicity. The reason how TLR4 becomes activated in the pathophysiology of AD is unclear. These findings further support a role of TLR4 in neuroinflammation in AD. Microglial activation in AD pathophysiology is discussed as a two-edged sword. [29]

It has been demonstarted that Aβ1–40 administration induced an increase in TNF-α expression and oxidative alterations in prefrontal cortex and hippocampus. Likewise, Aβ1– 40 led to activation of both JNK (c-Jun-NH2-terminal kinase)/c-Jun and nuclear factor-κB, resulting in iNOS upregulation in both brain structures. [29] It has been shown that the anti-TNF-α antibody reduced all of the molecular and biochemical alterations promoted by Aβ1–40. These results provide new insights in Mouse models of AD, revealing TNF-α and iNOS as central mediators of Aβ action. These pathways might be targeted for AD drug development. [29]

Tumor necrosis factor-α (TNF-α) is a cytokine thought to play a central role in the self-propagation of neuroinflammation. TNF-α regulates many cellular processes, including inflammation, differentiation, and cell death through activation of TNF receptor 1 (TNFR1) or TNFR2. The transduction pathways activated by TNF-α include mitogen-activated protein kinases (MAPKs) and IκB kinase, which control gene expression through transcriptional factors such as activator protein-1 (AP-1) and nuclear factor-κB (NF-κB). Regarding the CNS, microglia and astrocytes are believed to be the primary sources of TNF-α. Evidence indicates the presence of increased levels of TNF-α in the brain and plasma of AD patients and an upregulation of TNFR1 have been detected in the AD brain. Aβ has been shown to interact in a synergistic manner with cytokines to induce neuronal damage via reactive oxygen species (ROS)- and NO-dependent pathways. [30] Numerous animal models have been used to evaluate the role of inflammation in the course of AD. An experimental model that mimics the progression of AD was developed using an intracerebroventricular injection of Aβ in mice. The cross talk between TNF-α and iNOS is probably mediated by activation of two major intracellular pathways: c-Jun-NH2-terminal kinase (JNK)/c-Jun and NF- κB. According to the results, they suggested that TNF-α and iNOS as important mediators of Aβ-induced cognitive impairment. TNF-α signaling effectors include JNK and c-Jun that might also contribute to iNOS promoter activity. [29]

6. Aβ and age

The glycation hypothesis of aging suggests that modification of proteins by glucose (the ''Maillard reaction'') leads to the development of ''advanced glycation end-products''

(AGEs). [31] In the human brain, AGEs accumulate in neuronal perikarya of the hippocampus and parahippocampus, as well as in reactive astroglia in brains after the third decade of age. In AD, this effect is twofold: AGEs accumulate extracellularly on β-amyloid plaques and intracellulary in neurons and astrocytes. The binding of AGEs to its receptor, RAGE (receptor for advanced glycation endproducts), activates NADPH-oxidase, a central participant in the production of superoxide radicals. Superoxide and its conversion product, hydrogen peroxide, were shown to activate redoxsensitive transcription factors such as NF-κB and activator protein 1 (AP-1) resulting in the upregulation of cytokines such as interleukin (IL)-1, IL-6, tumor necrosis factor (TNF-α) and inducible nitric oxide synthase (iNOS). Interestingly, RAGE is also activated by Aβ, the major pro-inflammatory peptide present in amyloid plaques in AD and HMGB1/amphoterin, a novel pro-inflammatory ligand released from dying cells. TNF-α and NO were chosen as relevant biomolecules due to their role in augmenting inflammation and/or inducing cell death. TNF-α (cachexin or cachectin) is a cytokine involved in systemic inflammation that upregulates other NF-κB-regulated cytokines and is also a member of a group of cytokines that stimulate the acute phase reaction. TNF-α is also able to induce apoptotic cell death. [31]

Although the exact target of the polyphenols along the pro-inflammatory signal cascades is not known in detail, it is most likely suggested that they interfere with the NF-κB pathway somewhere upstream of kinases phosphorylating the inhibitor of κB, IκB. There are two signaling pathways leading to the activation of NF-κB known as the canonical pathway (or classical) and the noncanonical pathway (or alternative pathway). [31] The common regulatory step in both of these cascades is activation of an IκB kinase (IκK) complex consisting of catalytic kinase subunits (IκKa and/or IκKb) and the regulatory nonenzymatic scaffold protein NEMO. Activation of NF-κB dimers is due to IκK-mediated phosphorylation-induced proteasomal degradation of the IκB inhibitor enabling the active NF-κB transcription factor subunits to translocate to the nucleus and induce target gene expression. In the canonical (or classical) activation pathway, the complex consisting of IκK-b and IκK-g/NEMO phosphorylates two critical serine residues in IκB-a. IκB-a can then be targeted for ubiquitination and degradation. Some non-canonical pathways of IκK-independent activation of NF-κB stipulate the selective activation of NF-κB subunits. [31]

7. Deregulation of ıntracellular signallings due to Aβ

The studies suggest that various intracellular signaling pathways are deregulated in AD brains or during Aβ-induced neuronal apoptosis. For example, activation of stress-related kinases c-Jun N-terminal kinase (JNK) and p38 is associated with neuronal death in AD Mouse model. [32] Glycogen synthase kinase 3 (GSK-3) has also been implicated in Aβ-induced neurotoxicity.

Deregulation of distinct signaling pathways leads to aberrant phosphorylation of cellular proteins and has a profound effect on the progression of AD. [32]

They reported the identification of signal transducer and activator of transcription 3 (STAT3) as a potential key player in AD pathophysiology. STAT3 is a transcription factor that is typically associated with cytokine signaling during neuronal differentiation, inflammation, and malignancies. Interestingly, they found that tyrosine phosphorylation of STAT3, which is required for the activation of this transcription factor, is markedly elevated in neurons treated with Aβ *in vitro* or *in vivo* as well as in the brains of APP/PS1 transgenic mice. Inhibition of STAT3 activation or reduced STAT3 expression significantly attenuates Aβ-induced neuronal cell death. Moreover, activation of a tyrosine kinase Tyk2 is required for the Aβ-induced tyrosine phosphorylation of STAT3 and neuronal cell death. Notably, elevation of STAT3 tyrosine phosphorylation is evident in postmortem samples of AD brains. These observations collectively raise an intriguing possibility that STAT3 signaling is involved in neuronal apoptosis observed in AD patients. [32]

8. Interactions between Aβ and microglia

Activated microglia secrete various humoral substances (cytokines, free radicals) which influence neurons and glia. The inhibition of C3 conversion resulted in the lack of Aβ opsonisation and prevented microglia from Aβ clearance and, as a result, doubled the amyloid burden in murine brains. [33] The following may be responsible for the inconsistency in the results of experiments on microglia behaviour in contact with Aβ:

- immunomodulation of astroglia,
- immunomodulation of neurons,
- senescence of microglia.

Microglia activation is followed by astrocyte activation. Astrocytes phagocyte and degrade Aβ. *In vivo* experiments suggest that the coexistence of microglia and astrocytes diminishes the ability of microglia to digest and degrade plaques and Aβ. Therefore, activated astrocytes may exert a regulative effect (negative feedback) on the phagocytic activity of microglia. Another factor influencing microglia activation is the neuronal expression of cyclooxygenase-2 (COX-2). COX-2 participates in prostaglandin production and its expression is usually elevated in places of inflammation. [33]

In AD, initially COX-2 expression is evident in pyramidal neurons particularly involved in AD. COX-2 expression rises at the onset of the disease and then declines in the advanced stages of AD. Of note, the expression of COX-2 correlated positively with the level of prostaglandin E2 (PGE2) in cerebrospinal fluid (CSF). CSF PGE2 levels are clearly higher in people with mild dementia and decrease in the late stages of AD. [33]

Together with astrocytes, microglia have the ability to bind and take up Aβ in vitro and in vivo, being important players for the deposition and removal of Aβ, although there are also reports suggesting that Aβ formation occurs independently of microglial cells. [34] Microglial cells express several pattern-recognition receptors, which allow them to remove potentially toxic molecules such as Aβ. These receptors include scavenger receptors (SR) class A (SR-A), class B type I, low-density lipoprotein receptor-related protein (LRP), cluster of differentiation 36 (CD36), receptor for end glycation product, mannose receptor, and SR-MARCO. [34]

In fact, microglial cells secrete multiple cytokines such as interleukin-1b (IL1b), tumor necrosis factor (TNF-α), interleukin 10 (IL10), and transforming growth factor-b (TGFβ) as well as short-lived cytotoxic factors such as superoxide (O_2^{-2}) and NO^-, which contribute to neurotoxicity. [34] It has been suggested that TGFβ1 produced by astrocytes and hippocampal cells prevents induction of reactive oxygen species (ROS) and NO^- production by inflammatory mediators (lipopolysaccharide [LPS] 1 interferon-γ [IFNγ]) and neurotoxicity in vitro and that the modulation of microglia is at least partially mediated by the activation of the ERK pathway. TGFβ superfamily signaling plays important roles in a diverse set of cellular responses, including cell proliferation, differentiation, extracellular matrix remodeling, and embryonic development. TGFβ1 signaling is mediated by cell surface type I and type II receptors, which phosphorylates the two R-Smad proteins Smad2 and Smad3 downstream. Phospho-Smad2/3 forms a complex with the common mediator Smad4 that binds to a Smad-binding element (SBE) in the nucleus with a large number of transcription coregulators to activate gene promoter. They showed that the TGFβ1 Smad3 pathway is involved in modulation of microglial cell activity through its effects on expression of SRs, NO^- secretion, and phagocytosis. Microglial cell activation can be initiated by various signal transduction pathways, including nuclear factor-jB, JAK/STAT, and p38 pathways, which are activated by several inflammatory mediators and Aβ. [34]

9. Aβ and apoptosis

Apoptosis, or programmed cell death, is a highly regulated process involved in embryonic development, developmental tissue remodeling and normal cell turnover. [35] However, when dysregulation occurs in apoptotic pathways, excessive or insufficient cell death can lead to diseases such as cancers, autoimmune syndromes and/or neurodegenerative diseases. Caspases are a family of intracellular cysteine-aspartic proteases that are not only essential for triggering programmed cell death, but have also been shown to play key roles in non-apoptotic pathways, such as differentiation and proliferation of diverse cell types, axon guidance and synaptic activity and plasticity. Caspases are divided into long prodomain caspases (caspases-2, -8, -9 and -10), which are initiators of apoptosis, and short prodomain caspases (caspases-3, -6, -7 and -14), which are generally termed the effectors of apoptosis. However, some caspases, including caspase-3 (Casp3) and caspase-6 (Casp6), appear to function as both initiators and effectors. Aberrant activation of caspases has been implicated in several neurodegenerative diseases, such as AD, HD, various ataxias and amyotrophic lateral sclerosis [35].

Apoptosis is a cell death program that is central to cellular and tissue homeostasis, and is involved in many physiological and pathological processes. [36] Apoptosis is characterized morphologically by a series of events that include cytoplasmic shrinkage, chromatin condensation, nuclear and cellular fragmentation, and the formation of apoptotic bodies. Although caspases are the main players involved in apoptosis, there are other molecules involved in the progression of the apoptotic cascade that are relevant to AD. The neuronal death in AD may result directly and/or indirectly from the triggering insults caused by Aβ toxicity, glutamate excitotoxicity, long-lasting oxidative stress, DNA damage, and elevation of intracellular calcium levels. Thus, the mode of cell death in AD remains a matter of controversy, and it is possible that both apoptotic and non-apoptotic cell death coexist in the brains of affected patients. [36]

Previously, it was generally considered that apoptotic neuronal death in chronic neurodegenerative disease, e.g., AD, Parkinson's disease, etc., is associated with classical caspase mediated cell death. However, in part, it was suggested that the caspase-independent pathway might also participate in the pathogenesis of the disease. Cross talk is extensive between different cell death pathways, which include multiple types of caspase-dependent and caspase-independent programmed cell death. [36]

Cells undergo apoptosis through two major pathways, the extrinsic pathway (death receptor pathway) and the intrinsic pathway (the mitochondrial pathway). These two pathways can be linked by caspase-8-activated truncated Bid formation. Very recently, death receptor 6 (DR6) was shown to be involved in the neurodegeneration observed in Alzheimer disease. DR6, also known as TNFRSF21, is a relatively new member of the death receptor family, and it was found that DR6 induces apoptosis when it is overexpressed. However, how the death signal mediated by DR6 is transduced intracellularly is not known. To this end, in a study they have examined the roles of caspases, apoptogenic mitochondrial factor cytochrome c, and the Bcl-2 family proteins in DR6-induced apoptosis. In their study results demonstrated that Bax translocation is absolutely required for DR6-induced apoptosis. On the other hand, they found inhibition of caspase-8 and knockdown of Bid have no effect on DR6-induced apoptosis. Their results strongly suggest that DR6-induced apoptosis occurs through a new pathway that is different from the type I and type II pathways through interacting with Bax. [37]

Different studies reported both necrotic and apoptotic mechanisms for Aβ-mediated neurotoxicity. In particular, oxidative-mediated DNA damage, with a pattern indicative of apoptosis, was found in AD brain, which is consistent with several lines of experimental evidence linking oxidative stress and neuronal apoptosis. [38] Apoptosis is induced by micromolar concentrations of Aβ in cultured CNS neurons, however, physiological nanomolar concentrations of Aβ1-40 and Aβ1-42 are insufficient to initiate significant apoptosis in cultures of human fetal neurons. In fact, both Aβ peptides downregulate "bcl-2", a key anti- apoptotic protein, while only Aβ1-42 upregulates "bax", a protein known to promote apoptotic cell death. Interestingly, Aβ treated neurons exposed to different levels of oxidative stress, unable to increase apoptosis in control neurons, show 10-20 times more apoptotic-mediated DNA-damage, suggesting that Aβ renders the neurons vulnerable to age-dependent oxidative stress and neurodegeneration. Other links between oxidative stress and apoptotic neuronal cell death in AD have been described. Apoptosis induced by 4-HNE is prevented in cells that overexpress "bcl-2" or by incubation with glutathione, which binds 4-HNE. Also, PC12 cells expressing a mutated presenilin-1 gene, which accounts for the majority of cases of inherited early onset forms of AD are more susceptible to apoptosis induced by micromolar concentrations of Aβ and to oxidative stress induced by nerve growth factor with- drawal. [38]

Microglial activation can lead to microglial apoptosis, which may serve to remove highly reactive and possibly neurotoxic microglia. [39] However the loss of microglia may have consequences for future recovery, protection and repair. P53, a nuclear phosphoprotein transcription factor, is critical for activating the expression of genes involved in cell-cycle arrest and stress-induced apoptosis. In neurodegenerative diseases the expression of p53 is significantly increased in glial cells, and microglial numbers fall. P53 is a transcription factor, the activation of which promotes cellular apoptosis through the normal cell cycle. [39]

P53 also activates the expression of genes involved in stress-induced apoptosis and the apoptotic pathways implicated in neurodegenerative diseases which may arise from inappropriate p53 activation. Changes in p53 expression occur in glial cells in neurological conditions; p53 expression increases predominantly in glial cells in Alzheimer's disease. The sustained reactivity of microglia is implicated in the pathology of many neurodegenerative diseases and microglia may secrete substances which compromise neighbouring cells. Increased microglial reactivity can lead to microglial apoptosis. This apoptosis results from microglial stress and is triggered by nitric oxide-dependent mitochondrial depolarization and caspase activation. Whilst microglial apoptosis may serve to limit the number of reactive microglia in the brain, the processes of microglial stress and apoptosis can in themselves result in the release of pro-apoptotic species such as soluble Fas ligand which can trigger bystander cell apoptotic cascades. Microglial numbers significantly decrease in aged human brain and in Alzheimer's brain and such loss may restrict the ability of the brain to recover from injury. Apoptotic changes in microglia precede changes in neurons or other glia in models of neurodegenerative disease. As microglia secrete neurotrophins important for neuronal survival and regeneration, the apoptosis of microglia may impact on brain health. They examined the role p53 plays in mediating microglial apoptosis following microglial activation with the Alzheimer peptides amyloid beta and chromogranin A, as well as with the activator lipopolysaccharide. [39]

Taken together, these results suggest that mitochondrial energy metabolism might be impaired by Aβ through down-regulation of mitochondrial proteins and activity. [40] In addition, the interaction between NO and cytochrome *c* oxidase controls mitochondrial production of hydrogen peroxide, which has been shown to be implicated in cellular redox signaling. In a study they used synthetic Aβ1–42 to impair the function of complexes I and IV in CP epithelial cells and to investigate whether ROS generation was also altered. [40] Their results support the hypothesis that Aβ1–42 interferes with oxidative phosphorylation, which results in oxidative stress, and demonstrate that ROS generation is secondary to mitochondrial damage. The results of the study also show that Aβ1–42-treated CP epithelial cells have an increased expression of caspases 3 and 9. [40] This result is consistent with a recent study, where APP transfected cells showed a significant increase in the expression and activity of caspases 3 and 9. The data suggest that the excessive generation of ROS would be responsible for initiating the apoptotic cell death process by up-regulating caspase signaling, as previously demonstrated. In view of the results from their *in vitro* and *in vivo* studies, they proposed that Aβ-induced mitochondrial dysfunction provides an important source of ROS, which could ultimately initiate a programmed cell death pathway. In CP from APP/PS1 mice and AD patients, this pathway involves high levels of MMP-9, increased caspases expression and cell loss. [40]

Previous studies found that expression levels of Bcl-2 family proteins, such as Bax, Bak, Bad, Bcl-2, Bim, Bcl-w and Bcl-x are altered in the vulnerable neurons in AD. [41] They demonstrated that oligomeric Aβ altered the expression levels of Bcl-2, Bim and Bax, and that the genetic or pharmacological ablation of Bax activity suppresses oligomeric Aβ-mediated neurotoxicity in both ex vivo and in vivo. These results clearly indicate that Bax has an essential role in the induction of neuronal cell death caused by oligomeric Aβ. [41] In healthy cells, Bax is located in the cytosol or loosely associated to mitochondria and endoplasmic reticulum. Bax translocation to the mitochondria, which occurs in cells with apoptotic stresses, is thought to lead to mitochondrial dysfunction and release of cytochrome c and subsequent apoptosis. Before its translocation to mitochondria, Bax changes its conformation that exposes the N-terminal residues. This conformational change is believed to be necessary for membrane insertion of Bax at mitochondria and multimerization of Bax. They demonstrated that oligomeric Aβ induced the N-terminal exposure of Bax in neurons and that the inhibition of this event by BIP rescues neurons from oligomeric Aβ's neurotoxicity, suggesting the activation of Bax by its conformational change is a key element of oligomeric Aβ-induced neurotoxicity. Although the molecular mechanism(s) of Bax activation has not been clearly defined, multiple pro-apoptotic proteins (e.g.,Bim) and anti-apoptotic proteins (e.g., Bcl-2) are known to regulate the activation of Bax thorough heterodimerization. These data strongly suggest that Bim might be an upstream regulator of Bax activation in oligomeric Aβ-induced neurotoxicity and the pathological role of Bim and Bax in neuronal cell loss in AD. [41]

As the activation of JNK by Aβ has been shown and the active form of JNK has been reported to be increased in vulnerable neurons in AD, it is plausible that the activation of JNK and subsequent activation of Bim/Bax-mediated apoptosis pathway might be the mechanism causing neuronal cell death in oligomeric Aβ treated neurons and AD. [41]

As the chronic administration of resveratrol also protected animals from Aβ-induced neuronal loss, it is reasonably speculated that the improvement in spatial memory by resveratrol might be ascribed to its effectiveness in reducing the levels of oxidative stress and the Aβ-induced neuronal loss. [42] The activation of iNOS gene by Aβ is controlled by the transcription factor NF-κB, which is known to regulate iNOS transcription by binding to the regulatory region of iNOS gene. In addition, Aβ treatment was reported to result in the activation of NF-κB in various brain regions and cell types, and resveratrol was shown to markedly attenuate the Aβ-induced NFκB nuclear translocation. Based on these, it is suggested that the regulation pathway triggered by resveratrol is to decrease the Aβ accumulation, which in turn suppresses Aβ-induced NF-κB translocation, or activation, and leads to the downregulation of iNOS. [42]

Considering the strong correlation between Aβ-induced oxidative stress and cytotoxicity, ROS produced in mitochondria may leak to the cytoplasm, leading to oxidative stress and the initiation of apoptosis via the activation of apoptosis signaling. [43] It is well established that the ratio of Bcl-2/Bax is crucial in the apoptosis of the mitochondrial pathway. Bcl-2 is a potent cell death suppressor, and its overexpression prevents cell death. However, Bax is a death-promoting factor, and its translocation to the mitochondrial membrane may lead to the loss of mitochondrial membrane potential and an increase in mitochondrial permeability. Increased mitochondrial permeability results in the egress of cytochrome *c* from the mitochondria and the subsequent activation of procaspase-3 to caspase-3, which eventually leads to apoptosis. Aβ treatment significantly decreased the Bcl-2/Bax protein expression ratio and increased caspase-3 activity, in agreement with previous reports. [43]

Classic programmed cell death is more frequently associated with a death program that requires gene transcription and protein synthesis, whereas apoptosis is generally independent of protein synthesis and represents a posttranslational response of host cells. Apoptosis is characterized by a requirement for specific proteolysis driven by caspases, although it is also reported that caspases (caspase 9 in particular) participate in nonapoptotic cell death. [35]

The name caspase is a contraction of cysteinedependent aspartate-specific protease; their enzymatic properties are governed by a dominant specificity for substrates containing Asp and by the use of a Cys side chain for catalyzing peptide bond cleavage. Mammals contain two biologically distinct caspase subfamilies: One of these participates in the processing of proinflammatory cytokines, and the other is required to elicit and execute the apoptotic response during programmed cell death. [35]

The intrinsic pathway responds primarily to cellular stress (ionizing radiation, cytotoxic drugs, etc.) as well as some neurodevelopmental cues, with the mitochondrion acting as an important integrator. Activation of the apical protease caspase 9 occurs when it is driven into a catalytic conformation by its cofactor Apaf-1, which itself requires prior binding to cytochrome c. The extrinsic apoptosis pathway is triggered through the extracellular ligation of death receptors by their cognate ligands, resulting in receptor clustering, adapter recruitment, and activation of the apical protease caspase 8. [35]

The in vivo models offer the advantage of allowing neuronal death to proceed in a more physiologic setting, where the different components of the nervous system are intact. The in vivo models, however, do not adequately allow determination of the specific caspases necessary to execute neuronal death in each disease. [35] Elucidation of the specific caspase pathways is best approached in the cell culture models, with which biochemical studies can be more easily performed. Cell culture models include both primary neuronal cultures and cell lines. Both are valid models, as long as their limitations are appreciated. Cell lines offer the advantage of providing large amounts of homogenous material in which expression levels of the different components of the death pathways can be easily manipulated. Results from cell lines must normally be validated in vivo in the cell that they are modeling. After establishment of the potential caspase pathways in the cell culture models, the in vivo and human samples can be analyzed. [35] Caspases are a family of cysteine proteases that cleave their substrates after aspartic residues. They are usually synthesized as inactive zymogens that are proteolytically cleaved into subunits at the onset of apoptosis and function as active caspases after reconstitution to molecular heterodimers. [45] Caspases are composed of three domains including an N-terminal prodomain, a large subunit, and a small subunit. The apoptotic-associated caspases include initiator caspases, such as caspases 2, 8, 9, and 10, that activate

http://dx.doi.org/10.5772/54718

downstream executioner caspases, resulting in an amplification of cascade activity. The initiator caspases consist of long N-terminal prodomains that contain caspase recruitment domains (CARDs) in caspase 2 and caspase 9, or death effector domains (DEDs) in caspase 8 and caspase 10. Another set of caspases, termed the executioner caspases, consists of caspases 3, 6, and 7 that function to directly cleave crucial cellular protein substrates that result in cell destruction. [45] The executioner caspases contain short prodomains or have no prodomains. Apoptotic injury during Alzheimer's disease may require caspase-mediated pathways. A strong body of evidence supports the premise that caspase activation is involved in the pathological process of Alzheimer's disease. The elevation of caspase genes including caspases 1, 2, 3, 5, 6, 7, 8, and 9 has been observed in human postmortem brains from Alzheimer's disease patients. In the brains of Alzheimer's patients, single neurons with DNA fragmentation have been shown to contain cytoplasmic immunoreactivity for active caspase 3, implying that apoptotic injury results during Alzheimer's disease. In addition, activation of caspase 3 was found to occur in the parahippocampal gyrus in brains from patients with mild forms of Alzheimer's disease. Caspase 3 immunoreactivity was also co-localized with paired helical filaments in neurons, suggesting that caspase 3 activation may contribute to the formation of neurofibrillary tangles. [45]

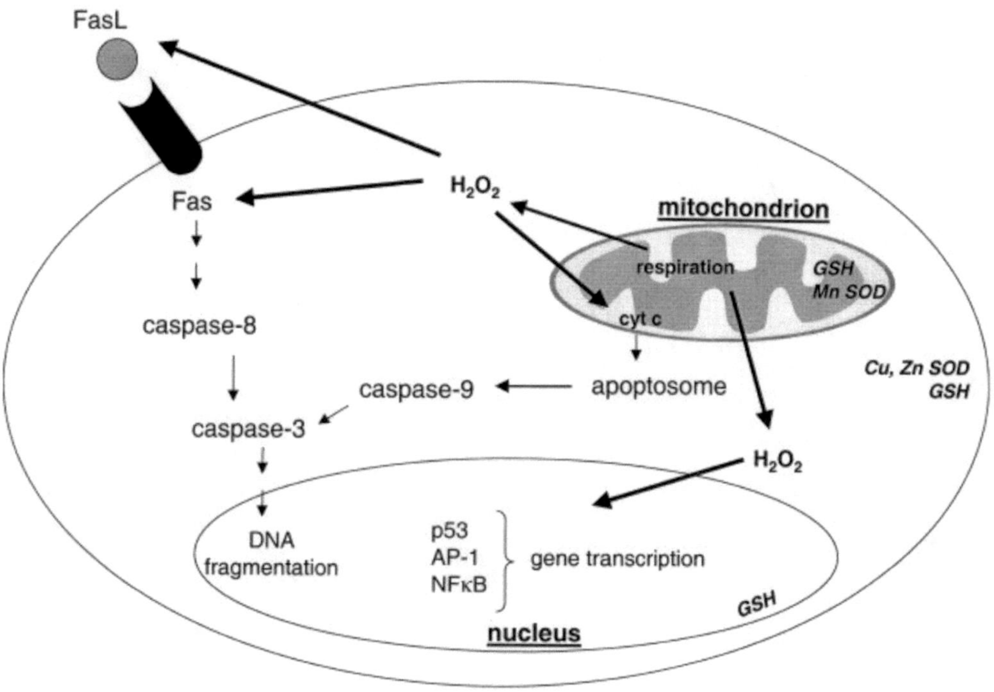

Figure 3. Intracellular sources of ROS and their interaction with the apoptotic pathway. [Chandra J. 2000, ref 26]

As Aβ peptides are used to mimic AD in animal models, and because sporadic AD is known to arise mostly in older ages, we designed a study to investigate the acute effects of Aβ 1-42 injection in aged rats suggesting the onset of sporadic AD. In the light of the current literature, we investigated not only the effect of Aβ 1-42 injection on aged rat brain, but also age related changes in lipid peroxidation, nNOS and iNOS expression and caspase 3 in which involves apoptotic process as an apoptosis marker. In this study, a prominent increase of caspase 3 activity in hippocampus has been shown in Aβ 1-42 injected aged rats. [24] This result suggests that apoptotic mechanism triggers neuronal death in hippocampus, and results a significant decrement nNOS expression consequently in Aβ 1-42 injected aged rats. Another explanation of these results is that because of possible neuronal death by the way of caspase-3, there may not be enough neurons remained to cause lipid peroxidation. This suggests that acute effect of Aβ 1-42 result with increase in caspase 3 activity which is seen before the oxidative stress-dependent neurotoxic effects. In this study Aβ 1-42 lead to a counter effect on nNOS expression in young adults and aged rats. The results of this study suggest that the aged rat brain does not successfully offset the oxidative stress. [24] We suggest that the relationship between aging, NOS-mediated ROS-dependent toxicity of beta amyloid toxicity and apoptotic events should be bring out into the open this vicious cycle.

Abbreviations

ROS: Reactive oxygen species

AD: Alzheimer's disease

Aβ: Beta amyloid peptide

NO: Nitric oxide

NOS: Nitric oxide synthase

CA: Cornu ammonis

H_2O_2: Hydrogen peroxide

$ONOO^-$: Peroxynitrite

APP: Amyloid precursor protein

RNS: Reactive nitrogen species

GADPH: Glucose 6-phosphate dehydrogenase

MAPK: Mitogen activated protein kinase

AP-1: Activated protein

NFκB: Nuclear factor kapa B

CNS: Central nervous system

AGE: Advanced glycation end product

IκB: Inhibitor of κB

http://dx.doi.org/10.5772/54718

IκBK: Inhibitor of κB kinase

JNK: c-Jun N-terminal kinase

GSK-3: Glycogen synthase kinase 3

STAT3: Signal transducer and activator of transcription 3

Tyk2: tyrosine kinase 2

SR: Scavenger receptor

LRP: Low-density lipoprotein receptor related protein

TGF: Transforming growth factor

SBE: Smad binding element

HD: Huntington disease

PD: Parkinson disease

DR6: Death receptor 6

SOD: Superoxide dismutase

GSH: Glutathione

Author details

Ferihan Cetin*

Address all correspondence to: ferihan@yahoo.com

Izmir University Faculty of Medicine, Department of Physiology, Medical Park Hospital, Izmir, Turkey

References

[1] Beckman, K. B, & Ames, B. N. The free radical theory of aging matures. Physiol Rev. (1998). , 78, 547-581.

[2] Sastre, J, & Pallardo, F. V. Mitochondrial oxidative stress plays a key role in aging and apoptosis. IUBMB life (2000). , 49427-435.

[3] Fiala, M, Cribbs, D. H, Rosenthal, M, & Bernard, G. Phagocytosis of amyloid-beta and inflammation: two faces of innate immunity in Alzheimer's disease. J Alzheimers Dis. (2007). , 11(4), 457-63.

[4] Yamada, K, & Nabeshima, T. Animal models of Alzheimer's disease and evaluation of anti-dementia drugs. Pharmacol. Therap. (2000). , 88-93.

[5] Camandola, S, Poli, G, & Mattson, M. P. Lipid Peroxidation Product 4-hydroxynonenal increases AP-1 binding activity through caspase activation in neurons. J Neurochem. (2000). , 74(1), 159-68.

[6] Stepanichev, M. Y, Onufriev, M. V, Yakovlev, A. A, Khrenov, A. I, & Peregud, D. I. Amyloid-β (25-35) increases activity of neuronal NO-synthase in rat brain. Neurochemistry International (2008). , 52-1114.

[7] Law, A, Gauthier, S, & Quiron, R. Say NO to Alzheimer's disease: putative links between nitric oxide and dementia of the Alzheimer's type. Brain Res. Rev. (2001). , 35-73.

[8] Xie, X, Wang, H-T, Li, H-L, Gao, X-H, Ding, J, & Zhao, H-H. Ginsenoside Rb1 protects PC12 cells against β-amyloid-induced cell injury Mol Med Reports (2010). , 3, 635-639.

[9] Christen, Y. Oxidative stress and Alzheimer disease. Am J Clin Nutr (2000).

[10] Lovell, M. A, Ehmann, W. D, Butler, S. M, & Markesberry, W. R. Elevated thiobarbituric acid-reactive substances and antioxidant enzyme activity in the brain in Alzheimer's disease. Neurology (1995). , 45-1594.

[11] Machiavelli, L. I, Poliandri, A. H, Quinteros, F. A, Cabilla, J. P, & Duvilanski, B. H. Reactive oxygen species are key mediators of the nitric oxide apoptotic pathway in anterior pituitary cells. Nitric Oxide Mar (2007). , 16(2), 237-46.

[12] Vina, J, Lloret, A, Vallés, S. L, Borrás, C, Badía, M. C, Pallardó, F. V, & Sastre, J. Mitochondrial oxidant signalling in Alzheimer's disease. J Alzheimers Dis. (2007). , 11(2), 175-81.

[13] Feng, Z, Qin, C, Chang, Y, & Zhang, J. Early melatonin supplementation alleviates oxidative stress in a transgenicmouse model of Alzheimer's disease. Free Rad Biol & Med (2006). , 40-101.

[14] Thorns, V, Lawrence, H. L, & Masliah, E. nNOS Expressing Neurons in the Entorhinal Cortex and Hippocampus Are Affected in Patients with Alzheimer's Disease. Exper Neurol (1998). , 150-14.

[15] Norris, P. J, Faull, R. L, & Emson, P. C. Neuronal nitric oxide synthase (nNOS) mRNA expression and NADPH-diaphorase staining in the frontal cortex, visual cortex and hippocampus of control and Alzheimer's disease brains. Brain Res Mol Brain Res. (1996).

[16] Koliatsos, V. E, Kecojevic, A, Troncoso, J. C, Gastard, M. C, Bennett, D. A, & Schneider, J. A. Early involvement of small inhibitory cortical interneurons in Alzheimer's disease. Acta Neuropathol (2006). , 112-147.

[17] Butterfield, D. A, & Lauderback, C. M. Lipid peroxidation and protein oxidation in Alzheimer's Disease brain: potential causes and consequences involving Amyloid β-

Peptide-associated free radical oxidative stress. Free Rad Biol Med. (2002). , 32(11), 1050-1060.

[18] Jhoo, J. H, Kim, H-C, Nabeshima, T, Yamada, K, Shin, E-J, Jhoo, W-K, & Kim, W. Amyloid (1-42)-induced learning and memory deficits in mice: involvement of oxidative burdens in the hippocampus and cerebral cortex. Behav Brain Res (2004). , 155, 185-196.

[19] Siles, E, Martinez-lara, E, Canuelo, A, Sánchez, M, Hernández, R, & López-ramos, J. C. M, Age related changes of the nitric oxide system in the brain. Brain Res. November (2002). , 956(2), 385-92.

[20] Koppal, T, Drake, J, Yatin, S, Jordan, B, Varadarajan, S, Bettenhausen, L, & Butterfield, D. A. Peroxynitrite-induced alterations in synaptosomal membrane proteins: insight into oxidative stress in Alzheimer's Disease. J. Neurochem. (1999). , 72, 310-317.

[21] Malinski, T. Nitric oxide and nitro-oxidative stress in Alzheimer's Disease. J.Alz. Disease. May (2007). , 11(2), 207-18.

[22]] Maccioni, R. B, Muñoz, J. P, & Barbeito, L. The Molecular Bases of Alzheimer's Disease and Other Neurodegenerative Disorders. Archives of Medical Research (2001). , 32, 367-381.

[23] Weldon, D. T, Rogers, S. D, Ghilardi, J. R, Finke, M. P, Cleary, J. P, Hare, O, Esler, E, Maggio, W. P, Mantyh, J. E, & Fibrillar, P. W. Amyloid Induces Microglial Phagocytosis, Expression of Inducible Nitric Oxide Synthase, and Loss of a Select Population of Neurons in the Rat CNS In Vivo The Journal of Neuroscience, March 15, (1998). , 18(6), 2161-2173.

[24] Cetin, F, Yazihan, N, Dincer, S, & Akbulut, K. G. The The Effect of Intracerebroventricular Injection of Beta Amyloid Peptide (1-42) on Caspase 3 Activity, Lipid Peroxidation and NOS expression in Young Adult and Aged Rat Brain. Turkish Neurosurgery (2012). date accepted May 17.DOİ. :10.5137/JTN.5855-12.1, 1019-5149.

[25] Markesbery William ROxidative stress hypothesis in Alzheimer's Disease. Free Radical Biology & Medicine, (1997). , 23(1), 134-147.

[26] Chandra, J, Samali, A, & Orrenius, S. Triggering and modulation of apoptosis by oxidative stres. Free Radical Biology & Medicine, (2000). Nos. 3/4, , 29, 323-333.

[27]] Calabrese, V, Cornelius, C, Rizzarelli, E, Owen, J. B, Dinkova-kostova, A. T, & Butterfield, D. A. Nitric Oxide in Cell Survival: A Janus Molecule. Antioxidants & Redox Signaling (2009). , 11(11)

[28] Spuch, C, Ortolano, S, & Navarro, C. New Insights in the Amyloid-Beta Interaction withMitochondria. Journal of Aging Research Article ID 324968, 9 pages doi: 10.1155/2012/324968, 2012

[29] Walter, S, Letiembre, M, Liu, Y, Heine, H, Penke, B, Hao, W, Bode, B, & Manietta, N. Jessica Walter J., Schulz-Schäffer W. and Faßbender K., Role of the Toll-Like Receptor

4 in Neuroinflammation in Alzheimer's Disease. Cell Physiol Biochem (2007). , 20, 947-956.

[30] Medeiros, R, Prediger, R. D. S, Passos, G. F, Pandolfo, P, Duarte, F. S, Franco, J. L, Dafre, A. L, Giunta, G. D, Figueiredo, C. P, Takahashi, R. N, Campos, M. M, & Calixto, J. B. Connecting TNF-β Signaling Pathways to iNOS Expression in a Mouse Model of Alzheimer's Disease: Relevance for the Behavioral and Synaptic Deficits Induced by Amyloid β Protein. Neurobiology of Disease, The Journal of Neuroscience, May 16, (2007). , 27(20), 5394-5404.

[31] Chandler, D, Woldu, A, Rahmadi, A, Shanmugam, K, Steiner, N, Wright, E, Benavente-garci, a O, Schulz, O, Castillo, J, & Munch, G. Effects of plant-derived polyphenols on TNF-α and nitric oxide production induced by advanced glycation endproducts. Mol. Nutr. Food Res. (2010). SS150, 141.

[32] Wan, J, Fu, A. K. Y, & Ip, F. C. F. Ho-Keung Ng, Hugon J., Page G., Wang J.H., Kwok-On Lai, Wu Z., and Ip N.Y., Tyk2/STAT3 Signaling Mediates β-Amyloid-Induced Neuronal Cell Death: Implications in Alzheimer's Disease. Neurobiology of Disease The Journal of Neuroscience, May 19, (2010). , 30(20), 6873-6881.

[33] Wojtera, M, Sobów, T, Kloszewska, I, Liberski, P. P, Brown, D. R, & Sikorska, B. Expression of immunohistochemical markers on microglia in Creutzfeldt-Jakob disease and Alzheimer's disease: morphometric study and review of the literature. Folia Neuropathol (2012). , 50(1), 74-84.

[34] Juan, E, Tichauer, J. E, & Bernhardi, R. Transforming Growth Factor-β Stimulates β-Amyloid Uptake by Microglia Through Smad3-Dependent Mechanisms. Journal of Neuroscience Research (2012). , 90, 1970-1980.

[35] Uribe, V, Wong, B.K.Y, Graham, R.K, Cusack, C.L, Skotte, N.H, Pouladi, M.A, Xie, Y, Feinberg, K, Ou, Y, Ouyang, Y, & Deng, . ., Rescue from excitotoxicity and axonal degeneration accompanied by age-dependent behavioral and neuroanatomical alterations in caspase-6-deficient mice. Human Molecular Genetics, 2012; Vol. 21, No. 9 1954-1967

[36] Lee, J-H, & Cheon, . ., Evidence of early involvement of apoptosis inducing factor-induced neuronal death in Alzheimer brain. Anatomy and Cell Biolog.2012; pISSN 2093-3665 eISSN 2093-3673. http://dx.doi.org/10.5115/acb.2012.45.1.26

[37] Zeng, L, Li, T, Xu, D. C, Liu, J, Mao, G, Cui, M. Z, Fu, X, & Xu, X. Death Receptor 6 Induces Apoptosis Not through Type I or Type II Pathways, but via a Unique Mitochondria-dependent Pathway by Interacting with Bax Protein. J Biol Chem. 2012 Aug 17; Epub (2012). Jul 3., 287(34), 29125-33.

[38] Miranda, S, Opazo, C, & Larrondo, L. F. MunÄ oz F.J., Ruiz F., Leighton F., Inestrosa N.C., The role of oxidative stress in the toxicity induced by amyloid b- peptide in Alzheimer's disease. Progress in Neurobiology (2000). , 62, 633-648.

[39] Davenport, C. M, Sevastou, I. G, Hooper, C, Pocock, J. M, & Inhibiting, P. Pathways in microglia attenuates microglial evoked neurotoxicity following exposure to Alzheimer peptides. Journal of Neurochemistry (2010). , 112, 552-563.

[40] Vargas, T, Ugalde, C, Spuch, C, Antequera, D, Moránc, M. J, Martín, M. A, Ferrer, I, Bermejo-pareja, F, & Carro, E. Aβ accumulation in choroid plexus is associated with mitochondrial-induced apoptosis. Neurobiology of Aging (2010). , 31, 1569-1581.

[41] Kudo, W, Lee, H-P, Smith, M. A, Zhu, X, Matsuyama, S, & Lee, H-g. Inhibition of Bax protects neuronal cells from oligomeric Aβ neurotoxicity. Cell Death and Disease (2012). e309; doi:10.1038/cddis.2012.43

[42] Huang, T-C, & Lu, K-T. Peter Wo Y-Y., Wu Y-J., Yang Y-L., Resveratrol Protects Rats from Aβ-induced Neurotoxicity by the Reduction of iNOS Expression and Lipid Peroxidation. PLoS ONE December (2011). e 29102, 6(12)

[43] XiaxieHai-Taowang, Chun-Lili, Xu-Hong Gao, Jin-Landing, Hai-Huazhao and Yong-Lil, Ginsenoside Rb1 protects PC12 cells against β-amyloid-induced cell injury. Molecular Medicine REPORTS (2010). , 3, 635-639.

[44] Troy, C. M, & Salvesen, G. S. Caspases On The Brain. Journal of Neuroscience Research (2002). , 69, 145-150.

[45] Chonga, Z. Z, Lia, F, & Maiese, K. Stress in the brain: novel cellular mechanisms of injury linked to Alzheimer's disease. Brain Research Reviews (2005). , 49, 1-21.

Chapter 5

Alterations of Mitochondria and Golgi Apparatus Are Related to Synaptic Pathology in Alzheimer's Disease

Stavros J. Baloyannis

Additional information is available at the end of the chapter

http://dx.doi.org/10.5772/56079

1. Introduction

Alzheimer's disease (AD) is an insidiously progressive severe presenile and senile dementia, involving a number of cellular and biochemical mechanisms. AD affects millions of humans as the most common cause of cognitive decline worldwide, in addition to being a main medical challenge for aging population. From the clinical point of view, AD is mostly characterized by age-dependent inexorably progressing cognitive decline, affecting memory primarily associated with behavioral and mood disorders, which increasingly appear as the disease advances [1]. From the neuropathological point of view, AD is mostly characterized by selective neuronal loss [2, 3], marked synaptic alterations [4–6], morphological mitochondrial abnormalities [7, 8], tau pathology [9] resulting in neurofibrillary tangles (NFT) composed of hyperphosphorylated tau [10], inflammatory responses and by extracellular extensive deposits of polymers of Aβ peptide, in the form of neuritic plaques, which are a main hallmark of AD [11, 12]. These are dispersed in the neocortex, the hippocampus, and many subcortical structures, which play an important role in cognition. In addition, AD is characterized ultrastructurally by organelle pathology involving mostly the microtubules, the mitochondria, and Golgi apparatus [13].

Most studies have revealed that the main pathological criteria for AD, namely the neuritic plaques and neurofibrillary tangles, can account for 40%–70% of the cognitive impairment seen in advanced age, though additional cerebrovascular changes [14, 15] contribute greatly in plotting the dramatic profile of AD.

The two main hypotheses of AD - the amyloid cascade hypothesis, introduced in 1991 [16, 17] and the Tau protein hypothesis, are still subjects of extensive research and debate.The production and accumulation of Aβ peptide, a pathogenic factor leading to AD development, are the result of the post-translational proteolysis of the APP [18], by concerted actions of β- and γ-secretases [19].

The amyloidogenic pathway for APP is initiated by β- site amyloid precursor protein-cleavage enzyme 1 (BACE- 1), resulting in the generation of the intermediate product sAPPβ [20]. γ -Secretase activity is substantial for the cleavage of the transmembrane domain, releasing the Aβ peptide and the APP intracellular domain. Generation of Aβ peptide may occur in the endoplasmic reticulum (ER), trans-Golgi network [21], in lysosomes and on the surface of the cell, whereas its intracellular accumulation has been mostly detected in the majority of neurons in the endoplasmic reticulum, the mitochondria [22], the lysosomes, the multivesicular bodies, associated with synaptic pathology [23]. Many risk factors may affect APP protein metabolism and Aβ peptide production, mainly in late-onset AD. In addition changes in cellular protein homeostasis and aspects of protein folding or misfolding [24] are also linked to AD pathogenesis [25].

All the biochemical phenomena, which may occur within the spectrum of pathogenetic mechanisms in Alzheimer's disease affect the brain metabolic activity reasonably, since increasing evidence from functional neuroimaging plead in favor of the global and regional disruptions in brain metabolism in advanced cases of AD [26].

From the etiological point of view, it would be hypothesized that the multiple genetic loci [27, 28], associated with familial Alzheimer's disease would plead in favor of the heterogeneity of the disease and support the idea that the phenomenological profile of Alzheimer's disease may be the final consequence of various metabolic, neurochemical, and morphological alterations, based on a broad genetic background [29]. Although the majority of familial or inherited AD, which manifests at an early age, are often associated with mutations in AβPP [30], the numerous sporadic ones, which manifests usually at later stages of the life, are proved to be multifactorial, including induced expression of AβPP [31] by pathological stimuli, environmental factors, as well as deprivation of trophic factors. The eventual accumulation of Aβ peptide at synaptic terminals may be associated with synaptic damage, resulting in cognitive decline in patients with AD [32]. Moreover the increased risk of AD in sporadic cases, whenever a maternal relative is afflicted with the disease, pleads reasonably in favor of a maternally derived predisposition, which might be related to mutations of mitochondrial DNA (mtDNA) [33, 34].

1.1. Mitochondria in Alzheimer's disease

Mitochondria are highly dynamic ATP-generating organelles, which play an essential role in many cellular functions, such as alteration of reduction-oxidation potential of cells, free radical scavenging, intracellular calcium regulation and activation of apoptotic process. Mitochondria are unique amongst cellular organelles, since they dispose their own, spiral, double-stranded DNA (mtDNA), which is mostly inherited from the maternal line. The number of mitochondria is very high in neurons and especially in synaptic terminals, since they are the major energy generators for the cell biological processes and the synaptic activity, through tricarboxylic cycle and oxidative phosphorylation. The shape and size of mitochondria are not stable, since they undergo continual fission and fusion leading to their fragmentation or elongation accordingly.

http://dx.doi.org/10.5772/56079

Mitochondrial dysfunction might contribute to Aβ neurotoxicity and is also associated with oxidative stress, which may play an important role in the early stages of pathogenetic mechanisms in AD [35-37], presumably prior to the onset of the cognitive dysfunction, since a substantial body of evidence suggests that mitochondria play a crucial role in ageing-related neurodegenerative diseases [38].

Mitochondria may be the target for amyloid precursor protein (APP) and Aβ peptide, which might play an important role in impairing mitochondrial dynamics [39]. During AD processes accumulation of APP occurs mostly in the mitochondrial import channels, inducing mitochondrial functional impairment [40]. APP could not be processed to generate Aβ peptide locally [41] although a fraction of active γ-secretase is associated with mitochondria [42].

In the mitochondria, Aβ peptide uptake is mediated by the translocase, which is located in the outer mitochondrial membrane (TOM) [43]. Then Aβ peptide is accumulated mostly in the outer mitochondrial membrane, the inter membrane and the matrix and interacts with large number of proteins inside mitochondria, leading eventually to mitochondrial dysfunction, whenever substantial amount of molecules of Aβ peptide would be produced near mitochondria [44].

It is important to emphasize that mitochondrial alterations are associated with synaptic loss in AD patients, even before amyloid plaques are detected [32, 45]. Morphological and morphometric studies revealed that at early stages of AD the number of mitochondria in synaptic terminals is dramatically decrease and their structural pattern changes [45]. That modification might be attributed to enhanced nitrosative stress, generated by Aβ peptide, leading to mitochondrial fission, which is followed by mitochondrial depletion, resulting in synaptic degeneration eventually [46].

1.2. Golgi apparatus in Alzheimer's disease

Golgi apparatus plays an important role in the pathogenesis of AD [13, 47], since it is associated with protein trafficking. All newly synthesized proteins, which are used for fast axoplasmic transport are processed practically through the vesicles and the cisternae of Golgi complex [48]. From the first its visualization by Camillo Golgi, in 1898, Golgi apparatus has been subject of intense morphological and neurochemical research.

The electron microscopy study of the mammalian Golgi apparatus has revealed that it consists of stapled cisternae, which serve for the modification of newly synthesized proteins and lipids. At the entrance site of the Golgi apparatus, namely the cis-Golgi, numerous clusters of vesicles and tubular structures form an intermediate chain between the smooth endoplasmic reticulum and the Golgi stack. The exit site, the so called trans-Golgi network (TGN) is the main site of sorting proteins to distinct cellular destinations. Bi-directional traffic between the Golgi apparatus and the endosomal system sustains the functions of the trans-Golgi network (TGN) in secretion and organelle biogenesis [49].

The function of the Golgi complex consists mainly on vesicular transport, involving constant membrane fission and fusion, mediated by GTPases, coat proteins, Rabs, tethers and SNARE proteins, respectively, as it was documented from studies on glycosylation enzymes [50]. The activity of γ-secretase, which consists of presenilins (PSs) [51], nicastrin [52,53], pen-2 [54] and the aph proteins [54,55], is closely related with the function of Golgi complex, since it requires the presenilin-dependent trafficking of nicastrin, through the Golgi apparatus [56].

It was hypothesized that the passage of nicastrin and other components of the γ-secretase complex through Golgi apparatus is essential for the molecular stabilization and the protease activity [56]. In addition APP, which is normally synthesized in the endoplasmic reticulum (ER), is transported to trans-Golgi network (TGN) for trafficking to the cell surface [57, 58], or to synaptic terminals. APP is transported by fast axonal transport, been recycled back for further trafficking or final storing within the lysosomal system [59], in view that TGN generates transport vesicles bound for distinct domains of the plasma membrane and early endosomes. Whereas a small proportion of APP molecules are delivered to the plasma membrane and then cleaved by α-secretase into non-amyloidogenic fragments, the majority of APP molecules undergo degradation, following amyloidogenic pathway in the trans-Golgi network [59].

2. Material and methods

2.1. Patients

We studied the hippocampus, the acoustic and the visual cortices, the thalamus, the globus pallidus, the locus coeruleus, the red nucleus, the hypothalamus and many regions of the cerebellar cortex in ten brains of patients who suffered from AD, four men and six women, aged 62–87 years, who fulfilled the clinical, neuropsychological, and laboratory diagnostic criteria of AD.

The mean education of the patients was 15.2 years, and all of them spoke their native language fluently. Screening procedures were applied, which included medical history, medical examination, cardiological investigation, physical neurologic assessment, psychiatric and neuropsychological examinations. All the patients underwent EEG, carotid duplex Doppler, computerized tomography (CT) scanning and magnetic resonance imaging (MRI) of the brain, and single-photon emission computed tomography (SPECT).

The mental status of the patients was assessed by Mini mental State Examination (MMSE) and dementia rating scale (DRS) [60] and ADAS-COX test.

The cause of death of the patients was heart arrest, following to cardiac infarct one to seven months after the final neurological assessment. The postmortem examination of each one of the cases was performed within 6 h after death.

2.2. Electron microscopy

Small samples (2×2×2 mm) from the hippocampus, the acoustic and the visual cortices, the thalamus, the globus pallidus, the locus coeruleus, the red nucleus, the hypothalamus and from many regions of the cortex of the cerebellar hemispheres and the vermis were excised and immediately immersed in Sotelo's fixing solution, composed of 1% paraformaldehyde,

2.5% glutaraldehyde in cacodylate buffer 0.1 M, adjusted at pH 7.35. Then they were postfixed by immersion in 1% osmium tetroxide for 30 min at room temperature and dehydrated in graded alcohol solutions and propylene oxide.

Thin sections were cut in a Reichert ultratome, contrasted with uranyl acetate and lead citrate, and studied in a Zeiss 9aS electron microscope.

We studied the morphology of the mitochondria, the Golgi apparatus, and the synapses and we proceeded to morphometric estimations at electron microscope on micrographs of a standard magnification of 56. 000 X.

2.3. Light microscope, Golgi staining, Golgi-Nissl method

The remaining parts of the above-mentioned areas of the brain and the cerebellum were processed for silver impregnation techniques, according to rapid Golgi method.

Thus, after a four-week fixation in formalin they were immersed in potassium dichromate (7 g potassium dichromate in 300 mL water) for 10 days. Then they were immersed in 1% silver nitrate for 10 days. Following a rapid dehydration in graded alcohol solutions, the specimens were embedded in paraffin and cut, some of them at 100 μ and some at 25 μ, alternatively. Many sections of 25 μ were stained also with methylene blue, according to Golgi-Nissl method. All the sections were mounted in permount, between two cover slips and were studied in a Zeiss Axiolab Photomicroscope.

We estimated the dendritic arborization, the morphology and the number of the dendritic branches, and the morphology of the dendritic spines in light microscope on sections stained according to rapid Golgi and Golgi-Nissl methods

2.4. Statistical analysis

Statistical analysis was based on the *t*-test on the basis of 5000 mitochondria and 600 Golgi apparatus from 30 specimens of AD brains and 30 specimens of normal control brains.

3. Results

3.1. Silver impregnation techniques

The silver impregnation technique or black reaction (*reazione near*) according to Golgi [61] is a simple and easy histological procedure that enables the visualization of the three-dimensional morphology of neurons and glial cells. Santiago Ramón y Cajal has been applying Golgi technique extensively for the histological analysis of the CNS, defending successfully the "neuron doctrine" and sharing with Camillo Golgi the Nobel Prize in 1906. After 140 years from its first application, the Golgi technique continues to remain a very useful and valuable method in neuropathology for the morphological and morphometric estimation of neuronal circuits at the early stages of the degenerative processes of the brain [62].

The application of silver impregnation technique in our specimens revealed neuronal loss and marked abbreviation of the dendritic arborization in all the layers of the acoustic and the visual cortices, the hippocampus, the thalamus, the globus pallidus, the locus coeruleus, the red nucleus, the hypothalamus (Fig.1), the cerebellar cortex (Fig.2) and the vermis of the cerebellum (Fig.3). The layer I, of the acoustic and visual cortices, which includes Cajal-Retzius cells, which normally protrude very long horizontal axonal profiles with substantial number of collaterals [63. 64], was practically empty of neurons in patients who suffered from AD, in contrast to normal controls.

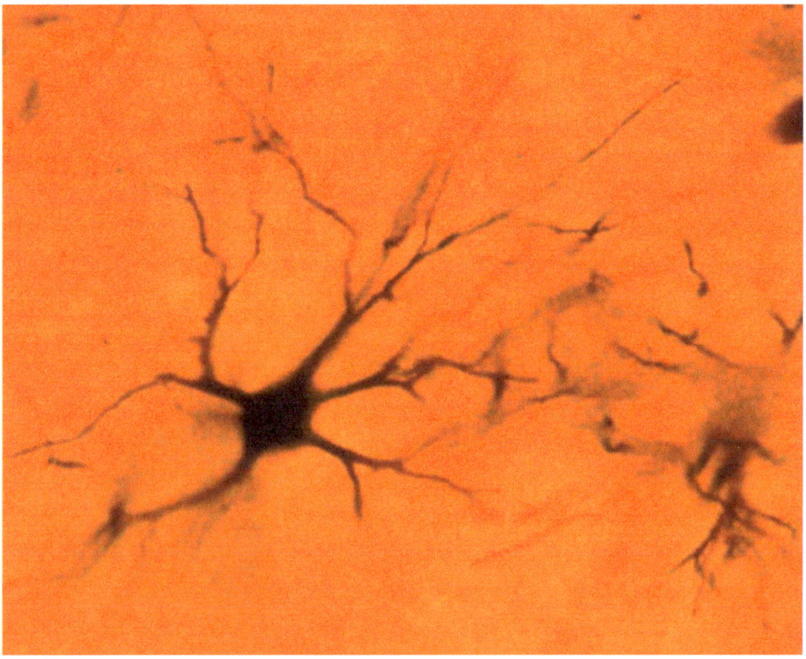

Figure 1. Neuron from the Hypothalamus of a case of AD, showing abbreviation of dendritic arborization and marked loss of dendritic spines (Golgi staining 2,400X)

Loss of tertiary dendritic branches was also noticed in the acoustic and visual cortices in all of the specimens. Abbreviation of the dendritic arborization was mostly prominent in neurons of layers III and V of the acoustic and visual cortices, the pyramidal neurons of the hippocampus, the polyhedral neurons of the locus coeruleus and in Purkinje cells of the cerebellar cortex, which demonstrated also a marked decrease of the number of dendritic spines (Fig.3) in comparison with the normal controls.

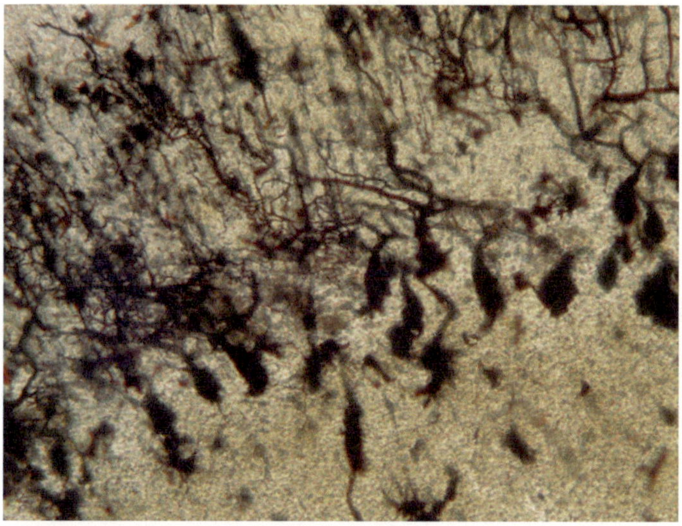

Figure 2. Purkinje cells from the cerebellar hemisphere of a case of AD, demonstrating marked abbreviation of the dendritic arborization and considerable loss of dendritic spines (Golgi staining 2,000X).

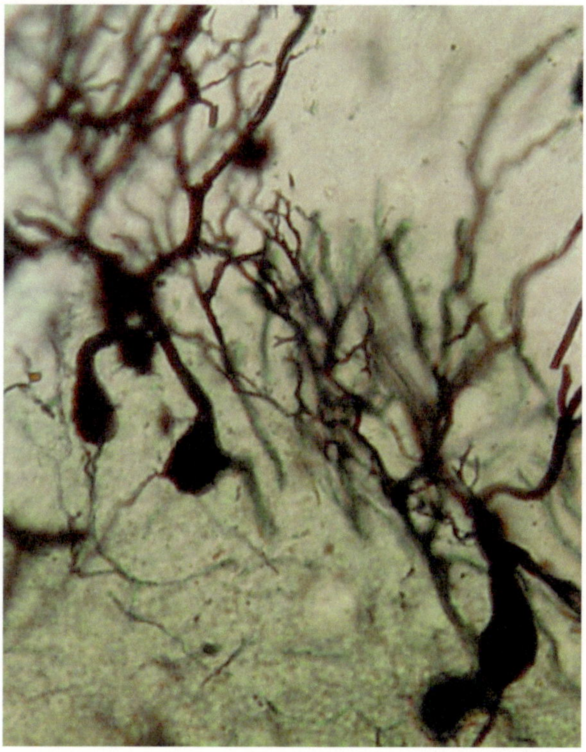

Figure 3. Purkinje cells from the vermis of the cerebellum of a case of AD, showing dramatic reduction of dendritic branches and loss of dendritic spines (Golgi staining 3,100X)

In addition, the axonal collaterals in layers III, IV, V, and VI of the acoustic and visual cortices were dramatically decreased in comparison with the normal controls.

The decrease of the branches of the apical dendrites of the cortical neurons as well as decrease in spine density was widespread phenomena seen in the large majority of neurons of the acoustic (Fig.4) and the visual cortices, in the hippocampus, the thalamus, the globus pallidus, the red nucleus, the locus coeruleus, the hypothalamus and the cerebellar cortex (Figs 1,2).

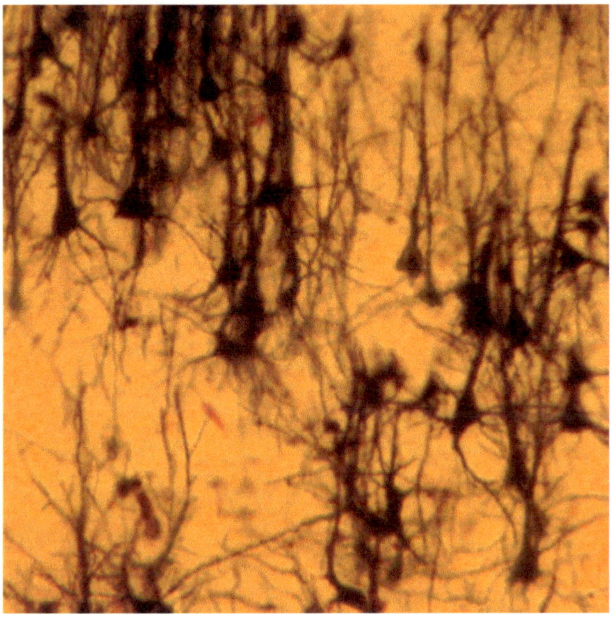

Figure 4. Neurons from the acoustic cortex of a case of AD, showing marked decrease of tertiary dendritic branches and tremendous loss of spines (Golgi staining 2,400X).

3.2. Electron microscopy

Electron microscopy is the most valuable and precise method for the morphological and morphometric study of the cell organelles, the synapses, the dendritic spines as well as the neuron- glial relationships in the CNS both in health and disease.

In our study, the electron microscopy revealed pathological alterations of the dendritic spines and impressive decrease in spine density in the secondary and tertiary dendritic branches in all of the layers of the acoustic and visual cortices.

The reduction in spine size was prominent in neurons of layers II, III, and V of the acoustic cortex. A substantial number of dendritic spines demonstrated large multivesicular bodies, abnormal spine apparatus, and mitochondria, which were characterized by marked morphological alterations. Morphological alterations of the dendritic spines were also seen in the pyramidal neurons of the hippocampus, the large polyhedral neurons of the thalamus, the globus pallidus, the polyhedral neurons of the locus coeruleus as well as the Purkinje cells of the cerebellar hemispheres (Fig.5). Giant elongated spines were mostly seen in the hippocampus and in the Purkinje cells of the cerebellum. In a large number of presynaptic terminals of the acoustic and visual cortices of patients who suffered from AD, the ultrastructural study has revealed an considerable polymorphism and pleomorphism of the synaptic vesicles, which were dramatically decreased in number in comparison with normal controls.

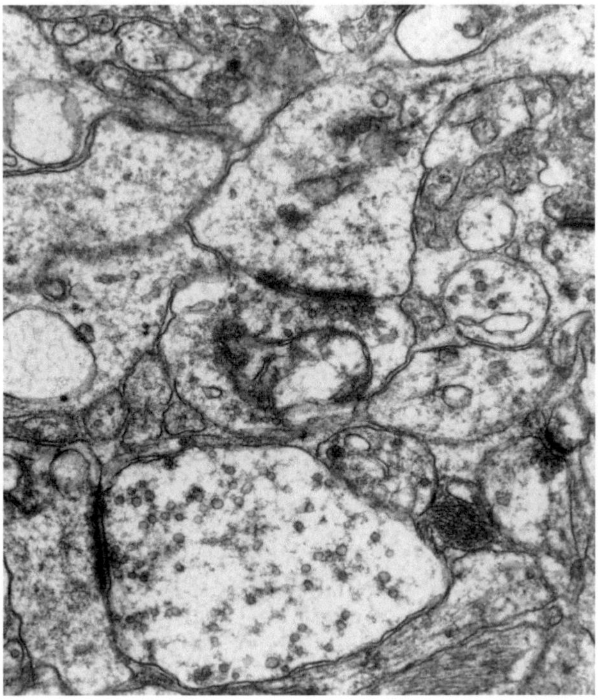

Figure 5. Synaptic alterations in the cerebellar cortex in a case of AD. Impressive poverty of synaptic vesicles is noticed at the presynaptic terminals associated with mitochondrial alterations and disruption of the spinal apparatus (Electron micrograph 128,000X).

Substatial poverty of the synaptic vesicles was particularly seen in the presynaptic terminals in layers III, IV, and V of the acoustic and visual cortices, as well as in the mossy fibers of the cerebellar cortex. Decrease of the number of synaptic vesicles associated with polymorphism of the remained vesicles was noticed in the hippocampus, the thalamus, the locus coeruleus, and the parallel and climbing fibers of the cerebellar cortex.

Mitochondrial pathology was demonstrated in the majority of the dendritic spines in all of the specimens. That consisted of substantial change of mitochondrial shape and size, fragmentation of cristae, and accumulation of osmiophilic material in a considerable number of mitochondrial profiles (Fig.6). Many dendritic branches included mitochondria, which showed an unusual polymorphic arrangement of the cristae, which either showed a concentric configuration or they were arranged in a parallel way to the long axis of the organelle. Some Purkinje cell dendrites

(Fig.6) and a substantial number of climbing fibers included very large elongated mitochondria. Small round mitochondria intermixed with dense bodies were seen in association with fragmentation or dilatation of the cisternae of the Golgi apparatus in the soma of a considerable number of neurons of the visual cortex (Fig.7), the hippocampus, the locus coeruleus, the red nucleus, the polyhedral neurons of globus pallidus, and the Purkinje cells in AD brains.

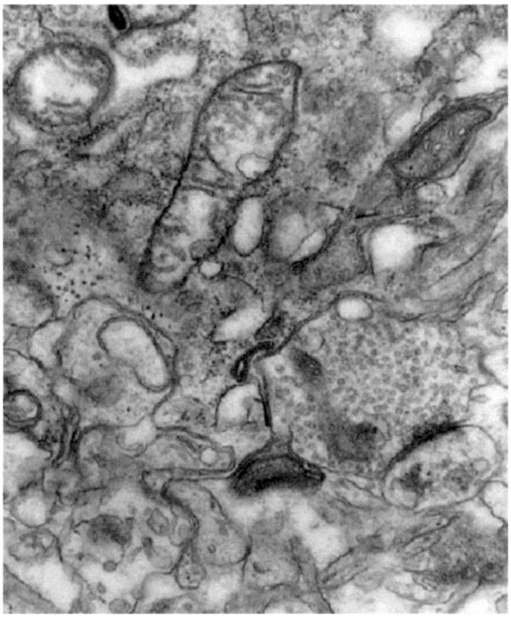

Figure 6. Abnormal mitochondria in a dendritic profile of Purkinje cell in a case of AD. The disruption of the cristae is a prominent phenomenon (Electron micrograph 128,000X).

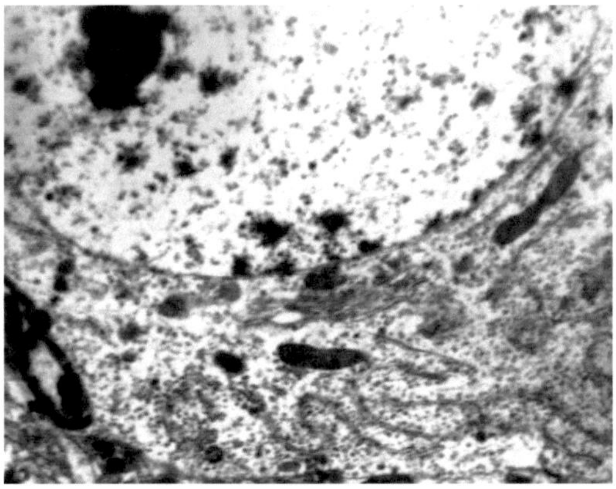

Figure 7. Elongated mitocondria and mitochondria in fusión, intermixed with dense bodies and dilated cisternae of Golgi apparatus in a case of AD (Electron micrograph 25,000X).

It is worth to emphasize that morphological alterations of the mitochondria were also seen in the soma of astrocytes, the perivascular processes, and the astrocytic sheaths in AD brains, in contrast to normal controls.

From the morphometric point of view the ellipsoid mitochondria of the dendritic spines in normal control brains appear to have an average diameter of 650 ± 250 nm and a mean axial ratio of 1.9 ± 0.2. The round or global mitochondria appeared to have in normal controls a mean radius of 350 nm. In AD brains, the ellipsoid mitochondria of the neurons in acoustic and visual cortices appear to have an average diameter of 480 ± 250 nm and a mean axial ratio of 1.7 ± 0.2. The round mitochondria appear to have a mean radius of 280 nm (Chart.1).

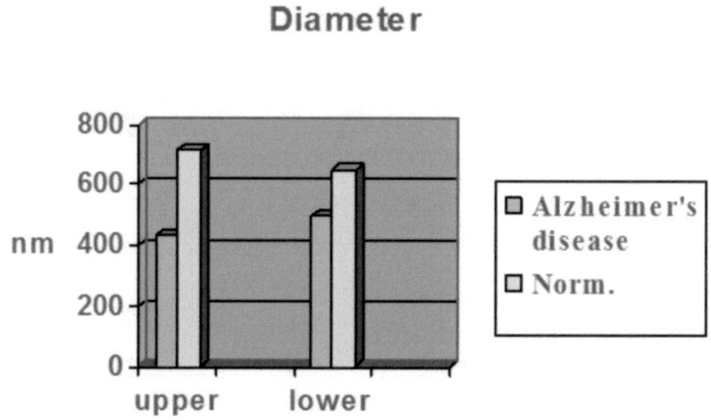

Chart 1. Decrease of the diameter of mitochondria in the visual cortex in Alzheimer's cases in comparison with normal controls.

In the majority of Purkinje cells of the cerebellum, in the hippocampal neurons and in neurons of the parietal, frontal, acoustic and visual cortices the Golgi apparatus was mostly fragmented and atrophic (Fig.8) in comparison with normal controls.

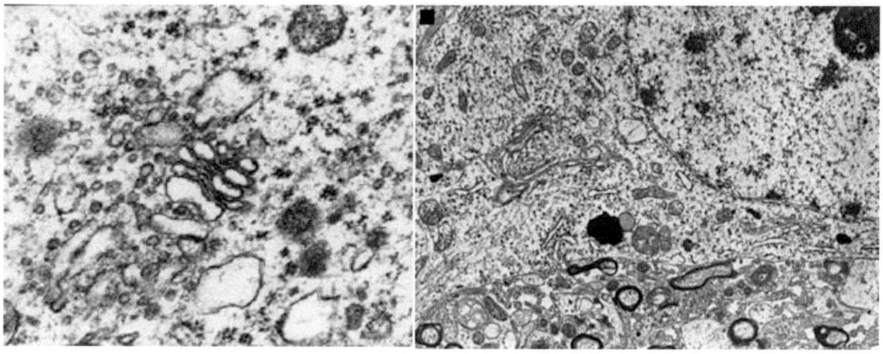

Figure 9. Fragmentation of the cisternae of the Golgi apparatus in a Purkinje cell of the cerebellar cortex of a case of AD (left) (Electron micrograph 128,000). Normal control (right) (Electron micrograph 65,000X)

It is important to underline that the fragmentation of the Golgi apparatus was seen in neurons which did not showed any tau pathology, such as accumulation of intracellular NFTs, and were located in areas with minimal deposits of Aβ peptide. However the atrophy and the fragmentation of Golgi apparatus coexisted with mitochondrial alterations and dendritic and spinal pathology in the large majority of neurons (Fig.9).

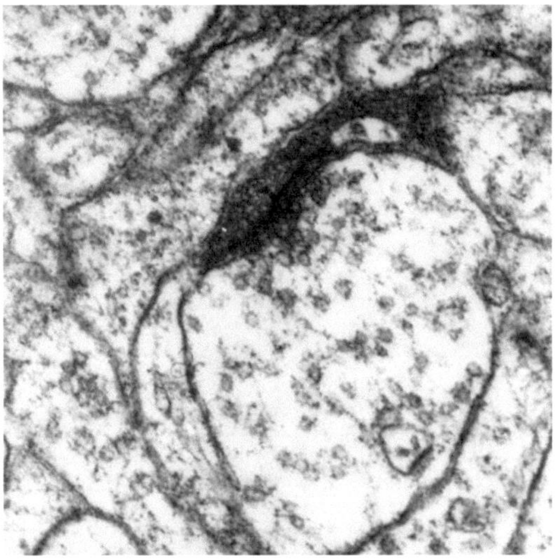

Figure 9. Degeneration of dendritic spine in the visual cortex of a case of AD (Electron micrograph 130,000X)

4. Discussion

The mitochondria, which are the only nonnuclear constituents of the cell with their own DNA (mtDNA), having machinery for synthesizing RNA and proteins, are critical to homeostasis of the cell, by virtue of providing most of the energy for cellular processes, since energy, realized by oxidative phosphorylation, comes through the mitochondria, which generate most of the cell's supply of ATP. Mitochondria are also critical regulators of cell apoptosis, as being involved in a considerable number of neurodegenerative diseases [65, 66],

From the morphological point of view the shape and size of the mitochondria are highly variable [67], depending on fission and fusion [68]. Their morphology is occasionally controlled by cytoskeletal elements, namely the neurofilaments and the microtubules [69]. The change of the mitochondrial shape occurs mostly through their move to axons, dendrites, and synaptic terminals via anterograde transport [70]. During the various neuronal processes approximately one-third of the mitochondria are in motion along microtubules and actin filaments [71–73]. Mitochondrial motility and accumulation are coordinated, since mitochondria are transported to regions where ATP consumption and necessity for energy are particularly high, as it occurs in the synapses, which have high energy demand reasonably, for serving neuronal communication [74].

Mitochondrial alterations and dysfunction have been reported in several neurodegenerative diseases [75] mostly associated with oxidative damage [76-78] and vascular lesions [79]. Oxidative stress is mostly related with the accumulation of Aβ peptide in the neocortex [80, 81], playing an important role in the pathogenesis of AD [82], since it is not only involved in the formation of senile plaques and in damage to the proteins of NFT [83], but also induces extensive damage to the cytoplasm of neuronal populations vulnerable to death [84].

It is also well documented that Aβ peptide may increase mitochondrial reactive oxygen species (ROS) production [85, 86], causing further impairment of mitochondrial function [87], since the lack of histones in mitochondrial DNA renders them a vulnerable target to oxidative stress. In major examples of neurodegenerative diseases, there is strong evidence that mitochondrial dysfunction occurs early and acts causally in disease pathogenesis. Mutations in mitochondrial DNA and oxidative stress, on the other hand, may contribute to ageing [88, 89], which is the substantial biological background for the majority of the neurodegenerative diseases [65].

Mitochondrial dysfunction has been associated with energy crisis of the cell and excitotoxic cell death and is considered to be of substantial importance in the cascade of phenomena, which eventually lead to apoptosis. Some observations in early cases of AD [90] indicate that morphological alterations of the mitochondria and oxidative damage may be one of the earliest events.

The morphological alteration of the mitochondria seen in subcortical centers, such as in the thalamus, the globus pallidus, the red nucleus, the hypothalamus and the locus coeruleus, pleads in favor of a generalized mitochondrial dysfunction in AD, which may be associated with wide neuronal loss and synaptic alterations, seriously affecting the mental faculties, which are basically related to extensive neural networks [91] and synaptic activity. Moreover, an impressive number of disease-specific proteins interact with mitochondria. Well-documented studies [92] demonstrate that a significant amount of the N-terminal domain of APP targeted the mitochondria of cortical neurons and select regions of the brain of a transgenic mouse model for AD. The accumulation of trans membrane-arrested APP blocked protein translocation, disrupted mitochondrial function, and impaired brain energy metabolism.

In AD it may be considered that mitochondria-associated Aβ peptide may directly cause neurotoxicity [93, 94]. Mitochondrial dysfunction, therefore, might be a hallmark of amyloid-beta-induced neuronal toxicity in Alzheimer's disease [95]. The binding site for amyloid beta peptide has been identified as alcohol dehydrogenase in the matrix space of the organelle. Recent evidence also suggest that PS1, PS2, APP, and γ-secretase activity are not homogeneously distributed in the ER, but rather are enriched in mitochondria-associated ER membranes (ER-MAMs or MAMs), which is a dynamic sub-compartment of the ER, which is connected with mitochondria [96]. Mitochondria and ER are closely connected in several functions such as transfer of Calium, lipid metabolism, the control of apoptosis and autophagy [96]

Many morphological alterations of AD could be well linked to mitochondria changes, since blockage of mitochondrial energy production shifts APP metabolism to the production of more amyloidogenic forms of amyloid [97]. In addition amyloid beta peptide promotes permeability transition pore in brain mitochondria [85, 98]. It is important to mention that many protein systems are also essential in mitochondrial function and morphological integrity as well as in binding to the cytoskeleton [99]. Mitochondrial porin is an outer-membrane protein that forms regulated channels (Voltage-Dependent Anionic Channels) between the mitochondrial intermembrane space and the cytosol [100]. Porin may play an important role in binding to neurofilaments and microtubules, since porin-rich domains contain most of the binding sites for MAP2 [101, 102]. In addition, preselinin-2 modulates endoplasmic reticulum-mitochondrial interactions [103], a fact that would plead in favor of the crucial role that mitochondria play in the pathogenetic cascade of AD.

Recent studies reported increased mitochondrial fission and decreased fusion, due to increased amyloid beta (Aβ) interaction with the mitochondrial fission protein Drp 1, inducing increased mitochondrial fragmentation, impaired axonal transport of mitochondria and synaptic degeneration in AD [104]. In addition, the interaction of the voltage-dependent anion channel 1 protein (VDAC1) with Aβ peptide and phosphorylated tau block mitochondrial pores, leading to mitochondrial dysfunction in AD [105].

The number of the mitochondria varies, according to energy state of the cell. Some evidence suggests that the mitochondria redistribute towards the dendritic profiles, in response to stimulation as a manifestation of synaptic plasticity [106]. Normally, a limited number of dendritic spines contain mitochondria, which are mostly small and round, which are increased in number inside the dendritic branches during the synaptogenesis. Decrease in energy metabolism and altered cytochrome c oxidase (CytOX) activity are among the earliest detectable defects in AD [107], affecting presumably neuronal plasticity and synaptogenesis. Some observations suggest that mitochondrial cytochrome c oxidase may be inhibited by a dimeric conformer of $A\beta 35$, a phenomenon which further emphasizes the role of the $A\beta$ peptide on the mitochondrial dysfunction in AD [108].

Among the ongoing therapeutic efforts [109], those targeting basic mitochondrial processes, such as energy metabolism, free-radical generation, or specific interactions of disease-related proteins with mitochondria, hold great promise. On the basis of the mitochondrial pathology, in the pathogenetic spectrum in AD, new strategies inducing protection to mitochondria by the administration of efficient antioxidant factors could be introduced in the treatment of early cases of AD.

Golgi apparatus, on the other hand plays a very important role in posttranslational modifications, transport, and targeting of large number of proteins, which participate in axoplasmic transport or are transported to plasma membrane, to lysosomes, to synaptic terminals and dendritic spines. A substantial body of evidence suggest that Golgi complex is involved in the pathogenesis of amyotrophic lateral sclerosis (ALS) [110-112] and AD, as it is well documented by highly specific immunocytochemistry techniques [47, 113].

The size of the Golgi apparatus may be an index of neuronal activity. Thus the fragmentation of the cisternae of Golgi apparatus may be associated with impaired trafficking of proteins to synapses and dendritic spines resulting in synaptic degeneration and cognitive impairment eventually. It is well documented that the trans-Golgi network (TGN) is the major sorting structure of the secretory pathway and the main site of intersection with the endo-lysosomal system [48, 49]. Current data clearly suggest that perturbations to the endosomal retrograde sorting pathway promote the production of Aβ. The recent discovery of an integral membrane protein, Gamma-secretase activating protein (GSAP) [114,115],which associates with γ-secretase, APP and promotes the production Aβ peptide may provide an important link for understanding how γ-secretase is directed to APP and help to clarify the site(s) of Aβ production. GSAP might be also an ideal target for designing γ-secretase modulators in an attempt for treating AD [116,117].

Author details

Stavros J. Baloyannis[1,2]

1 Department of Neurology, School of Medicine, Aristotle University of Thessaloniki, Greece

2 Institute for research on Alzheimer's disease, Thessaloniki, Greece

References

[1] Alzheimer's Association. Alzheimer's disease facts and figures. Alzheimer's and Dementia. 2010; 6: 158–194.

[2] Wisniewski H M, Wegiel J, Kotula L. Some neuropathological aspects of Alzheimer's disease and its relevance to other disciplines. Neuropathology and Applied Neurobiology, 1996; 22: 3–11.

[3] Duyckaerts C, Delatour B,. Potier M C. Classification and basic pathology of Alzheimer disease. Acta Neuropathologica, 2009; 118: 5–36.

[4] Baloyannis S, Costa V, Arnaoutoglou A, Arnaoutoglou H. Synaptic alterations in the molecular layer of the cerebellum in Alzheimer's disease. Neuropathology and Applied Neurobiology 1996; 22: 78–79.

[5] Baloyannis S J, Manolidis S L, Manolidis L S. The acoustic cortex in Alzheimer's disease. Acta Oto-Laryngologica. 1992; 494: 1–13.

[6] Baloyannis S J, Manolidis S L, Manolidis L S. Synaptic alterations in the vestibule-cerebellar system in Alzheimer's disease- a Golgi and electron microscope study. Acta Oto-Laryngolo-gica 2000; 120: 247–250.

[7] Baloyannis S J, Costa V. Michmizos D. Mitochondrial alterations in Alzheimer's disease. American Journal of Alzheimer's Disease and other Dementias. 2004; 19: 89–93.

[8] Baloyannis S J, Baloyannis J S. Mitochondrial alterations in Alzheimer's disease. Neurobiology of Aging. 2004; 25: 405–406.

[9] Iqbal K, Liu F, Gong C X, Grundke-Iqbal I. Tau in Alzheimer disease and related tauopathies. Current Alzheimer Research.2010; 7: 656–664.

[10] Mattson M P. Pathways towards and away from Alzheimer's disease. Nature. 2004; 430: 631–639.

[11] Dickson D M. The pathogenesis of senile plaques. Journal of Neuropathology and Experimental Neurology1997; 56: 321–339.

[12] Gandy S. The role of cerebral amyloid beta accumulation in common forms of Alzheimer disease. Journal of Clinical Investigation. 2005; 115: 1121–1129.

[13] Baloyannis S. The Golgi apparatus of Purkinje cells in Alzheimer's disease. in Neuropathology Back to the Roots, J. Bohl, (Ed)., pp. 1–10, Shaker Vertag, Aachen, Germany, 2002.

[14] Dolan D, Troncoso J, Crain B, Resnick S, Zonderman A, O'Brien R. Age, dementia and Alzheimer's disease in the BLSA. Brain. 2010; 133: 2225–2231.

[15] Baloyannis SJ, Baloyannis IS The vascular factor in Alzheimer's disease: A study in Golgi technique and electron microscopy. J Neurol Sci. 2012; 322:117-121.

[16] Hardy J, Allsop D. Amyloid deposition as the central event in the aetiology of Alzheimer's disease. Trends Pharmacol. Sci. 1991; 12: 383–388.

[17] Hardy J, Selkoe DJ. The amyloid hypothesis of Alzheimer's disease: progress and problems on the road to therapeutics. Science 2002; 297:353–356

[18] Tanzi RE, Bertram L. Twenty years of the Alzheimer's disease amyloid hypothesis: A genetic perspective. Cell. 2005; 120:545–555.

[19] Selkoe D J. Alzheimer's disease: genes, proteins, and therapy. Physiol. Rev. 2001; 81: 741–766.

[20] Greenfield J, Tsai J, Gouras G, Hai B, Thinakaran G, Checler F, Sisodia S, Greengard P, Xu H. Endoplasmic reticulum and trans-Golgi network generate distinct populations of Alzheimer β-amyloid peptides. Proc. Natl. Acad. Sci. U. S. A. 1999; 96: 742–747.

[21] Takahashi R, Milner T, Li F, Nam E, Edgar M, Yamaguchi H, Beal M, Xu H, Greengard P, Gouras G. Intraneuronal Alzheimer A42 accumulates in multivesicular bodies and is associated with synaptic pathology. Am. J. Pathol. 2002; 161: 1869–1879.

[22] Caspersen C, Wang N, Yao Y, Sosunov A, Chen X, Lustbader J W, Xu H W, Stern D, McKhann G, Yan S D. Mitochondrial A: a potential focal point for neuronal metabolic dysfunction in Alzheimer's disease. FASEB J. 2005;19: 2040–2041.

[23] Selkoe DJ. Soluble oligomers of the amyloid beta-protein impair synaptic plasticity and behavior. Behav. Brain Res. 2008; 192:106–113.

[24] Dobson CM Protein folding and misfolding. Nature 2003; 426:884–890.

[25] Morawe T, Hiebel C, Kern A, Behl C Protein Homeostasis, Aging and Alzheimer's Disease. Molecular Neurobiology. 2012; 46: 41-54.

[26] Ishii K, Sasaki M, Kitagaki H, Yamaji S, Sakamoto S, Matsuda K, *et al.* Reduction of cerebellar glucose metabolism in advanced Alzheimer's disease. J Nucl Med 1997:38: 925–928.

[27] Price D L, Sisodia S S. Mutant genes in familial Alzheimer's disease and transgenic models. Annual Review of Neuroscience. 1998; 21: 479–505.

[28] Tanzi R E. A genetic dichotomy model for the inheritance of Alzheimer's disease and common age-related disorders. Journal of Clinical Investigation. 1999; 104: 1175–1179.

[29] Caruso C, Franceschi C, Licastro F. Genetics of neurodegenerative disorders. The New England Journal of Medicine.2003; 349: 193–194.

[30] Hashimoto Y, Niikura T, Ito Y, Nishimoto I. Multiple mechanisms underlie neurotoxicity by different types of Alzheimer's disease mutations of amyloid precursor protein. Journal of Biological Chemistry. 2000; 275: 34541–34551.

[31] Selkoe D J. Alzheimer's disease results from the cerebral accumulation and cytotoxicity of amyloid beta-protein. Journal of Alzheimer's Disease.2001; 3: 75–80.

[32] Reddy P H, Beal M F.Amyloid beta, mitochondrial dysfunction and synaptic damage: implications for cognitive decline in aging and Alzheimer's disease. Trends in Molecular Medicine. 2008; 14: 45–53.

[33] Shoffner J M, Brown MD, Torroni A, et al. Mitochondrial DNA variants observed in Alzheimer disease and Parkinson disease patients. Genomics, 1993; 17: 171–184.

[34] Hirai K, Aliev G, Nunomura A, et al. Mitochondrial abnormalities in Alzheimer's disease. Journal of Neuroscience. 2001; 21: 3017–3023.

[35] Lin MT, Beal MF. Mitochondrial dysfunction and oxidative stress in neurodegenerative diseases. Nature 2006; 443: 787–795.

[36] Manczak M, Anekonda T S, Henson E, Park B S, Quinn J, Reddy P H. Mitochondria are a direct site of A beta accumulation in Alzheimer's disease neurons: implications for free radical generation and oxidative damage in disease progression. Human Molecular Genetics 2006; 15: 1437–1449.

[37] Sheng B, Wang X, Su B, Lee HG, Casadesus G, Perry G, *et al.* Impaired mitochondrial biogenesis contributes to mitochondrial dysfunction in Alzheimer's disease. J Neurochem 2012; 120: 419–429.

[38] Beal MF, Hyman B T, Koroshetz W. Do defects in mitochondrial energy metabolism underlie the pathology of neurodegenerative diseases? Trends in Neurosciences 1993; 16:125–131.

[39] Lin M T, Beal M F. Alzheimer's APP mangles mitochondria. Nat. Med. 2006; 12: 1241–1243.

[40] Anandatheerthavarada H K, Biswas G, Robin M A, Avadhani N G. Mitochondrial targeting and a novel transmembrane arrest of Alzheimer's amyloid precursor protein impairs mitochondrial function in neuronal cells. Journal of Cell Biology. 2003; 161: 41–54

[41] Pagani L, Eckert A. Amyloid-Beta Interaction with Mitochondria. International Journal of Alzheimer's Disease Volume 2011, Article ID 925050, 12 pages doi: 10.4061/2011/925050.

[42] Hansson C A, Fryckman S, Farmery M. R, Tjernberg L O, Nilsberth C, Pursglove S E, Ito A, Winblad B, Cowburn R F, Thyberg J, Ankarcrona, M. Nicastrin, presenilin,APH-1, and PEN-2 form active γ-secretase complexes in mitochondria J. Biol. Chem. 2004; 279: 51654–51660.

[43] Petersen H, Alikhani CA, Behbahani N, Wiehager H, Pavlov B, Alafuzoff I, Leinonen V, Ito A, Winblad B, Glaser E, Ankarcrona M. The amyloid beta peptide is imported into mitochondria via the TOM import machinery and localized to mitochondrial cristae. Proc. Natl. Acad. Sci. U.S.A. 2008; 105:13145–13150.

[44] Caspersen C, Wang N, Yao Y, Sosunov A, Chen X, Lustbader J W, Xu H W, Stern D, McKhann G, Yan S D. Mitochondrial Aβ: a potential focal point for neuronal metabolic dysfunction in Alzheimer's disease. FASEB J. 2005;19: 2040–2041.

[45] Baloyannis SJ. Mitochondria are related to synaptic pathology in Alzheimer's disease. Int J Alzheimers Dis. 2011; 2011:305395. Epub 2011 Sep 12

[46] Cho D H, Nakamura T, Fang J. et al., S-nitrosylation of Drp1 mediates beta-amyloid-related mitochondrial fission and neuronal injury. Science. 2009; 324:102–105.

[47] Stieber A, Mourelatos Z, Gonatas N K. In Alzheimer's Disease the Golgi Apparatus of a Population of Neurons without neurofibrillary Tangles Is Fragmented and Atrophic. American Journal of Pathology. 1996; 148: 415-426.

[48] Hammerschlag R, Stone GC, Bolen FA, Lindsey JD, Ellisman MH. Evidence that all newly synthesized proteins destined for fast axonal transport pass through the Golgi apparatus. J Cell Biol. 1982; 93:568-575

[49] Burd C G. Physiology and Pathology of Endosome-to-Golgi Retrograde Sorting Traffic 2011; 12: 948–955.

[50] Duncan JR, Kornfeld S. Intra cellular movement of two mannose 6-phosphate receptors: return to the Golgi apparatus. J Cell Biol. 1988; 106: 617–628.

[51] Zhang Z, Nadeau P, Song W, Donoviel D, Yuan M, Bernstein A, Yankner BA. Presenilins are required for gamma-secretase cleavage of beta-APP and trans-membrane cleavage of Notch-1. Nat Cell Biol. 2000; 2: 463-465.

[52] Chung H M, Struhl G. Nicastrin is required for Presenilin mediated trans-membrane cleavage in Drosophila. Nat Cell Biol. 2001; 3: 1129-1132.

[53] Hu Y, Ye Y, Fortini M E. Nicastrin is required for gamma secretase cleavage of the Drosophila notch receptor. Dev Cell 2002; 2: 69-78.

[54] Francis R, McGrath G, Zhang J, Ruddy D A, Sym M, Apfeld J, Nicoll M, Maxwell M, Hai B, Ellis M C. et al. aph-1 and pen-2 are required for Notch pathway signaling, gamma-secretase cleavage of beta APP, and presenilin protein accumulation. Dev Cell. 2002; 3: 85-97.

[55] Goutte C, Tsunozaki M, Hale V A, Priess J R. APH-1 is a multipass membrane protein essential for the Notch signaling pathway in Caenorhabditis elegans embryos. Proc. Natl. Acad. Sci. US A 2002;99: 775-779.

[56] Herreman An, Van Gassen G, Bentahir M, Nyabi O, Craessaerts K. Mueller U, Annaert W, De Strooper B. g-Secretase activity requires the presenilin-dependent trafficking of nicastrin through the Golgi apparatus but not its complex glycosylation. Journal of Cell Science. 2003; 116:1127-1136.

[57] Sisodia SS. Beta-amyloid precursor protein cleavage by a membrane bound protease. Proc Natl Acad Sci USA 1992; 89:6075–6079.

[58] Vetrivel KS, Thinakaran G. Amyloidogenic processing of beta-amyloid precursor protein in intracellular compartments, Neurology 2006;66: 69-73.

[59] Zheng L, Cedazo-Minguez A, Hallbeck M, Jerhammar F, Marcusson J, Terman A. Intracellular distribution of amyloid beta Peptide and its relationship to the lysosomal system. Translational neurodegeneration 2012, 19:1-7.

[60] Mattis S., Dementia Rating Scale Professional Manual, Psychological Assessment Resources, Odessa, Fla, USA, 1988.

[61] Pannese E. The Golgi stain: invention, diffusion and impact on neurosciences. J Hist Neurosci. 1999; 8:132- 140.

[62] Baloyannis SJ. Morphological and morphometric alterations of Cajal-Retzius cells in early cases of Alzheimer's disease: a Golgi and electron microscope study. Int J Neurosci. 2005; 115:965-80.

[63] Marín-Padilla M. Cajal-Retzius cells and the development of the neocortex. Trends in Neurosciences. 1998; 21: 64–71.

[64] Marín-Padilla M. Three-dimensional structural organization of layer I of the human cerebral cortex: a Golgi study. Journal of Comparative Neurology.1990; 299: 89–105.

[65] Beal MF. Mitochondrial dysfunction in neurodegenerative diseases. Biochimica et Biophysica Acta.1998; 1366: 211–223.

[66] Mizuno Y, Ikebe S I, Hattori N.et al. Role of mitochondria in the etiology and pathogenesis of Parkinson's disease. Biochimica et Biophysica Acta. 1995; 1271: 265–274.

[67] Bereiter-Hahn J, Vöth M. Dynamics of mitochondria in living cells: shape changes, dislocations, fusion, and fission of mitochondria. Microscopy Research and Technique.1994; 27:198–219.

[68] Chen H, McCaffery JM, Chan DC. Mitochondrial fusion protects against neurodegeneration in the cerebellum. Cell. 2007; 130: 548-562.

[69] Knowles M K, Guenza M G, Capaldi R A, Marcus A H. Cytoskeletal-assisted dynamics of the mitochondrial reticulum in living cells. Proceedings of the National Academy of Sciences USA. 2002; 99: 14772–14777.

[70] Hollenbeck PJ, Saxton WM. The axonal transport of mitochondria. Journal of Cell Science. 2005; 118: 5411–5419.

[71] Krendel M, Sgourdas G, Bonder EM. Disassembly of actin filaments leads to increased rate and frequency of mitochondrial movement along microtubules. Cell Motility and the Cytoskeleton. 1998; 40: 368–378.

[72] Leterrier J F, Rusakov D A, Nelson B D, Linden M. Interactions between brain mitochondria and cytoskeleton: evidence for specialized outer membrane domains involved in the association of cytoskeleton-associated proteins to mitochondria in situ and in vitro. Microscopy Research and Technique. 1994; 27: 233–261.

[73] Lifshitz J, Janmey PA, Linden M, McIntosh TK, Leterrier J F. Mechanisms of mitochondria-neurofilament interactions. The Journal of Neuroscience. 2003; 23: 9046–9058.

[74] Brown M R, Sullivan P G, Geddes J W. Synaptic mitochondria are more susceptible to Ca2+ overload than nonsynaptic mitochondria. Journal of Biological Chemistry. 2006; 281:11658–11668.

[75] Mattson M P, Gleichmann M, Cheng A. Mitochondria in neuroplasticity and neurological disorders. Neuron. 2008; 60: 748–766.

[76] Baloyannis S. Oxidative stress and mitochondria alterations in Alzheimer's disease. Neurobiology of Aging. 21: 264. 2000.

[77] Pereira C, Santos M S, Oliveira C. Involvement of oxidative stress on the impairment of energy metabolism induced by Abeta peptides on PC12 cells: protection by antioxidants. Neurobiology of Disease. 1999; 6: 209–219.

[78] Zhu X, Perry G, Moreira P I. et al. Mitochondrial abnormalities and oxidative imbalance in Alzheimer disease. Journal of Alzheimer's Disease. 2006; 9: 147–153.

[79] Aliev G, Smith M A, Seyidova D. et al. The role of oxidative stress in the pathophysiology of cerebrovascular lesions in Alzheimer's disease. Brain Pathology. 2002; 12:21–35.

[80] Arias C, Montiel T, Quiroz-Baez R, Massieu L. Beta-Amyloid neurotoxicity is exacerbated during glycolysis inhibition and mitochondrial impairment in the rat hippocampus in vivo and in isolated nerve terminals: implications for Alzheimer's disease. Experimental Neurology 2002; 176:163–174.

[81] Nunomura A, Perry G, Aliev G. et al. Oxidative damage is the earliest event in Alzheimer's disease. Journal of Neuropathology and Experimental Neurology 2001; 60: 759–767.

[82] Aliev G. Oxidative stress induced-metabolic imbalance, mitochondrial failure, and cellular hypoperfusion as primary pathogenetic factors for the development of Alzheimer disease which can be used as a alternate and successful drug treatment strategy: past, present and future.CNS and Neurological Disorders—Drug Targets. 2011; 10: 147–148.

[83] Hugon J, Esclaire F, Lesort M, Kisby G, Spencer P. Toxic neuronal apoptosis and modifications of tau and APP gene and protein expressions. Drug Metabolism Reviews. 1999; 31: 635–647.

[84] Moreira P I, Cardoso S M, Santos M S, Oliveira C R. The key role of mitochondria in Alzheimer's disease. Journal of Alzheimer's Disease 2006; 9: 101–110.

[85] Moreira PI, Santos MS, Moreno A, Oliveira C. Amyloid beta-peptide promotes permeability transition pore in brain mitochondria. Bioscience Reports. 2001; 21: 789–800.

[86] Maurer I, Zierz S, Moller HJ. A selective defect of cytochrome c oxidase is present in brain of Alzheimer disease patients. Neurobiology of Aging. 2000; 21: 455–462.

[87] Mecocci P, Cherubini A, Beal M F. et al. Altered mitochondrial membrane fluidity in AD brain. Neuroscience Letters.1996; 207: 129–132.

[88] Luo Y, Bond J D, Ingram VM. Compromised mitochondrial function leads to increased cytosolic calcium and to activation of MAP kinases. Proceedings of the National Academy of Sciences USA 1997; 94: 9705–9710.

[89] Hsin-Chen Lee, Yau-Huei Wei. Mitochondria and Aging. Advances in Experimental Medicine and Biology. 2012; 942: 311-327.

[90] Baloyannis SJ. Mitochondrial alterations in Alzheimer's disease. Journal of Alzheimer's Disease, 2006; 9: 119–126.

[91] Mesulam M M. Large-scale neurocognitive networks and distributed processing for attention, language, and memory. Annals of Neurology. 1990; 28: 597–613.

[92] Choia K, Kima M, Jea A, Ryua K, Chaea H, Kweona H, Leea C. A Three-Dimensional Study of Ultrastructural Variation of Abnormal Mitochondria in APP/PSEN1 Trans-

genic Mouse. Brain Microscopy and Microanalysis. 2012; 18 (Supplement S2): 212-213.

[93] Eckert A, Schmitt K, Gotz J. Mitochondrial dysfunction, the beginning of the end in Alzheimer's disease? Separate and synergistic modes of tau and amyloid beta toxicity. Alzheimer's Research and Therapy, 2011; 3:15.

[94] Spuch C, Ortolano S, Navarro C. New Insights in the Amyloid-Beta Interaction with Mitochondria. Journal of Aging Research Volume 2012, Article ID 324968. 9 pages doi: 10. 1155/ 2012/324968

[95] de Brito OM, Scorrano L. An intimate liaison: spatial organization of the endoplasmic reticulum-mitochondria relationship. EMBO J 2010; 29: 2715–2723.

[96] De Strooper Bart, Scorrano L. Close encounter: mitochondria, endoplasmic reticulum andAlzheimer's disease The EMBO Journal.2012; 31: 4095–4097.

[97] Crouch P J, Blake R,. Duce J A. et al. Copper-dependent inhibition of human cytochrome c oxidase by a dimeric conformer of amyloid-β1-42. Journal of Neuroscience 2005; 25: 672–679.

[98] Moreira P I, Santos M S, Moreno A, Rego A C, Oliveira C. Effect of amyloid beta-peptide on permeability transition pore: a comparative study. Journal of Neuroscience Research. 2002; 69: 257–267.

[99] Truscott K, Pfanner N, Voos W. Transport of proteins into mitochondria. Reviews of Physiology, Biochemistry and Pharmacology. 2001; 143: 81–136.

[100] Summersa WAT, Wilkinsb JA, Dwivedib RC, Ezzatib P, Courta DA. Mitochondrial dysfunction resulting from the absence of mitochondrial porin in Neurospora crassa. Mitochondrion. 2012;12: 220–229.

[101] Reddy PH. Is the mitochondrial outer membrane protein VDAC1 therapeutic target for Alzheimer's disease? Biochimica et Biophysica Acta (BBA) - Molecular Basis of Disease2013;1832: 67–75.

[102] Calkins M J, Reddy PH. Assessment of newly synthesized mitochondrial DNA using BrdU labeling in primary neurons from Alzheimer's disease mice: Implications for impaired mitochondrial biogenesis and synaptic damage. Biochimica et Biophysica Acta (BBA) - Molecular Basis of Disease. 2011; 1812:1182–1189.

[103] Zampese E, Fasolato C, Kipanyula J, Bortolozzi M, Pozzan T, Pizzo P. Presenilin 2 modulates endoplasmic reticulum (ER)—mitochondria interactions and Ca^{2+} cross-talk. Proceedings of the National Academy of Sciences USA. 2011; 7: 2777–2782.

[104] Manczak M, Reddy P H. Abnormal interaction between the mitochondrial fission protein Drp1 and hyperphosphorylated tau in Alzheimer's disease neurons: implications for mitochondrial dysfunction and neuronal damage. Hum. Mol. Genet. 2012; 21: 2538-2547.

[105] Manczak M, Reddy PH. Abnormal interaction of VDAC1 with amyloid beta and phosphorylated tau causes mitochondrial dysfunction in Alzheimer's disease. Hum Mol Genet. 2012; 21: 5131-5146.

[106] Li Z, Okamoto K.-I, Hayashi Y, Sheng M. The importance of dendritic mitochondria in the morphogenesis and plasticity of spines and synapses. Cell 2004; 119: 873–887.

[107] Cardoso S, Proenca M, Santos S, Santana I, Oliveira C. Cytochrome c oxidase is decreased in Alzheimer's disease platelets. Neurobiology of Aging 2004; 25:105–110.

[108] Lynch T, Cherny RA, Bush A I. Oxidative processes in Alzheimer's disease: the role of Ab-metal interactions. Experimental Gerontology 2000; 35: 445–451.

[109] He G, Luo W, Li P, Remmers C, Netzer WJ, Hendrick J, Bettayeb K, Flajolet M, Gorelick F, Wennogle LP, Greengard P. Gamma-secretase activating protein is a therapeutic target for Alzheimer's disease. Nature 2010; 467:95–98.

[110] Gonatas NK, Stieber A, Mourelatos Z, Chen Y, Gonatas JO, Appel SH, Hays AP, Hickey WF, Hauw JJ. Fragmentation of the Golgi apparatus of motor neurons in amyotrophic lateral sclerosis. Am J Pathol. 1992, 140:731-737.

[111] Mourelatos Z, Hirano A, Rosenquist A, Gonatas NK. Fragmentation of the Golgi apparatus of motor neurons in amyotrophic lateral sclerosis (ALS): clinical studies in ALS of Guam and experimental studies in deafferented neurons and in f3, f-iminodiproprionitrile axonopathy. Am J Pathol 1994, 144:1288-1300.

[112] Mourelatos Z, Yachnis A, Rorke L, Mikol J, Gonatas NK. The Golgi apparatus of motor neurons in amyotrophic lateral sclerosis. Ann Neurol. 1993, 33:608-615.

[113] Mourelatos Z, Adler H, Hirano A, Donnenfeld H, Gonatas JO, Gonatas NK. Fragmentation of the Golgi apparatus of motor neurons in amyotrophic lateral sclerosis revealed by organelle-specific antibodies. Proc Natl Acad Sci USA. 1990, 87:4393-4395.

[114] Deatherage CL, Hadziselimovic A, Sanders C R. Purification and Characterization of the Human γ-Secretase Activating Protein Biochemistry. 2012; 51: 5153–5159.

[115] Satoh J, Tabunoki H, Ishida T, Saito Y, Arima K. Immunohistochemical characterization of γ-secretase activating protein expression in Alzheimer's disease brains Neuropathology and Applied Neurobiology. 2012; 38: 132–141.

[116] Borgegard T, Jureus A, Olsson F, Rosqvist S, Sabirsh A, Rotticci D, Paulsen K, Klintenberg R, Yan H, Waldman M, Stromberg K, Nord J, Johansson J, Regner A, Parpal S, Malinowsky D, Radesater A-C, Li T, Singh R, Eriksson H, Lundkvist J. First and second generation gamma-secretase modulators (GSMs) modulate Abeta production through different mechanisms. The Journal of Biological Chemistry. 2012; 287: 11810-11819.

[117] Borgegård T, Gustavsson S, Nilsson C, Parpal S, Klintenberg R, Berg A-L, Rosqvist S, Serneels L, Svensson S, Olsson F, Jin S, Yan H, Wanngren J, Jureus A, Ridderstad-Wollberg A, Wollberg P, Stockling K, Karlström H, Malmberg Å, Lund J, Arvidsson PI, De Strooper B, Lendah U, Lundkvist J. Alzheimer's Disease: Presenilin 2-Sparing γ-Secretase Inhibition Is a Tolerable Aβ Peptide-Lowering Strategy. The Journal of Neuroscience. 2012; 32: 17297-17305.

Chapter 6

Caspases in Alzheimer's Disease

Yan Zhang

Additional information is available at the end of the chapter

http://dx.doi.org/10.5772/54627

1. Introduction

In AD, a significant synaptic loss ranging from 20% to 50% is reported. Biochemistry, electron microscopy and immunocytochemistry have shown a decrease in synaptic density, presynaptic terminals, synaptic vesicle and synaptic protein markers in AD brains compared with the normal aged controls (Terry et al., 1991; Geula, 1998; Larson et al., 1999; Yao et al., 1999; Ashe, 2000; Baloyannis et al., 2000; Terry, 2000; Masliah, 2001; Masliah et al., 2001; Price et al., 2001; Scheff and Price, 2001; Scheff et al., 2001; Stephan et al., 2001; Callahan et al., 2002; Chan et al., 2002; Dodd, 2002). Although synaptic loss is remarkable in AD, it is not specific to AD. Reduction in synaptic density is also found in Pick's disease, Huntington's disease, Parkinson's disease as well as in vascular dementia (Geula, 1998; Larson et al., 1999; Yao et al., 1999; Ashe, 2000; Baloyannis et al., 2000; Terry, 2000; Masliah, 2001; Masliah et al., 2001; Price et al., 2001; Scheff and Price, 2001; Scheff et al., 2001; Stephan et al., 2001; Callahan et al., 2002; Chan et al., 2002; Dodd, 2002).

Since one of the most important physiological functions of synapses is to release and accept neurotransmitters, the changes of activity of these neurotransmitters in neurodegenerative diseases have also been intensively studied (Terry, 2000). In AD, most significant lesions happen in the cholinergic, adrenergic and serotoninergic systems (Davies and Maloney, 1976; Geula, 1998; Larson et al., 1999; Yao et al., 1999; Ashe, 2000; Baloyannis et al., 2000; Terry, 2000; Masliah, 2001; Masliah et al., 2001; Price et al., 2001; Scheff and Price, 2001; Scheff et al., 2001; Stephan et al., 2001; Callahan et al., 2002; Chan et al., 2002; Dodd, 2002). Some other peptidergic neurotransmitters also decrease in AD, such as somatostatin, neuropeptide Y and substance P (Terry, 2000).

Synaptic loss might be one of the first events in AD development (Terry et al., 1991; Terry, 2000; Selkoe, 2002). Decrease in presynaptic terminals, synaptic vesicle and synaptic protein markers occur in very early stage of AD (Ashe, 2000; Terry, 2000; Masliah et al.,

2001; Price et al., 2001; Scheff et al., 2001; Callahan et al., 2002; Chan et al., 2002; Dodd, 2002). In the transgenic mice with FAD mutations, synaptophysin, marker for presynaptic protein, decreases before the appearance of Aβ deposits and formation of plaques (Hamos et al., 1989; Masliah et al., 1989; Selkoe, 2002). Most important, the decline of function of synaptic transmission occurs even before synaptic structural changes (Masliah, 2001; Scheff and Price, 2001; Chan et al., 2002; Selkoe, 2002). Long-term potentiation (LTP) is commonly accepted as a measurement for capacity of synaptic plasticity, which is the basis of learning, memory and complex information processing. The incidence and duration of LTP formation are used as an indication for formation and maintenance of working memory. Several lines of FAD mutant transgenic mice show a decline in the formation of LTP and synaptic excitation before the appearance of synaptic loss, plaques and other AD pathology (Geula, 1998; Ashe, 2000; Masliah, 2001; Masliah et al., 2001; Scheff and Price, 2001; Callahan et al., 2002; Chan et al., 2002; Selkoe, 2002). In summary, synaptic loss seems to appear earlier than all other pathological markers and the functional loss of synapses may be responsible for the initiation of cognitive decline in AD patients.

2. Neuronal loss in AD

Synaptic loss and degeneration induce neuronal dysfunction and cell body loss. Neuronal loss in the cerebral cortex and the hippocampus is a hallmark feature of AD. Some of AD patients at late stage of the disease can have a severe decrease in brain volume and weight due to either neuronal loss or atrophy (Smale et al., 1995; Cotman and Su, 1996; Gomez-Isla et al., 1996; Gomez-Isla et al., 1997; Li et al., 1997; Su et al., 1997; Gomez-Isla et al., 1999). Assumption-based and design-based unbiased stereological cell counting show decreased density of neurons in the cerebral cortex, the entorhinal cortex, the association cortex, the basal nucleus of Meynert, the locus coeruleus and the dorsal raphe of AD brains (Bondareff et al., 1982; Lippa et al., 1992; Gomez-Isla et al., 1996; Gomez-Isla et al., 1997; Gomez-Isla et al., 1999; Colle et al., 2000). Profound neuronal loss is especially observed in the entorhinal cortex in the mild AD brains (Gomez-Isla et al., 1996; Gomez-Isla et al., 1997; Gomez-Isla et al., 1999). Besides AD, significant neuronal loss is also observed in the entorhinal cortex in very mild cognitive impairment patient brains (Gomez-Isla et al., 1996; Gomez-Isla et al., 1997; Gomez-Isla et al., 1999). These data suggest that neuronal loss may be one of the early events before formation of SPs and NFTs in AD development.

The loss of cholinergic neurons in AD is widely studied. The hippocampus and cortex receive major cholinergic input from the basal forebrain nuclei (Hohmann et al., 1987). Decrease of choline acetyltransferase activity and acetylcholine synthesis correlate well with the degree of cognitive impairment in AD patients (Mesulam, 1986; Hohmann et al., 1987; Pearson and Powell, 1987). Cholinergic neuronal lesion can be detected in the patients that have showed clinical memory loss symptoms for less than 1 year (Whitehouse et al., 1981; Whitehouse et al., 1982; Francis et al., 1993; Weinstock, 1997). However, markers for dopamine, γ-aminobutyric acid (GABA), or somatostatin are not altered (Whitehouse et al., 1981; Whitehouse et al., 1982; Francis et al., 1993). These results suggest that cholinergic neuronal loss is probably one of the early events in AD. Besides the main pathology discussed above, some other pathologies of AD include granulovacuolar degeneration, cerebral amyloid angiopathy, blood-brain barrier disorder, white matter lesions, neuropil thread and gliosis (Jellinger, 2002a; Jellinger, 2002b, c; Jellinger and Attems, 2003).

As discussed above, stereological cell counting shows that densities of neurons in the AD cerebral cortex, the entorhinal cortex, the association cortex, the basal nucleus of Meynert, the locus coeruleus and the dorsal raphe decrease significantly compared to the age-matched non-AD controls (Bondareff et al., 1982; Lippa et al., 1992; Gomez-Isla et al., 1996; Gomez-Isla et al., 1997; Gomez-Isla et al., 1999; Colle et al., 2000). Neuronal cell loss is one of the first events during AD development. In the mild AD patient brains, remarkable neuronal cell loss of more than 40% is seen in the entorhinal cortex (Gomez-Isla et al., 1996; Gomez-Isla et al., 1997). Even in the mild cognitive impairment patient brains, significant neuronal loss is also observed in the entorhinal cortex (Gomez-Isla et al., 1996). Furthermore, the degree of neuronal loss correlates better with the clinical dementia level in AD than other pathology.

It was thought until recently that neuronal loss is mainly due to passive neurotrophic factor withdrawal. In 1988, Martin et al. (1988) showed that sympathetic neuronal death could be prevented by inhibiting RNA and protein synthesis, indicating that some of the neuronal death might be actively programmed (apoptotic) instead of passive (necrotic).

3. Apoptosis

Apoptosis, or programmed cell death (PCD), is a term proposed by Kerr, Wyllie and Currie in 1972 (Kerr et al., 1972) to describe a common type of cell death characterized by membrane blebbing, cell shrinkage, protein fragmentation, chromatin condensation and DNA degradation followed by rapid engulfment of corpses by surrounding cells (Kerr et al., 1972). It rapidly cleans out dysfunctional cells, limits toxic effects, saves energy and recycles molecules for future *de novo* synthesis.

Two major apoptotic pathways in mammalian cells are mediated through either death receptors or mitochondria (Figure 1). The so-called extrinsic pathway is initiated by death receptor CD95 (Apo-1/Fas), or other death receptors, such as tumor necrosis factor (TNF) receptor and tumor necrosis factor related apoptosis inducing ligand (TRAIL) receptor. CD95 is linked to pro-caspase-8 by an adapter factor FADD. Pro-caspase-8 has a death effecter domain (DED) which binds to the death domain (DD) on death receptor adapter FADD, and a caspase activation and recruitment domain (CARD), which binds to other downstream caspases and further processes the downstream caspases. Ligand binding signals the activation of pro-caspase-8 to form a tetramer of active caspase-8. Caspase-8 then mediates the cleavage of pro-caspase-3 and initiates the caspase activation cascade, which leads to protein and DNA cleavage and final termination of the cells. In this pathway, caspase-8 activation can be prevented by its natural inhibitors, such as cellular FADD-like interlukin-1-β-converting enzyme (FLICE/caspase-8)-inhibitory proteins (c-FLIPs) (Irmler et al., 1997; Thome et al., 1997) and apoptosis repressor with caspase recruitment domain (ARC) (Koseki et al., 1998) (Figure 1).

The intrinsic pathway is triggered mainly by internal insults such as DNA damage. Damaging insults such as UV irradiation activate tumor suppression gene product p53, a transcriptional factor. There are several hypotheses for p53 activation mechanism. First, stress-activated protein kinases, such as DNA-dependent protein kinase (DNA-PK), phosphorylates p53. This phosphorylation prevents p53 from degradation. For example, DNA-PK can be activated by DNA damage, and then phosphorylate p53 at Ser-15 in the N terminal, which prevents the interaction between p53 and its inhibitory protein MDM-2. In addition to phosphorylation, dephosphorylation, such as the one caused by 14-3-3 at Ser-376, can also enable DNA binding of p53 and activate its function. The second model states that p53 is constitutively active and is regulated by the negative regulator MDM-2. MDM-2 protein can bind to p53 and send it out of the nucleus for degradation. Interestingly, the MDM-2 gene can be activated by p53, therefore, p53 is negatively self-regulated. After activation, p53 acts as a transcriptional factor controlling the expression of certain genes. These genes are involved in cell cycle control (eg. p21, GADD45, 14-3-3, CyclinD1, CyclinG), DNA repair (eg. GADD45, p21), apoptosis (eg. Bax, Bcl-2, FASL, DR5), angiogenesis (eg. TSP-1, BAI1) and cellular stress response (eg. TP53TG1, CSR, PIG3).

During apoptosis, p53 activates transcription of the pro-apoptotic Bax and, at the same time, transcriptionally represses the anti-apoptotic Bcl-2. A family of Bcl-2 proteins is implicated in apoptosis. This family contains three subgroups of proteins, some of them are pro-apoptotic while some are anti-apoptotic. The Group I proteins, such as Bcl-2, have a transmembrane domain and conserved Bcl-2 homology (BH) 1-4 domains. The Group II lacks the BH4 domain, such as Bax, while in the Group III, only the BH3 domain is in common, such as Bid and Bik (Hengartner, 2000). Bax is a pro-apoptotic protein causing the depolarization of mitochondrial membrane and release of cytochrome c from the mitochondria to the cytosol. The detailed mechanism of Bax leading to cytochrome c release is unknown. Bax is located in the cytosol as monomers and upon the apoptotic stimulation, Bax oligomerizes and translocates to the mitochondria. There are several models suggested to explain how Bax oligomers cause intermembrane protein cytochrome c release (Degli Esposti and Dive, 2003). First, Bax oligomers may form a pore structure on the mitochondria outer membrane leading to cytochrome c release. Second, interaction between Bax and other mitochondrial proteins, such as voltage dependent anion selective channel (VDAC) and adenosine nucleotide transporter (ANT) may induce pore formation by VDAC and ANT, through which cytochrome c is released. Third, the pore may form on the membrane by low-selective ion channels and induce cytochrome c release through these channels (Degli Esposti and Dive, 2003). Cytochrome c, together with the adapter molecule Apaf-1 and pro-caspase-9, forms an apoptosome that cleaves pro-caspase-3 into its active form and initiates apoptosis. Bcl-2, the other member of Bcl-2 family in the Group I, is an anti-apoptotic protein preventing Bax-mediated cytochrome c release efficiently.

The two apoptotic pathways cross at Bid, a pro-apoptotic protein from Bcl-2 family Group III. Bid can be cleaved by active caspase-8 and the truncated Bid translocates to the mitochondrial membrane, increases mitochondrial outer membrane permeability, facilitates pore formation and potentiates cytochrome c release on the mitochondrial outer membrane (Figure 1) (Hengartner, 2000).

This apoptosis machinery is self-amplifying. For example, second mitochondria-derived activator of caspase/direct IAP-binding protein with low pI (Smac/DIABLO) and apoptosis-inducing factor (AIF) proteins (Hengartner, 2000; Cregan et al., 2002) are released from the mitochondria with cytochrome c to facilitate apoptosis. In addition, recent studies showed that caspase-3, -6, -7 and –8 can initiate cytochrome c release by activating cytosolic factors (Figure 1). Since cytochrome c acts as an initiator for the caspase activation cascade, this self-amplified loop facilitates cellular apoptosis (Figure 1) (Bossy-Wetzel and Green, 1999).

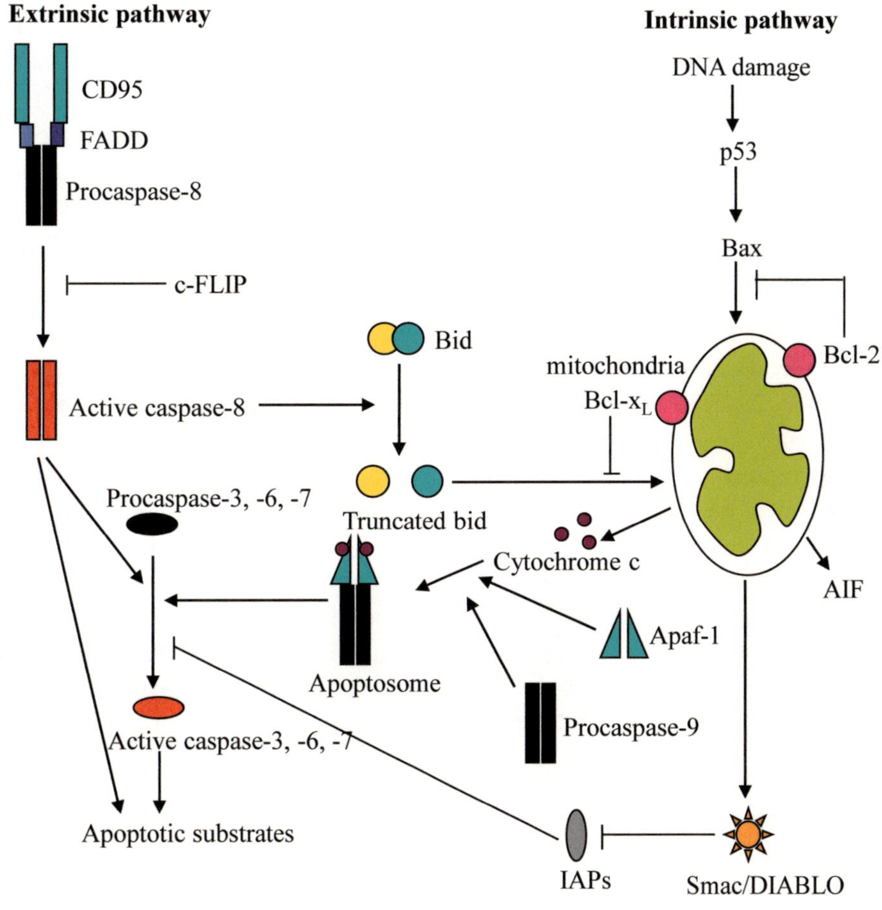

Figure 1. Schematic drawing of two major pathways involved in apoptosis. Schematic digram showing the two major pathways mediating apoptosis. The extrinsic pathway is mediated by death receptors, such as FADD, and caspase-8 activation. The intrinsic pathway is induced by DNA damage and mediated by caspase-9. IAP: inhibitor of apoptosis protein, Smac/DIABLO: second mitochondria-derived activator of caspase/direct IAP-binding protein with low pI, AIF: apoptosis inducing factor.

4. Apoptosis involvement in neuronal cell loss of AD

There is evidence for apoptosis involvement in neuronal loss in AD, but the evidence so far is not sufficient to support a significant role for apoptosis in the neuronal cell loss in AD. Evidence of apoptosis in AD is as follows. First, overexpression of FAD-related mutations causes apoptosis in the transfected cell lines, cultured neurons and transgenic mice. For example, overexpression of FAD mutations of APP^{V642I}, APP^{V642F} and APP^{V642G} in COS or F11 cells increases number of apoptotic cells as determined by DNA fragmentation and terminal dUTP nick end labeling (TUNEL) staining assay, which can be inhibited by anti-apoptotic protein Bcl-2 overexpression (Yamatsuji et al., 1996). These results support the role of FAD mutations in inducing apoptosis. Similarly, the data from transgenic mice confirm the above observations. Transgenic mice overexpressing FAD mutant APP^{V717F} develop neuritic dystrophy similar to some pathological features in AD patients (Games et al., 1995; Holcomb et al., 1998). The degenerating neurons in these mice also show typical apoptotic features, such as chromatin segmentation and condensation, and positive TUNEL staining (Nijhawan et al., 2000). However, in these studies, the FAD mutant proteins are normally overexpressed far beyond the physiological levels. However, FAD neurons do not necessarily undergo apoptosis. In the mutant PS1 expressing neurons, increased apoptosis is not reported (Bursztajn et al., 1998). Also, there is no neuronal loss found in mutant PS1 transgenic mice (Takeuchi et al., 2000).

Second, some studies indicate apoptosis in AD patient brains using *in situ* detection of DNA fragmentation by TUNEL staining (Su et al., 1994; Dragunow et al., 1995; Lassmann et al., 1995; Smale et al., 1995; Anderson et al., 1996; Su et al., 1996; Troncoso et al., 1996; Gervais et al., 1999; Anderson et al., 2000). However, in the AD brain tissues, some TUNEL-positive neurons show typical apoptotic morphology whereas some do not, suggesting degenerating neurons in AD may undergo both apoptosis and passive cell death, necrosis (Su et al., 1994; Troncoso et al., 1996; Lucassen et al., 1997; Yuan and Yankner, 2000). It is now commonly accepted that TUNEL staining sometimes is not specific to apoptosis (Stadelmann et al., 1998). The staining of TUNEL may indicate increased vulnerability of cells to a secondary insult, not necessarily undergoing apoptosis. On the other hand, the number of apoptotic neurons is difficult to measure precisely due to the chronic nature, relatively long progress of the disease and rapid clearance mechanism of dead cells.

Third, there are reports of changes of expression of apoptosis related proteins, such as p53, Bcl-2 and Bcl-x_L, in AD brains (Paradis et al., 1996; Kitamura et al., 1997; MacGibbon et al., 1997; Su et al., 1997; Cotman, 1998; Torp et al., 1998; Tortosa et al., 1998). For example, pro-apoptotic protein p53 is increased in AD brains (Kitamura et al., 1997), while anti-apoptotic proteins Bcl-2 and Bcl-x_L are decreased in AD brains (Kitamura et al., 1998; Tortosa et al., 1998). Also, another pro-apoptotic protein Bax is increased in AD brains (Paradis et al., 1996; Kitamura et al., 1997; MacGibbon et al., 1997; Su et al., 1997; Cotman, 1998; Torp et al., 1998; Tortosa et al., 1998). However, the regulation of these pro- or anti-apoptotic proteins could be primary or secondary response to insults. On the other hand, the upregulation of either pro-

http://dx.doi.org/10.5772/54627

or anti-apoptotic proteins could be explained by either the neurons undergoing apoptosis or neurons responding against apoptotic insults to prevent initiation of apoptosis.

Therefore, in summary, to date, there is no strong evidence showing significant involvement of apoptosis in AD neuronal loss. Since caspases, a family of cysteinyl proteases, play an important role in cell death, especially in apoptosis as discussed in the previous section (Thompson, 1995; Strasser et al., 2000; Yuan and Yankner, 2000), it is of interest to identify which caspase is responsible for human neuronal cell loss, how it is regulated, and whether it can be inhibited. In addition, caspase activation may be easier to use for identification of apoptosis since it is an upstream event of DNA fragmentation. Therefore, the apoptotic cells have not been cleared yet.

5. Caspase involvement in apoptosis and APP metabolism in AD

5.1. Caspases

Caspases (cysteinyl aspartate-specific proteases) belong to a cysteinyl protease family that cleaves specifically after an aspartic acid. To date, 14 caspases (11 of them are found in human) have been identified in mammals. The connection between apoptosis and caspases was first reported by Yuan et al. (1993) that caspase-1 is a homolog to CED-3, a gene regulating cell death in *Caenorhaditis elegans* (Yuan et al., 1993). The important role of caspases in apoptosis is also supported by the strong correlation between caspase activity and apoptosis in various cell types. Furthermore, caspase inhibition prevents apoptosis both *in vitro* and *in vivo* (Yuan et al., 1993; Kuida et al., 1995; Schwartz and Milligan, 1996; Alnemri, 1997; Thornberry, 1997; Li and Yuan, 1999; Yuan and Yankner, 2000).

Inactive caspases contain a pro-domain, a large subunit and a small subunit. According to their pro-domain structure and function, caspases are divided into "inflammatory", "initiator" and "effecter" caspases (Figure 2A) (Nicholson, 1999; Hengartner, 2000). Caspases are normally present as inactive precursors in cells. After receiving apoptotic signals, caspase pro-enzymes undergo proteolytic processing to remove the N terminal pro-domain and cleave between large and small subunits to produce the active form of a tetrameric enzyme formed by 2 copies of the large subunit and 2 copies of small subunit. To date, three caspase activation pathways are known in mammalian cells: recruitment-activation, trans-activation and autoactivation (Nicholson, 1999). Recruitment-activation is triggered by death receptors of the tumor necrosis factor receptor family. The so-called initiator caspases, namely caspase-2, -8, -9 and –10 (Figure 3A), are thought to be directly activated through the signals from death receptor (Boldin et al., 1996; Muzio et al., 1996). In addition, more recent data show that the initiator caspase-8, -9 and –10 can be activated by homodimerization of their monomeric zymogens, a so called "proximity-induced activation" (Boatright et al., 2003). Trans-activation occurs through downstream or executioner caspases, caspase-3, -6 and –7 that can be activated by direct proteolysis by their upstream initiator caspases. By such trans-activation cascade, apoptosis is well controlled and regulated (Darmon et al., 1995; Martin et al., 1996; Andrade et al., 1998). Caspase activation can also occur by activation of the dormant enzyme molecule by the already active one (autoactivation). The supporting evidence of this mechanism comes from the observation that arginine-glycine-aspartate (RGD) motif-containing peptides can induce caspase-3 autoactivation by triggering conformational changes of pro-caspase-3 (Buckley et al., 1999). A similar mechanism has been suggested for pro-caspase-8 and –2 activation (Hengartner, 2000).

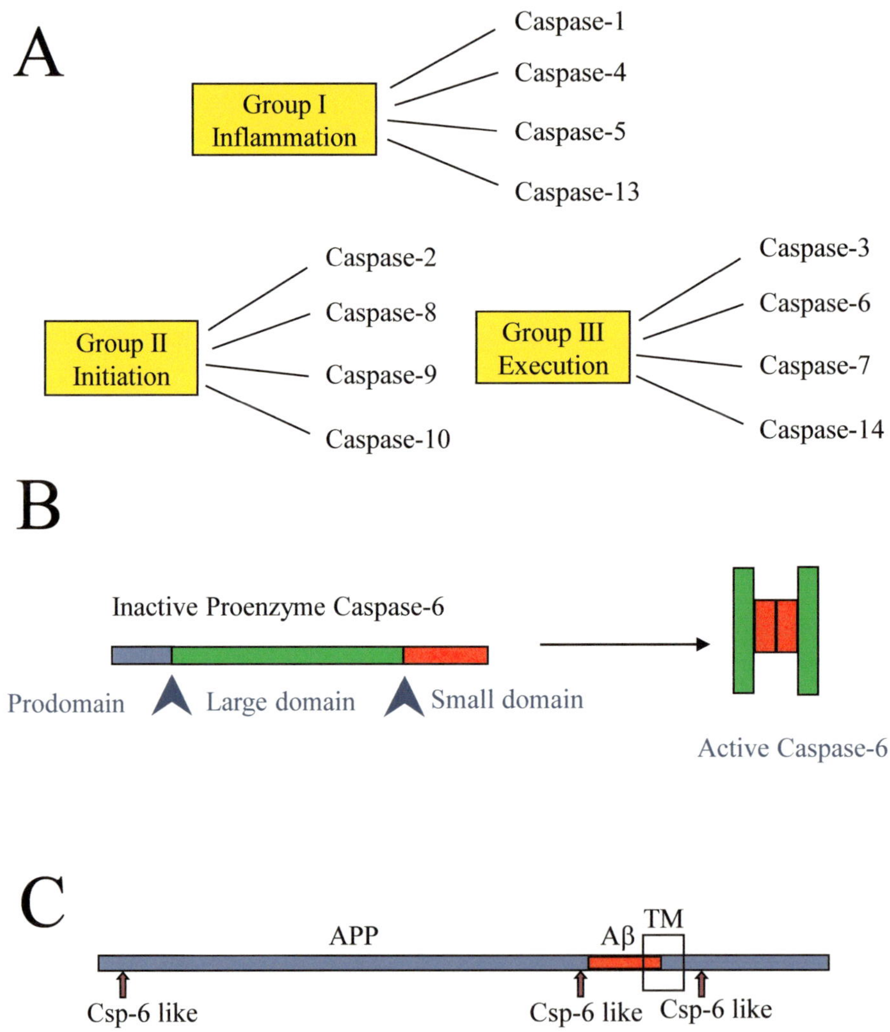

Figure 2. Caspases are cysteinyl proteases responsible for protein degradation during apoptosis. A. Schematic diagram of caspase category according to function. There are three groups of caspases according to their basic functions: inflammation, initiation and execution. B. Schematic drawing of pro-caspase-6 activation into active caspase-6. Caspase-6 activation by cleavage at the sites between pro-domain and large subunit (p20) as well as large subunit and small subunit (p10). Arrow head: cleavage. C. Schematic drawing of caspase-6-like cleavage sites on APP. There are three caspase-6-like cleavage sites on APP. Arrow: cleavage. TM: transmembrane domain.

After activation, caspases recognize four amino acid substrate sites as their targets and cleave the C terminal to an obligatory aspartic acid (XXXD). According to their specific substrates, caspases are divided into 3 groups: caspase-1, -4, -5 and –13 (substrates: WEHD and YVAD); caspase-2, -3 and -7 (substrate: DEXD) and caspase-6, -8, –9 and -10 (substrates: (I, V, L)EXD) (reviewed by (Thornberry, 1997)). Once activated, caspases cleave downstream substrates in a highly specific and rapid manner. More than 250 substrates are found including downstream caspases or apoptosis-related proteins (e.g. Bid, Bcl-2), structural proteins (e.g. lamins, actin, fodrin, gelsolin), DNA repair proteins (e.g. PARP, p21) and some other proteins involved in neurodegenerative diseases (eg. APP, tau, PSs, Huntingtin) (reviewed by (Bounhar et al., 2002).

Most of the morphological changes in apoptosis described by Kerr et al. (1972) are caused by caspases that are activated specifically in PCD. Caspase cleavage of nuclear lamins results in nuclear shrinking and blebbing (McCarthy et al., 1997; Sakahira et al., 1998). Loss of cell structure may be due to caspase cleavage of cytoskeletal proteins, such as fodrin (Vanags et al., 1996; Janicke et al., 1998) and gelsolin (Kothakota et al., 1997). DNA fragmentation is also caused by caspase-activated DNase (CAD), which is activated by caspases through removing the inhibitory subunit (ICAD) from the inactive CAD enzyme complex (Hengartner, 2000).

5.2. Involvement of caspases in neuronal loss in AD

In general, the evidence supporting the involvement of caspases in neuronal loss in AD is still not conclusive. The involvement of caspases in AD is first suggested by the finding that caspases, acting as proteases, are involved in PSs and APP metabolism and Aβ peptide generation in AD. Caspase-3 directly cleaves PSs during apoptosis (Kim et al., 1997). Caspase-3, -6, -7, -8 and –9 can cleave APP and generate Aβ or Aβ-containing fragments, therefore, giving a possibility of Aβ accumulation in AD (Barnes et al., 1998; Gervais et al., 1999; LeBlanc et al., 1999; Pellegrini et al., 1999; Weidemann et al., 1999). In chick motor neurons, caspase-3 cleaves APP and generates Aβ products (Barnes et al., 1998). In human 293 cells, caspase-9 cleaves APP at the C terminal and produces a "C31" peptide, which is cytotoxic to cells (Lu et al., 2000). Caspase-3 cleaves APP in NT-2 cells and is involved in Aβ formation (Gervais et al., 1999). APP is a caspase substrate in staurosporine-treated NT-2 cells and Fas-treated human Jurkat cells (Pellegrini et al., 1999). In addition, caspase inhibitors can prevent the formation of Aβ (Barnes et al., 1998; Gervais et al., 1999; LeBlanc et al., 1999).

Second, more direct proof of caspase involvement in AD comes from immuno-detection of active caspases in AD brain tissues, although the evidence is not sufficient enough to be conclusive. Some studies have shown the activation of caspase-8 in AD brains (Rohn et al., 2001; Rohn et al., 2002), while others found decreased level of caspase-8 in AD brains (Engidawork et al., 2001a). In yet another study, both inactive and active caspase-8 immunoreactivity are not changed in AD compared to control brains (Engidawork et al., 2001b). The cleavage fragment of caspase-9 is also detected in AD but not in the control brains (Lu et al., 2000; Goyal, 2001; Rohn et al., 2002), but the alteration of two caspase-9 activation co-factors, Apaf-1 and cytochrome c, is not detected (Engidawork et al., 2001b). Furthermore, there is recent evidence showing that pro-caspase-9 is activated through dimerization, but not cleavage (Boatright et al., 2003). Among all caspases, caspase-3 is the most intensively studied since the caspase-3 knockouts develop abnormal brains with significantly excessive numbers of neurons (Cregan et al., 1999; Keramaris et al., 2000; Simpson et al., 2001; Fernando et al., 2002). Some studies report increased caspase-3-like immunoreactivity in AD brains (Masliah et al., 1998; Gervais et al., 1999). However, the protein and mRNA levels of caspase-3 do not appear altered in AD compared to control brains (Desjardins and Ledoux, 1998; LeBlanc et al., 1999). Active caspase-3 is detected in granulovacuolar degeneration, an aging associated pathology that is not necessarily specific to AD (Stadelmann et al., 1999; Roth, 2001). Given that apoptosis results in a rapid clearance of dysfunctional cells, only small amount of caspase activation can be detected at a certain time window. Therefore, the extensive detection of active caspase-3 in some studies may be due to lack of immunospecificity of the caspase-3 antibody. Furthermore, although caspase-3 is critical for apoptosis in many cell types, it does not have significant role in the human neuronal loss in AD (Desjardins and Ledoux, 1998; LeBlanc et al., 1999; Selznick et al., 1999; Stadelmann et al., 1999).

Interestingly, LeBlanc et al. have shown that caspase-6 is activated in serum deprivation induced cell death of human neurons in primary cultured (LeBlanc et al., 1999). Therefore, could caspase-6 be the responsible caspase in human neuronal cell death in AD?

5.3. Caspase-6 is activated during human neuronal cell death

5.3.1. Introduction to caspase-6

Caspase-6 (Mch-2), located on human chromosome 4q25, is an "effecter" caspase with a short pro-domain. It recognizes VEID substrates and cleaves after the amino acid D. Its common substrates include APP (LeBlanc et al., 1999), cytoskeleton proteins, such as keratin 18 (Caulin et al., 1997), focal adhesion kinase (Gervais et al., 1998), tau (LeBlanc et al., 1999), β-catenin (Van de Craen et al., 1999), vimentin (Byun et al., 2001) and desmin (Chen et al., 2003), nuclear proteins, such as lamin A (Ruchaud et al., 2002), lamin B (Slee et al., 2001), PARP (Fernandes-Alnemri et al., 1995), DNA topoisomerase I (Samejima et al., 1999) and emerin (Columbaro et al., 2001), several transcriptional factors, such as SATB1, and AP-2α (Galande et al., 2001; Nyormoi et al., 2001). It is highly expressed in the heart, lung, liver, kidney and testis in murine tissues. There is immunodetectable caspase-6 in human brain and neurons (LeBlanc et al., 1999; Zheng et al., 1999; Harrison et al., 2001). Caspase-6 can be activated by caspase-1, -3, -7, -8 and –11 (Fernandes-Alnemri et al., 1995; Chinnaiyan et al., 1996; Orth et al., 1996). Pro-caspase-6 is a ~ 34 kDa protein, that can be cleaved into ~20 kDa (p20) and ~10 kDa (p10) fragments. The p20 and p10 fragments form a tetramer, which is the active form of the enzyme (Figure 3C) (Fernandes-Alnemri et al., 1995). Caspase-6 knockout mice do not show abnormal phenotype during development, which does not rule out the role of caspase-6 in cell death in later stage of life or under stress conditions (Zheng et al., 1999).

5.3.2. Caspase-6 involvement in human neuronal cell death and APP processing

Pro-caspase-6 decreases during apoptosis induced by serum deprivation in human neurons in primary cultures (LeBlanc et al., 1999). Moreover, caspase-6 active 10 kDa fragments is detected only in AD brains, and not in the normal aging control brains (LeBlanc et al., 1999),

http://dx.doi.org/10.5772/54627

although thus increase is not dramatic. Given that AD is a long progressive disease, at a certain postmortem time window, there is only limited amount of cell death where caspase activation can be detected. Meanwhile, in contrast to caspase-6, changes in the levels of pro- and active caspase-3 levels are not detectable in AD brains, suggesting that caspase-6, but not caspase-3, may be involved in human neuronal cell death (LeBlanc et al., 1999). Caspase-6 can also alter APP metabolism to generate Aβ-containing fragments. There are several caspase-6-like sites on APP_{695} (Figure 2C). However, incubating recombinant caspase-6 and APP_{695}-containing neuronal extract does not show APP cleavage. One of these cleavages at ^{591}VKMD^{594} generates a 6.5 kDa fragment denoted "Capp6.5" containing the Aβ sequence (Figure 2C) (LeBlanc et al., 1999). Although caspase-6 does not directly induce 4 kDa Aβ, pulse-chase experiments showed that this Capp6.5 fragment is able to generate 4 kDa Aβ in human neurons (Figure 2C) (LeBlanc et al., 1999). Caspase-6 can cleave APP close to β-secretase site at D^{653} to further generate $A\beta_{2\text{-}40}$ or $A\beta_{2\text{-}42}$ (Gervais et al., 1999). In the Swedish mutation of APP, which changes the VKMD^{653} sequence at the β-secretase site to VNLD^{653}, the caspase-6 cleavage of VNLD-AMC is 6 fold higher than the VKMD-AMC fluorogenic peptide *in vitro* (Gervais et al., 1999). Also, caspase-6 can cleave APP after the γ-secretase site at VEVD^{720}/A (Gervais et al., 1999). Therefore, caspase-6 may process APP similar to β- and γ-secretase activity. Direct microinjecting caspase-6 into human neurons induces dramatic cell death (Zhang et al., 2000). Taken together, the above evidence suggests that caspase-6 plays important role in human neuronal cell death, Aβ formation, and may be responsible for neuronal loss in AD (LeBlanc et al., 1999).

5.4. Inhibition of active caspases

5.4.1. Natural inhibitors to caspases

The natural inhibitors to caspases include Cowpox virus product cytokine response modifier A (crmA), FLIPs, protease inhibitor 9 (PI-9), p35, ARC and inhibitor of apoptosis proteins (IAPs). CrmA is a member of serpin family, a group of serine protease inhibitors. CrmA inhibits caspases by acting as a pseudosubstrate that binds to active caspases, such as caspase-1, -4, -5, -8 and –9 (Ray et al., 1992; Komiyana et al., 1994). Besides crmA, FLIPs inhibits caspase-8 by acting as the dominant negative form to suppress caspase-8 mRNA expression (Thornberry, 1997). The mammalian homolog of crmA is PI-9. PI-9 mRNA expression can be rapidly induced by estrogen in human liver (Kanamori et al., 2000). PI-9 is a granzyme B inhibitor (GBI). Granzyme B is a 30 to 32 kDa serine protease, which cleaves peptides at aspartyl residue in the killer T thymocytes and natural killer cells. Granzyme B is involved in the perforation of target cells and then initiation of proteolysis that leads to apoptosis. Although PI-9 can inhibit granzyme B and granzyme B-mediated apoptosis, *In vitro* experiments do not show that PI-9 inhibits active caspases (Bird et al., 1998; Bird, 1999).

p35 is a baculoviral protein that can block the defensive apoptotic response of insect cells to viral infection (Clem et al., 1991; Ekert et al., 1999). p35 inhibits CED-3 in *C. elegans* and mammalian caspase-1, -3, -6, -7, -8 and -10 (Ekert et al., 1999). P35 is cleaved at its P1 residue by caspases, and the cleaved fragment forms an inhibitory complex to block caspase activation (Zhou et al., 1998). ARC interacts with caspase-2, -8 and CED-3, but not caspase-1, -3, or –9. ARC inhibits caspase-8 enzyme activity in 293 cells, and further attenuates apoptosis induced by FADD through stimulation of death receptors coupled with pro-caspase-8 (Koseki et al., 1998).

IAPs were found in a search for viral genes with a similar function to p35. A group of cellular IAP homologs are found in yeast, *C. elegans*, *Drosophila* and vertebrates (Ekert et al., 1999). To date, the IAP family contains about a dozen proteins from viruses, *Drosophila*, mice and humans. All known IAPs share a baculovirus inhibitory repeat (BIR) domain, which contains a number of conserved residues including a zinc-binding region. Most of the IAPs also contain a RING zinc-binding finger motif at the C terminal. Both BIR motifs and RING finger are important for IAP function (Ekert et al., 1999). The neuronal apoptosis inhibitory protein (NAIP) in human was found by searching for mutations in spinal muscular atrophy (SMA), which is characterized by degeneration of the anterior horn cells in the spinal cord. The NAIP gene is deleted in the SMA patients. During development, excessive neurons are ultimately needed to send out axons, the neurons do not target properly undergo apoptosis. It is suggested that NAIP is involved by preventing apoptosis in the "successful" cells (Miller, 1997).

The most studied IAP is the X-linked IAP (XIAP). XIAP binds to active caspase-9 small subunit through its BIR3 domain and cleaves the small subunit to inactivate caspase-9 (Srinivasula et al., 2001). On the other hand, XIAP binds to active caspase-3 or –7 through BIR2 domain and mask the active site of these caspases (Huang et al., 2001; Riedl et al., 2001; Stennicke et al., 2002). In addition, evidence shows that in insects, some IAPs interact with apoptosis-related proteins, such as Grim, Reaper and Hid (Hay et al., 1995; Miller, 1997; Vucic et al., 1997; Vucic et al., 1998). IAPs can also inhibit caspase-3 directly and cytochrome c-induced caspase-9 (Deveraux et al., 1998). However, up to now, although IAPs may inhibit caspase-6 activation by blocking upstream caspase-9 or –3 activation (Deveraux et al., 1998), there is no evidence showing that mammalian IAPs directly inhibit active caspase-6 enzyme activity.

5.4.2. Synthetic inhibitors to active caspases

Synthetic caspase inhibitors function as pseudosubstrates for active caspases and therefore, they are competitive inhibitors of active caspases (Ekert et al., 1999). The N terminal blocking groups of the pseudosubstrate peptides are usually acetyl- (Ac-) or benzocarbonyl (Z-). The biochemical property of these synthetic inhibitors depends on the chemical group linked to pseudosubstrate peptides. Aldehyde (CHO-) group inhibitors are reversible since there is no covalent bond formed between these inhibitors and caspases. These CHO inhibitors have poor cell membrane permeability, which limits largely the use of these inhibitors on live cells and animals (Schotte et al., 1999; Bounhar et al., 2002). The inhibitors linked to methylketone (chloromethylketone, cmk or fluoromethylketone, fmk) irreversibly inhibit caspases due to the formation of thyomethylketone bonds with the cysteine in the active site of caspases (Bounhar et al., 2002). These inhibitors are membrane permeable, but have less specificity of inhibitory action to caspases (Schotte et al., 1999; Bounhar et al., 2002).

Although synthetic caspase inhibitors are widely used in research, they may not be the ideal candidates for disease treatment since these inhibitors cannot inhibit caspase activation in specific certain cell types. For example, in AD, caspase-6 is the key caspase responsible for neuronal loss. If the synthetic caspase-6 inhibitor is applied and it would inhibit active caspase-6 activity in all types of cells, which has a large potential to develop cancer in cells that proliferate. If a natural inhibitor to active caspase-6 can be activated somehow specifically in human neurons, the risk of oncogenesis in the brain would be greatly reduced.

Since neuronal loss is a striking feature of AD, decreasing or suppressing neuronal cell loss may benefit early AD patients in retaining cognitive capacities and prevent or delay disease progression. Caspases seem to play a significant role in human neuronal cell loss in AD, thus it is intriguing to determine if caspase activity can be inhibited after activation by neuroprotective agents.

Author details

Yan Zhang*

Address all correspondence to: yanzhang@pku.edu.cn

State Key Laboratory of Biomembrane and Membrane Biotechnology, College of Life Sciences, Peking University, Beijing, China

References

[1] Alnemri, E. S. (1997). Mammalian cell death proteases: a family of highly conserved aspartate specific cysteine proteases. J Cell Biochem , 64, 33-42.

[2] Alorainy, I. (2000). Senile scleral plaques: CT. Neuroradiology , 42, 145-148.

[3] Anderson, A. J, Stoltzner, S, Lai, F, Su, J, & Nixon, R. A. (2000). Morphological and biochemical assessment of DNA damage and apoptosis in Down syndrome and Alzheimer disease, and effect of postmortem issue archival on TUNEL. Neurobiol Aging , 21, 511-524.

[4] Anderson, A. J, Su, J. H, & Cotman, C. W. (1996). DNA damage and apoptosis in Alzheimer's disease: colocalization with c-Jun immunoreactivity, relationship to brain area, and effect of postmortem delay. J Neurosci , 16, 1710-1719.

[5] Andrade, F, Roy, S, Nicholson, D, Thornberry, N, Rosen, A, & Casciola-rosen, L. (1998). Granzyme B directly and efficiently cleaves several downstream caspase substrates: implications for CTL-induced apoptosis. Immunity , 8, 451-460.

[6] Arnold, S. E, Hyman, B. T, Flory, J, Damasio, A. R, & Van Hoesen, G. W. (1991). The topographical and neuroanatomical distribution of neurofibrillary tangles and neuritic plaques in the cerebral cortex of patients with Alzheimer's disease. Cereb Cortex , 1, 103-116.

[7] Ashe, K. H. (2000). Synaptic structure and function in transgenic APP mice. Ann N Y Acad Sci , 924, 39-41.

[8] Baloyannis, S. J, Manolidis, S. L, & Manolidis, L. S. (2000). Synaptic alterations in the vestibulocerebellar system in Alzheimer's disease--a Golgi and electron microscope study. Acta Otolaryngol , 120, 247-250.

[9] Barnes, N. Y, Li, L, Yoshikawa, K, Schwartz, L. M, Oppenhein, R. W, & Milligan, C. E. (1998). Increased production of amyloid precursor protein provides a substrate for caspase-3 in dying motoneurons. J Neurosci , 18, 5869-5880.

[10] Bird, C. H, Sutton, V. R, Sun, J. R, Hirst, C. E, Novak, A, Kumar, S, Trapani, J. A, & Bird, P. I. (1998). Selective regulation of apoptosis-the cytotoxic lymphocyte serpin protease inhibitor 9 protects against granzyme B-mediated apoptosis without perturbing the Fas cell death pathway. Mol Cell Biol , 18, 6387-6398.

[11] Bird, P. I. (1999). Regulation of pro-apoptotic leukocyte granule serine proteinases by intracellular serpins. Immunol Cell Biol , 77, 47-57.

[12] Boatright, K. M, Renatus, M, Scott, F. L, Sperandio, S, Shin, H, Pedersen, I. M, Ricci, J. E, Edris, W. A, Sutherlin, D. P, Green, D. R, & Salvesen, G. S. (2003). A unified model for apical caspase activation. Mol Cell , 11, 529-541.

[13] Boldin, M. P, Goncharov, T. V, Goltsev, Y. V, & Wallach, D. (1996). Involvement of MACH, a novel MORT1/FADD-interacting protease, in Fas/APO-1 and TNF receptor-induced cell death. Cell , 85, 803-815.

[14] Bondareff, W, Mountjoy, C. Q, & Roth, M. (1982). Loss of neurons of origin of the adrenergic projection to cerebral cortex (nucleus locus ceruleus) in senile dementia. Neurology , 32, 164-168.

[15] Bossy-wetzel, E, & Green, D. R. (1999). Caspases induce cytochrome c release from mitochondria by activating cytosolic factors. J Biol Chem , 274, 17484-17490.

[16] Bounhar, Y, & Tounekti, O. LeBlanc A ((2002). Monitoring Caspases in Neuronal Cell Death, 2nd Edition. Totowa: Humana Press Inc.

[17] Braak, H, & Braak, E. (1994). Pathology of Alzheimer's disease. In: Neurodegenerative Disease., Philadelphia: Saunders., 585-613.

[18] Buckley, S, Driscoll, B, Barsky, L, Weinberg, K, Anderson, K, & Warburton, D. (1999). ERK activation protects against DNA damage and apoptosis in byperoxic rat AEC2. Am J Physiol 277:LL166., 159.

[19] Bursztajn, S, De Souza, R, & Mcphie, D. L. (1998). Overexpression in neurons of human presenilin-1 familial Alzheimer disease mutant does not enhance apoptosis. J Neurosci , 18, 9790-9799.

[20] Byun, Y, Chen, F, Chang, R, Trivedi, M, Green, K. J, & Cryns, V. L. (2001). Caspase cleavage of vimentin disrupts intermediate filaments and promotes apoptosis. Cell Death Differ , 8, 443-450.

[21] Callahan, L. M, Vaules, W. A, & Coleman, P. D. (2002). Progressive reduction of synaptophysin message in single neurons in Alzheimer disease. J Neuropathol Exp Neurol , 61, 384-395.

[22] Caulin, C, Salvesen, G. S, & Oshima, R. G. (1997). Caspase cleavage of keratin 18 and reorganization of intermediate filaments during epithelial cell apoptosis. J Cell Biol , 138, 1379-1394.

[23] Chan, S. L, Furukawa, K, & Mattson, M. P. (2002). Presenilins and APP in neuritic and synaptic plasticity: implications for the pathogenesis of Alzheimer's disease. Neuromolecular Med , 2, 167-196.

[24] Chen, F, Chang, R, Trivedi, M, Capetanaki, Y, & Cryns, V. L. (2003). Caspase proteolysis of desmin produces a dominant-negative inhibitor of intermediate filaments and promotes apoptosis. J Biol Chem , 278, 6848-6853.

[25] Chinnaiyan, A. M, Orth, K, Rourke, O, Duan, K, Poirier, H, & Dixit, G. G. VM ((1996). Molecular ordering of the cell death pathway. Bcl-2 and Bcl-xL function upstream of the CED-3-like apoptotic proteases. J Biol Chem , 271, 4573-4576.

[26] Clem, R. J, Fechheimer, M, & Miller, L. K. (1991). Prevention of apoptosis by a baculovirus gene during infection of insect cells. Science , 254, 1388-1390.

[27] Colle, M. A, Duyckaerts, C, Laquerriere, A, Pradier, L, Czech, C, Checler, F, & Hauw, J. J. (2000). Laminar specific loss of isocortical presenilin 1 immunoreactivity in Alzheimer's disease. Correlations with the amyloid load and the density of tau-positive neurofibrillary tangles. Neuropathol Appl Neurobiol , 26, 117-123.

[28] Columbaro, M, Mattioli, E, Lattanzi, G, Rutigliano, C, Ognibene, A, Maraldi, N. M, & Squarzoni, S. (2001). Staurosporine treatment and serum starvation promote the cleavage of emerin in cultured mouse myoblasts: involvement of a caspase-dependent mechanism. FEBS Lett , 509, 423-429.

[29] Cotman, C. W. (1998). Apoptosis decision cascades and neuronal degeneration in Alzheimer's disease. Neurobiol Aging 19:S, 29-32.

[30] Cotman, C. W, & Su, J. H. (1996). Mechanism of neuronal death in Alzheimer's disease. Brain Pathol , 6, 493-506.

[31] Cregan, S. P, & Fortin, A. MacLaurin JG, Callaghan SM, Cecconi F, Yu SW, Dawson TM, Dawson VL, Park DS, Kroemer G, Slack RS ((2002). Apoptosis-inducing factor is involved in the regulation of caspase-independent neuronal cell death. J Cell Biol , 158, 507-517.

[32] Cregan, S. P. MacLaurin JG, Craig CG, Robertson GS, Nicholson DW, Park DS, Slack RS ((1999). Bax-dependent caspase-3 activation is a key determinant in apoptosis in neurons. J Neurosci 19:7860-7869., 53.

[33] Darmon, A. J, Nicholson, D. W, & Bleackley, R. C. (1995). Activation of the apoptotic protease CPP32 by cytotoxic T-cell-derived granzyme B. Nature , 377, 446-448.

[34] Davies, P, & Maloney, A. J. (1976). Selective loss of central cholinergic neurons in Alzheimer's disease. Lancet 2:1403.

[35] Defigueiredo, R. J, Cummings, B. J, Mundkur, P. Y, & Cotman, C. W. (1995). Color image analysis in neuroanatomical research: application to senile plaque subtype quantification in Alzheimer's disease. Neurobiol Aging , 16, 211-223.

[36] Degli Esposti MDive C ((2003). Mitochondrial membrane permeabilisation by Bax/Bak. Biochem Biophys Res Commun , 304, 455-461.

[37] Desjardins, P, & Ledoux, S. (1998). Expression of ced-3 and ced-9 homologs in Alzheimer's disease cerebral cortex. Neurosci Lett , 244, 69-72.

[38] Deveraux, Q. L, Roy, N, Stennick, H. R, Van Arsdale, T, Zhou, Q, Srinivasula, S. M, Alnemri, E. S, Salvesen, G. S, & Reed, J. C. (1998). IAPs block apoptotic events induced by caspase-8 and cytochrome c by direct inhibition of distinct caspases. EMBO J , 17, 2215-2223.

[39] Dodd, P. R. (2002). Excited to death: different ways to lose your neurones. Biogerontology , 3, 51-56.

[40] Dragunow, M, Faull, R. L, Lawlor, P, Beilharz, E. J, Singleton, K, Walker, E. B, & Mee, E. (1995). In situ evidence for DNA fragmentation in Huntington's disease striatum and Alzheimer's disease temporal lobes. Neuroreport , 6, 1053-1057.

[41] Ekert, P. G, Silke, J, & Vaux, D. L. (1999). Caspase inhibitors. Cell Death Differe , 6, 1081-1086.

[42] Engidawork, E, Gulesserian, T, Yoo, B. C, Cairns, N, & Lubec, G. (2001a). Alteration of caspases and apoptosis-related proteins in brains of patients with Alzheimer's disease. Biochem Biophys Res Commun , 281, 84-93.

[43] Engidawork, E, Gulesserian, T, Yoo, B. C, Cairns, N, & Lubec, G. (2001b). Alternation of caspase- and apoptosis-related proteins in brains of patients with Alzheimer's disease. Biochem Biophys Res Comm , 281, 84-93.

[44] Fernandes-alnemri, T, Litwack, G, & Alnemri, E. S. (1995). Mch2, a new member of the apoptotic Ced-3/Ice cysteine protease gene family. Cancer Res , 55, 2737-2742.

[45] Fernando, P, Kelly, J. F, Balazsi, K, Slack, R. S, & Megeney, L. A. (2002). Caspase 3 activity is required for skeletal muscle differentiation. Proc Natl Acad Sci U S A , 99, 11025-11030.

[46] Francis, P. T, Webster, M. T, Chessell, I. P, Holmes, C, Stratmann, G. C, Procter, A. W, Cross, A. J, Green, A. R, & Bowen, D. M. (1993). Neurotransmitters and second messengers in aging and Alzheimer's disease. Ann N Y Acad Sci , 695, 19-26.

[47] Galande, S, Dickinson, L. A, Mian, I. S, Sikorska, M, & Kohwi-shigematsu, T. (2001). SATB1 cleavage by caspase 6 disrupts PDZ domain-mediated dimerization, causing detachment from chromatin early in T-cell apoptosis. Mol Cell Biol , 21, 5591-5604.

[48] Games, D, Adams, D, Alesandrini, R, Barbour, R, & Berthelette, P. (1995). Alzheimer-type neuropathology in transgenic mice overexpression beta-amyloid precursor protein. Nature 373:523-527., 717F

[49] Garver, T. D, Harris, K. A, Lehman, R. A, Lee, V. M, Trojanowski, J. Q, & Billingsley, M. L. (1994). Tau phosphorylation in human, primate, and rat brain: evidence that a pool of tau is highly phosphorylated in vivo and is rapidly dephosphorylated in vitro. J Neurochem , 63, 2279-2287.

[50] Gervais, F. G, Thornberry, N. A, Ruffolo, S. C, Nicholson, D. W, & Roy, S. (1998). Caspases cleave focal adhesion kinase during apoptosis to generate a FRNK-like polypeptide. J Biol Chem , 273, 17102-17108.

[51] Gervais, FG, Xu, D, Robertson, GS, Vaillancourt, JP, Zhu, Y, & Le, J. H. , Zheng H, van Der Ploeg LHT, Ruffolo SC, Thornberry NS, Xanthoudakis S, Zamboni RJ, Roy S, Nicholson DW (1999) Involvement of caspases in proteolytic cleavage of Alzheimer's amyloid-b precursor protein and amyloidogenic Ab peptide formation. Cell 97:395-406.

[52] Geula, C. (1998). Abnormalities of neural circuitry in Alzheimer's disease: hippocampus and cortical cholinergic innervation. Neurology 51:Sdiscussion S65-17., 18-29.

[53] Glenner, G. G, & Wong, C. W. (1984). Alzheimer's disease: initial report of the purification and characterization of a novel cerebrovascular amyloid protein. biochem Biophys Res Comm , 120, 885-890.

[54] Gold, M. (2002). Tau therapeutics for Alzheimer's disease: the promise and the challenges. J Mol Neurosci , 19, 331-334.

[55] Gomez-isla, T, Growdon, W. B, Mcnamara, M, Newell, K, Gomez-tortosa, E, Hedley-whyte, E. T, & Hyman, B. T. (1999). Clinicopathologic correlates in temporal cortex in dementia with Lewy bodies. Neurology , 53, 2003-2009.

[56] Gomez-isla, T, Hollister, R, West, H, Mui, S, Growdon, J. H, Petersen, R. C, Parisi, J. E, & Hyman, B. T. (1997). Neuronal loss correlates with but exceeds neurofibrillary tangles in Alzheimer's disease. Ann Neurol , 41, 17-24.

[57] Gomez-isla, T, Price, J. L, & Mckeel, D. W. Jr., Morris JC, Growdon JH, Hyman BT ((1996). Profound loss of layer II entorhinal cortex neurons occurs in very mild Alzheimer's disease. J Neurosci , 16, 4491-4500.

[58] Goyal, L. (2001). Cell death inhibition: Keeping caspases in check. Cell 104:805.

[59] Hamos, J. E, Degennaro, L. J, & Drachman, D. A. (1989). Synaptic loss in Alzheimer's disease and other dementias. Neurology , 39, 355-361.

[60] Hardy, J. (2003). The Relationship between Amyloid and Tau. J Mol Neurosci , 20, 203-206.

[61] Harrison, D. C, Davis, R. P, Bond, B. C, Campbell, C. A, James, M. F, Parsons, A. A, & Philpott, K. L. (2001). Caspase mRNA expression in a rat model of focal cerebral ischemia. Brain Res Mol Brain Res , 89, 133-146.

[62] Hartig, W, Klein, C, Brauer, K, Schuppel, K. F, Arendt, T, Bruckner, G, & Bigl, V. (2000). Abnormally phosphorylated protein tau in the cortex of aged individuals of various mammalian orders. Acta Neuropathol (Berl) , 100, 305-312.

[63] Hay, B. A, Wassaman, D. A, & Rubin, G. M. (1995). Drosophila homologs of baculoirus inhibitor of apoptosis proteins function to block cell death. Cell , 83, 1253-1262.

[64] Hengartner, M. O. (2000). The biochemistry of apoptosis. Nature , 407, 770-776.

[65] Hohmann, G. F, Wenk, G. L, Lowenstein, P, Brown, M. E, & Coyle, J. T. (1987). Age-related recurrence of basal forebrain lesion-induced cholinergic deficits. Neurosci Lett , 82, 253-259.

[66] Holcomb, L, Gordon, M. N, Mcgowan, E, Yu, X, & Benkovic, S. (1998). Accelerate Alzheimer-type phenotype in transgenic mice carrying both mutant amyloid precursor protein and presenilin 1 transgenes. Nat Med , 4, 97-100.

[67] Huang, Y, Park, Y. C, Rich, R. L, Segal, D, Myszka, D. G, & Wu, H. (2001). Structural basis of caspase inhibition by XIAP: differential roles of the linker versus the BIR domain. Cell , 104, 781-790.

[68] Irmler, M, Thome, M, Hahne, M, Schneider, P, Hofmann, K, Steiner, V, Bodmer, J. L, Schroter, M, Burns, K, Mattmann, C, Rimoldi, D, French, L. E, & Tschopp, J. (1997). Inhibition of death receptor signals by cellular FLIP. Nature , 388, 190-195.

[69] Janicke, R. U, Ng, P, Sprengart, M. L, & Porter, A. G. (1998). Caspase-3 is required for alpha-fodrin cleavage but dispensable for cleavage of other death substrates in apoptosis. J Biol Chem , 273, 15540-15545.

[70] Jellinger, K. (2002a). Prevalence of Alzheimer's disease in very elderly people: a prospective neuropathological study. Neurology author reply 671-672., 58, 671-672.

[71] Jellinger, K. A. dementia: an update. J Neural Transm Suppl:, 1-23.

[72] Jellinger, K. A. (2002c). Alzheimer disease and cerebrovascular pathology: an update. J Neural Transm , 109, 813-836.

[73] Jellinger, K. A, & Attems, J. (2003). Incidence of cerebrovascular lesions in Alzheimer's disease: a postmortem study. Acta Neuropathol (Berl) , 105, 14-17.

[74] Kanamori, H, Krieg, S, & Mao, C. Di Pippo VA, Wang S, Zajchowski DA, Shapiro DJ ((2000). Proteinase inhibitor 9, an inhibitor of granzyme B-mediated apoptosis, is a primary estrogen-inducible gene in human liver cells. J Biol Chem , 275, 5867-5873.

[75] Keramaris, E, & Stefanis, L. MacLaurin J, Harada N, Takaku K, Ishikawa T, Taketo MM, Robertson GS, Nicholson DW, Slack RS, Park DS ((2000). Involvement of caspase 3 in apoptotic death of cortical neurons evoked by DNA damage. Mol Cell Neurosci , 15, 368-379.

[76] Kerr, J. E, Wyllie, A. H, & Currie, A. R. (1972). Apoptosis: a basic biological phenomenon with wide-ranging implications in tissue kinetics. Br J Cancer , 26, 239-257.

[77] Kim, T. W, Pettingell, W. H, Jung, Y. K, Kovacs, D. M, & Tanzi, R. E. (1997). Alternative cleavage of Alzheimer-associated presenilins during apoptosis by a caspase-3 family protease. Science , 277, 373-376.

[78] Kitamura, Y, Shimohama, S, Kamoshima, W, Matsuoka, Y, Nomura, Y, & Taniguchi, T. (1997). Changes of in the brains of patients with Alzheimer's disease. Biochem Biophys Res Commun 232:418-421., 53.

[79] Kitamura, Y, Shimohama, S, Kamoshima, W, Ota, T, Matsuoka, Y, Nomura, Y, Smith, M. A, Perry, G, Whitehouse, P. J, & Taniguchi, T. (1998). Alteration of proteins regulating apoptosis, Bcl-2, Bcl-x, Bax, Bak, Bad, ICH-1 and CPP32, in Alzheimer's disease. Brain Res , 780, 260-269.

[80] Komiyana, T, Ray, C. A, Pickup, D. J, Howard, A. D, Thornberry, N. A, Peterson, E. P, & Salvesen, G. (1994). Inhibitorion of interleukin-1-Beta converting enzyme by the cowpox virus serpin CrmA-an example of cross-class inhibition. J Biol Chem , 269, 19331-19337.

[81] Koseki, T, Inohara, H, Chen, S, Ez, N, & Are, G. an inhibitor of apoptosis expressed in skeletal muscle and heart that interacts selectively with caspases. Proc Natl Acad Sci USA , 95, 5156-5160.

[82] Kothakota, S, Azuma, T, Reinhard, C, Klippel, A, Tang, J, Chu, K, Mcgarry, T. J, Kirschner, M. W, Koths, K, Kwiatkowski, D. J, & Williams, L. T. (1997). Caspase-3-generated fragment of gelsolin: effector of morphological change in apoptosis. Science , 278, 294-298.

[83] Kuida, K, Lippke, J. A, Ku, G, Harding, M. W, Livingston, D. J, Su, M. S, & Flavell, R. A. (1995). Altered cytokine export and apoptosis in mice deficient in interleukin-1 beta converting enzyme. Science , 267, 2000-2003.

[84] Larson, J, Lynch, G, Games, D, & Seubert, P. (1999). Alterations in synaptic transmission and long-term potentiation in hippocampal slices from young and aged PDAPP mice. Brain Res , 840, 23-35.

[85] Lassmann, H, Bancher, C, Breitschopf, H, Wegiel, J, & Bobinski, M. (1995). Cell death in Alzheimer's disease evaluated by DNA fragmentation in situ. Acta Neuropathol , 89, 35-41.

[86] LeBlanc ALiu H, Goodyer C, Bergeron C, Hammond J ((1999). Caspase-6 role in apoptosis of human neurons, amyloidogenesis, and Alzheimer's disease. J Biol Chem , 274, 23426-23436.

[87] Lee VMYBalin BJ, Otvos LJ, Trojanowski JQ ((1991). A68: a major subunit of paired helical filaments and derivatized forms of normal tau. Science , 251, 675-678.

[88] Li, H, & Yuan, J. (1999). Deciphering the pathways of life and death. Curr Opin Cell Biol , 11, 261-266.

[89] Li, W. P, Chan, W. Y, Lai, H. W, & Yew, D. T. (1997). Terminal dUTP nick end labeling (TUNEL) positive cells in the different regions of the brain in normal aging and Alzheimer patients. J Mol Neurosci , 8, 75-82.

[90] Lippa, C. F, Hamos, J. E, Pulaski-salo, D, Degennaro, L. J, & Drachman, D. A. (1992). Alzheimer's disease and aging: effects on perforant pathway perikarya and synapses. Neurobiol Aging , 13, 405-411.

[91] Lu, D. C, Rabizadeh, S, Chandra, S, Shayya, R. F, Ellerby, L. M, Ye, X, Salvesen, G. S, Koo, E. H, & Bredesen, D. E. (2000). A second cytotoxic proteolytic peptide derived from amyloid b-protein precursor. Nature Med , 6, 397-404.

[92] Lucassen, P. J, Chung, W. C, Kamphorst, W, & Swaab, D. F. (1997). DNA damage distribution in the human brain as shown by in situ end labeling; area-specific differences in aging and Alzheimer disease in the absence of apoptotic morphology. J Neurophathol Exp Neuorl , 56, 887-900.

[93] MacGibbon GALawlor PA, Sirimanne ES, Walton MR, Connor B, Young D, Williams C, Gluckman P, Faull RL, Hughes P, Dragunow M ((1997). Bax expression in mammalian neurons undergoing apoptosis, and in Alzheimer's disease hippocampus. Brain Res , 750, 223-234.

[94] Martin, S. J, Finucane, D. M, Amarante-mendes, G. P, Brien, O, & Green, G. A. DR ((1996). Phosphatidylserine externalization during CD95-induced apoptosis of cells and cytoplasts requires ICE/CED-3 protease activity. J Biol Chem , 271, 28753-28756.

[95] Masliah, E. (2001). Recent advances in the understanding of the role of synaptic proteins in Alzheimer's Disease and other neurodegenerative disorders. J Alzheimers Dis , 3, 121-129.

[96] Masliah, E, Mallory, M, Alford, M, Deteresa, R, Hansen, L. A, & Mckeel, D. W. Jr., Morris JC ((2001). Altered expression of synaptic proteins occurs early during progression of Alzheimer's disease. Neurology , 56, 127-129.

[97] Masliah, E, Mallory, M, Alford, M, Tanaka, S, & Hansen, L. A. (1998). Caspase dependent DNA fragmentation might be associated with excitotoxicity in Alzheimer disease. J Neuropathol Exp Neurol , 57, 1041-1052.

[98] Masliah, E, Terry, R. D, Deteresa, R. M, & Hansen, L. A. (1989). Immunohistochemical quantification of the synapse-related protein synaptophysin in Alzheimer disease. Neurosci Lett , 103, 234-239.

[99] Masters, C. L, Simms, G, Weinman, N. A, Multhaup, G, Mcdonald, B. L, & Beyreuther, K. (1985). Amyloid plaque core protein in Alzheimer disease and Down syndrome. Proc Natl Acad Sci USA , 82, 4245-4249.

[100] Mccarthy, N. J, Whyte, M. K, Gilbert, C. S, & Evan, G. I. (1997). Inhibition of Ced-3/ICE-related proteases does not prevent cell death induced by oncogenes, DNA damage, or the Bcl-2 homologue Bak. J Cell Biol , 136, 215-227.

[101] Mckhann, G, Drachman, D, Folstein, M, Katzman, R, Price, D. L, & Stadlan, E. M. (1984). Clinical diagnosis of Alzheimer's disease: report of the NINCDS-ADRDA Work Group under the auspices of Department of Health and Human Services Task Force on Alzheimer's disease. Neurology , 34, 939-944.

[102] Mesulam, M. M. (1986). Alzheimer plaques and cortical cholinergic innervation. Neuroscience , 17, 275-276.

[103] Michaelis, M. L, Dobrowsky, R. T, & Li, G. (2002). Tau neurofibrillary pathology and microtubule stability. J Mol Neurosci , 19, 289-293.

[104] Miller, L. K. (1997). Baculovirus interaction with host apoptotic pathways. J Cell Physiol , 173, 178-182.

[105] Mori, H, Takio, k, Ogawara, M, & Selkie, D. (1992). Mass spectrometry of purified amyloid b protein in Alzheimer's disease. J Biol Chem , 267, 17082-17086.

[106] Morris, J. C. McKeel DWJ, Storandt M, Rubin EH, Price JL, Grant EA, Ball MJ, Berg L ((1991). Very mild Alzheimer's disease: informant-based clinical, psychometric, and pathologic distinction from normal aging. Neurology , 41, 469-478.

[107] Muzio, M, Chinnaiyan, A. M, Kischkel, F. C, Rourke, O, Shevchenko, K, Ni, A, Scaffidi, J, Bretz, C, Zhang, J. D, Gentz, M, Mann, R, Krammer, M, Peter, P. H, Dixit, M. E, & Flice, V. M. a novel FADD-homologous ICE/CED-3-like protease, is recruited to the CD95 (Fas/APO-1) death-inducing signaling complex. Cell , 85, 817-827.

[108] Nicholson, D. W. (1999). Caspase structure, proteilytic substrates, and function during apoptotic cell death. Cell Death Differe , 6, 1028-1042.

[109] Nijhawan, D, Honarpour, N, & Wang, X. (2000). Apoptosis in neural development and disease. Annu Rev Neurosci , 23, 73-87.

[110] Nyormoi, O, Wang, Z, Doan, D, Ruiz, M, Mcconkey, D, & Bar-eli, M. (2001). Transcription factor AP-2alpha is preferentially cleaved by caspase 6 and degraded by proteasome during tumor necrosis factor alpha-induced apoptosis in breast cancer cells. Mol Cell Biol , 21, 4856-4867.

[111] Orth, K, Rourke, O, Salvesen, K, & Dixit, G. S. VM ((1996). Molecular ordering of apoptotic mammalian CED-3/ICE-like proteases. J Biol Chem , 271, 20977-20980.

[112] Paradis, E, Douillard, H, Koutroumanis, M, & Goodyer, C. LeBlanc A ((1996). Amyloid beta peptide of Alzheimer's disease downregulates Bcl-2 and upregulates bax expression in human neurons. J Neurosci , 16, 7533-7539.

[113] Pearson, R. C, & Powell, T. P. (1987). Anterograde vs. retrograde degeneration of the nucleus basalis medialis in Alzheimer's disease. J Neural Transm Suppl , 24, 139-146.

[114] Pellegrini, L, Passer, B. J, Tabaton, M, Ganjei, J. K, Adamio, D, & Alternative, L. nonsecretase processing of Alzheimer's b-amyloid precursor protein during apoptosis by caspase-6 and-8. J Biol Chem , 274, 21011-21016.

[115] Price, D. L, & Sisodia, S. S. (1998). Mutant genes in familial Alzheimer's disease and transgenic models. Annu Reve Neurosci , 21, 479-505.

[116] Price, J. L, & Mckeel, D. W. Jr., Morris JC ((2001). Synaptic loss and pathological change in older adults--aging versus disease? Neurobiol Aging , 22, 351-352.

[117] Ray, C. A, Black, R. A, Kronheim, S. R, Greensheet, T. A, Sleath, P. R, Salvesen, G. S, & Pickup, D. J. (1992). Viral inhibition of inflammation: cowpox virus encodes an inhibitor of the interleukin-1 beta converting enzyme. Cell , 69, 597-604.

[118] Riedl, S. J, Renatus, M, Schwarzenbacher, R, Zhou, Q, Sun, C, Fesik, S. W, Liddington, R. C, & Salvesen, G. S. (2001). Structural basis for the inhibition of caspase-3 by XIAP. Cell , 104, 791-800.

[119] Roder, H. (2003). Prospect of therapeutic approaches to tauopathies. J Mol Neurosci , 20, 195-202.

[120] Roher, A, Lowenson, J, Clarke, S, Woods, S, Cotter, R, Gowing, E, & Ball, M. J. (1993). beta-Amyloid-(1-42) is a major component of cerebrovascular amyloid deposits: implications for the pathology of Alzheimer's disease. Proc Natl Acad Sci USA , 90, 10836-10840.

[121] Rohn, T. T, Head, E, Nesse, W. H, Cotman, C. W, & Cribbs, D. H. (2001). Activation of caspase-8 in the Alzheimer's disease brain. Neurobiol Dis , 8, 1006-1016.

[122] Rohn, T. T, Rissman, R. A, Davis, M. C, Kim, Y. E, Cotman, C. W, & Head, E. (2002). Caspase-9 activation and caspase cleavage of tau in the Alzheimer's disease brain. Neurobiol Dis , 11, 341-354.

[123] Roth, K. A. (2001). Caspases, apoptosis, and Alzheimer disease: Causation, correlation, and confusion. J Neuropathol Exp Neurol , 60, 829-838.

[124] Ruchaud, S, Korfali, N, Villa, P, Kottke, T. J, Dingwall, C, Kaufmann, S. H, & Earnshaw, W. C. (2002). Caspase-6 gene disruption reveals a requirement for lamin A cleavage in apoptotic chromatin condensation. Embo J , 21, 1967-1977.

[125] Sakahira, H, Enari, M, & Nagata, S. (1998). Cleavage of CAD inhibitor in CAD activation and DNA degradation during apoptosis. Nature , 391, 96-99.

[126] Samejima, K, Svingen, P. A, Basi, G. S, Kottke, T, & Mesner, P. W. Jr., Stewart L, Durrieu F, Poirier GG, Alnemri ES, Champoux JJ, Kaufmann SH, Earnshaw WC ((1999). Caspase-mediated cleavage of DNA topoisomerase I at unconventional sites during apoptosis. J Biol Chem , 274, 4335-4340.

[127] Scheff, S. W, & Price, D. A. (2001). Alzheimer's disease-related synapse loss in the cingulate cortex. J Alzheimers Dis , 3, 495-505.

[128] Scheff, S. W, Price, D. A, & Sparks, D. L. (2001). Quantitative assessment of possible age-related change in synaptic numbers in the human frontal cortex. Neurobiol Aging , 22, 355-365.

[129] Schotte, P, Declercq, W, Van Huffel, S, Vandenabeele, P, & Beyaert, R. (1999). Non-specific effects of methyl ketone peptide inhibitors of caspases. FEBS Lett , 442, 117-121.

[130] Schwartz, L. M, & Milligan, C. E. (1996). Cold thoughts of death : the role of ICE proteases in neuronal cell death. Trends Neurosci , 19, 555-562.

[131] Selkoe, D. J. (2002). Alzheimer's disease is a synaptic failure. Science , 298, 789-791.

[132] Selznick, L. A, Holtzman, D. M, Han, B. H, Gokden, M, & Srinivassan, A. N. Johnson EMJ, Roth KA ((1999). In situ immunodetection of neuronal caspase-3 activation in Alzheimer disease. J Neurophathol Exp Neurol , 58, 1020-1026.

[133] Simpson, M. T. MacLaurin JG, Xu D, Ferguson KL, Vanderluit JL, Davoli MA, Roy S, Nicholson DW, Robertson GS, Park DS, Slack RS ((2001). Caspase 3 deficiency rescues peripheral nervous system defect in retinoblastoma nullizygous mice. J Neurosci , 21, 7089-7098.

[134] Slee, E. A, Adrain, C, & Martin, S. J. (2001). Executioner caspase-3,-6, and-7 perform distinct, non-redundant roles during the demolition phase of apoptosis. J Biol Chem , 276, 7320-7326.

[135] Smale, G, Nichols, N. R, Brady, D. R, & Finch, C. E. Horton WEJ ((1995). Evidence for apoptotic cell death in Alzheimer's disease. Exp Neurol , 133, 225-230.

[136] Srinivasula, S. M, Hegde, R, Saleh, A, Datta, P, Shiozaki, E, Chai, J, Lee, R. A, Robbins, P. D, Fernandes-alnemri, T, Shi, Y, & Alnemri, E. S. (2001). A conserved XIAP-interaction motif in caspase-9 and Smac/DIABLO regulates caspase activity and apoptosis. Nature , 410, 112-116.

[137] Stadelmann, C, Br, k W, Bancher, C, Jellinger, K, & Lassmann, H. (1998). Alzheimer disease: DNA fragmentation indicates increased neuronal vulnerability, but not apoptosis. J Neuropathol Exp Neurol , 57, 456-464.

[138] Stadelmann, C, Deckwerth, T, Srinivasan, A, Bancher, C, Br, k W, Jellinger, K, & Lassmann, H. (1999). Activation of caspase-3 in single neurons and autophagic granules of granulovacuolar degeneration in Alzheimer's disease. Am J Path , 155, 1459-1466.

[139] Stennicke, H. R, Ryan, C. A, & Salvesen, G. S. (2002). Reprieval from execution: the molecular basis of caspase inhibition. Trends Biochem Sci , 27, 94-101.

[140] Stephan, A, Laroche, S, & Davis, S. (2001). Generation of aggregated beta-amyloid in the rat hippocampus impairs synaptic transmission and plasticity and causes memory deficits. J Neurosci , 21, 5703-5714.

[141] Strasser, A, Connor, O, & Dixit, L. Apoptosis signaling. Annu Rev Biochem 69:217-245., 2000

[142] Su, J. H, Anderson, A. J, Cummings, B. J, & Cotman, C. W. (1994). Immunohistochemical evidence for apoptosis in Alzheimer's disease. Neuroreport , 5, 2529-2533.

[143] Su, J. H, Deng, G, & Cotman, C. W. (1997). Bax protein expression is increased in Alzheimer's brain: correlations with DNA damage, Bcl-2 expression, and brain pathology. J NeuropatholExp Neurol , 56, 86-93.

[144] Su, J. H, Satou, T, Anderson, A. J, & Cotman, C. W. (1996). Up-regulation of Bcl-2 is associated with neuronal DNA damage in Alzheimer's disease. Neuroreport , 7, 437-440.

[145] Takeuchi, A, Irizarry, M. C, & Duff, K. (2000). Age-related amyloid beta deposition in transgenic mice overexpressing both Alzheimer mutant presenilin 1 and amyloid beta precursor protein Swedish mutant is not associated with global neuronal loss. Am J Path , 157, 331-339.

[146] Terry, R. D. (2000). Cell death or synaptic loss in Alzheimer disease. J Neuropathol Exp Neurol , 59, 1118-1119.

[147] Terry, R. D, Masliah, E, & Salmon, D. P. (1991). Physical basis of cognitive alterations in Alzheimer's disease: Synaptic loss is a major correlate of cognitive impairment. Ann Neurol , 30, 572-580.

[148] Thome, M, Schneider, P, Hofmann, K, Fickenscher, H, Meinl, E, Neipel, F, Mattmann, C, Burns, K, Bodmer, J. L, Schroter, M, Scaffidi, C, Karammer, P. H, Peter, M. E, & Tachopp, J. (1997). Viral FLICE-inhibitory proteins (FLIPs) prevent apoptosis induced by death receptors. Nature , 386, 517-521.

[149] Thompson, C. S. (1995). Apoptosis in the pathogenesis and treatment of disease. Science , 2667, 1456-1462.

[150] Thornberry, N. A. (1997). The caspase family of cysteine proteases. Br Med Bull , 53, 478-490.

[151] Torp, R, Su, J. H, Deng, G, & Cotman, C. W. (1998). GADD45 is induced in Alzheimer's disease, and protects against apoptosis in vitro. Neurobiol Dis , 5, 245-252.

[152] Tortosa, A, Lopez, E, & Ferrer, I. (1998). Bcl-2 and Bax protein expression in Alzheimer's disease. Acta Neuropathol (Berl) , 95, 407-412.

[153] Troncoso, J. C, Sukhov, R. R, Kawas, C. H, & Koliatsos, V. E. (1996). In situ labeling of dying cortical neurons in normal aging and in Alzheimer's disease: correlations with senile plaques and disease progression. J Nuropathol Exp Neurol , 55, 1134-1142.

[154] Tseng, B. P, Esler, W. P, Clish, C. B, Stimson, E. R, Ghilardi, J. R, Vinters, H. V, Mantyh, P. W, Lee, J. P, & Maggio, J. E. (1999). Deposition of monomeric, not oligomeric, Abeta mediates growth of Alzheimer's disease amyloid plaques in human brain preparations. Biochemistry , 38, 10424-10431.

[155] Urbanc, B, Cruz, L, Buldyrev, S. V, Havlin, S, Irizarry, M. C, Stanley, H. E, & Hyman, B. T. (1999). Dynamics of plaque formation in Alzheimer's disease. Biophys J , 76, 1330-1334.

[156] Van de Craen MBerx G, Van den Brande I, Fiers W, Declercq W, Vandenabeele Proteolytic cleavage of beta-catenin by caspases: an in vitro analysis. FEBS Lett 458:167-170., 1999.

[157] Vanags, D. M, Porn-ares, M. I, Coppola, S, Burgess, D. H, & Orrenius, S. (1996). Protease involvement in fodrin cleavage and phosphatidylserine exposure in apoptosis. J Biol Chem , 271, 31075-31085.

[158] Vucic, D, Kaiser, W. J, Harvey, A. J, & Miller, L. K. (1997). Inhibition of reaper-induced apoptosis by interaction with inhibitor of apoptosis proteins (IAPs). Proc Natl Acd Sci USA , 94, 10183-10188.

[159] Vucic, D, Kaiser, W. J, & Miller, L. K. (1998). Inhibitor of apoptosis proteins physically interact with and block apoptosis induced by Drosophila proteins hid and grim. Mol Cell Biol , 18, 3300-3309.

[160] Weidemann, A, Paliga, K, Drwang, U, Reinhard, F. B, Schuckert, O, Evin, G, & Masters, C. L. (1999). Proteolytic processing of the Alzheimer/s disease amyloid precursor protein within its cytoplasmic domain by caspase-like proteases. J Biol Chem , 274, 5823-5829.

[161] Weinstock, M. (1997). Possible role of the cholinergic system and disease models. J Neural Transm Suppl , 49, 93-102.

[162] Whitehouse, P. J, Price, D. L, Clark, A. W, Coyle, J. T, & Delong, M. R. (1981). Alzheimer disease: evidence for selective loss of cholinergic neurons in the nucleus basalis. Ann Neurol , 10, 122-126.

[163] Whitehouse, P. J, Price, D. L, Struble, R. G, Clark, A. W, Coyle, J. T, & Delon, M. R. (1982). Alzheimer's disease and senile dementia: loss of neurons in the basal forebrain. Science , 215, 1237-1239.

[164] Yamatsuji, T, Okamoto, T, Takeda, S, Murayama, Y, Tanaka, N, & Nishinoto, I. (1996). Expression of APP mutant causes cellular apoptosis as Alzheimer trait-linked phenotype. EMBO J 15:498-509., 642

[165] Yao, P. J, Morsch, R, Callahan, L. M, & Coleman, P. D. (1999). Changes in synaptic expression of clathrin assembly protein AP180 in Alzheimer's disease analysed by immunohistochemistry. Neuroscience , 94, 389-394.

[166] Yuan, J, Shaham, S, Ledoux, S, Ellis, H. M, & Horvitz, H. R. Elegans cell death gene ced-3 encodes a protein similar to mammalian interleukin-1beta-converting enzyme. Cell , 75, 641-652.

[167] Yuan, J, & Yankner, B. A. (2000). Apoptosis in the nervous system. Nature , 407, 802-809.

[168] Zhang, Y, & Goodyer, C. LeBlanc A ((2000). Selective and protracted apoptosis in human primary neurons microinjected with active caspase-3,-6,-7, and-8. J Neurosci , 20, 8384-8389.

[169] Zheng, T. S, Hunot, S, Kuida, K, & Flavell, R. A. (1999). Caspase knockouts: matters of life and death. Cell Death Differe , 6, 1043-1053.

[170] Zhou, Q, Krebs, J. F, Snipas, S. J, Price, A, Alnemri, E. S, Tomaselli, K. J, & Salvesen, G. S. (1998). Interaction of the baculovirus anti-apoptotic protein with caspase-specificity, kinetics, and characterization of the caspase/p35 complex. Biochemistry 37:10757-10765., 35.

Chapter 7

Brain Reserve Regulators in Alzheimer's Disease

Ivana Delalle

Additional information is available at the end of the chapter

http://dx.doi.org/10.5772/53658

1. Introduction

Brain reserve refers to the ability of the brain to tolerate pathological changes such as those seen in AD before manifesting clinical signs and symptoms [1-3]. Neurotrophic factors (NTFs), most notably Brain Derived Neurotrophic Factor (BDNF) and its receptor Tyrosine kinase B (TrkB), regulate synaptic plasticity and functional efficiency in adulthood [4-6] and thus may influence brain reserve. BDNF/TrkB signaling affects memory formation and retention [7,8], determines neurite length [9,10], and governs regeneration upon neuronal injury [11,12] by modifying neuronal cytoskeleton. Abnormalities in the neuronal cytoskeleton are well documented in AD. However, how these abnormalities affect AD progression remains unclear. In *Drosophila*, neurodegeneration stems directly from mutations in alpha and beta subunits of the actin capping protein (CP), demonstrating that a mutation in a gene encoding an actin cytoskeleton regulator can lead to demise of neurons [13]. Further, a causative role for actin cytoskeleton abnormalities in neurotoxicity has been documented in a *Drosophila* tauopathy model [14].

Important evidence that cytoskeletal abnormalities are critically involved in the pathogenesis of neurodegeneration stems from the studies demonstrating the effect of apolipoprotein E isoform ε4 (ApoE ε4), the well-documented genetic risk factor for the most common form of AD, late-onset AD [15], on neuronal cytoskeleton. In the United States, the ApoE ε4 allele occurs in 60% of AD patients. ApoE ε4 inhibits neurite outgrowth in cultured neuronal cells [16] and correlates with the simplification of dendritic branching patterns in the brains of AD patients [17]. ApoE ε4 dose inversely correlates with dendritic spine density in dentate gyrus neurons of both AD and aged normal controls [18]. Overexpression and neuron-specific proteolytic cleavage of ApoE ε4 result in tau hyperphosphorylation in neurons of transgenic mice, suggesting a role of ApoE ε4 in cytoskeletal destabilization and the development of AD-related neuronal deficits [19,20]. Humanized ApoE ε4 knock-in homozygous transgenic mice exhibit cognitive deficits before the onset of age-dependent neuropathology including AD-associated neurofibrillary tangles and neuritic plaques [21,22].

While the relationships between BDNF gene polymorphisms and AD are not yet fully understood [23-25], there is compelling evidence that epigenetic regulation connects BDNF/TrkB signaling with learning and memory. Exercise restored TrkB in ApoE ε4 mice to the level observed in ε3 mice and increased synaptophysin (a marker of synaptic function) in ε4 mice; hippocampal BDNF levels were similarly increased in both ε3 and ε4 mice after exercise [26]. Exposure to an enriched environment for three to four weeks also caused dramatic increase in BDNF mRNA in mouse hippocampus [27]. Understanding the regulation of BDNF/TrkB signaling in AD pathogenesis, particularly in individuals carrying ApoE ε4, could be of great clinical and public health importance because BDNF is inducible and may be one of the key molecules mediating the beneficial effect of certain lifestyle measures (environmental enrichment, increased aerobic physical activity, lower caloric intake) [28-30] on the risk of developing dementia.

2. Neuronal cytoskeleton regulator actin capping protein ß2 (Capzb2) and BDNF/TrkB signaling

As hyperphosphorylated tau gives rise to neurofibrillary tangles in AD, dystrophic neurites, marked by reduced length and poor branching, become apparent. In parallel, perisomatic proliferation of dendrites and sprouting of distal dystrophic neurites take place[31]. These morphological changes in neurons during AD progression indicate major cytoskeletal reorganization raising the possibility that microtubules and microfilaments may represent a target for pathobiological mechanisms underlying AD. The presence of growth cone-like structures on distal ends of dystrophic neurites suggests that regenerative response accompanies cytoskeleton degeneration in AD [31].

Changes in growth cone morphology, motility, and direction of growth are controlled by interactions between F-actin and microtubules and their associated proteins [32]. The growth cone morphology is characterized by lamellipodia, which are the veil-like extensions at the periphery, and filopodia, which are narrow, spiky extensions coming from the periphery of the growth cone. Interestingly, APP concentrates in lamellipodia where it is proposed to play a role in growth cone motility and neurite outgrowth [33]. Upon acute neuronal injury, the first critical steps that initiate regenerative response are microtubule polymerization and F-actin cytoskeleton rearrangement leading to the formation of a motile growth cone [34]. Actin cytoskeleton regulator CP (F-actin capping protein, CapZ) is an α/β heterodimer that binds the barbed end of F-actin thus blocking the access of actin monomers to the fast growing end. Both mammalian and *Drosophila* CP subunits play a critical role in the organization and dynamics of lamellipodia and filopodia in non-neuronal cells [35]. One of the mammalian β-subunit isoforms, Capzb2, is predominantly expressed in the brain [36]. Capzb2 not only caps F-actin barbed end but also binds βIII-tubulin directly, affecting the rate and the extent of microtubule polymerization in the presence of tau [37]. Moreover,

Capzb2 - βIII-tubulin interaction is indispensable for normal growth cone morphology and neurite length (Figure 1) [37].

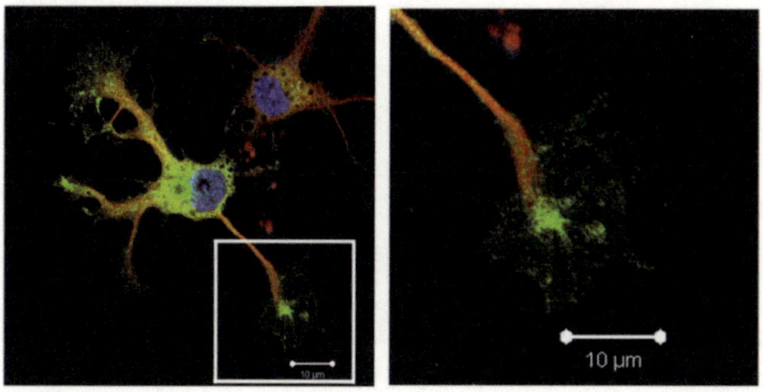

Figure 1. [37]: Capzb2-EGFP (green) expression in mouse hippocampal neurons. In addition to soma and processes, Capzb2 is expressed in growth cones (red- ß-tubulin, blue- nuclei).

Interestingly, the interaction between actin capping protein and ß-tubulin has been uncovered in a mass spectrometry screen for the alterations in protein-target binding *in vivo* in response to spatial learning [38], a process that requires BDNF [39].

In line with the previously documented increased cytoskeletal reorganization including dendritic proliferation and sprouting in neurons of AD patients [40,41,31], we recently demonstrated increased expression of Capzb2 (Figure 2) and TrkB in mid-stages (Braak and Braak III-IV, BBIII-IV) AD pathology[42].

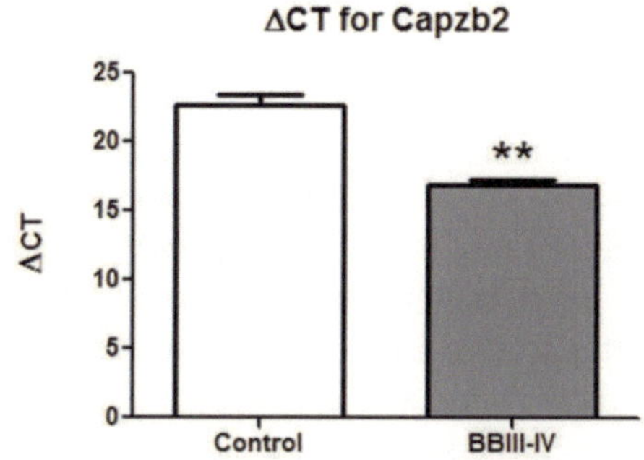

Figure 2. [42]: Hippocampal pyramidal neurons from a control case contain less Capzb2 mRNA (higher ΔCT) than the neurons from Braak and Braak III-IV AD cases (**$p<0.01$, Student's t test).

BDNF binding to the TrkB receptor initiates intracellular cascades involving cell survival, growth, and differentiation via mitogen-activated protein kinase (MAPK), phosphatidylinositol 3-kinase (PI3K), and phospholipase C-g (PLCγ) signaling pathways, as recently reviewed [43]. PI3K and MAPK simultaneous triggering alters both actin and microtubule dynamics needed for dendrite branching [43]. BDNF has been shown to promote growth of undifferentiated dendrites and axons in cultured hippocampal pyramidal neurons [44], a process that requires Capzb2 [37]. Thus, the expression of Capzb2 may represent one of the likely downstream read-outs for BDNF-TrkB neuronal signaling. In a rat model of dementia there is activity-dependent, synapse-specific regulation of CapZ redistribution possibly important in both maintenance and remodeling of synaptic connections receiving spatial and temporal patterns of inputs [45].

3. Increased expression of TrkB and Capzb2 accompanies preserved cognitive status in early AD pathology

Recent study compared mRNA (Figure 3) and protein (Figure 4) expression of BDNF, TrkB and Capzb2 in samples of neuropathologically normal and cognitively intact subjects (controls), with samples of persons with AD-related pathological changes who were cognitively intact prior to death (Clinical Dementia Rating zero, CDR0), and samples of persons with AD-related pathological changes as well as early clinical dementia (CDR0.5 – 1) [46]. This approach was possible due to the existence of a unique sample of Framingham Heart Study (FHS) participants who have undergone repeated antemortem cognitive testing and brain imaging [47,48]. All FHS participants in the FHS have undergone screening cognitive tests (an MMSE) once in two years and have also had a more detailed cognitive assessment examining multiple cognitive domains once in 1974-75, once in 1999-2004 and at least twice thereafter. The presence or absence of dementia in all FHS participants is defined using DSM-IV criteria that require impairment in memory and in at least one other area of cognitive function, as well as documented functional disability. AD is defined using NINCDS-ADRDA criteria for definite, probable or possible AD[49]. All FHS participants are invited to become brain donors and the nearly 700 persons who have accepted this invitation undergo a detailed neuropsychological testing [50,51], at least once every 2 years beyond age 75 years. Persons who screen positive or are otherwise referred (by self, family or treating physicians) undergo detailed neurological and neuropsychological assessment, informant interview (with a physician administered CDR) and a review of hospital records, nursing home notes, brain imaging and laboratory tests. A structured family interview (including Blessed Dementia and Hachinski scales) [52,53] is conducted with the next-of-kin based on which a retrospective CDR score is assigned after the participant dies. The retrospective CDR is very similar to the retrospective collateral dementia interview validated by Davis and colleagues (1991)[54]. A final clinical decision regarding the presence or absence of dementia, diagnosis of dementia type and date of onset/diagnosis is made by a clinical consensus panel including behavioral neurologists and neuropsychologists who review all available records including records at the time of death. All deaths are reviewed to assign a cause of death and to determine if dementia was present or absent at the time of death. The neuropathological report is generated prior to a final clinico-pathological conference during which the clinical diagnoses and pathological findings are discussed.

Hippocampi from selected FHS cases were used to determine whether specifically vulnerable population of CA1 neurons shows a compensatory response to the neuropathological changes of Alzheimer Disease (AD) and whether that response depends on an up-regulation of the BDNF pathway. The expression of TrkB and Capzb2 in CA1 hippocampal neurons of individuals with preserved cognitive status (CDR 0) and initial neurofibrillary tangle formation was increased in comparison to cognitively intact individuals without any neurofibrillary tangles (Figure 3) [46]. In contrast, BDNF expression remained unchanged, raising the possibility that the up-regulated TrkB expression in CDR0 individuals is responsible for the increase in BDNF/TrkB signaling tapping the brain reserve (Figure 3) [46]. In the group of individuals with more advanced tangle formation and early to mild dementia (CDR 0.5-1), the increase in TrkB expression and the unchanged expression of BDNF might have been insufficient to provide adequate brain reserve (Figure 3) [46].

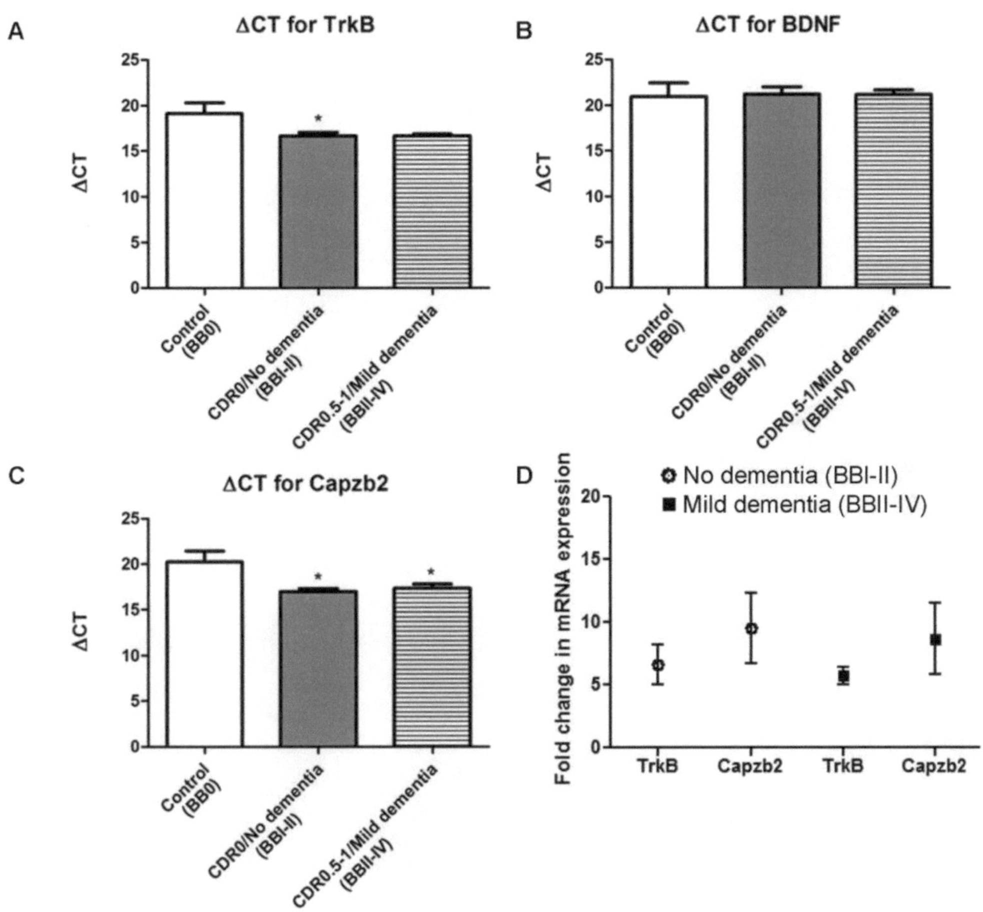

Figure 3. [46]: TrkB, BDNF, and Capzb2 mRNAs expression in control, CDR 0 (no dementia) and CDR 0.5-1 (mild dementia) subjects. TrkB mRNA expression is significantly increased (lower ΔCT) in subjects with early AD pathology (BBI-II) but no dementia (A). BDNF mRNA expression is similar in all groups examined (B). Capzb2 mRNA is significantly increased (lower ΔCT) in cases with AD pathology (C). Fold-increases of mean mRNA expression of TrkB and Capzb2 in cases with AD pathology in comparison to controls (D).

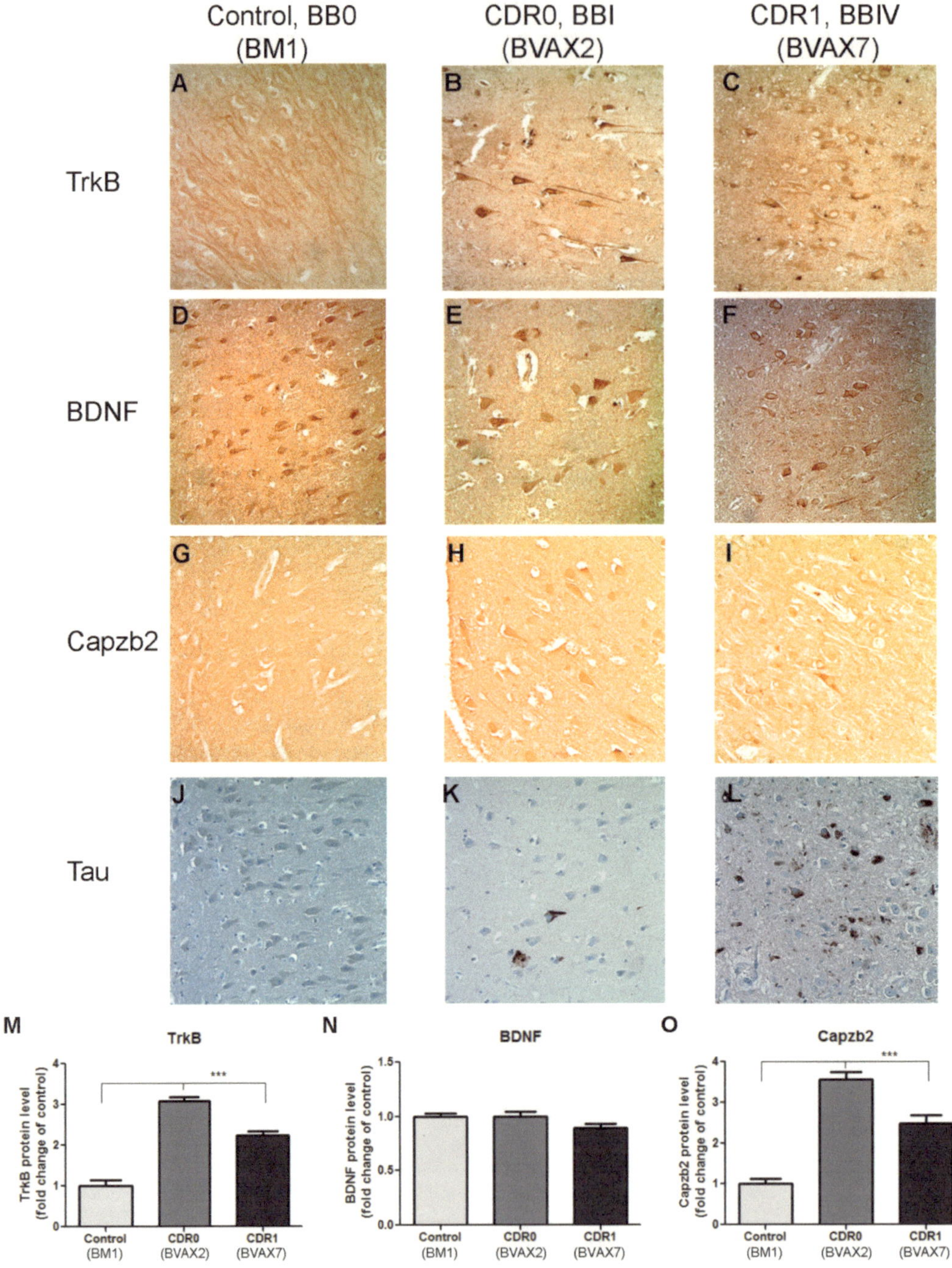

Figure 4. [46]: Immunohistochemistry for TrkB (A-C), BDNF (D-F), and Capzb2 (G-I) in representative individuals from control, CDR0, and CDR1 groups reflects established trends in mRNA expression. Immunohistochemistry for tau highlights intensity of neurofibrillary changes in a CDR0 subject (K) and in a CDR1 subject (L), while the control is free of neuropathology (J).

In light of the reported restoration of learning and memory functions in AD animal models upon BDNF gene delivery [55], exogenous intervention to boost BDNF/TrkB signaling might appear a compelling therapy in early AD. However, the experiments by Frank et al. (1996) suggest that the exposure of developing and adult rodent hippocampal neurons to BDNF *in vitro* and *in vivo* results in long-term functional desensitization to BDNF and down regulation of TrkB mRNA [56]. It is possible that BDNF/TrkB signaling is differentially regulated in healthy vs. diseased hippocampal neurons. Nevertheless, the reported increase in TrkB mRNA expression in astrocytes occasionally associated with senile plaques in hippocampi of AD brains raises concerns that the administration of neurotrophic factors could promote gliosis and plaque formation [57]. Importantly, if the observed increase in TrkB expression in cognitively intact FHS subjects with initial formation of neurofibrillary tangles constitutes brain reserve, down regulation of TrkB might represent a potentially harmful side-effect of exogenous BDNF delivery.

4. Conclusion

One in five persons currently 65 years old will develop clinical Alzheimer's dementia in their lifetime. However, postponing the onset of clinical disease by as little as five years could halve individual risk and population burden of disease [58,59]. Since the timing of clinical dementia onset is determined not only by the pace of pathological changes but also by brain reserve, that postponement might be possible. The study of CA1 hippocampal neurons in FHS participant brain donors[46] adds to the emerging evidence that the BDNF/TrkB pathway may be involved in the compensatory response to early AD pathology, i.e. it may underlie the biology of cognitive reserve. Consequently, an epigenetic enhancement of BDNF/TrkB signaling in persons with early cognitive changes associated with AD pathology (mild cognitive impairment, MCI, due to AD pathology)[60] and in persons with no clinical symptoms but with biomarker evidence of AD pathology (so-called preMCI due to AD pathology) [61] may be beneficial in delaying the onset of clinical dementia. The lifestyle modifications that are thought to reduce the risk of developing clinical AD, such as intake of docosahexaenoic acid (DHA) and increased exercise, appear to interact with BDNF-related synaptic plasticity[62]. As reviewed by Sananbenesi and Fischer (2009)[63], deregulation of "plasticity genes", in particular synaptic plasticity genes, accompanies aging, a major risk for AD. Histone deacetylase inhibitors (HDACs) and environmental enrichment have been shown to reinstate learning behavior and improve memory in a CK-p25 mouse model of neurodegeneration[64], whereas altered histone acetylation is associated with age-dependent memory impairment in mice[65]. These findings make deciphering of epigenetic signatures in preserved vs. failing human cognitive functions urgent and necessary for the development of rational interventions in the progression of AD [66,67]. The prevention of clinical AD will likely require a multi-dimensional approach and the modulation of the BDNF/TrkB pathway, calibrated to each individual's needs, might be one facet of this multi-dimensional approach.

Summary

During the progression of Alzheimer's disease (AD), hippocampal neurons show degenerative as well as regenerative changes, possibly influenced by genes that may modify brain reserve, the ability of the brain to tolerate pathological changes in AD before manifesting clinical signs and symptoms. Recent data suggest that the expression of these genes in the hippocampal neurons correlates with the cognitive function. Identifying molecules that may promote regenerative potential and/or increase brain reserve provides novel targets for interventions in late-onset AD.

Author details

Ivana Delalle

Department of Pathology and Laboratory Medicine, Boston University School of Medicine, Boston, USA

References

[1] Valenzuela, M. J, & Sachdev, P. (2006). Brain reserve and cognitive decline: a non-parametric systematic review. Psychol Med , 36, 1065-1073.

[2] Riley, K. P, Snowdon, D. A, Desrosiers, M. F, & Markesbery, W. R. (2005). Early life linguistic ability, late life cognitive function, and neuropathology: findings from the Nun Study. Neurobiol Aging , 26, 341-347.

[3] Snowdon, D. A, Kemper, S. J, Mortimer, J. A, Greiner, L. H, Wekstein, D. R, et al. (1996). Linguistic ability in early life and cognitive function and Alzheimer's disease in late life. Findings from the Nun Study. JAMA , 275, 528-532.

[4] Waterhouse, E. G, & Xu, B. (2009). New insights into the role of brain-derived neurotrophic factor in synaptic plasticity. Mol Cell Neurosci , 42, 81-89.

[5] Minichiello, L. (2009). TrkB signalling pathways in LTP and learning. Nat Rev Neurosci , 10, 850-860.

[6] Cowansage, K. K, Ledoux, J. E, & Monfils, M. H. (2009). Brain-Derived Neurotrophic Factor: A Dynamic Gatekeeper of Neural Plasticity. Curr Mol Pharmacol.

[7] Rex, C. S, Lin, C. Y, Kramar, E. A, Chen, L. Y, Gall, C. M, et al. (2007). Brain-derived neurotrophic factor promotes long-term potentiation-related cytoskeletal changes in adult hippocampus. J Neurosci , 27, 3017-3029.

[8] Lu, Y, Christian, K, & Lu, B. (2008). BDNF: a key regulator for protein synthesis-dependent LTP and long-term memory? Neurobiol Learn Mem , 89, 312-323.

[9] Miyamoto, Y, Yamauchi, J, Tanoue, A, Wu, C, & Mobley, W. C. (2006). TrkB binds and tyrosine-phosphorylates Tiam1, leading to activation of Rac1 and induction of changes in cellular morphology. Proc Natl Acad Sci U S A , 103, 10444-10449.

[10] Luo, L. (2000). Rho GTPases in neuronal morphogenesis. Nat Rev Neurosci , 1, 173-180.

[11] Goutan, E, Marti, E, & Ferrer, I. (1998). BDNF, and full length and truncated TrkB expression in the hippocampus of the rat following kainic acid excitotoxic damage. Evidence of complex time-dependent and cell-specific responses. Brain Res Mol Brain Res , 59, 154-164.

[12] Avwenagha, O, Campbell, G, & Bird, M. M. (2003). Distribution of GAP-43, beta-III tubulin and F-actin in developing and regenerating axons and their growth cones in vitro, following neurotrophin treatment. J Neurocytol , 32, 1077-1089.

[13] Delalle, I, Pfleger, C. M, Buff, E, Lueras, P, & Hariharan, I. K. (2005). Mutations in the Drosophila orthologs of the F-actin capping protein alpha- and beta-subunits cause actin accumulation and subsequent retinal degeneration. Genetics , 171, 1757-1765.

[14] Fulga, T. A, Elson-schwab, I, Khurana, V, Steinhilb, M. L, Spires, T. L, et al. (2007). Abnormal bundling and accumulation of F-actin mediates tau-induced neuronal degeneration in vivo. Nat Cell Biol , 9, 139-148.

[15] Li, Y, & Grupe, A. (2007). Genetics of late-onset Alzheimer's disease: progress and prospect. Pharmacogenomics , 8, 1747-1755.

[16] Nathan, B. P, Chang, K. C, Bellosta, S, Brisch, E, Ge, N, et al. (1995). The inhibitory effect of apolipoprotein E4 on neurite outgrowth is associated with microtubule depolymerization. J Biol Chem , 270, 19791-19799.

[17] Arendt, T, Schindler, C, Bruckner, M. K, Eschrich, K, Bigl, V, et al. (1997). Plastic neuronal remodeling is impaired in patients with Alzheimer's disease carrying apolipoprotein epsilon 4 allele. J Neurosci , 17, 516-529.

[18] Ji, Y, Gong, Y, Gan, W, Beach, T, Holtzman, D. M, et al. (2003). Apolipoprotein E isoform-specific regulation of dendritic spine morphology in apolipoprotein E transgenic mice and Alzheimer's disease patients. Neuroscience , 122, 305-315.

[19] Tesseur, I, Van Dorpe, J, & Spittaels, K. Van den Haute C, Moechars D, et al. ((2000). Expression of human apolipoprotein E4 in neurons causes hyperphosphorylation of protein tau in the brains of transgenic mice. Am J Pathol , 156, 951-964.

[20] Brecht, W. J, Harris, F. M, Chang, S, Tesseur, I, Yu, G. Q, et al. (2004). Neuron-specific apolipoprotein e4 proteolysis is associated with increased tau phosphorylation in brains of transgenic mice. J Neurosci , 24, 2527-2534.

[21] Wang, C, Wilson, W. A, Moore, S. D, Mace, B. E, Maeda, N, et al. (2005). Human apoE4-targeted replacement mice display synaptic deficits in the absence of neuropathology. Neurobiol Dis , 18, 390-398.

[22] Klein, R. C, Mace, B. E, & Moore, S. D. Sullivan PM Progressive loss of synaptic integrity in human apolipoprotein E4 targeted replacement mice and attenuation by apolipoprotein E2. Neuroscience , 171, 1265-1272.

[23] Riemenschneider, M, Schwarz, S, Wagenpfeil, S, Diehl, J, Muller, U, et al. (2002). A polymorphism of the brain-derived neurotrophic factor (BDNF) is associated with Alzheimer's disease in patients lacking the Apolipoprotein E epsilon4 allele. Mol Psychiatry , 7, 782-785.

[24] Lee, J, Fukumoto, H, Orne, J, Klucken, J, Raju, S, et al. (2005). Decreased levels of BDNF protein in Alzheimer temporal cortex are independent of BDNF polymorphisms. Exp Neurol , 194, 91-96.

[25] Forlenza, O. V, Diniz, B. S, Teixeira, A. L, Ojopi, E. B, Talib, L. L, et al. Effect of brain-derived neurotrophic factor Val66Met polymorphism and serum levels on the progression of mild cognitive impairment. World J Biol Psychiatry , 11, 774-780.

[26] Nichol, K, Deeny, S. P, Seif, J, Camaclang, K, & Cotman, C. W. (2009). Exercise improves cognition and hippocampal plasticity in APOE epsilon4 mice. Alzheimers Dement , 5, 287-294.

[27] Kuzumaki, N, Ikegami, D, Tamura, R, Hareyama, N, Imai, S, et al. Hippocampal epigenetic modification at the brain-derived neurotrophic factor gene induced by an enriched environment. Hippocampus , 21, 127-132.

[28] Verghese, J, Lipton, R. B, Katz, M. J, Hall, C. B, Derby, C. A, et al. (2003). Leisure activities and the risk of dementia in the elderly. N Engl J Med , 348, 2508-2516.

[29] Larson, E. B, Wang, L, Bowen, J. D, Mccormick, W. C, Teri, L, et al. (2006). Exercise is associated with reduced risk for incident dementia among persons 65 years of age and older. Ann Intern Med , 144, 73-81.

[30] Pasinetti, G. M, Zhao, Z, Qin, W, Ho, L, Shrishailam, Y, et al. (2007). Caloric intake and Alzheimer's disease. Experimental approaches and therapeutic implications. Interdiscip Top Gerontol , 35, 159-175.

[31] Mckee, A. C, Kowall, N. W, & Kosik, K. S. (1989). Microtubular reorganization and dendritic growth response in Alzheimer's disease. Ann Neurol , 26, 652-659.

[32] Dent, E. W, & Gertler, F. B. (2003). Cytoskeletal dynamics and transport in growth cone motility and axon guidance. Neuron , 40, 209-227.

[33] Sabo, S. L, Ikin, A. F, Buxbaum, J. D, & Greengard, P. (2003). The amyloid precursor protein and its regulatory protein, FE65, in growth cones and synapses in vitro and in vivo. J Neurosci , 23, 5407-5415.

[34] Spira, M. E, Oren, R, Dormann, A, & Gitler, D. (2003). Critical calpain-dependent ultrastructural alterations underlie the transformation of an axonal segment into a growth cone after axotomy of cultured Aplysia neurons. J Comp Neurol , 457, 293-312.

[35] Mejillano, M. R, Kojima, S, Applewhite, D. A, Gertler, F. B, Svitkina, T. M, et al. (2004). Lamellipodial versus filopodial mode of the actin nanomachinery: pivotal role of the filament barbed end. Cell , 118, 363-373.

[36] Schafer, D. A, Korshunova, Y. O, Schroer, T. A, & Cooper, J. A. (1994). Differential localization and sequence analysis of capping protein beta-subunit isoforms of vertebrates. J Cell Biol , 127, 453-465.

[37] Davis, D. A, Wilson, M. H, Giraud, J, Xie, Z, Tseng, H. C, et al. (2009). Capzb2 interacts with beta-tubulin to regulate growth cone morphology and neurite outgrowth. PLoS Biol 7: e1000208.

[38] Nelson, T. J, & Backlund, P. S. Jr., Alkon DL ((2004). Hippocampal protein-protein interactions in spatial memory. Hippocampus , 14, 46-57.

[39] Linnarsson, S, Bjorklund, A, & Ernfors, P. (1997). Learning deficit in BDNF mutant mice. Eur J Neurosci , 9, 2581-2587.

[40] Scheibel, A. B, & Tomiyasu, U. (1978). Dendritic sprouting in Alzheimer's presenile dementia. Exp Neurol , 60, 1-8.

[41] Scheibel, A. B. (1979). Dendritic changes in senile and presenile dementias. Res Publ Assoc Res Nerv Ment Dis , 57, 107-124.

[42] Kao, P. F, Davis, D. A, Banigan, M. G, Vanderburg, C. R, Seshadri, S, et al. Modulators of cytoskeletal reorganization in CA1 hippocampal neurons show increased expression in patients at mid-stage Alzheimer's disease. PLoS One 5: e13337.

[43] Grande, I, Fries, G. R, Kunz, M, & Kapczinski, F. (2010). The role of BDNF as a mediator of neuroplasticity in bipolar disorder. Psychiatry Investig , 7, 243-250.

[44] Labelle, C, & Leclerc, N. (2000). Exogenous BDNF, NT-3 and NT-4 differentially regulate neurite outgrowth in cultured hippocampal neurons. Brain Res Dev Brain Res , 123, 1-11.

[45] Kitanishi, T, Sakai, J, Kojima, S, Saitoh, Y, Inokuchi, K, et al. Activity-dependent localization in spines of the F-actin capping protein CapZ screened in a rat model of dementia. Genes Cells.

[46] Kao, P. F, Banigan, M. G, Vanderburg, C. R, Mckee, A. C, Polgar, P. R, et al. (2012). Increased Expression of TrkB and Capzb2 Accompanies Preserved Cognitive Status in Early Alzheimer Disease Pathology. J Neuropathol Exp Neurol , 71, 654-664.

[47] Farmer, M. E, White, L. R, Kittner, S. J, Kaplan, E, Moes, E, et al. (1987). Neuropsychological test performance in Framingham: a descriptive study. Psychol Rep , 60, 1023-1040.

[48] Au, R, Seshadri, S, Wolf, P. A, Elias, M, Elias, P, et al. (2004). New norms for a new generation: cognitive performance in the framingham offspring cohort. Exp Aging Res , 30, 333-358.

[49] Mckhann, G, Drachman, D, Folstein, M, Katzman, R, Price, D, et al. (1984). Clinical diagnosis of Alzheimer's disease: report of the NINCDS-ADRDA Work Group under the auspices of Department of Health and Human Services Task Force on Alzheimer's Disease. Neurology , 34, 939-944.

[50] Morris, J. C, Weintraub, S, Chui, H. C, Cummings, J, Decarli, C, et al. (2006). The Uniform Data Set (UDS): clinical and cognitive variables and descriptive data from Alzheimer Disease Centers. Alzheimer Dis Assoc Disord , 20, 210-216.

[51] Weintraub, S, Salmon, D, Mercaldo, N, Ferris, S, Graff-radford, N. R, et al. (2009). The Alzheimer's Disease Centers' Uniform Data Set (UDS): the neuropsychologic test battery. Alzheimer Dis Assoc Disord , 23, 91-101.

[52] Blessed, G, Tomlinson, B. E, & Roth, M. (1968). The association between quantitative measures of dementia and of senile change in the cerebral grey matter of elderly subjects. Br J Psychiatry , 114, 797-811.

[53] Hachinski, V. C, Iliff, L. D, & Zilhka, E. Du Boulay GH, McAllister VL, et al. ((1975). Cerebral blood flow in dementia. Arch Neurol , 32, 632-637.

[54] Davis, P. B, White, H, Price, J. L, Mckeel, D, & Robins, L. N. (1991). Retrospective postmortem dementia assessment. Validation of a new clinical interview to assist neuropathologic study. Arch Neurol , 48, 613-617.

[55] Nagahara, A. H, Merrill, D. A, Coppola, G, Tsukada, S, Schroeder, B. E, et al. (2009). Neuroprotective effects of brain-derived neurotrophic factor in rodent and primate models of Alzheimer's disease. Nat Med , 15, 331-337.

[56] Frank, L, Ventimiglia, R, Anderson, K, Lindsay, R. M, & Rudge, J. S. (1996). BDNF down-regulates neurotrophin responsiveness, TrkB protein and TrkB mRNA levels in cultured rat hippocampal neurons. Eur J Neurosci , 8, 1220-1230.

[57] Connor, B, Young, D, Lawlor, P, Gai, W, Waldvogel, H, et al. (1996). Trk receptor alterations in Alzheimer's disease. Brain Res Mol Brain Res , 42, 1-17.

[58] Seshadri, S, Wolf, P. A, Beiser, A, Au, R, Mcnulty, K, et al. (1997). Lifetime risk of dementia and Alzheimer's disease. The impact of mortality on risk estimates in the Framingham Study. Neurology , 49, 1498-1504.

[59] Seshadri, S, & Wolf, P. A. (2007). Lifetime risk of stroke and dementia: current concepts, and estimates from the Framingham Study. Lancet Neurol , 6, 1106-1114.

http://dx.doi.org/10.5772/53658

[60] Albert, M. S, Dekosky, S. T, Dickson, D, Dubois, B, Feldman, H. H, et al. (2011). The diagnosis of mild cognitive impairment due to Alzheimer's disease: recommendations from the National Institute on Aging-Alzheimer's Association workgroups on diagnostic guidelines for Alzheimer's disease. Alzheimers Dement , 7, 270-279.

[61] Sperling, R. A, Aisen, P. S, Beckett, L. A, Bennett, D. A, Craft, S, et al. (2011). Toward defining the preclinical stages of Alzheimer's disease: recommendations from the National Institute on Aging-Alzheimer's Association workgroups on diagnostic guidelines for Alzheimer's disease. Alzheimers Dement , 7, 280-292.

[62] Wu, A, Ying, Z, & Gomez-pinilla, F. (2008). Docosahexaenoic acid dietary supplementation enhances the effects of exercise on synaptic plasticity and cognition. Neuroscience , 155, 751-759.

[63] Sananbenesi, F, & Fischer, A. (2009). The epigenetic bottleneck of neurodegenerative and psychiatric diseases. Biol Chem , 390, 1145-1153.

[64] Fischer, A, Sananbenesi, F, Wang, X, Dobbin, M, & Tsai, L. H. (2007). Recovery of learning and memory is associated with chromatin remodelling. Nature , 447, 178-182.

[65] Been, E, Barash, A, Pessah, H, & Peleg, S. (2010). A new look at the geometry of the lumbar spine. Spine (Phila Pa 1976) 35: E , 1014-1017.

[66] Fischer, A, Sananbenesi, F, Mungenast, A, & Tsai, L. H. (2010). Targeting the correct HDAC(s) to treat cognitive disorders. Trends Pharmacol Sci , 31, 605-617.

[67] Stilling, R. M, & Fischer, A. (2011). The role of histone acetylation in age-associated memory impairment and Alzheimer's disease. Neurobiol Learn Mem , 96, 19-26.

Chapter 8

Cholesterol and Alzheimer's Disease

Iuliana Nicola-Antoniu

Additional information is available at the end of the chapter

http://dx.doi.org/10.5772/55502

1. Introduction

Cholesterol plays a central role in the brain's metabolism: the fact that the brain accounts for only 2% of the body mass and brain cholesterol represents 25% of the total body cholesterol speaks for itself. Overall, the brain is the organ with the highest content of cholesterol in the body.

Direct analysis of brain cholesterol metabolism is further complicated by the separation of brain cholesterol from plasma cholesterol owing to the blood-brain barrier.

It is commonly assumed that all brain cholesterol originates from in situ neo-synthesis. This conclusion is based mainly on studies tracking the incorporation of tritiated water into the pool of sterols contained in the brain.

Most brain cholesterol is unesterified (free) and is found within the specialized membranes of myelin. Since myelin has a very slow turnover rate, myelin-associated cholesterol is virtually immobilized.

The remaining brain cholesterol is found in neurons, glial cells and extracellular lipoproteins, and these pools of cholesterol participate in cholesterol homeostatis of the CNS. Considering that the large mass of cholesterol sequestered into myelin membranes, makes the analysis of cholesterol distribution in the brain (brain cholesterol) technically challenging.

Direct quantification of plasma cholesterol in the brain, which is very difficult, has thus far yielded negative results.

The membrane concentration of cholesterol is maintained within extremely fine variation limits owing to numerous homeostasis mechanisms. These mechanisms can be altered genetically, by environment factors, through aging or dietary induced.

The studies carried out throughout the years have shown cholesterol's vital importance for the brain:

Here are just a few examples:

- It is a limiting factor in the ability to form synapses. The "factor" searched for since 1997, that acts on the glial cells, stimulating them to increase synapse formation, was identified in 2001. It proved to be cholesterol.
- Synapses formed in the presence of cholesterol rich glial cells proved to be more effective and functional. When neurons deprived of this glial secretion were exposed to a solution of cholesterol, synapse formation increased by twelve times.
- THUS, cholesterol helps us think, learn and memorize by regulating the plasticity of synapses.
- Cholesterol has also been discovered to play an important role in forming what are called *lipid rafts,* areas in the plasma membrane of cells that anchor certain proteins important to cell signaling. Several of the proteins anchored in these *rafts* are responsible for stimulating and guiding the growth of nerve axons.
- It is the main regulator of the structure of lipids and neuronal membrane fluidity.

The interplay between Alzheimer's disease and cholesterol is very controversial, being supported by some authors and denied by others.

2. The involvement of cholesterol in the generation and deposit of amyloid beta

Although it is not completely elucidated, today it is generally acknowledged that the debut and evolution of AD's molecular mechanism consists in the overproduction and accumulation of toxic amyloid beta proteins.

Numerous studies show the direct relation between the cholesterol levels and the amyloid volume at brain level. High cholesterol level (more than 5.8 mmol/L) is significantly related to the brain plaques associated with Alzheimer's disease in autopsied people; there wasn't found any link between high cholesterol and the tangles that develop in the brain (plaques and tangles both known to be trademark signs of Alzheimer's disease)

Of the other part, a series of prospective studies did not support the hypothesis according to which high levels of cholesterol represent a risk factor for Alzheimer's disease.

- Cholesterol and the formation of the β-amyloid precursor protein

The amyloid processing of the amyloid precursor protein takes place only in certain areas of the cell membrane and is favored by its high cholesterol content.

Membrane rafts and isoprenylation play an important role in transforming the amyloid precursor protein at gamma-secretase level.

Lipid rafts are heterogenous, cholesterol and sphingolipid-rich membrane microdomains that mediate compartmentalized cellular processes by clustering receptors and signalling molecules. These dynamic lipid–protein assemblies are enriched in saturated glycerophospholipids and protein molecules with a high inherent affinity for ordered lipid domains.

Raft lipids are believed to be held together by relatively weak covalent bonds, establishing a dynamic equilibrium of raft and non-raft regions within the plasma membrane. The density, size, duration and exact composition of the rafts varies based on the cell type. In average they have a 50 nm diameter (between 10-100 nm), each comprising approximately 20 protein molecules. Theoretically, a cell may have approximately 1,000,00 membrane rafts, representing more than half of the total membrane surface.

When activated, membrane rafts have been shown to function as a concentrating platform for a variety of signal transduction molecules. During activation, several rafts cluster forming large platforms in order to allow the functional proteins to concentrate and interact. An especially important aspect is that this concentration is cholesterol dependant. Thus, membrane rafts have a central role in regulating a few cellular processes, such as membrane sorting, trafficking and signal transduction.

Even clearer evidence shows that amyloid processing of APP takes place at raft level, especially due to the presence of the active functional pool of BACE 1 and gamma-secretase at the level of these micro-domains. An even more supported idea is that the decreased association of these proteins at raft level would be beneficial for AD. When supporting this theory, the possibility of interfering with bodily functions must be taken into account.

Although, APP, BACE1 and presenile domains are present both in raft areas, as well as in membrane areas without rafts, APP processing at raft level seems to be predominantly amyloidogenic, while outside the raft level, the APP processing is predominantly non amyloidogenic, on the alpha-secretase pathway.

Cholesterol decrease does not favour the association of BACE1 with the lipid rafts, which correlates with the decrease of amyloidogenesis. In contrast, the acute exposure of cells to cholesterol stimulates the co clustering of APP and BACE1 at raft level and their fast endocytosis.

Besides gamma-secretase, the beta-secretase component seems to be located at membrane raft level. Cholesterol depletion abrogates this localization.

Thus, we can draw the conclusion that the production of cholesterol-influenced amyloid is determined, at least partially, at BACE1 level present in lipid rafts. Moreover, APP's association with rafts stimulates the formation of amyloid.

Genetic, metabolic and biochemical studies have shown that intracellular cholesterol distribution, rather than total cholesterol levels, regulates APP processing and β-amyloid generation.

At cellular level, the highest concentration of cholesterol is at plasmatic membrane level, just like in the endocytic recycling compartment. Because the blood-brain barrier prevents any exchange of lipoproteins between the serum and the brain, most of the brain cholesterol is synthesized de novo de novo, at glial level.

The excess free cholesterol is transformed by acyl-conezyme A: cholesterol acyltransferase (ACAT) resulting with the intracellular accumulation of lipid droplets or trans-membrane efflux in the extra-cellular environment.

ACAT is essential for the regulation of intracellular cholesterol homeostasis and distribution of cholesterol throughout the body. In the small intestine and liver it also regulates the secretion of chylomicrons and very large-density lipoproteins (VLDL).

Mammals, including humans, express two different isoforms of ACAT, called ACAT-1 and ACAT-2. Whereas ACAT-1 is almost uniformly distributed among several tissues, including the brain, ACAT-2 is selectively expressed in the intestine and liver. Both forms of ACAT are ER resident enzymes, allosterically regulated by cholesterol available in the ER membrane.

Acyl-coenzyme A cholesterol acyltrasferase (ACAT) catalyzes the formation of cholesteryl-esters from cholesterol and long-chain fatty acids. ACAT controls the dynamic equilibrium between these two forms of cellular cholesterol, ultimately affecting cholesterol homeostasis. This dynamic equilibrium ultimately regulates the generation of β-amyloid (Aβ). A selective increase in cholesteryl-esters is sufficient to up-regulate the generation of Aβ and increase the steady-state levels of β-APP CTFs (C-terminal excerpt). It has been shown that at neuron level, the ACAT competitive inhibitors reduce both cholesteryl-ester and Aβ biosynthesis in a dose-dependant manner, while increasing free cholesterol. Similar results were obtained with agents that block delivery of free cholesterol to ACAT.

How free cholesterol and cholesteryl-ester distribution affects the Aβ synthesis is not yet clear. HOWEVER, the participation of free cholesterol in cellular membranes must be also taken into account because altered cholesteryl-ester levels modulate the free cholesterol pool. Even undetectable changes in free cholesterol levels may affect APP processing.

Second, studies have shown that ACAT regulates ALL three cleavages of APP. Thus, altered cholesterol distribution affects either the activity of all three secretases, APP itself, or an-yet-unidentified protetin that controls APP processing.

The increase of cholesteryl-ester level in the cell cultures increases the release of Abeta, while the pharmacological inhibition of ACAT reduces the formation of cholesteryl-esters, as well as Aβ. The genetic ablation of ACAT1 in the mouse model with AD reduces the formation of AD as well as cognitive decline.

The ACAT1 ablation also increases the oxy-cholesterol levels and 24S-hydrocholesterol, thus suggesting a potential reduction role of amyloidogenesis for these cholesterol metabolites. THUS, a possible mechanism is that the excess brain cholesterol resulted from ACAT1 ablation can be transformed in 24S-hydroxycholesterol and in this form cross the blood-brain barrier to the periphery, reducing the brain cholesterol level. The corroborated data suggests that the equilibrium (report) between free cholesterol and cholesteryl-esters is the key element for controlling amyloidogenesis.

3. Isoprenylation

Abeta in turn regulates cholesterol metabolism. Abeta 40 supresses the mevalonate pathway by inhibiting HMG CoA reductase, thus decreasing the cholesterol level.

The HMG-CoA reductase pathway, also called the mevalonate pathway, leads to cholesterol synthesis, as well as supplies indispensable lipids, such as isoprenoids, to eukaryotic cells.

(The statins that block the HMG-CoA reductase pathway can thus manifest their effects through a cholesterol independent mechanism).

Long-chain isoprenoids participate in membrane organization and proteic glycosylation, as well as in mitochondrial oxygen consumption.

The short-chain isoprenoids (farnesylpyrophosphate-FPP) and metabolite or geranylgeranyl-pyrophosphate (GGPP) are used for the isoprenylation of complex proteins, including nuclear lamins and GTPases.

Isoprenylation of proteins, respectively farnsylation and geranylgeranylation influence the signalling capacity of the respective proteins.

Recent studies indicate that AD has a metabolism interference at FPP and GGPP level, consequently affecting signalling through GTPases. This is relevant for AD because signalling through GTPases controls multiple aspects of amyloidogenesis, including trafficking of APP, BACE1 and the secretase complex.

- Cholesterol and intracellular accumulation of amyloid beta

Intracellular amyloid beta induces the increase of oxidative stress through mitochondrial perturbation.

Recent studies evince that the specific mitochondrial cholesterol pool sensitizes neurons to cell death (induced by oxidative stress) as well as at caspase-independent apoptosis. This is due to due to selective mitochondrial GSH (mGSH) depletion induced by cholesterol-mediated perturbation of mitochondrial membrane dynamics.

"MGSH replenishment by permeable precursors such as glutatione ethyl ester protected against Ab-mediated neurotoxicity and inflammation"

Thus, mitochondrial cholesterol determines amyloid beta neurotoxicity by regulating mitochondrial GSH.

In the relation between CHOLESTEROL-AMYLOID it is essential to analyze the hypercholesterolemia *subtypes.*

The increased levels of serum cholesterol are the result of different factors that should be taken into account. For instance, familial hypercholesterolemia involves a dysfunction of LDL receptors. On the one hand, cholesterol levels in the blood increase because they cannot be received into cells, and on the other, the absence of properly functioning LDL receptors could be causing other intracellular problems. Thus this more likely results from a specific *defect of receptors*, rather than from high cholesterol, or even a *deficiency of intracellular cholesterol*.

The role of the LDL receptor-related protein is so much more important and disputed now that we know that its associated proteins are responsible in both increased free brain cholesterol and increased beta-amyloid in Alzheimer's disease. They are also responsible for bringing apolipoprotein-E-associated cholesterol into cells. Apparently, the deficiency or dysfunction of LRP could be a factor that results in both increased free brain cholesterol and increased beta-amyloid, which could be accidental.

4. Tau pathology and cholesterol

Together with amyloid deposits, the second defining element of AD from a histopathological point of view are the intraneuronal neurofibrillary tangles, formed from hyperphosphorylation of Tau protein.

In contrast with APP and secretases, which are membrane bound, tau is a protein that stabilizes microtubules, which are found in cytoplasm.

However there is an interaction between cholesterol and its pathology.

- The Aβ signalling pathway perturbs pathways involving lipid metabolizing enzymes ultimately affecting tau phosphorylation
- The cholesterol levels are a key parameter controlling Aβ-induced tau proteolysis by calpain and proteolytic cleavage of tau by this protease, but also by caspases. These seem to be the early steps leading to tau pathology.
- A pool of hyperphosphorylated tau is present in lipid rafts, along with APP metabolites, BACE1, the γ-secretase complex and ApoE. Thus, evincing that significant crosstalk may exist between Aβ and tau at the raft interface.
- Kinases implicated in tau phosphorylation, such as Cdk5 and GSK-3β, are activated on cellular membranes and thus dysregulation of lipid metabolism may affect the activity of these kinases.
- The aggregate treatment pathway is also influenced by the lipidic metabolism. Cdk5 phosphorylates the lipid kinase Vps34, whose product PtdIns3P, may regulate the clearance of tau aggregates by stimulating the autophagy pathway
- More and more theories support that the propagation of the tau pathology is similar to prion-like infections, by crossing cell membranes, case in which the importance of the cell MEMBRANE's functionality comes forefront.

http://dx.doi.org/10.5772/55502

5. HDL colesterol and AD

HDL is one of the main protein carriers in the brain. It can cross the brain-blood barrier. It is difficult to estimate to what extent its serum value reflects its brain concentration. Studies carried out throughout the years regarding the correlation between cholesterol HDL – AD have not allowed to reach a decisive conclusion. Some authors say that the HDL association is more relevant with stroke, and stroke is associated with AD.

Other authors have found an interplay between the high levels of HDL cholesterol and the presence of plaques and intraneuronal neurofibrillary tangles (study carried out in 2001 by Launer on "Japanese-American men".)

Until now, the data offered by the studies do not allow to make a recommendation regarding the HDL cholesterol levels for preventing AD. We have no reasonable argument for boosting the HDL levels to try to prevent AD.

It should be considered to keep cholesterol under control (within the recommended values) in order to reduce the risk of heart diseases. This has sense because by reducing the risk of heart disease, you also reduce the risk of AD.

Guidelines recommend an optimal HDL level of 60 mg/dL or higher, under 40 mg/dL for men and under 50 mg/dL for women.

6. APOE- cholesterol and AD

ApoE is one of the major plasma apolipoproteins and the principal cholesterol carrier in the brain.

ApoE encodes a 34kDa protein that is an essential regulator of the brain cholesterol metabolism and triglycerides in the body. It mediates the capturing of lipoprotein particles from the brain via associated receptor for LDL (LRP) and VLDL.

In humans, there are three common alleles of the ApoE gene: ε2, ε3 and ε4. The protein isoforms produced by these alleles differ in the amino acids at positions 112 and/or 158: E2 (Cys112, Cys158), E3 (Cys112, Arg158), which is the most common, and E4 (Arg112,Arg158), which is present in at least one copy in less than 25% of the population.

Peripheral apolipoprotein E is synthesized in the liver, while apolipoprotein E from the brain is synthesized in situ, especially by astrocytes.

It has been confirmed that APOE ε4 allele is the most prevalent risk factor for the development of sporadic AD.

The risk for Alzheimer's disease conferred by APOE ε4 increases in a dose-dependant manner; individuals that are homozygous for APOE ε4 alleles are 8 times more likely to develop AD than are homozygotes for APOE ε3. Less than 2% of the population is homozygous for APOE ε4. This is neither necessary nor sufficient to cause AD; it only increases risk for the disease.

The mechanisms through which APOE leads to the development of the disease are partially unknown.

ApoE may alter brain cholesterol homeostasis by modifying lipoprotein-particle formation. In the plasma, ApoE4 is associated with VLDL particles, which contain more cholesterol, whereas ApoE3 is associated with HDL. Subjects homozygous for the ApoE ε4 allele have higher levels of cholesterol in the plasma and 25-hydroxycholesterol in the cerebrospinal fluid. 25-hydroxycholesterol is a catabolic derivative of cholesterol and represents the major metabolic route for cholesterol clearance from the brain. The lipoproteins produced in the brain are very different from the particles found in the plasma, in what concerns composition as well density or other properties.

As ApoE4 shows differential preference for VLDL in the plasma, it is possible that different ApoE isoforms modify brain cholesterol homeostasis by preferentially associating with specific lipoprotein particles. The predominant nature of Apoe in brain lipoproteins would accentuate small differences in lipoprotein affinity for ApoE isoforms. The role of apoE in maintaining cholesterol homeostasis in the brain may contribute to the increased risk for AD associated with APOE ε4.

ApoE may up-regulate the rate of Aβ generation by increasing cellular cholesterol. After receptor-mediated internalization and enzymatic digestion of the lipoproteins, cholesterol is released to cellular membranes. APOEA tend to contain more cholesterol. The increased cholesterol content of cellular membranes promotes the increased production of amyloid-beta from its precursor, APP.

Epidemiologic studies suggest that high levels of cholesterol may contribute to the pathogenesis of AD. Individuals with elevated levels of plasma cholesterol have an increased susceptibility to AD, apparently influenced by the APOE ε4 genotype. Moreover, AD patients have increased levels of total serum and low density lipoprotein (LDL) cholesterol along with reduced levels of apoA/high-density lipoprotein (HDL) in their plasma, as compared to age-matched controls. This is strengthened by the significantly decreased lecithin cholesterol acyltransferase activity (LCAT) in AD patients. LCAT is an enzyme found in plasma that catalyzes an acyltransferase reaction on lipoprotein-associated cholesterol and is a key step in reverse cholesterol transport in humans (the process that eliminates cholesterol from peripheral cells).

APOE may mediate the internalization of amyloid-beta by binding to the proteins associated to the LDL receptor.

LRP is a multi-ligand receptor, a member of the LDL receptor family, with many common structural motifs and functional particularities, such as the high-affinity binding activity for LDL particles. LRP's main protein ligand is APOE, but it also binds other molecules such as α2-macroglobulin and APP751/750 containing the KPI domain.

LRP may be linked to the degradation of secreted amyloid-beta by facilitating the internalization of Aβ bound to APOE. The internalization of Aβ mediated by LRP is more likely followed by its intracellular aggregation, rather than degradation, suggesting that LRP might be involved in the process of Aβ deposition.

Soluble Aβ interacts with APOE associated with lipoparticles and under-goes receptor-mediated endocytosis. The lipoproteins are enzymatically digested in the lysosomal compartment, releasing cholesterol to the cell. A fraction of APOE and Aβ undergoes degradation at lysosomal level. The rest of APOE remains associated with Aβ and promotes its aggregation into amyloid fibrils and is then secreted back in the extracellular milieu.

The internalization of Aβ is not necessarily followed by its degradation. Amyloid aggregates from the endocytic compartment may be secreted in a more toxic fibrillar form. Finally, APOE may contribute to the aggregation of amyloid-beta through its internalization.

Moreover, the non-lypidic form of APOE seems to have a high-affinity binding activity to Aβ and favour the formation of Aβ fibrils rather than APOE3 isoforms.

7. Cholesterol — Common risk factor for AD and atherosclerosis

Epidemiologic studies indicate that people with risk factors such as high blood pressure, diabetes, cerebrovascular disease and high cholesterol are two times more likely to develop Alzheimer disease than those without vascular risk factor.

The causal chain between the high plasma cholesterol level and atherosclerosis is well defined.

We can discuss a risk factor profile for sporadic cases of AD, with late-onset, which account for 90-95% of all cases. In elderly patients that suffer from AD there is an obvious link between this disease and vascular risk factors and atherosclerosis. However, the nature of this link remains partially speculative. Some authors have suggested that AD occurs as a secondary event related to atherosclerosis of extracranial or intracranial vessels with secondary cerebral hypoperfusion or small cerebral strokes. The toxic effects of vascular risk factors on susceptible areas of the brain, such as the temporal lobe, have also been discussed.

Another approach is that both AD and atherosclerosis are common among elderly persons. They are similar with regard to the long prodromal period when specific, clinically "silent" lesions accumulate that manifest according to the symptomatology plan when the disease is already after many years of evolution. However, this fact does not impede us from considering them as two independent diseases with convergent evolution. This idea is supported by epidemiological observations, pathological elements and the answer to common therapy for both diseases.

The APOE risk factor is also associated with atherosclerosis. In cell cultures, APOE is linked with the decreased cholesterol efflux from macrophages, as well as from neurons and astrocytes. At macrophage level, APOE promotes foam cell formation, at neuronal level it promotes the increased APP processing for forming Aβ.

Is has also been evinced that APOE 4 has a more reduced antioxidant capacity than its isoform APOE3. The pathogenic strain of both atherosclerosis and AD is the increase of the oxidative stress associated with the production of reactive oxygen and nitrogen species that oxidize

• ApoEe 4 polmorphism
• Hypercholesterolemia
• High blood pressure
• Hyperhomocysteinemia
• Diabetes mellitus
• Metabolic syndrome
• Smoking
• Systemic inflammatory response
• High level of fats and obesity

Table 1. Common risk factors for AD and atherosclerosis

amino acids and lipids. The loss of the antioxidant protection conferred by APOE may lead to increased alterations produced by oxidative stress.

Epidemiologic studies suggest that AD patients have increased levels of total serum and low density lipoprotein (LDL) cholesterol along with reduced levels of apoA/high-density lipoprotein (HDL) in their plasma, as compared to age-matched controls. LCAT is an enzyme found in plasma that catalyzes an acyltransferase reaction on lipoprotein-associated cholesterol and is a key step in reverse cholesterol transport in humans (the process that eliminates cholesterol from peripheral cells).

The same metabolic profile with high plasma cholesterol level, high LDL cholesterol and low HDL cholesterol is found with atherosclerosis patients.

8. Predictive value of cholesterol based on AGE

The study carried out in 2010 on Swedish women has not evinced any increase in AD risk associated with high plasma cholesterol values between the ages of 40 and 60. This finding contradicts several previous studies which did suggest a role for elevated plasma cholesterol at middle age in the later development of AD.

However, this study has evinced another association of cholesterol level to DA based on age. Namely, women whose cholesterol decreased the most from middle age to old age were more than twice (x2!) as likely to develop AD as women whose cholesterol levels increased or stayed the same between the same age intervals.

Rapidly declining cholesterol late in life (over 60) appears to be associated with increased frailty and may be an early sign of dementia.

It seems that this is due to the fact that 10 years earlier people develop symptoms of dementia, they tend to become more frail. They forget to eat and start to lose weight, which can impact cholesterol levels.

http://dx.doi.org/10.5772/55502

People with high cholesterol in their early 40s are more likely to develop Alzheimer's disease than those with low cholesterol. High levels of high-density lipoprotein-"good cholesterol" appear to be associated with a reduced risk for Alzheimer disease in older adults.

9. Statins and the evolution of AD

Is statin treatment protective?

Statins have a pleiotropic effect – they act on cholesterol, as well as on isoprenylation. They block the HGM-Co A reductase pathway and thus manifest their effects through a cholesterol independent mechanism.

10. Diet and the evolution of Alzheimer's disease

The usefulness of hyper or hypo-cholesterolemic diets in preventing AD is also another controversial issue. Most of the studies are carried out on rodents: 1998 studies found that the hypercholesterolemic diet lowers beta-amyloid at cerebral level, while 2000 studies found the opposite.

11. Conclusions

Although the link between cholesterol and AD remains an open issue, that still has many unresolved aspects, the studies have found strong evidence that cholesterol is a factor in the pathogenesis of AD.

Cholesterol is involved in the development of AD owing to its intervention, at different levels, on the formation and deposit of amyloid-beta and the genesis of intraneuronal neurofibrillary tangles, also favoring the atherogenesis process.

Based on these data and knowing cholesterol's essential role both at cerebral and body level, as well as the relative difficulty to estimate the exact link between the plasma cholesterol and the brain cholesterol level, it is important to maintain throughout your entire life, in correlation with age and sex, the cholesterol concentration (and its fractions) within the recommended limits in order to prevent cardio-vascular diseases.

It is also important to avoid the drastic "correction" of cholesterol, sometimes even under normal levels, especially in the case of elderly persons, in order to prevent Alzheimer's disease, considering that cholesterol is an essential substance for the entire body.

Author details

Iuliana Nicola-Antoniu

Departement of Neurology,"Colentina" Clinical Hospital, Bucharest, Romania

References

[1] Bu. Apolipoprotein E and its receptors in Alzheimer,s disease:patways,pathogenesis and therapy. Nat Rev Neurosci. 2008;9:333 – 344

[2] Casserly I, Topol E. Convergence of atherosclerosis and Alzheiemr's disease:inflammation,cholesterol,and misfolded proteins.Lancet 2004;363:1139-46

[3] Chang TY,Chang CC,Lu X&Lin S Catalysis of ACAT may be completed with the plane of the membrane. A working ipothesis. J Lipig Res.2001;42:1933-1938

[4] Cole S, Vassar R. Isoprenoids and Alzheiemr's disease: a complex realtionship. Neuro Dis 2006; 22:209 -22

[5] Colell A,Fernandez A,Fernandez-Checa JC. Mitochondria,cholesterol and amyloid beta peptide; a dangerous tri in Alzheimer,s disease. J Bioenerg Biomembr.2009;41(5): 417-23

[6] Cordy JM, Hooper NM, Turner AJ. The involvement of lipid rafts in Alzheimer's disease. Mol Mem Bio.2006; 23:111-22

[7] Di Paolo G,Kim TW,Linking lipids to Alzheiemr,s disease:cholesterol and beyond, Nat Rev Neurosci,2011;12(5):284-96

[8] Dietschy JM & Turley SD. Cholesterol metabolism in the brain. Curr. Opin. Lipiol 2001;12:105- 112

[9] Frears ER, Stephens DJ,Walters CE, Davies H&Austen BM. The role of cholesterol in the biosyntesis of beta-amyloid. Neuroreport 1995;10:1699-1705

[10] Goodman Brenda, High cholesterol predicts brain-clagging protein deposits on autopsy,MA, Neurology,sept 2011

[11] Hartmann T,Kuchenbecker J, Grimm MO. Alzheiemr's disese: the lipid connection. J Neurochem,2007;103(Suppl 1):159-170

[12] Hoffman A,Ott A, Breteler MM et alAtherosclerosis,apolipoprotein E and prevalence of dementia and Alzheimer's disease in the Rotterdam study. Lancet 1997;349:151 54

[13] Ivanhoe Newswere,Study links high cholesterol and Alzheimer's-Neurology,sept 2011

[14] Kim J,Bassak JM,Holtzman DM. The role af apolipoprotein E in Alzheimer's disease.Nuron.2009;63:287 -303

[15] Kivipelto M,Helkala EL,Laakso MP,et al.Midlife vascular risk factors and Alzheimer's disease in latter life:longitudinal,populational base3d study.BMJ 2001;322:1447-51

[16] Kojoro E,GimplG,Lammich S, Marz W,Fahrenholz F. Low cholesterol stimulates the nonamyloidogenic pathway by its effct on the alpha-secretase Alzheimer's disease AM 10 Proc Natl Acad Sci USA 2001;98:5815 -5820

[17] Lingwood D,Simons K.Lipid rafts as a membrane-orhganisind principle. Science, 2010;327: 46-50

[18] Nicholson AM,Ferreira A. Increased membrane cholesterol might render mature hipocampal neurons more susceptible to the beta-amyloid-induced calpain activation and tau toxicity. J Neurosci 2009;29:4640 -4651

[19] Puglielli L et al. Acyl-coenzyme A:cholesterol acyltranferase modulate tehe generation of the amyloid beta-peptide. Nat.Cell Biol,2001;3:905 – 912

[20] Puglielli L, Tanzi R, Kovacs D. Alzheimer's diasease: the closterol connection. Nature Publishing Group,2003

[21] Refolo LM,Malestre B,La Francois J et al. Hypercolesterolemia accelerates the Alzheimer's amyloid pathology in a trangenic mouse model. Neurobiol Dis 2000;7:321-31

[22] Runz H,et al.Inhibition of intracellular cholesterol transport alters presenilin localization and amyloid precursor protein processing in neuronal in neuronal cells. J Neurosci,2001;22:1679- 1689

[23] Salynn Boyls,Mielke,Cholesterol level doesn't predict Alzheiemr's in old age,new study finds,MM Neurology, Nov. 23,2010;vol 75 pp1888-1895

[24] Simons M,Keller P,Dichgans J Schulz JB. Cholesterol and Alzheimer's disease:is there a link? Neurology,2001;57:1089 -93

[25] Sparks DL,Scheff SW,Hunsanker JC, Liu H,Landers T, Gross DR. Induction of Alzheimer -like beta-amyloid immnureactivity in the brain of rabbits with dietary cholesterol. Exp Neurol.1994;126;88-94

[26] Tall AR.Cholesterol efflux pathways and other potential mechanisms involved in the athero-protective effect of high density lipoproteins. J Intern Med 2008;263:256 -273

[27] de la Torre JC. Alzheimer disease as a vascular disorder:nosological evidence. Stroke 2002;33:1152-62

[28] Vance JE,Hayashi H,Karten B.Cholesterol homeostasis in neurons and glial cells. Semin Cell Dev Biol.2005;16:193-212

[29] Vetrivel KS,Thinakaran G. Membrane rafts in Alzheimer's disease beta-amyloid production. Biochim Biophy Acta. 2010

Section 2

Therapeutic Aspects of Alzheimer

Chapter 9

Emerging Therapeutic Strategies in Alzheimer's Disease

Tomohiro Chiba

Additional information is available at the end of the chapter

http://dx.doi.org/10.5772/55293

1. Introduction

Alzheimer's disease (AD) is the most common cause of dementia in mid- to late-life. It currently affects about 10% of individuals older than 65 years old, counting for more than 25 million people in the world (Chiba et al., 2007; Huang and Mucke, 2012; Mattson, 2004). A century has passed since the famous neurologist Alois Alzheimer first described about a 51-year-old female patient with severe progressive memory deficit, brain atrophy, senile plaques (SPs, or neuritic plaques), and neurofibrillary tangles (NFTs) in 1906 (1987). SPs and NFTs are abnormal protein aggregates consisting of extracellular amyloid β protein (Aβ) and intracellular hyperphosphorylated microtubule associated protein tau (Braak and Braak, 1991; Perrin et al., 2009). The worst affected areas in AD brains are the olfactory bulb, the cerebral neocortex, and the hippocampus. SPs and NFTs are spatially and temporally disjointed: SPs occur in the cerebral neocortex, preceding the occurrence of NFTs, which is predominant in the entorhinal cortex, by about 10 years (Fig. 1). The onset of mild dementia, or currently described as mild cognitive impairment (MCI), is better correlated with significant synaptic and neuronal loss, which is about 10-15 years behind the occurrence of NFTs.

Knowledge of AD has considerably expanded in the last two decades with the progress in molecular biology and genetics although curative therapy for AD is not yet available. Most AD cases occur sporadically (sporadic AD or SAD), while about 1% of AD cases are inherited in an autosomal dominant manner (familial AD, FAD). In 1984, Glenner and Wong first purified and sequenced Aβ (Glenner and Wong, 1984), which was followed by the identification of amyloid precursor protein (APP) as a source of Aβ (Kang et al., 1987). Genetic analysis of FAD then revealed that mutations in APP co-segregate with FAD (Chartier-Harlin et al., 1991; Goate et al., 1991). Consequently, drug candidates have been developed for AD based on a putative pathogenic hypothesis that increase in Aβ production and aggregation, which can be accelerated by the mutations in genes related to FAD, results in tau hyperphosphorylation and neuronal death. This is termed the "amyloid cascade" hypothesis (Hardy and

Higgins, 1992; Reitz, 2012). In this review, therapeutic strategies for AD will be discussed from a viewpoint of neuronal death and neuroprotection.

2. Molecular pathogenesis of Alzheimer's Disease (AD)

In this section, the overview of molecular pathogenesis of AD will be discussed. This is important to elaborate therapeutic strategies for AD. The current knowledge of pathogenic mechanisms for AD can be classified into two major categories, namely the "amyloid cascade" hypothesis and the alternative hypotheses. Recently, pathogenic roles of signal transducer and activator of transcription 3 (Stat3) and related intracellular signaling pathways in neurons has been described, which is attracting attention of AD researchers (Chiba et al., 2009a; Chiba et al., 2009b; Nicolas et al., 2012). In addition, genome-wide association studies (GWAS) have been carried out rigorously to seek for novel genes and loci related AD. These unbiased global genetic studies are now providing novel insights into both canonical and alternative pathogenic mechanisms for AD.

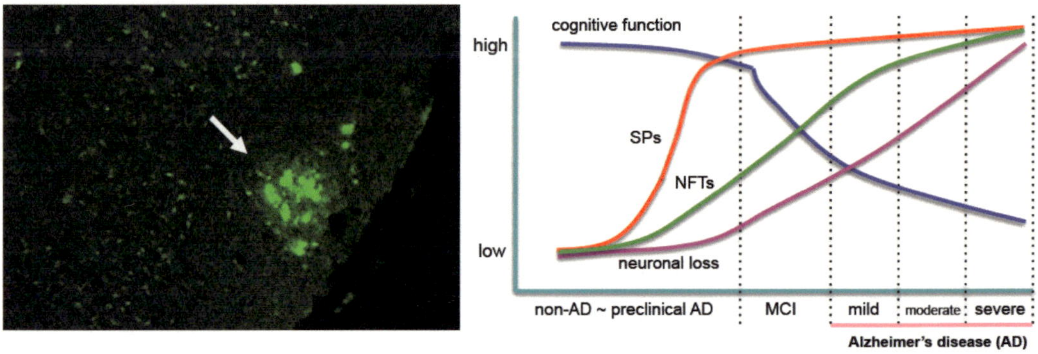

Figure 1. Pathological and clinical features of Alzheimer's disease (AD). (left) Senile plaques (SPs) in the cerebral cortex of an AD model mouse at the age of 12 monthes were stained with Thioflavin T. (right) Clinical process of AD and its relationship with pathological hallmarks of AD (mild cognitive impairment, MCI; cognitive function [blue]; SPs [red]; neurofibrillary tangles, NFTs [green]; neuronal loss [purple]). SP formation precedes NFT formation, which is followed by neuronal loss. Cognitive decline occurs as a result of neuronal loss.

2.1. The "amyloid cascade" hypothesis

2.1.1. Causative genes for FAD and their roles

FAD, which accounts for up to 1% of total AD cases, usually occurs between the age of 40-65 years (early-onset AD, EOAD) and is inherited in an autosomal dominant manner (Bertram et al., 2010; Schellenberg and Montine, 2012). Genetic analysis has identified so far three causative genes for FAD: *amyloid precursor protein (APP)* on chromosome 21, *presenilin 1 (PSEN1)* on chromosome 14 (Sherrington et al., 1995), and *presenilin 2 (PSEN2)* on chromosome 1 (Rogaev et al., 1995).

http://dx.doi.org/10.5772/55293

APP is ubiquitously expressed type-I single transmembrane glycoprotein (Kang et al., 1987). From its primary structure, it is likely to be a cell surface receptor (Fig. 2A). APP undergoes sequential processing by three proteases: α-, β- and γ-secretase. β- and γ-cleavage generates Aβ, secretory APPβ (sAPPβ), and APP intracellular domain (AICD), whereas α- and γ-cleavage generates secretory APPα (sAPPα), AICD, and p3 fragment (De Strooper and Annaert, 2000; Kawasumi et al., 2002). Since β- and γ-cleavage generates Aβ, it is believed that initial cleavage by β-secretase is pathogenic and one by α-secreatese is non-pathogenic on the other hands. Val 642 Ile (V642I, numbering by a neuron-specific APP695 form) mutation within the transmembrane domain of APP was identified as the first FAD-linked mutation and is called as London-type mutation (Fig. 2B) (Chartier-Harlin et al., 1991; Goate et al., 1991). Then, several other types of mutations in APP, including K595N/M596L (Swedish type mutant or NL mutant), were identified (pathological impact of these mutations will be discussed later, see 2.1.3). It is notable that E618Q (Dutch type, numbering by APP695) mutation within Aβ sequence does not cause FAD but causes cerebral amyloid angiopathy called as hereditary cerebral hemorrhage with amyloidosis-Dutch type (HCHWA-D) (Fernandez-Madrid et al., 1991), while E618G (Arctic type, numbering by APP695) mutation at the same position causes FAD without severe cerebral amyloid angiopathy (Nilsberth et al., 2001). Recently, a rare recessive (A598V, numbering by APP695; A673V, numbering by a ubiquitous APP770 form) and a disease-resistant mutation (A598T, by APP695; A672T, by APP770) have been identified in APP at Ala 598, the second amino acid in Aβ (Di Fede et al., 2009; Jonsson et al., 2012).

PSEN1 and PSEN2 are highly homologous proteins consisting of 467 and 448 amino acid residues respectively with 8 or 9 transmembrane domains (Laudon et al., 2005; Marjaux et al., 2004) (Fig. 2C). They are ubiquitously expressed and localized in the endoplasmic reticulum (ER) and golgi apparatus. Mutations in the *PSEN1* gene are the most frequently involved in FAD accounting for about 10-20% of all FAD cases. More than one hundred mutations throughout entire *PSEN1* gene have been reported while about ten mutations have been reported in *PSEN2* (Bertram et al., 2010; Schellenberg and Montine, 2012). *PSEN1* and *PSEN2* are now regarded as the active core of the γ-secretase which cleaves the hydrophobic integral membrane domain of APP to generate Aβ. It is now widely recognized that γ-secretase, at least, involves four different proteins: PSEN, nicastrin, Aph-1, and Pen-2 (De Strooper, 2003; Takasugi et al., 2003). It should be noted that FAD-linked mutations in *PSEN1* and *PSEN2* induce neuronal death or enhance neuronal vulnerability to several toxic insults independent of the γ-secretase activity (Guo et al., 1996; Hashimoto et al., 2002a; Hashimoto et al., 2002b; Zhang et al., 1998).

2.1.2. *Tau-hyperphosphorylation in AD*

NFTs are comprised of paired helical filaments (PHFs), which is resulted from hyperphosphorylation of tau at Ser/Thr residues. NFT formation is one of the hallmarks of AD although tau dysfunction is not limited to AD but is widely observed in neurological disorders (usually termed as tauopathy) (Goedert et al., 1998; Johnson and Stoothoff, 2004). It is reported that the number of NFT correlates well with neuronal loss in AD brain and severity of dementia than that of SPs (Braak and Braak, 1991; Perrin et al., 2009). It is also notable that putative tau kinases

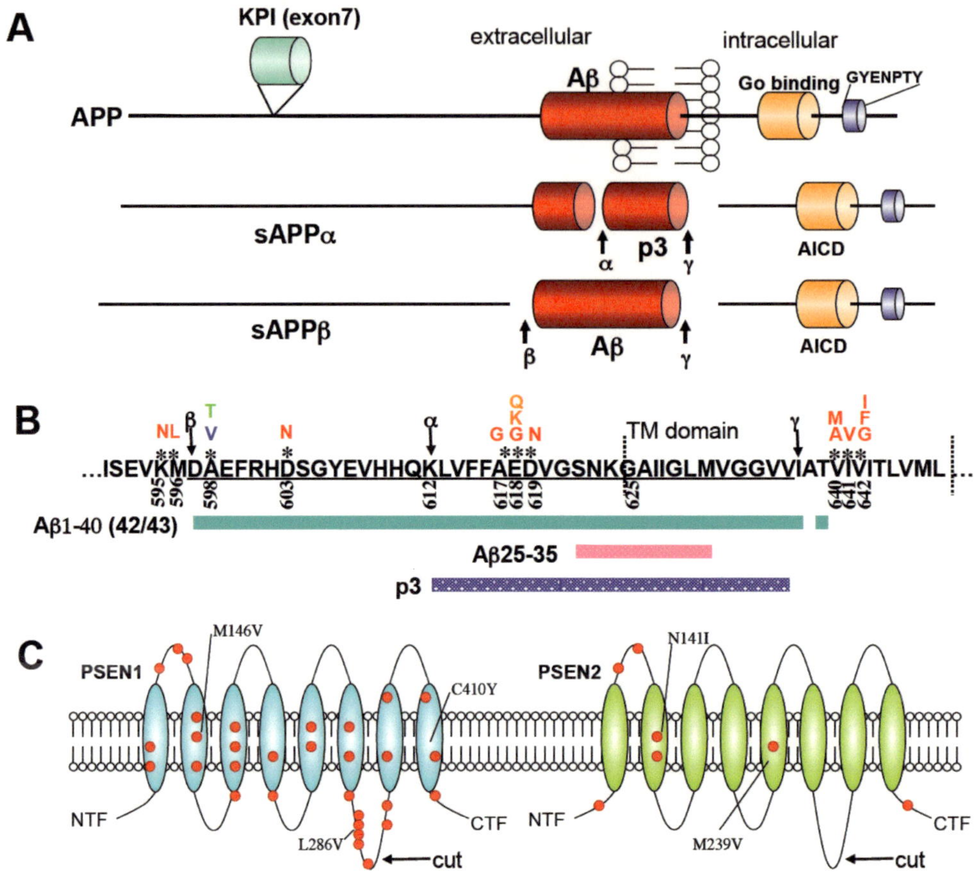

Figure 2. Familial AD (FAD) causative genes. (A) Proteolytic processing of APP. APP is consisting of extracellular, transmembrane and intracellular domains. There are several isoforms of APP with or without a Kunitz protease inhibitor (KPI) domain. Intracellular domain has signal transducing domains such as a G protein-binding motif (Go-binding domain) and an NPXY motif (GYENPTY) recognized by phosphotyrosine-binding domains. Sequential cleavage by α-/γ- or β-/γ-secretases produces soluble APP (sAPPα or sAPPβ, respectively), APP intracellular domain (AICD) and small peptides (Aβ or p3 fragment, respectively). (B) APP mutations were indicated in the Aβ coding region (amino acids). FAD mutations are indicated in red characters (numbering by a neuronal isoform of APP [APP695]); Swedish (K595N/M596N, NL mutation), London (V642I), Flemish (A617G, AD with strokes), Arctic (A618G), Iowa (A619N), German (V640A), French (V640M), Florida (I641V) and Indiana (V642F). Dutch type mutation (E618Q) is related to hereditary cerebral hemorrhage with amyloidosis, Dutch type (HCHWA-D, [orange]). E618K is also related to cerebral hemorrhage with amyloidosis. A598V [blue] is a rare recessive mutation and A598T [green] has been identified as a disease-resistant mutation. (C) Presenilin 1 (PSEN1) and 2 (PSEN2) were also schematically indicated with mutations (red dots). Autocatalytic cleavage of PSENs (arrow) into N- and C-terminal fragments is required for the activation of the γ-secretase.

including glycogen synthase kinase 3β (GSK3β), cyclin dependent kinase 5 (cdk5), c-Jun N-terminal kinase (JNK), p38 mitogen-activated protein kinase (p38-MAPK) and Calcium/calmodulin-dependent kinase II (CaMKII) are reported to be upregulated in AD (Ferrer et al., 2002; Ferrer et al., 2001; Sato et al., 2002; Takashima et al., 2001). These data suggest that the mechanism of NFT formation plays an important role in neuronal loss in AD brain. Genetic mutations in tau, however, cause frontotemporal dementia with parkinsonism linked to chromosome 17 (FTDP-17) rather than AD (Hutton et al., 1998; Lewis et al., 2000). Recently, however, several observations supporting the relation between tau and AD have been reported, which led to the "amyloid cascade" hypothesis for AD (Fig. 3).

2.1.3. Basis of the "amyloid cascade" hypothesis

The "amyloid cascade hypothesis" postulates that excessive formation of insoluble fibrillar Aβ, with consequent formation of SPs, is the initial event in AD pathogenesis (Hardy and Higgins, 1992; Reitz, 2012). Then, a neurotoxic cascade, including NFT formation, secondarily occurs, leading to synaptic and neuronal loss. The hypothesis is originally based on the two key observations: the detection of Aβ as a main constituent of SPs, and identification of the FAD-causative mutations in the Aβ precursor (*APP*) and γ-secretase genes (*PSEN1* and *PSEN2*) (Bertram et al., 2010; Chiba et al., 2007; Schellenberg and Montine, 2012). Aβ can vary in length at the c-terminus; Aβ1-40 (Aβ40, 40 amino acids) is the most prevalent, followed by Aβ1-42 (Aβ42). The latter has hydrophobic properties and aggregates more readily than Aβ40, which leads to the notion that Aβ42 is the toxic Aβ property. Mutations of all three FAD genes generally increase the ratio of Aβ42 to Aβ40 (Aβ42/Aβ40) and promote Aβ oligomerization and aggregation, followed by the synaptic and neuronal loss.

As already mentioned, SPs and NFTs are distributed independently of each other. Researchers, however, have postulated that NFT formation lies downstream from SP formation to integrate NFTs into the "amyloid cascade", based on the experimental observations showing the relationship between Aβ and NFT formation: (i) APP or PSEN1 transgene enhanced NFT formation in tau transgenic mice (Gotz et al., 2001; Lewis et al., 2001; Oddo et al., 2003), (ii) fetal rat hippocampal neurons and human cortical neurons treated with fibrillar Aβ display an increased degree of tau phosphorylation (Busciglio et al., 1995; Rapoport et al., 2002), (iii) reduction of endogenous levels of tau can ameliorate some of the behavioral and other dificits mediated by Aβ (Roberson et al., 2007), and (iv) mutations in the tau gene cause FTDP-17 with a tau pathology similar to that in AD without SP formation (Hutton et al., 1998; Lewis et al., 2000).

There are several objections to the "amyloid cascade" hypothesis. There is only a weak correlation between cerebral SPs and the severity of dementia. SPs and NFTs may be reactive products resulting from neurodegeneration in AD rather than being its cause. It remains unclear whether and how the deposition of Aβ leads to the formation of NFTs. These should be addressed in the future investigations.

2.2. Stat3 inactivation in the "amyloid casdade"

Signal transducer and activator of transcription 3 (Stat3) is an important mediator of cellular physiological functions such as cell proliferation, differentiation, and survival, mainly upon cytokine receptor stimulation (Chiba et al., 2009a; Stephanou and Latchman, 2005). Immuno-histochemical analysis using a specific antibody against phosphorylated (p-) or activated form of Stat3 revealed that p-Stat3 levels were significantly reduced in hippocampal neurons of clinically and pathologically diagnosed AD patients and several lines of AD model mice as compared with age-matched controls (Chiba et al., 2009b). Animal experiments further showed that (i) i.c.v. injection of toxic Aβ peptide reduces p-Stat3 in hippocampal neurons to induce memory impairment (a toxic Aβ gain of function effect) and that (ii) Aβ passive immunotherapy reduces cerebral Aβ burden and recovers cognitive function of Tg2576 mice in parallel with Stat3 activation in hippocampal neurons (a toxic Aβ loss of function effect). These data suggest that cerebral Aβ levels are inversely correlated with p-STAT3 levels in hippocampal neurons *in vivo* (Chiba et al., 2009b).

Aging, one of the most common risk factor for AD, seems to be one of the other factors responsible for the AD-related neuronal inactivation of Stat3 because p-Stat3 immunoreactivity in hippocampal neurons of young subjects was substantially higher than that of elder cognitively normal subjects in both humans and rodents (Chiba et al., 2009b). Aging-dependent reduction of p-Stat3 levels may be due to age-dependent decrease in endogenous neurotrophic factors, which play a role in sustaining neuronal p-Stat3 levels. In support of this idea, it is reported that endogenous levels of insulin-like growth factor I (IGF-I), which activates Stat3, decrease with aging and that this decrease may be linked to the pathogenesis of AD (Rollero et al., 1998).

Relationship between Stat3 and tau is yet to be elucidated. Stat3 binds to and inhibits stathmin, which depolymerizes microtubules, while tau binds to and stabilizes microtubules (Ng et al., 2006). Involvement of STAT3-mediated stathmin regulation in tau phosphorylation should be addressed in the future research. There are some reports describing Stat3 inactivation and cell death; i.e. Stat3 deletion sensitizes cells to oxidative stress (Barry et al., 2009; Sarafian et al.). Combined with the fact that Aβ induces neuronal death by inducing oxidative stress *in vitro* and *in vivo* (Butterfield et al., 2002; De Felice et al., 2007; Guglielmotto et al., 2009), Stat3 may sensitize neurons to Aβ neurotoxicity through oxidative stress.

In addition to the role of Stat3 in neuronal death, roles of Jak2/Stat3 pathway in synaptic plasticity have been reported. Activation of the Jak2/Stat3 pathway induces presynaptic transcriptional upregulation of cholinergic genes including choline acetyletransferase (ChAT) and vesicular acetylcholine transporter (VAChT) and postsynaptic sensitization of m_1-type muscarinic acetylcholine receptor (m_1-mAChR) to support cholinergic neurotransmission (Chiba et al., 2009b). The Jak2/Stat3 pathway also plays an essential role in the induction of NMDA-receptor dependent long-term depression (NMDAR-LTD) in the hippocampus (Nicolas et al., 2012).

2.3. Emerging genetic risk factors for AD

AD can be classified into early onset (EOAD, <65 years) and late onset (LOAD, >65 years) form. According to family history, AD can be also classified into FAD and sporadic (SAD) (Alves et al., 2010). Although aforementioned three FAD genes generally result in EOAD, there is a substantial genetic component in LOAD as well (an estimated heritability of 58-79%). Accordingly, *apolipoprotein E (APOE)* gene on chromosome 19 has also been shown to be a genetic risk factor for LOAD in the early 1990s (Bertram et al., 2010; Schellenberg and Montine, 2012). *APOE* contains three major alleles: ε2, ε3, and ε4. Inherited ε4 allele is reported to worsen the loss of neuronal function in AD patients and decrease the age of onset (Huang and Mucke, 2012;

http://dx.doi.org/10.5772/55293

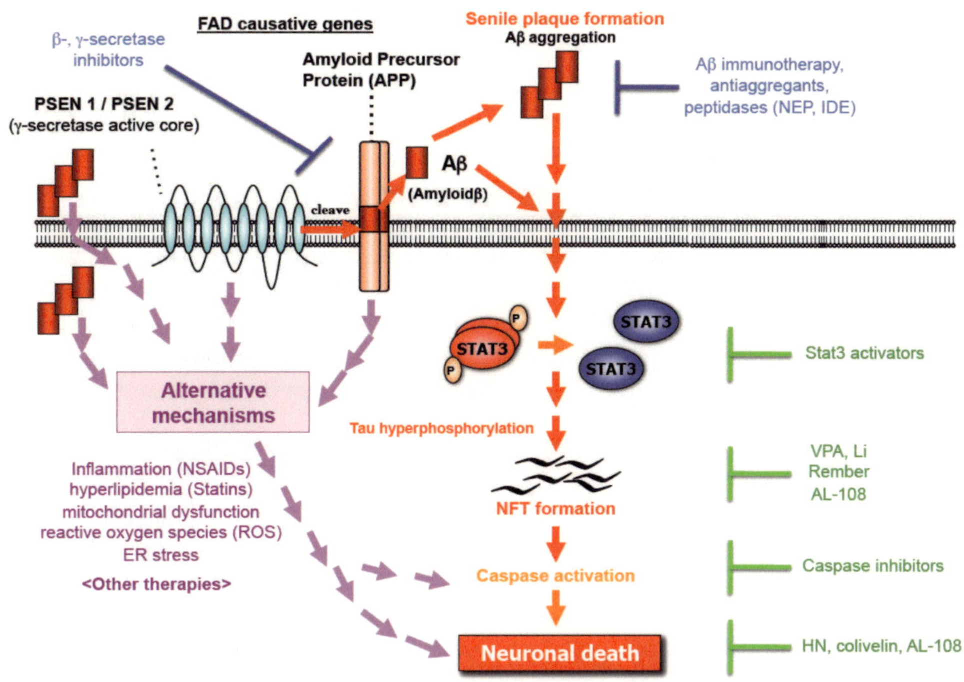

Figure 3. A schematic overview of the "amyloid cascade" hypothesis and therapeutic strategies. (Red arrows) The "amyloid cascade" begins with the proteolytic cleavage of APP by the γ-secretase. Aβ forms toxic oligomers or aggregates, inducing neuronal Stat3 inactivation, NFT formation, caspase activation and neuronal death. Therapies targeting the canonical "amyloid cascade" such as secretase inhibitors and immunotherapy are indicated in blue characters. Therapies targeting on the downstream pathways of the "amyloid cascade" are indicated in green characters. Alternative pathological mechanisms, which can be caused by intracellular Aβ, extracellular Aβ, or FAD mutants themselves, are also targeted (purple). (NEP, neprilysin; IDE, insulin degrading enzyme; VPA, valproic acid; HN, humanin).

Poirier, 2005). One copy of *APOE* ε4 increases the risk for AD fourfold and two copies further raise the risk tenfold. *APOE* is not a causative gene, i.e. *APOE* ε4 is neither necessary nor sufficient for LOAD. In addition to *APOE* itself, a variable-length poly-T (deoxythymidine homopolymer) polymorphism in the *TOMM40* gene, located in a region of strong linkage disequilibrium next to *APOE*, was reported to be associated with the age of onset of LOAD (Lutz et al., 2010; Roses et al.).

Genetic association studies on LOAD susceptibility loci and small nucleotide polymorphisms (SNPs) revealed two genes: *ubiquilin 1 (UBQLN1)* on chromosome 9 (Bertram et al., 2005) and *sortilin-related receptor (SORL1)* (Rogaeva et al., 2007). Identification of *UBQLN1* is intriguing since it not only interacts with PSEN1, PSEN2 and APP but also may play a role in the proteasome degradation of them (Mah et al., 2000; Massey et al., 2004). SORL1 is involved in both trafficking of APP from the cell surface into recycling pathways and processing of APP by γ-secretase. A recent meta-analysis of genetic data and GWAS supported that mutations in *SORL1* may play a role in LOAD although the effect on the AD risk is moderate (Schellenberg and Montine, 2012). On the other hand, no evidence for *UBQLN1* has been provided from GWAS.

Since 2009, several GWAS results have been published (Alves et al., 2010; Bertram, 2011; Eisenstein, 2011; Reitz, 2012; Schellenberg and Montine, 2012). In GWAS, researchers analyze millions of SNPs in affected and healthy individuals. There is a criticism that two many comparisons at the same time will just lead to a number of false positive associations, which cannot be reproduced by other studies. This is partially true. GWAS, however, have identified nine novel loci reproducibly associated with LOAD: (i) *clusterin (CLU)*, (ii) *phosphatidylinositol-binding clathrin assembly protein (PICALM)*, (iii) *complement receptor 1 (CR1)*, (iv) *bridging integrator 1 (BIN1)*, (v) *ATP-binding cassette, subfamily A, member 7 (ABCA7)*, (vi) *membrane-spanning 4-domains, subfamily A, members 4 and 6E (MS4A4/MS4A6E, MS4A cluster)*, (vii) *CD2-associated protein (CD2AP)*, (viii) *CD33 molecule (CD33)* and (ix) *EPH receptor A1 (EPHA1)* (Bertram, 2011). These genes significantly increase risk for LOAD although they rather have small effects on susceptibility to AD (within 1.5 times increase or decrease in odds ratio).

One of the important aims of GWAS is to identify novel pathogenic pathways for AD. Although Morgan, for example, classified risk genes identified from GWAS into three new pathogenic pathways (Morgan): immune system function (*CLU, CR1, ABCA7, MS4A cluster, CD33 and EPHA1*), cholesterol metabolism (*APOE, CLU and ABCA7*) and synaptic dysfunction (*PICALM, BIN1, CD33, CD2AP and EPHA1*). Others assume that most of risk genes are related to the "amyloid cascade", providing a solid support for the "amyloid cascade" hypothesis. This discrepancy is due to multiple functions of each risk gene. E.g. *CLU*, which is also known as *apolipoprotein-J (APOJ)*, helps *APOE* in cholesterol trafficking in the central nervous system and is also involved in Aβ aggregation and clearance. *CR1* is an important component of the innate immune response against infection and is also involved in the clearance of circulating Aβ. In summary, *APOE* is still the biggest risk gene for LOAD and detailed functional analyses are necessary for other novel risk genes to discuss novel or relevant pathogenic mechanisms for AD.

3. Clinically available drugs for AD

In this section, currently available drugs in AD clinics, such as cholinesterase inhibitors (ChEIs) and N-methyl-D-aspartate (NMDA) receptor antagonists will be discussed (Lleo et al., 2006; Mangialasche et al., 2010). More than 15 years have passed since the first ChEI, donepezil (Aricept®), was approved as a clinical drug for AD in the United States. Many clinical trials and follow-up surveys have revealed marginal to moderate effects of ChEIs and NMDA antagonists in AD patients (Riordan et al., 2011). They show only symptomatic effects although potential neuroprotective effects have been postulated.

3.1. Cholinesterase inhibitors (ChEIs)

Deteriorated cholinergic function such as loss of basal forebrain cholinergic neurons is one of the pathological features of AD (Bartus et al., 1982; Farrimond et al., 2012; Van der Zee et al.). Acetylcholine (ACh), which is one of neurotransmitters functioning in both central and peripheral nervous system, is synthesized from choline and acetyl coenzyme A (acetyl-CoA) by an enzyme ChAT in certain neurons. There are two major classes of ACh receptors (AChRs); i.e. ionotropic nicotinic AChR (nAChR) and metabotropic muscarinic AChR (mAChR). ACh in the synaptic cleft is rapidly degraded into two inactive metabolites choline and acetate by an enzyme, ChE. Thus, cholinergic neurotransmission can be improved with ChEIs via prevention of ACh degradation.

ChEIs, such as donepezil (Aricept®), galantamine (Razadyne®) and rivastigmine (Exelon®) are approved by the Food and Drug Administration (FDA) for the treatment of AD (Farrimond et al., 2012; Pettenati et al., 2003). Donepezil is a reversible ChEI with high specificity with few side effects and can be used for all stages of AD. Galantamine, which is approved for mild-to-moderate AD, has multiple functions such as inhibition of ChE, induction of ACh release and allosteric stimulation of nAChR. Rivastigmine, which is also for mild-to-moderate AD, suppresses both acetyl- and butyryl-ChE. Some placebo-controlled, double-blind trials have demonstrated that ChEI therapy results in significant improvement in cognitive performance of AD patients. Unfortunately, however, a long-term rondamized trial named 'AD2000' failed to prove therapeutic benefits of Donepezil (Courtney et al., 2004; Tariot et al., 2001; Winblad et al., 2006). Although ChEIs may slow worsening of AD symptoms to some extent, it should be noted that the effectiveness of ChEIs and how long they work, would vary from person to person. In addition, direct activation of acetylcholine receptors, such as m_1-mAChR and $\alpha7$ nAChR, is currently under development.

3.2. N-methyl-D-aspartate (NMDA) receptor antagonists

Excitotoxicity by excess amount of glutamatergic neurotransmission is also implicated in the pathogenesis of AD. Memantine (Namenda®) is a non-competitive, voltage-dependent and of moderate affinity N-methyl-D-aspartate (NMDA) receptor antagonist, preventing neuronal cells from excitotoxic death caused by a glutamate-induced excessive income of calcium ions. Memantine was approved by the FDA in 2003 for the treatment of moderate-to-severe AD since it improved cognitive function of AD patients who were receiving stable doses of a ChEI (Tariot et al., 2004). Serious side effects have not been reported to occur at high frequency. In addition to the NMDA antagonism, memantine is reported to decrease Aβ production (Alley et al., 2009; Ray et al., 2009), suppress synaptic dysfunction (Klyubin et al., 2009) and induce protein phosphatase-2A (PP2A)-mediated reduction of tau hyperphosphorylation (Chohan et al., 2006; Martinez-Coria et al., 2010).

3.3. Other supporting drugs

AD patients also suffer from neuropsychiatric symptoms such as apathy, depression, anxiety, psychosis, aggression and sleep disturbances, which are generally called as behavioral and psychological symptoms in dementia (BPSD) (Alves et al., 2010). When BPSD are severe and persist despite the use of ChEIs and memantine, pharmacological treatment will be started. For severe depression, antidepressive drugs such as sertraline, which is one of the selective serotonin reuptake inhibitors (SSRIs) used to treat major depression. Neuroleptic drugs such as risperidone, which is a dopamine antagonist and mainly used to treat schizophrenia, are used to treat aggression, agitation and psychosis. Anxiolytics such as loracepam and oxacepam (benzodiazepines) are also used to ameliorate anxiety and verbal problems. For sleeping disturbances, non-pharmacological interventions are common because sleeping drugs or sedative-hypnotic medications have only a limited efficacy and significant adverse effects (David et al., 2010; Shub et al., 2009). In addition, melatonin, which is an endogenous regulator of circadian rhythms and is used as a chronobiotic or soporific, showed no benefits in a multicenter, placebo-controlled trial for sleep disturbance in AD (Singer et al., 2003). These drugs are used to reduce BPSD and to improve patients' activities of daily living and quality of life.

4. Emerging therapeutic strategies

Finally, emerging therapeutic strategies will be discussed. For better understanding, strategies are first classified into two major categories: AD-specific and AD-non-specific disease modifying treatments (Table 1). As to AD-specific disease-modifying treatments, the amyloidogenic processes and their regulatory mechanisms are defined as the canonical "amyloid cascade". Strategies based on other findings related to the downstream pathways of the "amyloid cascade" are summarized in the other drugs based on alternative pathways. Drugs related to the downstream mechanisms from the amyloidogenesis including tau phosphorylation and Stat3 inactivation are classified into the alternative pathways here because the connection between the canonical "amyloid cascade" and the downstream mechanisms is still elusive. As to AD-non-specific treatments, regenerative therapy may be realized in the near future with an enormous progress in the field of stem cell biology.

4.1. AD-specific drugs targeting the canonical "amyloid cascade"

In the last 10 years, most pharmaceutical companies were trying hard to develop secretase inhibitors such as α-, β- and γ-secretase inhibitors to suppress amyloid beta production, the initial step of the "amyloid cascade" (Ghosh et al., 2012; Wolfe, 2012). A number of clinical trials of β-secretase inhibitors and γ-secretase inhibitors have been carried out or are ongoing.

Another major attempt has been the development of Aβ immunotherapy to remove amyloid deposits, which is also targeting the initial step of the cascade (Delrieu et al., 2012). Both active and passive immunization have been developed by utilizing Aβ peptide and its antigenic epitopes, or anti-Aβ antibodies.

4.1.1. Aβ immunotherapy to remove brain Aβ

Initial findings from a clinical trial of active Aβ immunotherapy

Aβ immunotherapy is an approach to remove accumulated Aβ in AD brains immunologically: Aβ vaccination therapy and passive immunization with anti-Aβ antibody. Schenk *et al.* reported that the Aβ vaccine named AN-1792, which contains Aβ42 peptide and adjuvants, significantly reduced amyloid plaques in brain of PD-APP mice (Schenk et al., 1999). With the evidence in transgenic mice, clinical trial was started in 2001. Phase II studies performed in

Europe and USA, however, were suspended since 6% of the subjects gave a sign of meningoencephalitis such as fever, vomiting, headache, loss of consciousness, and so on after the second vaccination (Orgogozo et al., 2003). Patients who received AN-1792 have been reported to show elevated levels of antibodies against Aβ (Hock et al., 2002) and some immunized patients resulted in reduction of amyloid deposits without significant decrease in both NFT formation and neuronal cell death (Nicoll et al., 2003).

As reported, there is a potential risk in the Aβ immunothrerapy that antibodies against APP induce neuronal cell death, which may lead to meningoencephalitis (Rohn et al., 2000; Sudo et al., 2000). Although it is reported that antibodies elevated in patients mainly recognize SPs, there is still a certain possibility that small fraction of elevated antibodies binds to APP and induces neuronal death. Another potential risk is that cytotoxic T cells, which might cause cellular toxicity on neurons, are also activated by active immunization. In agreement, there were a number of lymphocytic infiltration in brains of immunized AD patients (Nicoll et al., 2003).

Improvement of Aβ immunotherapy

Recently, however, several alternatives of Aβ immunotherapy have been proposed. Passive immunization with anti-Aβ monoclonal antibodies is first one (Dodart et al., 2002; Kotilinek et al., 2002). In this approach, it seems easier to control side-effects by using monoclonal antibody than non-specific activation of immune system by active immunization. Active immunization can be safer by specific targeting of immunogen to T-helper cells. Other types of immunization have been also developed. Hara *et al.* developed an oral vaccine using recombinant adeno-associated virus (AAV) vector encoding Aβ cDNA (Hara et al., 2004) and Okura *et al.* developed nonviral Aβ DNA vaccine (Okura et al., 2006). With these vaccines, serum antibodies against Aβ were elevated by ectopic Aβ expression without T cell proliferative response. Safety of these vaccines, however, should be carefully tested.

Improved active Aβ immunotherapy

New vaccines that selectively target B-cell epitopes (N-terminus of Aβ peptide) have been developed. CAD-106, consisting of Aβ1-6 peptide coupled to virus-like carrier particle Qβ (a T-helper cell epitope) could efficiently induce Aβ antibodies without induction of Aβ-specific T-cells (Wiessner et al., 2011). Similar strategy is employed in other vaccines: ACC-01 (Aβ1-6 donjugated to the mutated diphtheria toxin protein CRM19), V-950 (Aβ N-terminus with an aluminium-containing adjuvant with or without ISCOMATRIX), ACI-24 (Aβ1-15 closely apposed to the surface of the liposome), UB-311 (Aβ1-14 associated with the UBITh peptide, a T-helper cell epitope) (Mangialasche et al., 2010; Reitz, 2012). Another active immunization strategy is based on Affitopes, short peptides mimicking parts of native Aβ42 without its sequence identity. AD-01 and AD-02 mimick the N-terminal Aβ fragments. These vaccines are generally reported to be safe and well-tolerated in phase I studies. Results of phase II and III studies are awaited.

Passive Aβ immunotherapy

Passive immunotherapy is based on the administration of antibodies against Aβ. This can be achieved by both monoclonal antibodies and polyclonal immunoglobulins. In animal models, anti-Aβ antibodies are reported to prevent oligomer formation with reduced brain Aβ load. Several monoclonal antibodies are currently tested in clinical trials: bapineuzumab (AAB-001), solanezumab (LY-2062430), ponezumab (PF-04360365), GSK-933776, R-1450 (RO-4909832), and MABT-5102A (Mangialasche et al., 2010). A phase II study of bapineuzumab in patients with mild to moderate AD did not attain statistical significance on the primary efficacy endpoints in the overall study population (Salloway et al., 2009). They only found some statistically significant benefits in limited subpopulations without the APOE e4 allele. A phase III study of bapineuzumab finally again failed recently (Aug. 6, 2012: www.pfizer.com). Solanezumab, which mobilized brain Aβ in a phase II study (Farlow et al., 2012), also failed to slow cognitive decline in phase III clinical trials including more than 2,050 AD patients (Aug. 24, 2012: www.lilly.com). Ponezumab is a humanized monoclonal IgG2 antibody binding to the C-terminus of Aβ40 and a phase I trial showed that the antibody is well tolerated in AD patients (Freeman et al., 2012). Other antibodies are also currently tested in phase I and II studies.

Passive immunization can also be achieved by intravenous infusion of immunoglobins (IVIg), from healthy donors, which are assumed to include naturally occurring polyclonal antibodies against pathogenic Aβ (Britschgi et al., 2009; Dodel et al., 2002; Dodel et al., 2004; Fillit et al., 2009). IVIg is already approved for immune deficiency, meaning that it is safe and well tolerated. Preliminary data from a phase II study showed a positive effect on cognition (Relkin et al., 2009).

Active versus passive Aβ immunotherapy

Active immunotherapy will keep high antibody titers for a long period, enabling few follow-up observations and reduced costs. The control of the antibody concentrations and adverse effects are limited, however. Passive immunotherapy offers a good and rapid control of antibody properties and concentrations. In addition, passive immunotherapy could be more effective in elderly population with reduced immune responses. However, administration of antibodies is time- and money-consuming. The effects of active and passive Aβ immunotherapy are not so much different and unfortunately both immunotherapy are not successful so far.

4.1.2. γ-secretase and β-secretase inhibitors for reduction of Aβ production

Secretases have become the targets to control Aβ production and prevent the progress of AD since Aβ is generated from APP via sequential cleavage by β- and γ-secretases (Chiba et al., 2007; De Strooper and Annaert, 2000). This is the initial step in the canonical "amyloid cascade". Considering that most of the mutant *APP* and *PSEN1* result in increased Aβ42/Aβ40 ratio, abnormal γ-secretase function seems to be closely related to the pathogenesis of AD. In addition, the choice of the first cleavage by α- or β-secretase decides the generation of Aβ, which gives us the notion that β-cleavage inhibition and α-cleavage activation greatly reduce Aβ production.

β-secretase inhibitors

In 1999, β-site APP cleaving enzyme (BACE1), a membrane-anchored aspartyl protease, was reported to have β-secretase activity (John et al., 2003; Vassar et al., 1999). The BACE1 knock out mice studies showed that Aβ levels in brain was drastically reduced, and they remain healthy without any anomaly in clear contrast to that of PSEN knockout mice (Cai et al., 2001; Luo et al.,

2001). Consequently, it is assumed that β-secretase inhibitors are safer than γ-secretase inhibitors. Recently, however, BACE1/2 double knockout mice was generated and resulted in lethal phenotype, presumably because BACE1/2 have many substrates (including neuregulin-1, which is involved in myelination) required in the development (Dominguez et al., 2005).

Pioglitazone and rosiglitazone are thiazolidinediones, which control blood sugar by stimulating the nuclear peroxisome proliferator-activated receptor γ (PPARγ), clinically used for type II diabetes mellitus (DM). They turned out to be good BACE1 inhibitors: i.e. PPARγ activation by the thiazolidinediones suppresses BACE1 and APP expression (Mangialasche et al., 2010). In addition, pioglitazone and rosiglitazone promote Aβ degradation, which is competitively inhibited by insulin, by reducing insulin concentrations. Results from clinical studies are, however, disappointing (Miller et al., 2011). Neither pioglitazone nor rosiglitazone showed any efficacy on cognition in AD patients.

γ-secretase inhibitors

Development of γ-secretase inhibitors, which suppress the final step in amyloidgenesis, is one of the major issues in AD research. Transition state analogs of γ-secretase, such as L-685458 (Merk), inhibit the γ-secretase activity and decreases production of Aβ40 and Aβ42 (Shearman et al., 2000). Chemical compunds including pepstatin A, sulfonamide derivatives and benzodiazepines are also shown to inhibit the γ-secretase activity in mechanisms other than competitive inhibition (Tian et al., 2002). Since γ-secretase is also involved in processing of other membrane proteins including Notch, γ-secretase inhibitors may induce severe side effects. In agreement, the chronic administration of a γ-secretase inhibitor triggered abnormal blood cell differentiation and damage on digestive tracts (Searfoss et al., 2003). APP-specific γ-secretase inhibitors or γ-secretase modulators may resolve this problem.

Several γ-secretase inhibitors are currently tested in clinical studies: semagacestat (LY450139), begacestat (GSI-953), avagacestat (BMS-708163), PF-3084014, MK-0752, E-2012 and NIC5-15 (Mangialasche et al., 2010). Phase III trials for semagacestat, which inhibits Notch cleavage as well as APP cleavage, not only failed but also worsened clinical measures of cognition and activity of daily living with increased incidence of skin cancer (Cummings, 2010). Other Notch-sparing γ-secretase inhibitors (second-generation inhibitors) such as begacestat and avagacestat are now in phase I or II studies and they show reduction of plasma and/or cerebrospinal fluid (CSF) Aβ levels. PF-3084014, a γ-secretase inhibitor with high selectivity for APP, and NIC5-15, a Notch-sparing γ-secretase inhibitor with insulin sensitizing activity, showed some positive effects with good tolerance and now proceeded into phase II studies (Mangialasche et al., 2010). Effects of a γ-secretase modulator, tarenflurbil, will be discussed later (see 4.3.2.).

α-secretase activators

Upregulation of α-cleavage, which results in non-amyloidogenic cleavage of APP, can competitively inhibit β-cleavage, leading to downregulation of Aβ production and reciprocal upregulation of neuroprotective soluble APPα (sAPPα) secretion (Vingtdeux and Marambaud, 2012). α-Secretase is a member of the ADAM (a disintegrin and metalloprotease) family of proteases including ADAM10, ADAM17/TACE (TNFα converting enzyme), or ADAM9. There is a number of ways to activate α-secretase (Mangialasche et al., 2010): (i) activation of neurotransmitter receptors such as muscarinic, glutamate, γ-aminobutyric acid (GABA) (e.g. etazolate [SQ-20009, EHT-0202]) and serotonin receptors (e.g. SB-742457, PRX-03140, AVN-322 and RQ-00000009), (ii) steroid hormones such as estrogens and testosterones, and (iii) protein kinase C (PKC) activation (e.g. bryostatin-1). No conclusive results are published yet from clinical trials.

4.1.3. Drugs preventing Aβ aggregation, destabilizing Aβ oligomers and inducing Aβ clearance

Neurotoxic activity of Aβ is likely to be mediated by certain types of soluble oligomers (Di Carlo, 2010; Lesne et al., 2006; Schilling et al., 2008). Oligomerization and aggregation of Aβ further promote SP formation or accumulation of brain Aβ load. Therefore, compounds preventing Aβ aggregation or destabilizing Aβ oligomers seem to be promising drug candidates for AD. Compounds binding to Aβ monomers may prevent oligomerization and promote Aβ degradation, while compounds recognizing Aβ oligomers may neurtralize the neurotoxicity and facilitate Aβ clearance.

Tramiprosate (homotaurine, 3APS), which is one of the non-peptidic anti-aggregants binding to Aβ monomers, failed to show clinical efficacy in a phase III study (the Alphase study) (Aisen et al., 2011). An antifungal and antiprotozoal drug clioquinol (PBT1) (Tabira, 2001), which disrupts interactions between Aβ, copper and zinc, showed positive results in phase II studies, but further studies were halted due to manufacturing toxicity issues (Ritchie et al., 2003; Sampson et al., 2008). PBT2, a second-generation inhibitor without toxicity, also showed promising results in a phase II study (Lannfelt et al., 2008). Scyllo-inositol (ELND-005), an orally administered stereoisomer of inositol, binds to Aβ, inhibits Aβ aggregation and promotes dissociation of aggregates. Phase II studies, however, revealed serious adverse events among patients with high-dose treatments (Salloway et al., 2011). Epigallocatechin-3-gallate (EGCg), a polyphenol from green tea, preventing Aβ aggregation by binding to unfolded Aβ, is currently tested in phase II/III studies (Mandel et al., 2008; Rezai-Zadeh et al., 2005).

Aβ clearance itself is also a target of novel therapeutics, which is based on the fact that Aβ clearance from brains is impaired in AD patients, especially in those with *APOE* ε4. Aβ clearance can be achieved by local Aβ uptake and degradation in the CNS (Aβ degradation will be discussed in 4.1.4), or pumping out of Aβ through the blood-brain-barrier (BBB) from the brain to the plasma. Aβ clearance is facilitated by APOE, the transcription or expression levels of which are regulated by PPARγ and heterodimeric receptors consisting of liver X receptors (LXRs) and retinoid X receptors (RXRs) (Cramer et al., 2012; Huang and Mucke, 2012). Agonists of these receptors could be used to reduce Aβ load in AD brains. Aβ translocation through BBB is regulated by lipoprotein receptor related protein-1 (LRP-1), which is a receptor for APOE and α2-macroglobulin, and the receptor for advanced glycation endproducts (RAGE) (Deane et al., 2003; Deane et al., 2008). LRP-1 pumps Aβ out of the CNS across the BBB, while RAGE supports Aβ influx into the CNS. The soluble form of RAGE (sRAGE) competes with the membrane-linked RAGE, promoting removal of circulating Aβ. A phase II study on a RAGE inhibitor (TTP-488) is ongoing (Mangialasche et al., 2010). Lactoferrin, a globular glycoprotein found in various secretory fluids such as milk, saliva and tears, is known to stimulate LRP-1 (Ito et al., 2007). LRP-1 agonists are also candidates for AD therapy.

http://dx.doi.org/10.5772/55293

4.1.4. Drugs inducing Aβ degradation

An endopeptidase named neprilysin (NEP) was identified to degrade Aβ aggregates and regulate Aβ metabolism *in vivo* (Iwata et al., 2001; Iwata et al., 2000). It is a type II transmembranous ectoenzyme, and cleaves peptide bond of N-terminal hydrophobic amino acid residue in lower than 5kDa peptide. In knock out mice study, Aβ levels in brain elevated to twice as that in the control mice (Iwata et al., 2001), and NEP gets lower in old wild type mice brain (Iwata et al., 2002). Furthermore, the expression levels of NEP were decreased to the half levels in sporadic AD patients' brain as compared with healthy controls' (Yasojima et al., 2001a; Yasojima et al., 2001b). The cleavege of Aβ by NEP, however, is not so potent that NEP itself may be difficult to be clinically effective. Recently, Saito *et al.* have reported that somatostatin regulates brain Aβ42 through modulating proteolytic degradation catalyzed by NEP (Saito et al., 2005). Somatostatin and its receptor could also be utilized in the Aβ degradation therapy for AD.

Insulin degrading enzyme (IDE) is another enzyme degrading Aβ (Qiu et al., 1998). Overexpression of IDE in AD mouse models retarded or even completely prevented SP formation, while IDE knockout mice showed increased levels of Aβ and insulin (Farris et al., 2003; Leissring et al., 2003). Cabrol *et al.* performed high-throughput compound screening for small-molecule activator of IDE and found promising compound activating IDE by binding to its putative ATP-binding domain (Cabrol et al., 2009). Current investigations have further suggested that Aβ degradation is also mediated by multiple types of proteases including presequence peptidase, endothelin converting enzyme (ECE), angiotensin-converting enzyme (ACE), the uPA/tPA-plasmin system, transthyretin (TTR, gelsolin, α2-macroglobulin and matrix metalloproteinases (MMP-2 and 9) (Nalivaeva et al., 2012).

4.2. AD-specific drugs based on the alternative pathways

Drugs targeting the downstream pathways of the "amyloid cascade" have been also developed. These include tau inhibitors and neuronal death inhibitors. Tau inhibitors are either based on suppression of tau phosphorylation or inhibition of tau aggregation. Glycogen-synthase-kinase-3β (GSK3β) inhibitors are shown to reduce tau phosphorylation and methylene blue inhibits tau aggretation. Neuronal death can be suppressed by endogenous soluble factors such as leptin, AL-108 (NAP) and humanin (HN) as well as artificially modified small peptides such as colivelin (CLN) (Chiba et al., 2009a). Some of them activate Stat3, which is specifically inactivated in AD patients. AL-108 shows anti-Aβ activity and anti-tau activity at the same time.

Alternative therapeutic targets are also emerging. One of the major targets is related to the metabolic syndrome. Several lines of evidence supported that the metabolic syndrome increases the relative risk of AD (Misiak et al., 2012). Especially, there seems to be a link between type 2 diabetes mellitus (DM) and AD. Thiazolidinediones, commonly used for type 2 DM such as piaglitazone and rosiglitazone, are already mentioned focusing on their BACE1 inhibiting activity. In addition, there is epidemiological evidence that drugs used for high cholesterol (hypercholesterolemia) and high blood pressure also lower the risk of AD (Burgos et al., 2012; Davies et al., 2011).

Symptomatic treatments (= currently available)	
Treatments for AD-related dementia	Treatments for BPSD
1. **Cholinesterase inhibitors (ChEIs):** donepezil (Aricept®), galantamine (Razadyne®), rivastigmine (Exelon®) 2. **NMDA receptor antagonist:** memantine (Namenda®)	1. Anti-depresseive drugs: sertraline (SSRI) etc. 2. Neuroleptic: risperidone (atypical antipsychotics) etc. 3. Anxiolytics: loracepam, oxacepam (benzodiazepines) etc. 4. Sleep disturbance: non-pharmacological interventions
AD-specific Disease-modifying treatments	
Drugs targeting the canonical "amyloid cascade"	Drugs based on the alternative pathways
1. **Aβ immunotherapy (IT):** active IT: AN-1792 (f), CAD-106, ACC-01, V-950 etc. passive IT: bapineurzumab (f), solanezumab (f), IVIg etc. 2. **Secretase inhibitors:** suppression of Aβ production β-inhibitors: pioglitazone (f), rosiglitazone (f). γ-inhibitors: semagacestat (f), begacestat, avagacestat etc. α-activators: etazolate, SB-742457, bryostatin-1 etc. 3. **Aβ aggregation inhibitor:** tramiprosate (f), PBT2 etc. 4. **Aβ degradation:** Aβ degradase (NEP, IDE) activator	1. Drugs based on tau pathology: VPA (f), Li (f), Rember 2. Neuronal death inhibitors: caspase inhibitors (Q-VD-OPh), neuroprotective peptides (HN, colivelin, AL-108 etc.) 3. Stat3 activation therapy: cytokines, PTP inhibitors etc. 4. Prion hypothesis for AD 5. Drugs based on epidemiological findings in AD 5-1. NSAIDs: Flurizan (f) 5-2. Statins: atorvastatin (f), simvastatin (f) 5-3. Dimebon (f)
AD-non-specific Disease-modifying treatments	
Memory enhancing treatments	Regenerative treatments
1. Antioxidants: vitamin E (f), natural polyphenols 2. Neurotrophic factors: NGF, BDNF, bFGF, VEGF, HGF etc. 3. Other drugs: PDE9A inhibitor, DHA (f) etc.	1. Implantation of NSCs, NPCs, neurons 2. Activation of endogenous neurogenesis: BDNF etc.

Table 1. Therapeutic strategy for AD. Drugs which failed in clinical trials are indicated with "(f)".

4.2.1. Drugs based on tau pathology

In AD, abnormally hyperphosphorylated tau forms aggregates called NFT. This pathway can be inhibited by preventing either hyperphosphorylation or aggregation. Tau phosphorylation is regulated by the equilibrium between tau kinases (e.g. cdk5, JNK and GSK3β) and tau phosphatases (e.g. protein phosphatase 2A [PP2A]). Aggregated tau shows β-sheet structure similar to Aβ aggregates although tau locates only in the cytoplasm.

Valproate (valproic acid, VPA) is reported to suppress tau phosphorylation via inhibiting cdk5 and GSK3β (Hu et al., 2011). This is so far the only compound, which reached phase III studies, in this category. Unfortunately, VPA showed no efficacy on cognition (Mangialasche et al., 2010; Tariot and Aisen, 2009). Lithium (Li), as well as VPA, is a well-known drug for psychiatric disorder, inhibiting GSK3β. A small clinical study with Li, however, did not show any cognitive benefit or any change in biomarkers (Hampel et al., 2009). Regardless of these failures, several GSK3 inhibitors are under development. NP-031112 (NP-12) is one of those GSK3 inhibitors and is currently tested in a phase II study, the result of which have not been reported.

Methylene blue (Rember®), which is used as a redox indicator in analytical chemistry and as a dye for nuclear staining in histology, is recently attracting attention as an anti-aggregant for

http://dx.doi.org/10.5772/55293

tau (Schirmer et al., 2011). Rember also has antioxidant activity and supports mitochondrial function. A phase II study showed slower disease progression in patients receiving a middle-dose (60 mg) although the highest-dose (100 mg) failed to show its efficacy presumably due to drug formulation defects (Mangialasche et al., 2010). A phase III study is now on-going.

4.2.2. Neuronal death inhibitors

Neuronal death is directly implicated in the pathogenesis of AD (Rohn and Head, 2009). Neuronal loss, but not SPs, correlates with the cognitive impairment in AD. Consequently, it is supposed that neuronal death suppression will result in potent therapeutic effect or even a curative one. Neuronal death could be caused by not only toxic Aβ oligomers but also death signals activated by mutations in the FAD genes. Notably, the death signals can differ depending on the types of FAD genes and the types of mutations (Chiba et al., 2007; Kawasumi et al., 2002). Apoptosis is implicated in the neuronal loss related to AD: terminal deoxyuridine triphosphate nick endlabeling (TUNEL)-staining and caspase activation are observed in neurons of patients' brains.

Complicated mechanisms of neuronal loss

It was a milestone in AD research that Yamatsuji *et al.* first showed that expression of FAD-associated mutants of *APP* (V642I/F/G) induce apoptosis via a mechanism independent of Aβ because it suggested not only that there might be neurotoxic insults other than Aβ underlying AD pathogenesis but also that APP might have physiological function besides its role as a precursor of Aβ (Yamatsuji et al., 1996). Actually, multiple groups have confirmed that overexpression of FAD mutants of *APP* induces neuronal cell death by triggering intracellular death signaling cascades (Hashimoto et al., 2000; Zhao et al., 1997). In addition, a number of observations support the idea that APP might function as a cell-surface receptor inducing cell death signals. Given that APP-dimerization activates the intracellular death signals identical to that induced by FAD mutants of APP without ligand stimulation, it is likely that there is a natural ligand for APP to trigger intracellular death signals. In accordance with the idea, transforming growth factor β2 (TGFβ2) and death receptor 6 (DR6) are reported to be physiological ligands for APP triggering the fore-mentioned death signals (Hashimoto et al., 2005; Nikolaev et al., 2009).

FAD-linked mutants of *PSEN1* and *PSEN2* also enhance cell death in several cell lines and primary neurons. Mechanisms of death induced by mutants of *PSEN1* is likely to be distinct from that by *PSEN2*. *PSEN1* mutants induce calcium-dependent oxidative stress (Guo et al., 1996), destabilization of β-catenin (Zhang et al., 1998), down-regulation of Akt (Weihl et al., 1999), ER stress (Mattson et al., 1998), and activation of nitric oxide synthase (NOS)-mediated caspase-independent death signals (Hashimoto et al., 2002a), while PSEN2 mutants induce downregulation of Bcl-X(L) (Passer et al., 1999) and Bcl-2 (Araki et al., 2001), activation of NADPH oxidase and xanthine oxidase (XO) (Hashimoto et al., 2002b).

Activated caspases may serve as positive feedback regulators of death. APP is reported to be a substrate for caspase-3, which may contribute to Aβ formation and synaptic loss (Gervais et al., 1999). Tau is also a substrate for caspases and truncation of tau by caspases may lead to the formation of paired helical filaments (PHFs) and further NFTs (Gamblin et al., 2003).

Caspase inhibitors for AD

Evidence supports a role for executioner caspases including caspases-3, -6 and -7 in the pathogenesis of AD. Caspase activation can be prevented by peptide-based inhibitors such as Z-VAD-fmk and Z-DEVD-fmk (more specific to caspase-3). Although these inhibitors are potent and efficient *in vitro*, establishment of a proper drug delivery system and formulation is necessary for *in vivo* treatment of AD patients (Rohn and Head, 2009). An alternative small molecule, the quinolyl-valyl-O-methylaspartyl-[-2, 6-difluorophenoxy]-methyl ketone (Q-VD-OPh), has been developed to substitute Z-VAD-fmk (Caserta et al., 2003). Q-VD-OPh is not toxic to cells at high concentrations and is systemically active, demonstrating efficacy in animal models of Parkinson's disease (PD), Huntington's disease (HD) and stroke (Renolleau et al., 2007; Yang et al., 2004).

Another potential therapeutic strategy lies on upregulation of anti-apoptotic Bcl-2 protein. Small compounds inhibiting Bcl-2 have been synthesized for the treatment of cancer, while compounds activating Bcl-2 have not been obtained so far. In addition, Bcl-2 should not be activated systemically because of expected severe side effects such as tumorigenesis. Consequently, the delivery of *Bcl-2* gene by viral vectors, such as adenoviruses, AAV and lentiviruses, is considered. Local delivery of *Bcl-2* and its family genes by viral vectors are shown to be efficient in several animal models of neurodegeneration including cerebral ischemia, axotomy and amyotrophic lateral sclerosis (ALS) (Caleo et al., 2002; Kilic et al., 2002; Yamashita et al., 2001).

Another potential drug candidate is minocycline, which is reported to prevent mitochondrial release of cytochrome c and the following caspase-3 activation (Hashimoto, 2011). Minocycline is an orally available second-generation tetracycline, which can cross the BBB. It is reported that minocycline elicited therapeutic effects in animal models of ischemic brain injury, ALS, PD, HD and multiple sclerosis (Berger, 2000; Du et al., 2001; Zhu et al., 2002). Recent studies revealed that minocycline protects neurons and reduces Aβ deposition in AD mice although efficacy of minocycline in AD is yet to be carefully addressed (Choi et al., 2007; Seabrook et al., 2006).

Multi-spectrum neuroprotective factor, humanin and its derivatives

A functional screening for a death-suppressing factor, which antagonizes death induced by overexpression of V642I-APP, was carried out with a cDNA library established from occipital lobes of AD patients, which are relatively preserved regions in AD brains (Hashimoto et al., 2001b). As a result, cDNA encoding a novel 24 amino-acid peptide, termed humanin (HN), was identified (MAPRGFSCLLLLTSEIDLPVKRRA). Notably, HN specifically abolished death induced by AD-related neurotoxicity such as soluble oligomeric Aβ and *PSEN1*/*PSEN2* mutants as well as overexpressed *APP* mutants, but did not suppress neurotoxicity related to PD, HD and prion diseases (Hashimoto et al., 2001a; Hashimoto et al., 2001b). As a result of detailed structural characterization of HN, several types of HN derivatives with higher efficacy, such as S14G-HN (HNG), have been developed (Chiba et al., 2007; Hashimoto et al., 2001a). One of HN derivatives termed colivelin (SALLRSIPA-PAGASRLLLLTGEIDLP, a 26 amino-acid peptide) elicits 10^8-fold more potent effects than authentic HN (Chiba et al., 2005).

http://dx.doi.org/10.5772/55293

HN derivatives ameliorate cognitive deficits observed in several types of AD model mice, presumably through activating its receptor consisting of the cytokine receptor gp130 and the downstream intracellular signaling pathways including the Jak2/Stat3 pathway (Chiba et al., 2009a; Yamada et al., 2008).

Effects of HN on the metabolic syndrome including DM and atherosclerosis are also reported: (i) HN suppresses pancreatic β-cell death (Hoang et al., 2010), (ii) HN increases peripheral insulin sensitivity (Muzumdar et al., 2009), and (iii) HN protects endothelial cells from LDL-induced oxidative stress (Bachar et al., 2010; Oh et al., 2011). These findings suggest that HN may reduce risks for LOAD through improving glucose and lipid metabolisms.

Activity-dependent neurotrophic factor (ADNF) and NAP

ADNF-9 or SAL (SALLRSIPA, a 9 amino-acid peptide) is an active core domain of ADNF, which antagonizes various types of neurotoxicity, such as tetrodotoxin (TTX), oxidative stress, NMDA, Aβ, ALS and gp120 of human immunodeficiency virus (HIV) (Brenneman and Gozes, 1996; Chiba et al., 2004; Chiba et al., 2007; Chiba et al., 2006; Dibbern et al., 1997). ADNF-9 exerts a neuroprotective effect at extremely low concentrations, such as hundred femtomolar concentrations, while it loses its neuroprotective effect at 1 nM or greater concentrations. Although ADNF receptors have not been identified, ADNF-mediated prosurvival mechanisms have been reported to involve activation of (i) CREB, (ii) NFkB, (iii) CaMKIV, (iv) hsp60, (v) transcriptional up-regulation of IGF-I, and (vi) poly ADP-ribosylation (Chiba et al., 2007).

Through expression screening of proteins recognized by antiserum against ADNF, a gene-encoding, activity-dependent neurotrophic protein (ADNP) was identified (Bassan et al., 1999). An eight-amino-acid sequence termed NAP (NAPVSIPQ, an 8 amino-acid peptide) in ADNP shows homology with ADNF and is recognized by antiserum against ADNF. NAP exhibits ADNF-like neuroprotective activity against various insults. NAP and its relative peptides, such as ADNF-9, D-SAL, and D-NAP have been reported to bind to and stabilize tubulin (Gozes and Divinski, 2004). NAP suppressed zinc-mediated microtubule depolymerization in astrocytes by promoting microtubule assembly and reorganization (Gozes and Divinski, 2007; Vulih-Shultzman et al., 2007). Accordingly, NAP is reported to protect neurons from tau-related neurotoxicity.

AL-108 (Davunetide), an intranasal formulation of NAP, and AL-208, an intravenous formulation of NAP, have been developed for clinical use (Shiryaev et al., 2011). A phase II study was safe and well tolerated and had positive effects on cognition. Currently, a phase III study is on-going.

4.2.3. Stat3 activation therapy for AD

Stat3 activation is another option for AD therapy, which can be achieved by soluble factors activating Stat3 signals; i.e. activation of upstream kinases and suppression of endogenous Stat3 inhibitors or regulators (Chiba et al., 2009a). As mentioned above, HN and its derivatives activate the Jak2/Stat3 signaling pathway. There are also many types of cytokines activating Stat3, such as interleukin-6 (IL-6) family cytokines (IL-6, ciliary neurotrophic factor [CNTF], leukemia inhibitory factor [LIF] and cardiotrophin-1 [CT-1]), erythropoietin (EPO), IL-27, granulocyte-colony stimulating factor (G-CSF), and leptin. Administration of these soluble factors could be considered although the bioavailability and delivery of these cytokines into the CNS should be addressed. Stat3 is phosphorylated by cellular Tyr kinases such as Jaks and Src family kinases. Synthetic activators such as Src family activator (EPQYEEIPIYL, Src family activator from Santa Cruz Biothechnology, sc-3052) may activate Stat3 to suppress the pathogenesis of AD although it may bring a large risk of carcinogenesis.

There are several endogenous regulator of Stat3: protein Tyr phosphatases (PTPs) like Src homology region 2 domain-containing phosphatase-1 (SHP-1) and SHP-2, suppressor of cytokine signaling 3 (SOCS3) and protein inhibitor of activated Stat3 (PIAS3) (Chiba et al., 2009a; Hendriks et al., 2012; Stephanou and Latchman, 2005). There are a number of PTPs and some of them are involved in the dephosphorylation or inactivation of the Jak2/Stat3 signaling pathway. SOCS3 is transcriptionally induced by activated Stat3 as a negative feedback regulator. SOCS3 binds to and inhibits Jak2 to prevent Stat3 phosphorylation. PIAS3 is a nuclear protein inhibiting activated Stat3 via multiple mechanisms. Expression of PIAS3 seems to be epigenetically regulated. Regulation of PIAS3 may contribute to recover Stat3 phosphorylation in AD.

4.2.4. Drugs based on prion protein

Prion diseases such as Creutzfeldt-Jakob disease are transmitted from patients to others by infectious agents consisting of misfolded proteins. The prion hypothesis for AD, suspected during 1970s and 80s, is re-emerging based on the reports that AD pathology can be transmitted to mice as prions do (Eisele et al., 2009; Eisele et al., 2010). Recent findings support the notion that there is a considerable similarity between Aβ and prion protein: (i) Aβ aggregation has similar structure to prion protein aggregation (Nussbaum et al., 2012), (ii) Aβ oligomer binds to postsynaptic prion protein to impair neuronal function (Um et al., 2012), and (iii) Aβ aggregates infect like prions (Stohr et al., 2012). Accordingly, AD therapy targeting prion proteins or prophylaxis for AD based on the prion hypothesis may be possible.

4.3. AD-specific drugs based on epidemiological findings

Epidemiology, as well as genetics, has pointed out several important aspects of the pathogenesis of AD. Based on the findings, a number of clinical trials have been carried out.

4.3.1. Nonsteroidal Anti-Inflammatory Drugs (NSAIDs)

Anti-inflammatory agents have been attracting attentions based on the fact that there is severe astrogliosis in AD brains and that epidemiological study showed that long-term users of nonsteroidal anti-inflammatory drugs (NSAIDs) have the lower risk of AD (Etminan et al., 2003). Considering that there are also several NSAIDs without benefits for AD patients including rofecoxib (a selective cyclooxygenase-2 [COX-2] inhibitor), and naproxen (a mixed COX-1 and 2 inhibitor) (Aisen et al., 2003), there seems to be additional anti-AD mechanisms other than attenuation of inflammatory response in effective NSAIDs including ibuprofen and indomethacin. For example, some NSAIDs may directly modify the γ-secretase activity and reduce Aβ42 levels without any evidence of inhibition of Notch processing, which might results in severe side effect (Lim et al., 2000; Lleo et al., 2004; Weggen et al., 2001). Flurizan (Tarenflurbil or R-flurbiprofen) is originally developed as an NSAID and is shown to reduce toxic longer Aβ42 levels as a γ-secretase modifier. In 2008, Myriad Genetics, Inc. announced that an 18-month phase III study of Flurizan in patients with mild AD (the Act-Earil-AD trial), unfortunately failed to achieve significant disease-modifying effect and that they decided to discontinue development of Flurizan (www.myriad.com) (Green et al., 2009). It should be noted that several COX-2 inhibitors may increase the production of the toxic Aβ42 peptide (Kukar et al., 2005). Further basic study about how and which NSAIDs work on AD should be piled up and elaborate clinical trials are essential.

4.3.2. Inhibitors for cholesterol synthesis: Statins

High cholesterol level is now recognized as a risk factor for LOAD (Shobab et al., 2005). As already mentioned, *APOE*, which is involved in lipid metabolisms, is reported to be a risk factor for LOAD (Bertram, 2011; Schellenberg and Montine, 2012). In this line, it was reported that long-term taking of HMG-CoA reductase inhibitors (statins) lowered the risk of AD significantly (Jick et al., 2000; Wolozin et al., 2000). In APP transgenic mice, statins improved brain pathology (Refolo et al., 2001). The mechanism in detail is unclear, but one possible mechanism is that statins modulate secretases: activation of α-secretase and inhibition of β-secretase to exert its anti-AD effect (Kojro et al., 2001; Parsons et al., 2006). These facts and clinical safety of chronic use of statins led this therapy to clinical trials. Recently, no significant clinical benefit on cognition or global functioning was, unfortunately, reported for atorvastatin and simvastatin in phase III studies (Feldman et al., 2010; Sano et al., 2011).

4.3.3. Dimebon

Dimebon (latrepirdine) received a huge attention as a potential therapy for AD after a publication in the *Lancet* of a positive phase II study carried out in Russia (Doody et al., 2008; Jones, 2010). Dimebon is an orally available and well-tolerated drug, which used to be approved for clinical use in Russia as a non-selective anti-histamine drug. Dimebon is reported to elicit multiple anti-AD effects such as ChE inhibition, prevention of NMDA-mediated excitotoxicity and inhibition of mitochondrial permeability transition pore opening. The phase III study of dimebon, called the CONNECTION study, unfortunately, showed no clinical benefit on co-primary (cognition and global function) and secondary endpoints. Moreover, an additional phase III study called the CONCERT study again failed to show efficacy of dimebon (announcement from Pfizer and Medivation on Jan 17, 2012, www.medivation.com). Complete discrepancy between the results of phase II and phase III studies has brought researchers a huge confusion. Negative comments about the underlying rationale for the use of dimebon in AD are currently increasing because of the complete failure of dimebon in the phase III studies.

4.4. AD-non-specific drugs for dementia

AD-non-specific drugs are also possible. The therapeutic bases of these drugs lie on protection of neurons from aging-related toxicity such as oxidative stress, promotion of synaptic plasticity and regeneration of neural tissues using stem cell technologies.

4.4.1. Antioxidants

Antioxidants are assumed to trap toxic reactive oxygen species (ROS), which increase as aging. ROS is also present in the damaged neurons containing NFTs or close to SPs. The principal antioxidant strategy involves treatments with vitamin E (α-tocopherol), which resulted in benefit for AD patients in a randomized, placebo-controlled trial (Sano et al., 1997). Vitamin E, however, does not seem to be so effective because it failed to show reproducible efficacy in a double-blind study performed recently (Petersen et al., 2005). Natural polyphenolic compounds such as ginkgo biloba extracts, curcumin, green tea catechins and grape-seed oil extract (resveratrol) are also attracting attention as antioxidants (Aranda-Abreu et al., 2011).

4.4.2. Neurotrophic factors to promote synaptic plasticity

Neurotrophins are well-characterized "trophic" factors, which generally promote neuronal survival and plasticity (Chiba et al., 2007). Each factor has its own relevance in AD. Nerve growth factor (NGF), which is discovered in the 1950s to be the first neurotrophic factor, mainly expressed in the peripheral nervous system, but also plays a key role in stimulation, maintenance, and survival of basal forebrain cholinergic neurons, which are destroyed in AD. Brain-derived neurotrophic factor (BDNF), purified from porcine brain homogenates in 1982, is highly expressed in cortical and hippocampal structures and plays roles in neuronal survival, neurite outgrowth and synaptic plasticity. A SNP in the *BDNF* gene that results in Met substitution of Val 66 in the pro-domain (V66M-BDNF or BDNFMet) causes dysregulation in BDNF secretion, which is linked to memory impairment as well as to altered susceptibility to neuropsychiatric disorders, such as AD, PD, depression, eating disorder, and bipolar disorder (Hong et al., 2011; Nagata et al., 2012).

Basic fibroblast growth factor (bFGF), vascular endothelial growth factor (VEGF), and hepatocyte growth factor (HGF) are also considered to be neurotrophic or neuroprotective factors whose receptors belong to the tyrosine kinase receptor family. bFGF and HGF exhibit a neuroprotective effect against Aβ neurotoxicity (Hashimoto et al., 2004; Takeuchi et al., 2008). Genetic variations in the VEGF gene modifies risks of AD (Del Bo et al., 2009).

Clinical application of these factors seem to be relatively difficult because proteins are not stable and are not easily delivered through BBB. Clinical studies on NGF, however, are promising. NGF treatments were initially based on intracerebroventricular infusion, which counterbalanced the positive effects with adverse effects. Accordingly, other drug delivery systems are currently tested in clinical trials: gene therapy with AAV or genetically modified fibroblasts producing NGF, encapsulated-cell biodelivery, intranasal delivery and topical application on the ocular surface (Mangialasche et al., 2010; Tuszynski et al., 2005).

4.4.3. Other therapies promoting synaptic plasticity

Phosphodiesterase inhibitors

Phosphodiesterases (PDEs) such as PDE-2, -4, -5 and -9 are expressed in the brain and play a key role in synaptic plasticity (Domek-Lopacinska and Strosznajder, 2010). Cyclic GMP (cGMP) positively regulates synaptic plasticity in this scheme, suggesting that PDE should be suppressed to increase cGMP. Consequently, PDE9A inhibitors are reported to promote synaptic plasticity via activation of cGMP signaling pathways (Andreeva et al., 2001). PF-04447943 is a selective PDE9A inhibitor, increasing cGMP concentrations in the CSF of healthy volunteers, and is being tested in a phase II study among mild-to-moderate AD patients (Mangialasche et al., 2010).

Omega-3 polyunsaturated fatty acids (docosahexaenoic acid etc.)

Omega-3 polyunsaturated fatty acids, such as docosahexaenoic acid (DHA), are involved in neurite outgrowth, remodeling of membrane lipid rafts and neurogenesis (Aranda-Abreu et al., 2011). They are also reported to suppress tau hyperphosphorylation and Aβ aggregation. Omega-3 fatty acids may repair damages in neuronal membranes and restore lipid rafts for appropriate trafficking of membrane proteins, leading to promotion of synaptic activity. Some clinical trials have reported beneficial effects of DHA in elderly people with cognitive impairment but other studies resulted in no effects on AD patients (Quinn et al., 2010).

4.4.4. Neuroregenerative therapy

Adult neurogenesis is now generally recognized. In adult brains, neurogenesis occurs mainly in two regions of the CNS including the subventricular zone (SVZ) of the lateral ventricles and the subgranular zone (SGZ) of hippocampal dentate gyri (Rodriguez and Verkhratsky, 2011). Multipotent neural stem cells (NSCs), localized in these regions, undergo self-renewal and differentiation into neuronal progenitor cells (NPCs) or glial progenitor cells (GPCs) with a faster cell cycle, which ultimately differentiate into neurons or glia. Impaired neurogenesis is expected for AD patients with massive neuronal loss. There is, however, a prevalent controversy among neurogenesis in AD brains. In a number of animal models for AD, toxic Aβ oligomers seem to enhance neurogenesis (Jin et al., 2004a; Sotthibundhu et al., 2009) although there are still several inconsistent observations that neurogenesis is disturbed in AD models (Feng et al., 2001; Haughey et al., 2002; Rodriguez et al., 2008). In post mortem AD brains, reduction of NPCs in the SVZ (Ziabreva et al., 2006) and an increase in NPCs in the DG (Jin et al., 2004b) are reported inconsistently as well. Accordingly, further clarification is mandatory.

Regardless of the discussion on the neurogenesis in AD brains, neuroregeneration, which can be achieved by either enhancement of endogenous neurogenesis or implantation of neurons or their progenitors (cell therapy), is getting to be considered as a valid therapeutic strategy for AD. This is mainly due to the progress in stem cell biology and a number of successful observations in preclinical studies. NSCs can be cultured and expanded *in vitro*. Moreover, NSCs can be differentiated from embryonic stem cells (ESCs) or induced pluripotent stem cells (iPSs) established from AD patients themselves. Stem cell transplantation experiments have been carried out in animal models with some positive observations (Moghadam et al., 2009; Park et al., 2012; Wu et al., 2008; Yamasaki et al., 2007). These experiments, however, did not show significant regeneration or replacement of neural circuits by transplanted stem cells. Some of them used gene-modified stem cells with NGF or ChAT expression, supporting function of endogenous neurons. Delivery methods for NSCs/NPCs, cell viability and efficiency of engraftment should be considerably improved as well as resolving the safety issues. Endogenous neurogenesis is shown to be upregulated by soluble factors such as serotonin (5-HT) agonists and BDNF in rodents (Lee et al., 2002; Santarelli et al., 2003). Effects in humans should be carefully addressed.

5. Conclusion

Disease-modifying therapy for AD is not yet available despite vast efforts on drug development and plenty of candidate drugs. As shown in Table 1, failure rate of phase II and III clinical trials for AD are extremely high, meaning not only that current *in vitro* or pre-clinical models of AD can hardly predict the clinical efficacy but also that drugs, which showed only a mild effect in phase II studies, would eventually fail in phase III studies. Consequently, ChEIs and memantine are still in the center of clinical therapies for AD. The "amyloid cascade" hypothesis certainly gave us important insights into AD pathogenesis and provided a number of candidates, most of which are still under assessment in clinical trials. However, the results obtained from completed clinical trials are rather negative for the "amyloid cascade" hypothesis: e.g. Aβ immunotherapy and β-/γ-secretase inhibitors continue to fail in the trials. In addition, there are critical objections to the "amyloid cascade", which has not been properly answered: (i) about one third of the cases of a cognitively normal elder population showed AD-like brain pathology such as SPs and NFTs (Bennett et al., 2006), and (ii) post-mortem pathological analyses of AD brains with immunotherapy revealed that a certain population of patients with Aβ immunotherapy resulted in significant decrease in senile plaques without significant recovery of cognitive function (Gilman et al., 2005; Nicoll et al., 2003). Time might have come to further modify the "amyloid cascade", integrate alternative hypotheses into it, or reconstitute a novel hypothesis for AD, in order to develop clinically effective AD therapies.

Acknowledgements

This work was supported in part by a grant from the Japan Research Foundation for Clinical Pharmacology. I thank Drs. Ikuo Nishimoto (1956-2003), Sadakazu Aiso and Bernd Groner.

Author details

Tomohiro Chiba[1,2,3]

Address all correspondence to: chibatomohero@gmail.com

1 Georg-Speyer-Haus, Institute for Biomedical Research, Frankfurt am Main, Germany

2 Department of Anatomy, Keio University, School of Medicine, Tokyo, Japan

3 Department of Pathology, Kyorin University School of Medicine, Tokyo, Japan

References

[1] (1987). About a peculiar disease of the cerebral cortex. By Alois Alzheimer, 1907 (Translated by L. Jarvik and H. Greenson). Alzheimer Dis Assoc Disord *1*, 3-8.

[2] Aisen, P.S., Gauthier, S., Ferris, S.H., Saumier, D., Haine, D., Garceau, D., Duong, A., Suhy, J., Oh, J., Lau, W.C., *et al.* (2011). Tramiprosate in mild-to-moderate Alzheimer's disease - a randomized, double-blind, placebo-controlled, multi-centre study (the Alphase Study). Arch Med Sci *7*, 102-111.

[3] Aisen, P.S., Schafer, K.A., Grundman, M., Pfeiffer, E., Sano, M., Davis, K.L., Farlow, M.R., Jin, S., Thomas, R.G., and Thal, L.J. (2003). Effects of rofecoxib or naproxen vs placebo on Alzheimer disease progression: a randomized controlled trial. JAMA *289*, 2819-2826.

[4] Alley, G.M., Bailey, J.A., Chen, D., Ray, B., Puli, L.K., Tanila, H., Banerjee, P.K., and Lahiri, D.K. (2009). Memantine lowers amyloid-beta peptide levels in neuronal cultures and in APP/PS1 transgenic mice. J Neurosci Res *88*, 143-154.

[5] Alves, L., Correia, A.S., Miguel, R., Alegria, P., and Bugalho, P. (2010). Alzheimer's disease: a clinical practice-oriented review. Front Neurol *3*, 63.

[6] Andreeva, S.G., Dikkes, P., Epstein, P.M., and Rosenberg, P.A. (2001). Expression of cGMP-specific phosphodiesterase 9A mRNA in the rat brain. J Neurosci *21*, 9068-9076.

[7] Araki, W., Yuasa, K., Takeda, S., Takeda, K., Shirotani, K., Takahashi, K., and Tabira, T. (2001). Pro-apoptotic effect of presenilin 2 (PS2) overexpression is associated with down-regulation of Bcl-2 in cultured neurons. J Neurochem *79*, 1161-1168.

[8] Aranda-Abreu, G.E., Hernandez-Aguilar, M.E., Manzo Denes, J., Garcia Hernandez, L.I., and Herrera Rivero, M. (2011). Rehabilitating a brain with Alzheimer's: a proposal. Clin Interv Aging *6*, 53-59.

[9] Bachar, A.R., Scheffer, L., Schroeder, A.S., Nakamura, H.K., Cobb, L.J., Oh, Y.K., Lerman, L.O., Pagano, R.E., Cohen, P., and Lerman, A. (2010). Humanin is expressed in human vascular walls and has a cytoprotective effect against oxidized LDL-induced oxidative stress. Cardiovasc Res *88*, 360-366.

[10] Barry, S.P., Townsend, P.A., McCormick, J., Knight, R.A., Scarabelli, T.M., Latchman, D.S., and Stephanou, A. (2009). STAT3 deletion sensitizes cells to oxidative stress. Biochem Biophys Res Commun *385*, 324-329.

[11] Bartus, R.T., Dean, R.L., 3rd, Beer, B., and Lippa, A.S. (1982). The cholinergic hypothesis of geriatric memory dysfunction. Science *217*, 408-414.

[12] Bassan, M., Zamostiano, R., Davidson, A., Pinhasov, A., Giladi, E., Perl, O., Bassan, H., Blat, C., Gibney, G., Glazner, G., *et al.* (1999). Complete sequence of a novel pro-

tein containing a femtomolar-activity-dependent neuroprotective peptide. J Neurochem *72*, 1283-1293.

[13] Bennett, D.A., Schneider, J.A., Arvanitakis, Z., Kelly, J.F., Aggarwal, N.T., Shah, R.C., and Wilson, R.S. (2006). Neuropathology of older persons without cognitive impairment from two community-based studies. Neurology *66*, 1837-1844.

[14] Berger, A. (2000). Minocycline slows progress of Huntington's disease in mice. BMJ *321*, 70.

[15] Bertram, L. (2011). Alzheimer's genetics in the GWAS era: a continuing story of 'replications and refutations'. Curr Neurol Neurosci Rep *11*, 246-253.

[16] Bertram, L., Hiltunen, M., Parkinson, M., Ingelsson, M., Lange, C., Ramasamy, K., Mullin, K., Menon, R., Sampson, A.J., Hsiao, M.Y., *et al.* (2005). Family-based association between Alzheimer's disease and variants in UBQLN1. N Engl J Med *352*, 884-894.

[17] Bertram, L., Lill, C.M., and Tanzi, R.E. (2010). The genetics of Alzheimer disease: back to the future. Neuron *68*, 270-281.

[18] Braak, H., and Braak, E. (1991). Neuropathological stageing of Alzheimer-related changes. Acta Neuropathol *82*, 239-259.

[19] Brenneman, D.E., and Gozes, I. (1996). A femtomolar-acting neuroprotective peptide. J Clin Invest *97*, 2299-2307.

[20] Britschgi, M., Olin, C.E., Johns, H.T., Takeda-Uchimura, Y., LeMieux, M.C., Rufibach, K., Rajadas, J., Zhang, H., Tomooka, B., Robinson, W.H., *et al.* (2009). Neuroprotective natural antibodies to assemblies of amyloidogenic peptides decrease with normal aging and advancing Alzheimer's disease. Proc Natl Acad Sci U S A *106*, 12145-12150.

[21] Burgos, J.S., Benavides, J., Douillet, P., Velasco, J., and Valdivieso, F. (2012). How statins could be evaluated successfully in clinical trials for Alzheimer's disease? Am J Alzheimers Dis Other Demen *27*, 151-153.

[22] Busciglio, J., Lorenzo, A., Yeh, J., and Yankner, B.A. (1995). beta-amyloid fibrils induce tau phosphorylation and loss of microtubule binding. Neuron *14*, 879-888.

[23] Butterfield, D.A., Castegna, A., Lauderback, C.M., and Drake, J. (2002). Evidence that amyloid beta-peptide-induced lipid peroxidation and its sequelae in Alzheimer's disease brain contribute to neuronal death. Neurobiol Aging *23*, 655-664.

[24] Cabrol, C., Huzarska, M.A., Dinolfo, C., Rodriguez, M.C., Reinstatler, L., Ni, J., Yeh, L.A., Cuny, G.D., Stein, R.L., Selkoe, D.J., *et al.* (2009). Small-molecule activators of insulin-degrading enzyme discovered through high-throughput compound screening. PLoS One *4*, e5274.

[25] Cai, H., Wang, Y., McCarthy, D., Wen, H., Borchelt, D.R., Price, D.L., and Wong, P.C. (2001). BACE1 is the major beta-secretase for generation of Abeta peptides by neurons. Nat Neurosci *4*, 233-234.

[26] Caleo, M., Cenni, M.C., Costa, M., Menna, E., Zentilin, L., Giadrossi, S., Giacca, M., and Maffei, L. (2002). Expression of BCL-2 via adeno-associated virus vectors rescues thalamic neurons after visual cortex lesion in the adult rat. Eur J Neurosci *15*, 1271-1277.

[27] Caserta, T.M., Smith, A.N., Gultice, A.D., Reedy, M.A., and Brown, T.L. (2003). Q-VD-OPh, a broad spectrum caspase inhibitor with potent antiapoptotic properties. Apoptosis *8*, 345-352.

[28] Chartier-Harlin, M.C., Crawford, F., Houlden, H., Warren, A., Hughes, D., Fidani, L., Goate, A., Rossor, M., Roques, P., Hardy, J., *et al.* (1991). Early-onset Alzheimer's disease caused by mutations at codon 717 of the beta-amyloid precursor protein gene. Nature *353*, 844-846.

[29] Chiba, T., Hashimoto, Y., Tajima, H., Yamada, M., Kato, R., Niikura, T., Terashita, K., Schulman, H., Aiso, S., Kita, Y., *et al.* (2004). Neuroprotective effect of activity-dependent neurotrophic factor against toxicity from familial amyotrophic lateral sclerosis-linked mutant SOD1 in vitro and in vivo. J Neurosci Res *78*, 542-552.

[30] Chiba, T., Nishimoto, I., Aiso, S., and Matsuoka, M. (2007). Neuroprotection against neurodegenerative diseases: development of a novel hybrid neuroprotective peptide Colivelin. Mol Neurobiol *35*, 55-84.

[31] Chiba, T., Yamada, M., and Aiso, S. (2009a). Targeting the JAK2/STAT3 axis in Alzheimer's disease. Expert Opin Ther Targets *13*, 1155-1167.

[32] Chiba, T., Yamada, M., Hashimoto, Y., Sato, M., Sasabe, J., Kita, Y., Terashita, K., Aiso, S., Nishimoto, I., and Matsuoka, M. (2005). Development of a femtomolar-acting humanin derivative named colivelin by attaching activity-dependent neurotrophic factor to its N terminus: characterization of colivelin-mediated neuroprotection against Alzheimer's disease-relevant insults in vitro and in vivo. J Neurosci *25*, 10252-10261.

[33] Chiba, T., Yamada, M., Sasabe, J., Terashita, K., Aiso, S., Matsuoka, M., and Nishimoto, I. (2006). Colivelin prolongs survival of an ALS model mouse. Biochem Biophys Res Commun *343*, 793-798.

[34] Chiba, T., Yamada, M., Sasabe, J., Terashita, K., Shimoda, M., Matsuoka, M., and Aiso, S. (2009b). Amyloid-beta causes memory impairment by disturbing the JAK2/STAT3 axis in hippocampal neurons. Mol Psychiatry *14*, 206-222.

[35] Chohan, M.O., Khatoon, S., Iqbal, I.G., and Iqbal, K. (2006). Involvement of I2PP2A in the abnormal hyperphosphorylation of tau and its reversal by Memantine. FEBS Lett *580*, 3973-3979.

[36] Choi, Y., Kim, H.S., Shin, K.Y., Kim, E.M., Kim, M., Park, C.H., Jeong, Y.H., Yoo, J., Lee, J.P., Chang, K.A., *et al.* (2007). Minocycline attenuates neuronal cell death and improves cognitive impairment in Alzheimer's disease models. Neuropsychopharmacology *32*, 2393-2404.

[37] Courtney, C., Farrell, D., Gray, R., Hills, R., Lynch, L., Sellwood, E., Edwards, S., Hardyman, W., Raftery, J., Crome, P., *et al.* (2004). Long-term donepezil treatment in 565 patients with Alzheimer's disease (AD2000): randomised double-blind trial. Lancet *363*, 2105-2115.

[38] Cramer, P.E., Cirrito, J.R., Wesson, D.W., Lee, C.Y., Karlo, J.C., Zinn, A.E., Casali, B.T., Restivo, J.L., Goebel, W.D., James, M.J., *et al.* (2012). ApoE-directed therapeutics rapidly clear beta-amyloid and reverse deficits in AD mouse models. Science *335*, 1503-1506.

[39] Cummings, J. (2010). What can be inferred from the interruption of the semagacestat trial for treatment of Alzheimer's disease? Biol Psychiatry *68*, 876-878.

[40] David, R., Zeitzer, J., Friedman, L., Noda, A., O'Hara, R., Robert, P., and Yesavage, J.A. (2010). Non-pharmacologic management of sleep disturbance in Alzheimer's disease. J Nutr Health Aging *14*, 203-206.

[41] Davies, N.M., Kehoe, P.G., Ben-Shlomo, Y., and Martin, R.M. (2011). Associations of anti-hypertensive treatments with Alzheimer's disease, vascular dementia, and other dementias. J Alzheimers Dis *26*, 699-708.

[42] De Felice, F.G., Velasco, P.T., Lambert, M.P., Viola, K., Fernandez, S.J., Ferreira, S.T., and Klein, W.L. (2007). Abeta oligomers induce neuronal oxidative stress through an N-methyl-D-aspartate receptor-dependent mechanism that is blocked by the Alzheimer drug memantine. J Biol Chem *282*, 11590-11601.

[43] De Strooper, B. (2003). Aph-1, Pen-2, and Nicastrin with Presenilin generate an active gamma-Secretase complex. Neuron *38*, 9-12.

[44] De Strooper, B., and Annaert, W. (2000). Proteolytic processing and cell biological functions of the amyloid precursor protein. J Cell Sci *113 (Pt 11)*, 1857-1870.

[45] Deane, R., Du Yan, S., Submamaryan, R.K., LaRue, B., Jovanovic, S., Hogg, E., Welch, D., Manness, L., Lin, C., Yu, J., *et al.* (2003). RAGE mediates amyloid-beta peptide transport across the blood-brain barrier and accumulation in brain. Nat Med *9*, 907-913.

[46] Deane, R., Sagare, A., Hamm, K., Parisi, M., Lane, S., Finn, M.B., Holtzman, D.M., and Zlokovic, B.V. (2008). apoE isoform-specific disruption of amyloid beta peptide clearance from mouse brain. J Clin Invest *118*, 4002-4013.

[47] Del Bo, R., Ghezzi, S., Scarpini, E., Bresolin, N., and Comi, G.P. (2009). VEGF genetic variability is associated with increased risk of developing Alzheimer's disease. J Neurol Sci *283*, 66-68.

[48] Delrieu, J., Ousset, P.J., Caillaud, C., and Vellas, B. (2012). 'Clinical trials in Alzheimer's disease': immunotherapy approaches. J Neurochem *120 Suppl 1*, 186-193.

[49] Di Carlo, M. (2010). Beta amyloid peptide: from different aggregation forms to the activation of different biochemical pathways. Eur Biophys J *39*, 877-888.

[50] Di Fede, G., Catania, M., Morbin, M., Rossi, G., Suardi, S., Mazzoleni, G., Merlin, M., Giovagnoli, A.R., Prioni, S., Erbetta, A., *et al.* (2009). A recessive mutation in the APP gene with dominant-negative effect on amyloidogenesis. Science *323*, 1473-1477.

[51] Dibbern, D.A., Jr., Glazner, G.W., Gozes, I., Brenneman, D.E., and Hill, J.M. (1997). Inhibition of murine embryonic growth by human immunodeficiency virus envelope protein and its prevention by vasoactive intestinal peptide and activity-dependent neurotrophic factor. J Clin Invest *99*, 2837-2841.

[52] Dodart, J.C., Bales, K.R., Gannon, K.S., Greene, S.J., DeMattos, R.B., Mathis, C., DeLong, C.A., Wu, S., Wu, X., Holtzman, D.M., *et al.* (2002). Immunization reverses memory deficits without reducing brain Abeta burden in Alzheimer's disease model. Nat Neurosci *5*, 452-457.

[53] Dodel, R., Hampel, H., Depboylu, C., Lin, S., Gao, F., Schock, S., Jackel, S., Wei, X., Buerger, K., Hoft, C., *et al.* (2002). Human antibodies against amyloid beta peptide: a potential treatment for Alzheimer's disease. Ann Neurol *52*, 253-256.

[54] Dodel, R.C., Du, Y., Depboylu, C., Hampel, H., Frolich, L., Haag, A., Hemmeter, U., Paulsen, S., Teipel, S.J., Brettschneider, S., *et al.* (2004). Intravenous immunoglobulins containing antibodies against beta-amyloid for the treatment of Alzheimer's disease. J Neurol Neurosurg Psychiatry *75*, 1472-1474.

[55] Domek-Lopacinska, K.U., and Strosznajder, J.B. (2010). Cyclic GMP and nitric oxide synthase in aging and Alzheimer's disease. Mol Neurobiol *41*, 129-137.

[56] Dominguez, D., Tournoy, J., Hartmann, D., Huth, T., Cryns, K., Deforce, S., Serneels, L., Camacho, I.E., Marjaux, E., Craessaerts, K., *et al.* (2005). Phenotypic and biochemical analyses of BACE1- and BACE2-deficient mice. J Biol Chem *280*, 30797-30806.

[57] Doody, R.S., Gavrilova, S.I., Sano, M., Thomas, R.G., Aisen, P.S., Bachurin, S.O., Seely, L., and Hung, D. (2008). Effect of dimebon on cognition, activities of daily living, behaviour, and global function in patients with mild-to-moderate Alzheimer's disease: a randomised, double-blind, placebo-controlled study. Lancet *372*, 207-215.

[58] Du, Y., Ma, Z., Lin, S., Dodel, R.C., Gao, F., Bales, K.R., Triarhou, L.C., Chernet, E., Perry, K.W., Nelson, D.L., *et al.* (2001). Minocycline prevents nigrostriatal dopaminergic neurodegeneration in the MPTP model of Parkinson's disease. Proc Natl Acad Sci U S A *98*, 14669-14674.

[59] Eisele, Y.S., Bolmont, T., Heikenwalder, M., Langer, F., Jacobson, L.H., Yan, Z.X., Roth, K., Aguzzi, A., Staufenbiel, M., Walker, L.C., *et al.* (2009). Induction of cerebral

beta-amyloidosis: intracerebral versus systemic Abeta inoculation. Proc Natl Acad Sci U S A *106*, 12926-12931.

[60] Eisele, Y.S., Obermuller, U., Heilbronner, G., Baumann, F., Kaeser, S.A., Wolburg, H., Walker, L.C., Staufenbiel, M., Heikenwalder, M., and Jucker, M. (2010). Peripherally applied Abeta-containing inoculates induce cerebral beta-amyloidosis. Science *330*, 980-982.

[61] Eisenstein, M. (2011). Genetics: finding risk factors. Nature *475*, S20-22.

[62] Etminan, M., Gill, S., and Samii, A. (2003). Effect of non-steroidal anti-inflammatory drugs on risk of Alzheimer's disease: systematic review and meta-analysis of observational studies. BMJ *327*, 128.

[63] Farlow, M., Arnold, S.E., van Dyck, C.H., Aisen, P.S., Snider, B.J., Porsteinsson, A.P., Friedrich, S., Dean, R.A., Gonzales, C., Sethuraman, G., *et al.* (2012). Safety and biomarker effects of solanezumab in patients with Alzheimer's disease. Alzheimers Dement *8*, 261-271.

[64] Farrimond, L.E., Roberts, E., and McShane, R. (2012). Memantine and cholinesterase inhibitor combination therapy for Alzheimer's disease: a systematic review. BMJ Open *2*.

[65] Farris, W., Mansourian, S., Chang, Y., Lindsley, L., Eckman, E.A., Frosch, M.P., Eckman, C.B., Tanzi, R.E., Selkoe, D.J., and Guenette, S. (2003). Insulin-degrading enzyme regulates the levels of insulin, amyloid beta-protein, and the beta-amyloid precursor protein intracellular domain in vivo. Proc Natl Acad Sci U S A *100*, 4162-4167.

[66] Feldman, H.H., Doody, R.S., Kivipelto, M., Sparks, D.L., Waters, D.D., Jones, R.W., Schwam, E., Schindler, R., Hey-Hadavi, J., DeMicco, D.A., *et al.* (2010). Randomized controlled trial of atorvastatin in mild to moderate Alzheimer disease: LEADe. Neurology *74*, 956-964.

[67] Feng, R., Rampon, C., Tang, Y.P., Shrom, D., Jin, J., Kyin, M., Sopher, B., Miller, M.W., Ware, C.B., Martin, G.M., *et al.* (2001). Deficient neurogenesis in forebrain-specific presenilin-1 knockout mice is associated with reduced clearance of hippocampal memory traces. Neuron *32*, 911-926.

[68] Fernandez-Madrid, I., Levy, E., Marder, K., and Frangione, B. (1991). Codon 618 variant of Alzheimer amyloid gene associated with inherited cerebral hemorrhage. Ann Neurol *30*, 730-733.

[69] Ferrer, I., Barrachina, M., and Puig, B. (2002). Glycogen synthase kinase-3 is associated with neuronal and glial hyperphosphorylated tau deposits in Alzheimer's disease, Pick's disease, progressive supranuclear palsy and corticobasal degeneration. Acta Neuropathol *104*, 583-591.

[70] Ferrer, I., Blanco, R., Carmona, M., and Puig, B. (2001). Phosphorylated mitogen-activated protein kinase (MAPK/ERK-P), protein kinase of 38 kDa (p38-P), stress-activat-

ed protein kinase (SAPK/JNK-P), and calcium/calmodulin-dependent kinase II (CaM kinase II) are differentially expressed in tau deposits in neurons and glial cells in tauopathies. J Neural Transm *108*, 1397-1415.

[71] Fillit, H., Hess, G., Hill, J., Bonnet, P., and Toso, C. (2009). IV immunoglobulin is associated with a reduced risk of Alzheimer disease and related disorders. Neurology *73*, 180-185.

[72] Freeman, G.B., Lin, J.C., Pons, J., and Raha, N.M. (2012). 39-week toxicity and toxicokinetic study of ponezumab (PF-04360365) in cynomolgus monkeys with 12-week recovery period. J Alzheimers Dis *28*, 531-541.

[73] Gamblin, T.C., Chen, F., Zambrano, A., Abraha, A., Lagalwar, S., Guillozet, A.L., Lu, M., Fu, Y., Garcia-Sierra, F., LaPointe, N., *et al.* (2003). Caspase cleavage of tau: linking amyloid and neurofibrillary tangles in Alzheimer's disease. Proc Natl Acad Sci U S A *100*, 10032-10037.

[74] Gervais, F.G., Xu, D., Robertson, G.S., Vaillancourt, J.P., Zhu, Y., Huang, J., LeBlanc, A., Smith, D., Rigby, M., Shearman, M.S., *et al.* (1999). Involvement of caspases in proteolytic cleavage of Alzheimer's amyloid-beta precursor protein and amyloidogenic A beta peptide formation. Cell *97*, 395-406.

[75] Ghosh, A.K., Brindisi, M., and Tang, J. (2012). Developing beta-secretase inhibitors for treatment of Alzheimer's disease. J Neurochem *120 Suppl 1*, 71-83.

[76] Gilman, S., Koller, M., Black, R.S., Jenkins, L., Griffith, S.G., Fox, N.C., Eisner, L., Kirby, L., Rovira, M.B., Forette, F., *et al.* (2005). Clinical effects of Abeta immunization (AN1792) in patients with AD in an interrupted trial. Neurology *64*, 1553-1562.

[77] Glenner, G.G., and Wong, C.W. (1984). Alzheimer's disease: initial report of the purification and characterization of a novel cerebrovascular amyloid protein. Biochem Biophys Res Commun *120*, 885-890.

[78] Goate, A., Chartier-Harlin, M.C., Mullan, M., Brown, J., Crawford, F., Fidani, L., Giuffra, L., Haynes, A., Irving, N., James, L., *et al.* (1991). Segregation of a missense mutation in the amyloid precursor protein gene with familial Alzheimer's disease. Nature *349*, 704-706.

[79] Goedert, M., Crowther, R.A., and Spillantini, M.G. (1998). Tau mutations cause frontotemporal dementias. Neuron *21*, 955-958.

[80] Gotz, J., Chen, F., van Dorpe, J., and Nitsch, R.M. (2001). Formation of neurofibrillary tangles in P301l tau transgenic mice induced by Abeta 42 fibrils. Science *293*, 1491-1495.

[81] Gozes, I., and Divinski, I. (2004). The femtomolar-acting NAP interacts with microtubules: Novel aspects of astrocyte protection. J Alzheimers Dis *6*, S37-41.

[82] Gozes, I., and Divinski, I. (2007). NAP, a neuroprotective drug candidate in clinical trials, stimulates microtubule assembly in the living cell. Curr Alzheimer Res *4*, 507-509.

[83] Green, R.C., Schneider, L.S., Amato, D.A., Beelen, A.P., Wilcock, G., Swabb, E.A., and Zavitz, K.H. (2009). Effect of tarenflurbil on cognitive decline and activities of daily living in patients with mild Alzheimer disease: a randomized controlled trial. JAMA *302*, 2557-2564.

[84] Guglielmotto, M., Tamagno, E., and Danni, O. (2009). Oxidative stress and hypoxia contribute to Alzheimer's disease pathogenesis: two sides of the same coin. ScientificWorldJournal *9*, 781-791.

[85] Guo, Q., Furukawa, K., Sopher, B.L., Pham, D.G., Xie, J., Robinson, N., Martin, G.M., and Mattson, M.P. (1996). Alzheimer's PS-1 mutation perturbs calcium homeostasis and sensitizes PC12 cells to death induced by amyloid beta-peptide. Neuroreport *8*, 379-383.

[86] Hampel, H., Ewers, M., Burger, K., Annas, P., Mortberg, A., Bogstedt, A., Frolich, L., Schroder, J., Schonknecht, P., Riepe, M.W., *et al.* (2009). Lithium trial in Alzheimer's disease: a randomized, single-blind, placebo-controlled, multicenter 10-week study. J Clin Psychiatry *70*, 922-931.

[87] Hara, H., Monsonego, A., Yuasa, K., Adachi, K., Xiao, X., Takeda, S., Takahashi, K., Weiner, H.L., and Tabira, T. (2004). Development of a safe oral Abeta vaccine using recombinant adeno-associated virus vector for Alzheimer's disease. J Alzheimers Dis *6*, 483-488.

[88] Hardy, J.A., and Higgins, G.A. (1992). Alzheimer's disease: the amyloid cascade hypothesis. Science *256*, 184-185.

[89] Hashimoto, K. (2011). Can minocycline prevent the onset of Alzheimer's disease? Ann Neurol *69*, 739; author reply 739-740.

[90] Hashimoto, Y., Chiba, T., Yamada, M., Nawa, M., Kanekura, K., Suzuki, H., Terashita, K., Aiso, S., Nishimoto, I., and Matsuoka, M. (2005). Transforming growth factor beta2 is a neuronal death-inducing ligand for amyloid-beta precursor protein. Mol Cell Biol *25*, 9304-9317.

[91] Hashimoto, Y., Ito, Y., Arakawa, E., Kita, Y., Terashita, K., Niikura, T., and Nishimoto, I. (2002a). Neurotoxic mechanisms triggered by Alzheimer's disease-linked mutant M146L presenilin 1: involvement of NO synthase via a novel pertussis toxin target. J Neurochem *80*, 426-437.

[92] Hashimoto, Y., Kaneko, Y., Tsukamoto, E., Frankowski, H., Kouyama, K., Kita, Y., Niikura, T., Aiso, S., Bredesen, D.E., Matsuoka, M., *et al.* (2004). Molecular characterization of neurohybrid cell death induced by Alzheimer's amyloid-beta peptides via p75NTR/PLAIDD. J Neurochem *90*, 549-558.

[93] Hashimoto, Y., Niikura, T., Ito, Y., Kita, Y., Terashita, K., and Nishimoto, I. (2002b). Neurotoxic mechanisms by Alzheimer's disease-linked N141I mutant presenilin 2. J Pharmacol Exp Ther *300*, 736-745.

[94] Hashimoto, Y., Niikura, T., Ito, Y., and Nishimoto, I. (2000). Multiple mechanisms underlie neurotoxicity by different types of Alzheimer's disease mutations of amyloid precursor protein. J Biol Chem *275*, 34541-34551.

[95] Hashimoto, Y., Niikura, T., Ito, Y., Sudo, H., Hata, M., Arakawa, E., Abe, Y., Kita, Y., and Nishimoto, I. (2001a). Detailed characterization of neuroprotection by a rescue factor humanin against various Alzheimer's disease-relevant insults. J Neurosci *21*, 9235-9245.

[96] Hashimoto, Y., Niikura, T., Tajima, H., Yasukawa, T., Sudo, H., Ito, Y., Kita, Y., Kawasumi, M., Kouyama, K., Doyu, M., *et al.* (2001b). A rescue factor abolishing neuronal cell death by a wide spectrum of familial Alzheimer's disease genes and Abeta. Proc Natl Acad Sci U S A *98*, 6336-6341.

[97] Haughey, N.J., Nath, A., Chan, S.L., Borchard, A.C., Rao, M.S., and Mattson, M.P. (2002). Disruption of neurogenesis by amyloid beta-peptide, and perturbed neural progenitor cell homeostasis, in models of Alzheimer's disease. J Neurochem *83*, 1509-1524.

[98] Hendriks, W.J., Elson, A., Harroch, S., Pulido, R., Stoker, A., and den Hertog, J. (2012). Protein tyrosine phosphatases in health and disease. FEBS J.

[99] Hoang, P.T., Park, P., Cobb, L.J., Paharkova-Vatchkova, V., Hakimi, M., Cohen, P., and Lee, K.W. (2010). The neurosurvival factor Humanin inhibits beta-cell apoptosis via signal transducer and activator of transcription 3 activation and delays and ameliorates diabetes in nonobese diabetic mice. Metabolism *59*, 343-349.

[100] Hock, C., Konietzko, U., Papassotiropoulos, A., Wollmer, A., Streffer, J., von Rotz, R.C., Davey, G., Moritz, E., and Nitsch, R.M. (2002). Generation of antibodies specific for beta-amyloid by vaccination of patients with Alzheimer disease. Nat Med *8*, 1270-1275.

[101] Hong, C.J., Liou, Y.J., and Tsai, S.J. (2011). Effects of BDNF polymorphisms on brain function and behavior in health and disease. Brain Res Bull *86*, 287-297.

[102] Hu, J.P., Xie, J.W., Wang, C.Y., Wang, T., Wang, X., Wang, S.L., Teng, W.P., and Wang, Z.Y. (2011). Valproate reduces tau phosphorylation via cyclin-dependent kinase 5 and glycogen synthase kinase 3 signaling pathways. Brain Res Bull *85*, 194-200.

[103] Huang, Y., and Mucke, L. (2012). Alzheimer mechanisms and therapeutic strategies. Cell *148*, 1204-1222.

[104] Hutton, M., Lendon, C.L., Rizzu, P., Baker, M., Froelich, S., Houlden, H., Pickering-Brown, S., Chakraverty, S., Isaacs, A., Grover, A., *et al.* (1998). Association of mis-

sense and 5'-splice-site mutations in tau with the inherited dementia FTDP-17. Nature *393*, 702-705.

[105] Ito, S., Ohtsuki, S., Kamiie, J., Nezu, Y., and Terasaki, T. (2007). Cerebral clearance of human amyloid-beta peptide (1-40) across the blood-brain barrier is reduced by self-aggregation and formation of low-density lipoprotein receptor-related protein-1 ligand complexes. J Neurochem *103*, 2482-2490.

[106] Iwata, N., Takaki, Y., Fukami, S., Tsubuki, S., and Saido, T.C. (2002). Region-specific reduction of A beta-degrading endopeptidase, neprilysin, in mouse hippocampus upon aging. J Neurosci Res *70*, 493-500.

[107] Iwata, N., Tsubuki, S., Takaki, Y., Shirotani, K., Lu, B., Gerard, N.P., Gerard, C., Hama, E., Lee, H.J., and Saido, T.C. (2001). Metabolic regulation of brain Abeta by neprilysin. Science *292*, 1550-1552.

[108] Iwata, N., Tsubuki, S., Takaki, Y., Watanabe, K., Sekiguchi, M., Hosoki, E., Kawashima-Morishima, M., Lee, H.J., Hama, E., Sekine-Aizawa, Y., *et al.* (2000). Identification of the major Abeta1-42-degrading catabolic pathway in brain parenchyma: suppression leads to biochemical and pathological deposition. Nat Med *6*, 143-150.

[109] Jick, H., Zornberg, G.L., Jick, S.S., Seshadri, S., and Drachman, D.A. (2000). Statins and the risk of dementia. Lancet *356*, 1627-1631.

[110] Jin, K., Galvan, V., Xie, L., Mao, X.O., Gorostiza, O.F., Bredesen, D.E., and Greenberg, D.A. (2004a). Enhanced neurogenesis in Alzheimer's disease transgenic (PDGF-APPSw,Ind) mice. Proc Natl Acad Sci U S A *101*, 13363-13367.

[111] Jin, K., Peel, A.L., Mao, X.O., Xie, L., Cottrell, B.A., Henshall, D.C., and Greenberg, D.A. (2004b). Increased hippocampal neurogenesis in Alzheimer's disease. Proc Natl Acad Sci U S A *101*, 343-347.

[112] John, V., Beck, J.P., Bienkowski, M.J., Sinha, S., and Heinrikson, R.L. (2003). Human beta-secretase (BACE) and BACE inhibitors. J Med Chem *46*, 4625-4630.

[113] Johnson, G.V., and Stoothoff, W.H. (2004). Tau phosphorylation in neuronal cell function and dysfunction. J Cell Sci *117*, 5721-5729.

[114] Jones, R.W. (2010). Dimebon disappointment. Alzheimers Res Ther *2*, 25.

[115] Jonsson, T., Atwal, J.K., Steinberg, S., Snaedal, J., Jonsson, P.V., Bjornsson, S., Stefansson, H., Sulem, P., Gudbjartsson, D., Maloney, J., *et al.* (2012). A mutation in APP protects against Alzheimer's disease and age-related cognitive decline. Nature *488*, 96-99.

[116] Kang, J., Lemaire, H.G., Unterbeck, A., Salbaum, J.M., Masters, C.L., Grzeschik, K.H., Multhaup, G., Beyreuther, K., and Muller-Hill, B. (1987). The precursor of Alzheimer's disease amyloid A4 protein resembles a cell-surface receptor. Nature *325*, 733-736.

[117] Kawasumi, M., Hashimoto, Y., Chiba, T., Kanekura, K., Yamagishi, Y., Ishizaka, M., Tajima, H., Niikura, T., and Nishimoto, I. (2002). Molecular mechanisms for neuronal cell death by Alzheimer's amyloid precursor protein-relevant insults. Neurosignals *11*, 236-250.

[118] Kilic, E., Hermann, D.M., Kugler, S., Kilic, U., Holzmuller, H., Schmeer, C., and Bahr, M. (2002). Adenovirus-mediated Bcl-X(L) expression using a neuron-specific synapsin-1 promoter protects against disseminated neuronal injury and brain infarction following focal cerebral ischemia in mice. Neurobiol Dis *11*, 275-284.

[119] Klyubin, I., Wang, Q., Reed, M.N., Irving, E.A., Upton, N., Hofmeister, J., Cleary, J.P., Anwyl, R., and Rowan, M.J. (2009). Protection against Abeta-mediated rapid disruption of synaptic plasticity and memory by memantine. Neurobiol Aging *32*, 614-623.

[120] Kojro, E., Gimpl, G., Lammich, S., Marz, W., and Fahrenholz, F. (2001). Low cholesterol stimulates the nonamyloidogenic pathway by its effect on the alpha -secretase ADAM 10. Proc Natl Acad Sci U S A *98*, 5815-5820.

[121] Kotilinek, L.A., Bacskai, B., Westerman, M., Kawarabayashi, T., Younkin, L., Hyman, B.T., Younkin, S., and Ashe, K.H. (2002). Reversible memory loss in a mouse transgenic model of Alzheimer's disease. J Neurosci *22*, 6331-6335.

[122] Kukar, T., Murphy, M.P., Eriksen, J.L., Sagi, S.A., Weggen, S., Smith, T.E., Ladd, T., Khan, M.A., Kache, R., Beard, J., *et al.* (2005). Diverse compounds mimic Alzheimer disease-causing mutations by augmenting Abeta42 production. Nat Med *11*, 545-550.

[123] Lannfelt, L., Blennow, K., Zetterberg, H., Batsman, S., Ames, D., Harrison, J., Masters, C.L., Targum, S., Bush, A.I., Murdoch, R., *et al.* (2008). Safety, efficacy, and biomarker findings of PBT2 in targeting Abeta as a modifying therapy for Alzheimer's disease: a phase IIa, double-blind, randomised, placebo-controlled trial. Lancet Neurol *7*, 779-786.

[124] Laudon, H., Hansson, E.M., Melen, K., Bergman, A., Farmery, M.R., Winblad, B., Lendahl, U., von Heijne, G., and Naslund, J. (2005). A nine-transmembrane domain topology for presenilin 1. J Biol Chem *280*, 35352-35360.

[125] Lee, J., Duan, W., and Mattson, M.P. (2002). Evidence that brain-derived neurotrophic factor is required for basal neurogenesis and mediates, in part, the enhancement of neurogenesis by dietary restriction in the hippocampus of adult mice. J Neurochem *82*, 1367-1375.

[126] Leissring, M.A., Farris, W., Chang, A.Y., Walsh, D.M., Wu, X., Sun, X., Frosch, M.P., and Selkoe, D.J. (2003). Enhanced proteolysis of beta-amyloid in APP transgenic mice prevents plaque formation, secondary pathology, and premature death. Neuron *40*, 1087-1093.

[127] Lesne, S., Koh, M.T., Kotilinek, L., Kayed, R., Glabe, C.G., Yang, A., Gallagher, M., and Ashe, K.H. (2006). A specific amyloid-beta protein assembly in the brain impairs memory. Nature *440*, 352-357.

[128] Lewis, J., Dickson, D.W., Lin, W.L., Chisholm, L., Corral, A., Jones, G., Yen, S.H., Sahara, N., Skipper, L., Yager, D., *et al.* (2001). Enhanced neurofibrillary degeneration in transgenic mice expressing mutant tau and APP. Science *293*, 1487-1491.

[129] Lewis, J., McGowan, E., Rockwood, J., Melrose, H., Nacharaju, P., Van Slegtenhorst, M., Gwinn-Hardy, K., Paul Murphy, M., Baker, M., Yu, X., *et al.* (2000). Neurofibrillary tangles, amyotrophy and progressive motor disturbance in mice expressing mutant (P301L) tau protein. Nat Genet *25*, 402-405.

[130] Lim, G.P., Yang, F., Chu, T., Chen, P., Beech, W., Teter, B., Tran, T., Ubeda, O., Ashe, K.H., Frautschy, S.A., *et al.* (2000). Ibuprofen suppresses plaque pathology and inflammation in a mouse model for Alzheimer's disease. J Neurosci *20*, 5709-5714.

[131] Lleo, A., Berezovska, O., Herl, L., Raju, S., Deng, A., Bacskai, B.J., Frosch, M.P., Irizarry, M., and Hyman, B.T. (2004). Nonsteroidal anti-inflammatory drugs lower Abeta42 and change presenilin 1 conformation. Nat Med *10*, 1065-1066.

[132] Lleo, A., Greenberg, S.M., and Growdon, J.H. (2006). Current pharmacotherapy for Alzheimer's disease. Annu Rev Med *57*, 513-533.

[133] Luo, Y., Bolon, B., Kahn, S., Bennett, B.D., Babu-Khan, S., Denis, P., Fan, W., Kha, H., Zhang, J., Gong, Y., *et al.* (2001). Mice deficient in BACE1, the Alzheimer's beta-secretase, have normal phenotype and abolished beta-amyloid generation. Nat Neurosci *4*, 231-232.

[134] Lutz, M.W., Crenshaw, D.G., Saunders, A.M., and Roses, A.D. (2010). Genetic variation at a single locus and age of onset for Alzheimer's disease. Alzheimers Dement *6*, 125-131.

[135] Mah, A.L., Perry, G., Smith, M.A., and Monteiro, M.J. (2000). Identification of ubiquilin, a novel presenilin interactor that increases presenilin protein accumulation. J Cell Biol *151*, 847-862.

[136] Mandel, S.A., Amit, T., Kalfon, L., Reznichenko, L., Weinreb, O., and Youdim, M.B. (2008). Cell signaling pathways and iron chelation in the neurorestorative activity of green tea polyphenols: special reference to epigallocatechin gallate (EGCG). J Alzheimers Dis *15*, 211-222.

[137] Mangialasche, F., Solomon, A., Winblad, B., Mecocci, P., and Kivipelto, M. (2010). Alzheimer's disease: clinical trials and drug development. Lancet Neurol *9*, 702-716.

[138] Marjaux, E., Hartmann, D., and De Strooper, B. (2004). Presenilins in memory, Alzheimer's disease, and therapy. Neuron *42*, 189-192.

[139] Martinez-Coria, H., Green, K.N., Billings, L.M., Kitazawa, M., Albrecht, M., Rammes, G., Parsons, C.G., Gupta, S., Banerjee, P., and LaFerla, F.M. (2010). Memantine im-

proves cognition and reduces Alzheimer's-like neuropathology in transgenic mice. Am J Pathol *176*, 870-880.

[140] Massey, L.K., Mah, A.L., Ford, D.L., Miller, J., Liang, J., Doong, H., and Monteiro, M.J. (2004). Overexpression of ubiquilin decreases ubiquitination and degradation of presenilin proteins. J Alzheimers Dis *6*, 79-92.

[141] Mattson, M.P. (2004). Pathways towards and away from Alzheimer's disease. Nature *430*, 631-639.

[142] Mattson, M.P., Guo, Q., Furukawa, K., and Pedersen, W.A. (1998). Presenilins, the endoplasmic reticulum, and neuronal apoptosis in Alzheimer's disease. J Neurochem *70*, 1-14.

[143] Miller, B.W., Willett, K.C., and Desilets, A.R. (2011). Rosiglitazone and pioglitazone for the treatment of Alzheimer's disease. Ann Pharmacother *45*, 1416-1424.

[144] Misiak, B., Leszek, J., and Kiejna, A. (2012). Metabolic syndrome, mild cognitive impairment and Alzheimer's disease-The emerging role of systemic low-grade inflammation and adiposity. Brain Res Bull *89*, 144-149.

[145] Moghadam, F.H., Alaie, H., Karbalaie, K., Tanhaei, S., Nasr Esfahani, M.H., and Baharvand, H. (2009). Transplantation of primed or unprimed mouse embryonic stem cell-derived neural precursor cells improves cognitive function in Alzheimerian rats. Differentiation *78*, 59-68.

[146] Morgan, K. The three new pathways leading to Alzheimer's disease. Neuropathol Appl Neurobiol *37*, 353-357.

[147] Muzumdar, R.H., Huffman, D.M., Atzmon, G., Buettner, C., Cobb, L.J., Fishman, S., Budagov, T., Cui, L., Einstein, F.H., Poduval, A., *et al.* (2009). Humanin: a novel central regulator of peripheral insulin action. PLoS One *4*, e6334.

[148] Nagata, T., Shinagawa, S., Nukariya, K., Yamada, H., and Nakayama, K. (2012). Association between BDNF Polymorphism (Val66Met) and Executive Function in Patients with Amnestic Mild Cognitive Impairment or Mild Alzheimer Disease. Dement Geriatr Cogn Disord *33*, 266-272.

[149] Nalivaeva, N.N., Beckett, C., Belyaev, N.D., and Turner, A.J. (2012). Are amyloid-degrading enzymes viable therapeutic targets in Alzheimer's disease? J Neurochem *120 Suppl 1*, 167-185.

[150] Ng, D.C., Lin, B.H., Lim, C.P., Huang, G., Zhang, T., Poli, V., and Cao, X. (2006). Stat3 regulates microtubules by antagonizing the depolymerization activity of stathmin. J Cell Biol *172*, 245-257.

[151] Nicolas, C.S., Peineau, S., Amici, M., Csaba, Z., Fafouri, A., Javalet, C., Collett, V.J., Hildebrandt, L., Seaton, G., Choi, S.L., *et al.* (2012). The Jak/STAT pathway is involved in synaptic plasticity. Neuron *73*, 374-390.

[152] Nicoll, J.A., Wilkinson, D., Holmes, C., Steart, P., Markham, H., and Weller, R.O. (2003). Neuropathology of human Alzheimer disease after immunization with amyloid-beta peptide: a case report. Nat Med *9*, 448-452.

[153] Nikolaev, A., McLaughlin, T., O'Leary, D.D., and Tessier-Lavigne, M. (2009). APP binds DR6 to trigger axon pruning and neuron death via distinct caspases. Nature *457*, 981-989.

[154] Nilsberth, C., Westlind-Danielsson, A., Eckman, C.B., Condron, M.M., Axelman, K., Forsell, C., Stenh, C., Luthman, J., Teplow, D.B., Younkin, S.G., *et al.* (2001). The 'Arctic' APP mutation (E693G) causes Alzheimer's disease by enhanced Abeta protofibril formation. Nat Neurosci *4*, 887-893.

[155] Nussbaum, J.M., Schilling, S., Cynis, H., Silva, A., Swanson, E., Wangsanut, T., Tayler, K., Wiltgen, B., Hatami, A., Ronicke, R., *et al.* (2012). Prion-like behaviour and tau-dependent cytotoxicity of pyroglutamylated amyloid-beta. Nature *485*, 651-655.

[156] Oddo, S., Caccamo, A., Shepherd, J.D., Murphy, M.P., Golde, T.E., Kayed, R., Metherate, R., Mattson, M.P., Akbari, Y., and LaFerla, F.M. (2003). Triple-transgenic model of Alzheimer's disease with plaques and tangles: intracellular Abeta and synaptic dysfunction. Neuron *39*, 409-421.

[157] Oh, Y.K., Bachar, A.R., Zacharias, D.G., Kim, S.G., Wan, J., Cobb, L.J., Lerman, L.O., Cohen, P., and Lerman, A. (2011). Humanin preserves endothelial function and prevents atherosclerotic plaque progression in hypercholesterolemic ApoE deficient mice. Atherosclerosis *219*, 65-73.

[158] Okura, Y., Miyakoshi, A., Kohyama, K., Park, I.K., Staufenbiel, M., and Matsumoto, Y. (2006). Nonviral Abeta DNA vaccine therapy against Alzheimer's disease: long-term effects and safety. Proc Natl Acad Sci U S A *103*, 9619-9624.

[159] Orgogozo, J.M., Gilman, S., Dartigues, J.F., Laurent, B., Puel, M., Kirby, L.C., Jouanny, P., Dubois, B., Eisner, L., Flitman, S., *et al.* (2003). Subacute meningoencephalitis in a subset of patients with AD after Abeta42 immunization. Neurology *61*, 46-54.

[160] Park, D., Lee, H.J., Joo, S.S., Bae, D.K., Yang, G., Yang, Y.H., Lim, I., Matsuo, A., Tooyama, I., Kim, Y.B., *et al.* (2012). Human neural stem cells over-expressing choline acetyltransferase restore cognition in rat model of cognitive dysfunction. Exp Neurol *234*, 521-526.

[161] Parsons, R.B., Price, G.C., Farrant, J.K., Subramaniam, D., Adeagbo-Sheikh, J., and Austen, B.M. (2006). Statins inhibit the dimerization of beta-secretase via both isoprenoid- and cholesterol-mediated mechanisms. Biochem J *399*, 205-214.

[162] Passer, B.J., Pellegrini, L., Vito, P., Ganjei, J.K., and D'Adamio, L. (1999). Interaction of Alzheimer's presenilin-1 and presenilin-2 with Bcl-X(L). A potential role in modulating the threshold of cell death. J Biol Chem *274*, 24007-24013.

[163] Perrin, R.J., Fagan, A.M., and Holtzman, D.M. (2009). Multimodal techniques for diagnosis and prognosis of Alzheimer's disease. Nature *461*, 916-922.

[164] Petersen, R.C., Thomas, R.G., Grundman, M., Bennett, D., Doody, R., Ferris, S., Galasko, D., Jin, S., Kaye, J., Levey, A., *et al.* (2005). Vitamin E and donepezil for the treatment of mild cognitive impairment. N Engl J Med *352*, 2379-2388.

[165] Pettenati, C., Annicchiarico, R., and Caltagirone, C. (2003). Clinical pharmacology of anti-Alzheimer drugs. Fundam Clin Pharmacol *17*, 659-672.

[166] Poirier, J. (2005). Apolipoprotein E, cholesterol transport and synthesis in sporadic Alzheimer's disease. Neurobiol Aging *26*, 355-361.

[167] Qiu, W.Q., Walsh, D.M., Ye, Z., Vekrellis, K., Zhang, J., Podlisny, M.B., Rosner, M.R., Safavi, A., Hersh, L.B., and Selkoe, D.J. (1998). Insulin-degrading enzyme regulates extracellular levels of amyloid beta-protein by degradation. J Biol Chem *273*, 32730-32738.

[168] Quinn, J.F., Raman, R., Thomas, R.G., Yurko-Mauro, K., Nelson, E.B., Van Dyck, C., Galvin, J.E., Emond, J., Jack, C.R., Jr., Weiner, M., *et al.* (2010). Docosahexaenoic acid supplementation and cognitive decline in Alzheimer disease: a randomized trial. JAMA *304*, 1903-1911.

[169] Rapoport, M., Dawson, H.N., Binder, L.I., Vitek, M.P., and Ferreira, A. (2002). Tau is essential to beta -amyloid-induced neurotoxicity. Proc Natl Acad Sci U S A *99*, 6364-6369.

[170] Ray, B., Banerjee, P.K., Greig, N.H., and Lahiri, D.K. (2009). Memantine treatment decreases levels of secreted Alzheimer's amyloid precursor protein (APP) and amyloid beta (A beta) peptide in the human neuroblastoma cells. Neurosci Lett *470*, 1-5.

[171] Refolo, L.M., Pappolla, M.A., LaFrancois, J., Malester, B., Schmidt, S.D., Thomas-Bryant, T., Tint, G.S., Wang, R., Mercken, M., Petanceska, S.S., *et al.* (2001). A cholesterol-lowering drug reduces beta-amyloid pathology in a transgenic mouse model of Alzheimer's disease. Neurobiol Dis *8*, 890-899.

[172] Reitz, C. (2012). Alzheimer's disease and the amyloid cascade hypothesis: a critical review. Int J Alzheimers Dis *2012*, 369808.

[173] Relkin, N.R., Szabo, P., Adamiak, B., Burgut, T., Monthe, C., Lent, R.W., Younkin, S., Younkin, L., Schiff, R., and Weksler, M.E. (2009). 18-Month study of intravenous immunoglobulin for treatment of mild Alzheimer disease. Neurobiol Aging *30*, 1728-1736.

[174] Renolleau, S., Fau, S., Goyenvalle, C., Joly, L.M., Chauvier, D., Jacotot, E., Mariani, J., and Charriaut-Marlangue, C. (2007). Specific caspase inhibitor Q-VD-OPh prevents neonatal stroke in P7 rat: a role for gender. J Neurochem *100*, 1062-1071.

[175] Rezai-Zadeh, K., Shytle, D., Sun, N., Mori, T., Hou, H., Jeanniton, D., Ehrhart, J., Townsend, K., Zeng, J., Morgan, D., *et al.* (2005). Green tea epigallocatechin-3-gallate

(EGCG) modulates amyloid precursor protein cleavage and reduces cerebral amyloidosis in Alzheimer transgenic mice. J Neurosci *25*, 8807-8814.

[176] Riordan, K.C., Hoffman Snyder, C.R., Wellik, K.E., Caselli, R.J., Wingerchuk, D.M., and Demaerschalk, B.M. (2011). Effectiveness of adding memantine to an Alzheimer dementia treatment regimen which already includes stable donepezil therapy: a critically appraised topic. Neurologist *17*, 121-123.

[177] Ritchie, C.W., Bush, A.I., Mackinnon, A., Macfarlane, S., Mastwyk, M., MacGregor, L., Kiers, L., Cherny, R., Li, Q.X., Tammer, A., *et al.* (2003). Metal-protein attenuation with iodochlorhydroxyquin (clioquinol) targeting Abeta amyloid deposition and toxicity in Alzheimer disease: a pilot phase 2 clinical trial. Arch Neurol *60*, 1685-1691.

[178] Roberson, E.D., Scearce-Levie, K., Palop, J.J., Yan, F., Cheng, I.H., Wu, T., Gerstein, H., Yu, G.Q., and Mucke, L. (2007). Reducing endogenous tau ameliorates amyloid beta-induced deficits in an Alzheimer's disease mouse model. Science *316*, 750-754.

[179] Rodriguez, J.J., Jones, V.C., Tabuchi, M., Allan, S.M., Knight, E.M., LaFerla, F.M., Oddo, S., and Verkhratsky, A. (2008). Impaired adult neurogenesis in the dentate gyrus of a triple transgenic mouse model of Alzheimer's disease. PLoS One *3*, e2935.

[180] Rodriguez, J.J., and Verkhratsky, A. (2011). Neurogenesis in Alzheimer's disease. J Anat *219*, 78-89.

[181] Rogaev, E.I., Sherrington, R., Rogaeva, E.A., Levesque, G., Ikeda, M., Liang, Y., Chi, H., Lin, C., Holman, K., Tsuda, T., *et al.* (1995). Familial Alzheimer's disease in kindreds with missense mutations in a gene on chromosome 1 related to the Alzheimer's disease type 3 gene. Nature *376*, 775-778.

[182] Rogaeva, E., Meng, Y., Lee, J.H., Gu, Y., Kawarai, T., Zou, F., Katayama, T., Baldwin, C.T., Cheng, R., Hasegawa, H., *et al.* (2007). The neuronal sortilin-related receptor SORL1 is genetically associated with Alzheimer disease. Nat Genet *39*, 168-177.

[183] Rohn, T.T., and Head, E. (2009). Caspases as therapeutic targets in Alzheimer's disease: is it time to "cut" to the chase? Int J Clin Exp Pathol *2*, 108-118.

[184] Rohn, T.T., Ivins, K.J., Bahr, B.A., Cotman, C.W., and Cribbs, D.H. (2000). A monoclonal antibody to amyloid precursor protein induces neuronal apoptosis. J Neurochem *74*, 2331-2342.

[185] Rollero, A., Murialdo, G., Fonzi, S., Garrone, S., Gianelli, M.V., Gazzerro, E., Barreca, A., and Polleri, A. (1998). Relationship between cognitive function, growth hormone and insulin-like growth factor I plasma levels in aged subjects. Neuropsychobiology *38*, 73-79.

[186] Roses, A.D., Lutz, M.W., Amrine-Madsen, H., Saunders, A.M., Crenshaw, D.G., Sundseth, S.S., Huentelman, M.J., Welsh-Bohmer, K.A., and Reiman, E.M. A TOMM40 variable-length polymorphism predicts the age of late-onset Alzheimer's disease. Pharmacogenomics J *10*, 375-384.

[187] Saito, T., Iwata, N., Tsubuki, S., Takaki, Y., Takano, J., Huang, S.M., Suemoto, T., Higuchi, M., and Saido, T.C. (2005). Somatostatin regulates brain amyloid beta peptide Abeta42 through modulation of proteolytic degradation. Nat Med *11*, 434-439.

[188] Salloway, S., Sperling, R., Gilman, S., Fox, N.C., Blennow, K., Raskind, M., Sabbagh, M., Honig, L.S., Doody, R., van Dyck, C.H., *et al.* (2009). A phase 2 multiple ascending dose trial of bapineuzumab in mild to moderate Alzheimer disease. Neurology *73*, 2061-2070.

[189] Salloway, S., Sperling, R., Keren, R., Porsteinsson, A.P., van Dyck, C.H., Tariot, P.N., Gilman, S., Arnold, D., Abushakra, S., Hernandez, C., *et al.* (2011). A phase 2 randomized trial of ELND005, scyllo-inositol, in mild to moderate Alzheimer disease. Neurology *77*, 1253-1262.

[190] Sampson, E., Jenagaratnam, L., and McShane, R. (2008). Metal protein attenuating compounds for the treatment of Alzheimer's disease. Cochrane Database Syst Rev, CD005380.

[191] Sano, M., Bell, K.L., Galasko, D., Galvin, J.E., Thomas, R.G., van Dyck, C.H., and Aisen, P.S. (2011). A randomized, double-blind, placebo-controlled trial of simvastatin to treat Alzheimer disease. Neurology *77*, 556-563.

[192] Sano, M., Ernesto, C., Thomas, R.G., Klauber, M.R., Schafer, K., Grundman, M., Woodbury, P., Growdon, J., Cotman, C.W., Pfeiffer, E., *et al.* (1997). A controlled trial of selegiline, alpha-tocopherol, or both as treatment for Alzheimer's disease. The Alzheimer's Disease Cooperative Study. N Engl J Med *336*, 1216-1222.

[193] Santarelli, L., Saxe, M., Gross, C., Surget, A., Battaglia, F., Dulawa, S., Weisstaub, N., Lee, J., Duman, R., Arancio, O., *et al.* (2003). Requirement of hippocampal neurogenesis for the behavioral effects of antidepressants. Science *301*, 805-809.

[194] Sarafian, T.A., Montes, C., Imura, T., Qi, J., Coppola, G., Geschwind, D.H., and Sofroniew, M.V. Disruption of astrocyte STAT3 signaling decreases mitochondrial function and increases oxidative stress in vitro. PLoS One *5*, e9532.

[195] Sato, S., Tatebayashi, Y., Akagi, T., Chui, D.H., Murayama, M., Miyasaka, T., Planel, E., Tanemura, K., Sun, X., Hashikawa, T., *et al.* (2002). Aberrant tau phosphorylation by glycogen synthase kinase-3beta and JNK3 induces oligomeric tau fibrils in COS-7 cells. J Biol Chem *277*, 42060-42065.

[196] Schellenberg, G.D., and Montine, T.J. (2012). The genetics and neuropathology of Alzheimer's disease. Acta Neuropathol *124*, 305-323.

[197] Schenk, D., Barbour, R., Dunn, W., Gordon, G., Grajeda, H., Guido, T., Hu, K., Huang, J., Johnson-Wood, K., Khan, K., *et al.* (1999). Immunization with amyloid-beta attenuates Alzheimer-disease-like pathology in the PDAPP mouse. Nature *400*, 173-177.

[198] Schilling, S., Zeitschel, U., Hoffmann, T., Heiser, U., Francke, M., Kehlen, A., Holzer, M., Hutter-Paier, B., Prokesch, M., Windisch, M., *et al.* (2008). Glutaminyl cyclase in-

hibition attenuates pyroglutamate Abeta and Alzheimer's disease-like pathology. Nat Med *14*, 1106-1111.

[199] Schirmer, R.H., Adler, H., Pickhardt, M., and Mandelkow, E. (2011). "Lest we forget you--methylene blue...". Neurobiol Aging *32*, 2325 e2327-2316.

[200] Seabrook, T.J., Jiang, L., Maier, M., and Lemere, C.A. (2006). Minocycline affects microglia activation, Abeta deposition, and behavior in APP-tg mice. Glia *53*, 776-782.

[201] Searfoss, G.H., Jordan, W.H., Calligaro, D.O., Galbreath, E.J., Schirtzinger, L.M., Berridge, B.R., Gao, H., Higgins, M.A., May, P.C., and Ryan, T.P. (2003). Adipsin, a biomarker of gastrointestinal toxicity mediated by a functional gamma-secretase inhibitor. J Biol Chem *278*, 46107-46116.

[202] Shearman, M.S., Beher, D., Clarke, E.E., Lewis, H.D., Harrison, T., Hunt, P., Nadin, A., Smith, A.L., Stevenson, G., and Castro, J.L. (2000). L-685,458, an aspartyl protease transition state mimic, is a potent inhibitor of amyloid beta-protein precursor gamma-secretase activity. Biochemistry *39*, 8698-8704.

[203] Sherrington, R., Rogaev, E.I., Liang, Y., Rogaeva, E.A., Levesque, G., Ikeda, M., Chi, H., Lin, C., Li, G., Holman, K., *et al.* (1995). Cloning of a gene bearing missense mutations in early-onset familial Alzheimer's disease. Nature *375*, 754-760.

[204] Shiryaev, N., Pikman, R., Giladi, E., and Gozes, I. (2011). Protection against tauopathy by the drug candidates NAP (davunetide) and D-SAL: biochemical, cellular and behavioral aspects. Curr Pharm Des *17*, 2603-2612.

[205] Shobab, L.A., Hsiung, G.Y., and Feldman, H.H. (2005). Cholesterol in Alzheimer's disease. Lancet Neurol *4*, 841-852.

[206] Shub, D., Darvishi, R., and Kunik, M.E. (2009). Non-pharmacologic treatment of insomnia in persons with dementia. Geriatrics *64*, 22-26.

[207] Singer, C., Tractenberg, R.E., Kaye, J., Schafer, K., Gamst, A., Grundman, M., Thomas, R., and Thal, L.J. (2003). A multicenter, placebo-controlled trial of melatonin for sleep disturbance in Alzheimer's disease. Sleep *26*, 893-901.

[208] Sotthibundhu, A., Li, Q.X., Thangnipon, W., and Coulson, E.J. (2009). Abeta(1-42) stimulates adult SVZ neurogenesis through the p75 neurotrophin receptor. Neurobiol Aging *30*, 1975-1985.

[209] Stephanou, A., and Latchman, D.S. (2005). Opposing actions of STAT-1 and STAT-3. Growth Factors *23*, 177-182.

[210] Stohr, J., Watts, J.C., Mensinger, Z.L., Oehler, A., Grillo, S.K., DeArmond, S.J., Prusiner, S.B., and Giles, K. (2012). Purified and synthetic Alzheimer's amyloid beta (Abeta) prions. Proc Natl Acad Sci U S A *109*, 11025-11030.

[211] Sudo, H., Jiang, H., Yasukawa, T., Hashimoto, Y., Niikura, T., Kawasumi, M., Matsuda, S., Takeuchi, Y., Aiso, S., Matsuoka, M., *et al.* (2000). Antibody-regulated neuro-

toxic function of cell-surface beta-amyloid precursor protein. Mol Cell Neurosci *16*, 708-723.

[212] Tabira, T. (2001). Clioquinol's return: cautions from Japan. Science *292*, 2251-2252.

[213] Takashima, A., Murayama, M., Yasutake, K., Takahashi, H., Yokoyama, M., and Ishiguro, K. (2001). Involvement of cyclin dependent kinase5 activator p25 on tau phosphorylation in mouse brain. Neurosci Lett *306*, 37-40.

[214] Takasugi, N., Tomita, T., Hayashi, I., Tsuruoka, M., Niimura, M., Takahashi, Y., Thinakaran, G., and Iwatsubo, T. (2003). The role of presenilin cofactors in the gamma-secretase complex. Nature *422*, 438-441.

[215] Takeuchi, D., Sato, N., Shimamura, M., Kurinami, H., Takeda, S., Shinohara, M., Suzuki, S., Kojima, M., Ogihara, T., and Morishita, R. (2008). Alleviation of Abeta-induced cognitive impairment by ultrasound-mediated gene transfer of HGF in a mouse model. Gene Ther *15*, 561-571.

[216] Tariot, P.N., and Aisen, P.S. (2009). Can lithium or valproate untie tangles in Alzheimer's disease? J Clin Psychiatry *70*, 919-921.

[217] Tariot, P.N., Cummings, J.L., Katz, I.R., Mintzer, J., Perdomo, C.A., Schwam, E.M., and Whalen, E. (2001). A randomized, double-blind, placebo-controlled study of the efficacy and safety of donepezil in patients with Alzheimer's disease in the nursing home setting. J Am Geriatr Soc *49*, 1590-1599.

[218] Tariot, P.N., Farlow, M.R., Grossberg, G.T., Graham, S.M., McDonald, S., and Gergel, I. (2004). Memantine treatment in patients with moderate to severe Alzheimer disease already receiving donepezil: a randomized controlled trial. JAMA *291*, 317-324.

[219] Tian, G., Sobotka-Briner, C.D., Zysk, J., Liu, X., Birr, C., Sylvester, M.A., Edwards, P.D., Scott, C.D., and Greenberg, B.D. (2002). Linear non-competitive inhibition of solubilized human gamma-secretase by pepstatin A methylester, L685458, sulfonamides, and benzodiazepines. J Biol Chem *277*, 31499-31505.

[220] Tuszynski, M.H., Thal, L., Pay, M., Salmon, D.P., U, H.S., Bakay, R., Patel, P., Blesch, A., Vahlsing, H.L., Ho, G., *et al.* (2005). A phase 1 clinical trial of nerve growth factor gene therapy for Alzheimer disease. Nat Med *11*, 551-555.

[221] Um, J.W., Nygaard, H.B., Heiss, J.K., Kostylev, M.A., Stagi, M., Vortmeyer, A., Wisniewski, T., Gunther, E.C., and Strittmatter, S.M. (2012). Alzheimer amyloid-beta oligomer bound to postsynaptic prion protein activates Fyn to impair neurons. Nat Neurosci *15*, 1227-1235.

[222] Van der Zee, E.A., Platt, B., and Riedel, G. Acetylcholine: future research and perspectives. Behav Brain Res *221*, 583-586.

[223] Vassar, R., Bennett, B.D., Babu-Khan, S., Kahn, S., Mendiaz, E.A., Denis, P., Teplow, D.B., Ross, S., Amarante, P., Loeloff, R., *et al.* (1999). Beta-secretase cleavage of Alz-

heimer's amyloid precursor protein by the transmembrane aspartic protease BACE. Science *286*, 735-741.

[224] Vingtdeux, V., and Marambaud, P. (2012). Identification and biology of alpha-secretase. J Neurochem *120 Suppl 1*, 34-45.

[225] Vulih-Shultzman, I., Pinhasov, A., Mandel, S., Grigoriadis, N., Touloumi, O., Pittel, Z., and Gozes, I. (2007). Activity-dependent neuroprotective protein snippet NAP reduces tau hyperphosphorylation and enhances learning in a novel transgenic mouse model. J Pharmacol Exp Ther *323*, 438-449.

[226] Weggen, S., Eriksen, J.L., Das, P., Sagi, S.A., Wang, R., Pietrzik, C.U., Findlay, K.A., Smith, T.E., Murphy, M.P., Bulter, T., *et al.* (2001). A subset of NSAIDs lower amyloidogenic Abeta42 independently of cyclooxygenase activity. Nature *414*, 212-216.

[227] Weihl, C.C., Ghadge, G.D., Kennedy, S.G., Hay, N., Miller, R.J., and Roos, R.P. (1999). Mutant presenilin-1 induces apoptosis and downregulates Akt/PKB. J Neurosci *19*, 5360-5369.

[228] Wiessner, C., Wiederhold, K.H., Tissot, A.C., Frey, P., Danner, S., Jacobson, L.H., Jennings, G.T., Luond, R., Ortmann, R., Reichwald, J., *et al.* (2011). The second-generation active Abeta immunotherapy CAD106 reduces amyloid accumulation in APP transgenic mice while minimizing potential side effects. J Neurosci *31*, 9323-9331.

[229] Winblad, B., Kilander, L., Eriksson, S., Minthon, L., Batsman, S., Wetterholm, A.L., Jansson-Blixt, C., and Haglund, A. (2006). Donepezil in patients with severe Alzheimer's disease: double-blind, parallel-group, placebo-controlled study. Lancet *367*, 1057-1065.

[230] Wolfe, M.S. (2012). gamma-Secretase inhibitors and modulators for Alzheimer's disease. J Neurochem *120 Suppl 1*, 89-98.

[231] Wolozin, B., Kellman, W., Ruosseau, P., Celesia, G.G., and Siegel, G. (2000). Decreased prevalence of Alzheimer disease associated with 3-hydroxy-3-methyglutaryl coenzyme A reductase inhibitors. Arch Neurol *57*, 1439-1443.

[232] Wu, S., Sasaki, A., Yoshimoto, R., Kawahara, Y., Manabe, T., Kataoka, K., Asashima, M., and Yuge, L. (2008). Neural stem cells improve learning and memory in rats with Alzheimer's disease. Pathobiology *75*, 186-194.

[233] Yamada, M., Chiba, T., Sasabe, J., Terashita, K., Aiso, S., and Matsuoka, M. (2008). Nasal Colivelin treatment ameliorates memory impairment related to Alzheimer's disease. Neuropsychopharmacology *33*, 2020-2032.

[234] Yamasaki, T.R., Blurton-Jones, M., Morrissette, D.A., Kitazawa, M., Oddo, S., and LaFerla, F.M. (2007). Neural stem cells improve memory in an inducible mouse model of neuronal loss. J Neurosci *27*, 11925-11933.

[235] Yamashita, S., Mita, S., Arima, T., Maeda, Y., Kimura, E., Nishida, Y., Murakami, T., Okado, H., and Uchino, M. (2001). Bcl-2 expression by retrograde transport of adeno-

viral vectors with Cre-loxP recombination system in motor neurons of mutant SOD1 transgenic mice. Gene Ther *8*, 977-986.

[236] Yamatsuji, T., Matsui, T., Okamoto, T., Komatsuzaki, K., Takeda, S., Fukumoto, H., Iwatsubo, T., Suzuki, N., Asami-Odaka, A., Ireland, S., *et al.* (1996). G protein-mediated neuronal DNA fragmentation induced by familial Alzheimer's disease-associated mutants of APP. Science *272*, 1349-1352.

[237] Yang, L., Sugama, S., Mischak, R.P., Kiaei, M., Bizat, N., Brouillet, E., Joh, T.H., and Beal, M.F. (2004). A novel systemically active caspase inhibitor attenuates the toxicities of MPTP, malonate, and 3NP in vivo. Neurobiol Dis *17*, 250-259.

[238] Yasojima, K., Akiyama, H., McGeer, E.G., and McGeer, P.L. (2001a). Reduced neprilysin in high plaque areas of Alzheimer brain: a possible relationship to deficient degradation of beta-amyloid peptide. Neurosci Lett *297*, 97-100.

[239] Yasojima, K., McGeer, E.G., and McGeer, P.L. (2001b). Relationship between beta amyloid peptide generating molecules and neprilysin in Alzheimer disease and normal brain. Brain Res *919*, 115-121.

[240] Zhang, Z., Hartmann, H., Do, V.M., Abramowski, D., Sturchler-Pierrat, C., Staufenbiel, M., Sommer, B., van de Wetering, M., Clevers, H., Saftig, P., *et al.* (1998). Destabilization of beta-catenin by mutations in presenilin-1 potentiates neuronal apoptosis. Nature *395*, 698-702.

[241] Zhao, B., Chrest, F.J., Horton, W.E., Jr., Sisodia, S.S., and Kusiak, J.W. (1997). Expression of mutant amyloid precursor proteins induces apoptosis in PC12 cells. J Neurosci Res *47*, 253-263.

[242] Zhu, S., Stavrovskaya, I.G., Drozda, M., Kim, B.Y., Ona, V., Li, M., Sarang, S., Liu, A.S., Hartley, D.M., Wu, D.C., *et al.* (2002). Minocycline inhibits cytochrome c release and delays progression of amyotrophic lateral sclerosis in mice. Nature *417*, 74-78.

[243] Ziabreva, I., Perry, E., Perry, R., Minger, S.L., Ekonomou, A., Przyborski, S., and Ballard, C. (2006). Altered neurogenesis in Alzheimer's disease. J Psychosom Res *61*, 311-316.

Chapter 10

Dropping the BACE: Beta Secretase (BACE1) as an Alzheimer's Disease Intervention Target

Justin Read and Cenk Suphioglu

Additional information is available at the end of the chapter

http://dx.doi.org/10.5772/53603

1. Introduction

The β-site amyloid precursor protein cleaving enzyme 1 (BACE1) is an important regulator for the production of amyloid plaques, a characteristic of the Alzheimer's disease (AD) brain. The proteolytic cleavage of the amyloid precursor protein (APP), by BACE1, produces an insoluble amyloid-β (Aβ) fragment which has the ability to aggregate and migrate onto the dendrites and cell body of neuronal cells, initiating chronic immune responses of inflammation and microglia activation.

The cleavage of Aβ fragments trigger a feedback system that complements production numbers. This increases Aβ loading to such an extent that it exceeds the defences required for natural elimination. The fragments aggregate, developing into an insoluble plaque that has the ability to effect normal functioning by causing dysfunction. Without early identification and effective inhibition of this pathogenic pathway, the disease is anticipated to become more widespread with an aging population, in which AD is most prevalent.

Attempts to inhibit BACE1 have been relatively fruitless with most therapeutic trials being aborted in the early stages. A number of obstacles can be detrimental to the ability of an inhibitor like solubility, bioavailability, potency and effectiveness. In addition to the complexity, there are also a number of substrates cleaved by BACE1 which are important in other pathways like voltage gated sodium channels and axon myelination [1, 2]. This can create adverse reactions beyond the reduction of plaques.

Inhibitors of BACE1 have, so far, looked at active-site mimics that diverge from small and large molecules to short peptidic structures and expression modulators. Other approaches look to utilize technology with modelling software to determine the BACE1 3D structure and formulate an effective inhibitor via domain analysis. The underlying issue is translating an analytically based, site-directed mimic into a potential inhibitor with pharmaceutical integrity. This process is generally thwarted by the blood brain barrier (BBB), a specialized endothelium that separates systemic blood flow from the central nervous system (CNS). The aim is to fabricate an inhibitor that can pass through the BBB whilst maintaining structure and function.

The importance of BACE1 and the influence it has on AD, has been investigated thoroughly since it was first identified in 1999. The enzyme is an intricate part of Aβ cleavage and plaque formation instigating that inhibition could be the mechanism for relief in AD. In this chapter, we will summarize the structure and function of BACE1 and identify past attempts at its inhibition. The identification of important features regarding the protein-enzyme cleavage of APP will aid the understanding of the process and help theorize future perspectives of research.

2. Neurodegenerative disorders

Neurodegenerative disorders cover a wide range of brain conditions relating to the damage or death of neuronal cells [3]. Clinical characterisation suggests a regression in structure and function of the brain and central nervous system which is usually the final stage of a preceding period of neuronal dysfunction [4]. Specifically, dementia is of particular significance because of the devastating influence it bares on an ageing population and as the life expectancy of the general public increases, disease rates are predicted to escalate accordingly.

The burden of disease in relation to AD, the most predominant form of dementia, was calculated to be 26.6 million cases worldwide in 2006 [5]. This figure implicated 34% of the population over the age of 65 and 45% over the age of 85. The World Health Organization revised this figure in 2010 to incorporate dementia as a whole because of the difficulty to diagnose the varieties of neurodegenerative disorders [6]. The worldwide incidence was tallied at approximately 35.6 million with an estimated 7.7 million new cases annually instigating a new case arising every 4 seconds. The significance of this in regards to AD is that it covers 60-70% of dementia cases [6]. These figures could be inflated further because most cases go undiagnosed due to the requirement of post-mortem autopsy for confirmation.

The ripple effect of dementia extends far from those affected and into patient support networks. The worldwide costs are estimated to be US$604 billion annually and as the number of affected increases this number is expected to follow suit [6]. The chronic onset of the disease indicates an eventual requirement for long term care. The financial burdens relating to carers, as the disease evolves and symptoms increase with severity, the eventual requirement for long term formal care is inevitable [7]. AD patients specifically require increased supervision after diagnosis because of the increased risk of developing associated diseases like cardiovascular disease, diabetes, and bone weakening [8].

AD is largely defined by chronic symptoms of progressive neuronal and synaptic apoptosis in the cerebral cortex and subcortical regions of the brain [4]. The direct consequence is cellular atrophy, which includes degeneration in the temporal and parietal lobes, parts of the frontal cortex and cingulate gyrus [9, 10]. Progression of brain atrophy to well-defined brain structures results in symptoms of delusions, hallucinations, agitation, depression, anxiety, elation, apathy, disinhibition, irritability, aberrant motor behaviour and sleep disorders [11]. As the chronic nature of the disease progresses, the number of symptoms increases, becoming severely debilitating. Eventually, death results after long-term stress and reduction of brain structure and function [9].

Currently there are a variety of different intervention strategies being investigated to remedy these debilitating pathologies and focus to reduce the cause of neuronal cell death. Upwards of 100 irregular protein changes occur in a brain with AD, including hyperexpression, fragmentation and phosphorylation [12]. A number of these irregular protein modifications could be a result of degenerating neurons causing further damage to associated structures of the central nervous system [12]. The overall progression of AD is however, not restricted to the dysfunction of one mechanism. The number of different symptoms result from a conglomerate of sporadic cellular events that, as a consequence, stimulate the disease. The trigger or initial changes are not entirely clear and do not occur simultaneously which adds to the ambiguity of the disease.

Histopathological review of AD patients highlighted amyloid plaques and neurofibrillary tangles (NFT) as the two significant characteristics of cerebral regression identifying them as targets for the prevention of neuronal cell death [4, 13]. Investigation into the onset of NFTs implicate the tau protein as the leading cause [14]. The tau protein becomes hyperphosphorylated and releases from the intracellular microtubules decreasing structure and function and causing axons to become dishevelled and dedifferentiated. These subsequent microtubules bind together to become an insoluble fibre decreasing the ability of neurons to transmit action potentials along the axon and neurotransmitters across the synapse [15]. Alleviation from this facet of the disease is yet to be elucidated.

Amyloid plaque formation is characterized by an accumulation of amyloid-β (Aβ) sub-units on the cell membrane of neurons that, as a result, cause a decrease in cellular function [16]. The progressive damage of amyloid plaques cause neuronal apoptosis by activating the complement cascade and stimulating the membrane attack complex [17]. In developed cases of AD, where there is a high concentration of Aβ, significant damage to the physical structure of the brain can be a result of the immune response. The activation of the complement cascade involves microglia and astrocytes, which have both protective and destructive attributes. The eventual outcome is apoptosis because of the overwhelming immune response, which cannot be hindered by anti-inflammatory drugs [18]. The aggregations of Aβ deposits are neurotoxic, insoluble and become vastly distributed around the brain as they increase in numbers [19]. AD needs to be proactively prevented before amyloid plaque formation gains the ability to manipulate regular brain function and cause irreversible brain damage.

Closer investigation of the AD brain will encounter a plethora of imperative neuronal cell functions failures like synaptic failure [20], depletion of neurotransmitters [21], mitochondrial dysfunction [22], decreased cholesterol metabolism [23], reduction of neurotrophin [24] and axonal transport deficiencies [25] which can be classified as associated effects of the disease. These associated deficiencies become apparent with the onset of plaque formation, which precedes tau deconstruction [26]. The repercussions of tau mutations are a characteristic of frontotemporal dementia (FTD) and Parkinson's like defects rather than AD, which makes plaque formation the focus of this chapter [27].

3. Amyloid plaque formation

Amyloid plaques were originally purified in the early 80s and examined to contain peptides of approximately 40 amino acids that aggregated as oligomers, later to be generically named amyloid-beta (Aβ) [28]. Gene cloning and cDNA analysis of these monomers lead to the realization that the origins of this peptide remained part of a larger precursor protein [29]. This protein was later identified as the 695 amino acid, membrane bound cell receptor, amyloid precursor protein (APP), which contained the Aβ sequence in the extracellular domain [30]. It is the proteolytic cleavage, by that of multiple secretases, which releases the Aβ product.

Proteolytic processing of APP occurs by one of two pathways, the amyloidogenic (pathogenic) or the non-amyloidogenic (non-pathogenic). Transport to the membrane via endosomes is chaperoned by the intracellular adaptor protein, sorting nexin 17 (SNX17), where it becomes available for processing by the secretases [31]. The determinant of amyloidogenesis depends on the initial proteolytic cleavage in the extracellular space by either α- or β- secretase to create a soluble or insoluble fragment [19]. Cleavage of APP by the α-secretase, a protein investigated as part of the disintigrin and metalloprotease (ADAM) family, cleaves APP at the α-site releasing a soluble fragment sAPPα into the extracellular space [32]. This leaves the C-terminal fragment of 83 amino acid residues (C-83), which is abruptly cleaved by γ-secretase in the intramembrane space. This creates two subsequent fragments of the APP intracellular domain (AICD), released in the cytosol, and p3 which is released into the extracellular space (Figure 1).

The amyloidogenic pathway also utilises APP as a target. This pathway is much like that of the non-amyloidogenic pathway but instead α-secretase is substituted for β-secretase or beta site APP converting enzyme 1 (BACE1). This enzyme also cleaves APP in the extracellular space at the β-site, which is 18 amino acids towards the *N*-terminal, releasing a much shorter soluble APP-β (sAPPβ) fragment [33, 34]. The remaining C-terminal fragment of 99 amino acid residues (C-99) remains membrane bound until cleaved by γ-secretase. This releases two fragments of AICD and Aβ (Figure 1).

The non-amyloidogenic pathway has the ability to nullify the amyloidogenic pathway by simply having α-secretase cleave APP prior to that of BACE1. Since the α-site of APP is situated between that of β- and γ-, the shorter p3 fragment is produced instead of Aβ. The question over competition for the cleavage of APP is still debated but there is evidence suggesting that α-secretase nullification does not increase BACE1 activity *in vitro* [35]. The subsequent fragments of sAPPα and AICD from the non-amyloidogenic pathway suggest a purpose from the subsequent cleavage of APP. The sAPPα has shown to have neurotrophic and neuroprotective properties as well as promoting neurite expansion, synapse production and cell adhesion, while AICD has a role in p53 expression and caspase 3 activation, both associated with cell death, and in maintaining cellular actin dynamics [36-38]. This indicates that the non-amyloidogenic cleavage of APP is imperative to the maintenance of neuronal growth and function.

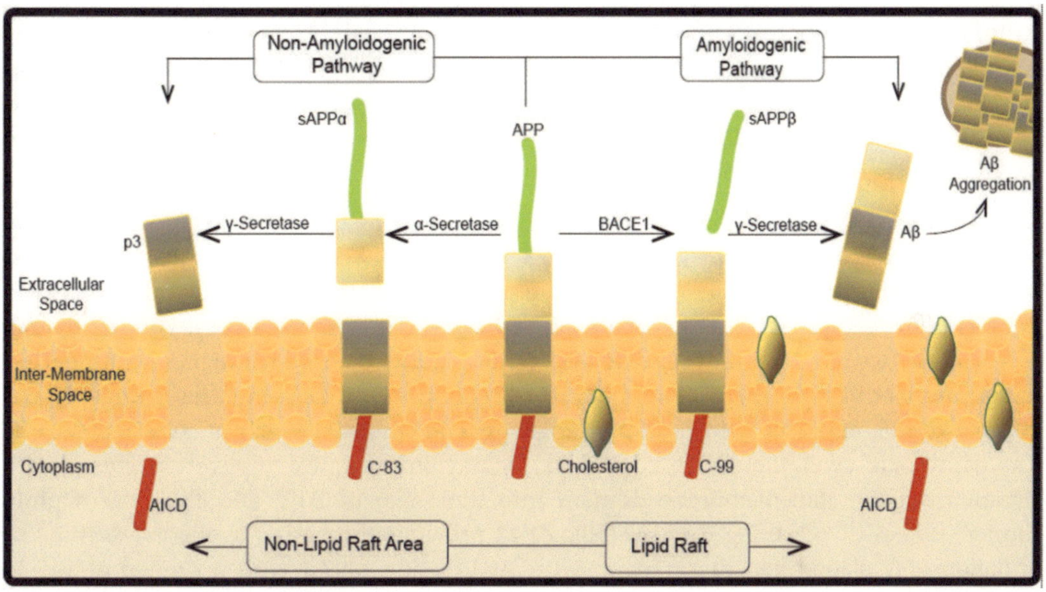

Figure 1. The cleavage of APP, depending whether by BACE1 or α-secretase, results in the production of an amyloid plaque. The non-amyloidogenic pathway (non-pathogenic) begins with α-secretase, which releases sAPPα externally from the endosome or cell membrane. The resulting C83 fragment is cleaved by γ-secretase in the intermembrane space releasing both the AICD and p3 fragments. The release of p3 into the extracellular space is not associated with plaque formation. Alternatively, the amyloidogenic (pathogenic) pathway begins with BACE1, instead of α-secretase, and cleaves APP in a lipid raft region of the membrane. The sAPPβ released is considerably shorter than sAPPα and is still released externally. The γ-secretase cleaves APP, the same as in the non-amyloidogenic pathway, but releases the 38-42 amino acid Aβ, and AICD. The externally released fragment, Aβ, has the capability to form an amyloid plaque by aggregation.

The underlying difference between the two processes is the release of the Aβ and p3 fragments. The p3 is a shorter bi-product of the overall APP cleavage that has no known function. However, the p3 fragment does not have the same ability to form stable oligomeric intermediates like that of Aβ, which poses no threat to synaptic function instigating that it is not the cause of amyloid plaques and is the reason for being the non-amyloidogenic pathway [39, 40]. This suggests that the longer Aβ peptide is the main neurotoxic fragment established from the APP fragment. The cleaved product becomes a peptide of 40 amino acid residues but this can be varied between 38 and 42 depending on where the γ-secretase cleaves APP.

3.1. Amyloid-β

The γ-secretase complex is composed of four proteins: either one of presenilin 1 (PS1) or presenilin 2 (PS2), nicastrin (NCT), anterior pharynx-defective phenotype 1 (Aph-1) and presenilin enhancer 2 (Pen-2) [41]. The complex formation is initiated with a sub complex that forms between NCT and Aph-1 which then binds to one of the PS proteins [42]. Pen-2 is used to activate the complex by selective binding [43]. Either PS can be used in this process, with a 67% amino acid homology, including two separate aspartate residues, asp257 and asp385, considered essential to catalytic ability, both have the ability to cleave APP [44, 45]. Consequently, the decrease in availability of the γ-secretase components results in a reduction of overall functionality, which can be targeted for use when considering inhibitors and the vulnerabilities of this complex [46]. Mutation to either the presenilins, whether it be PS1 or PS2, can be seen as a potential threat to the production of $A\beta_{40\text{-}42}$, as one can compensate for the other.

The γ-secretase, being the consistent piece of the APP cleavage puzzle, is actually responsible for the diseased state in which plaques are formed. There are upwards of 100 missense mutations identified in the presenilins, mostly creating the difference in cleaved fragments of APP [47]. The Aβ peptide created will be influenced with a varying overall length of between 38-42 amino acids [19]. The majority of these mutations influence a higher number of Aβ42 peptides, which have been found to be more amyloidogenic and neurotoxic [48, 49]. The wild-type presenilin generates Aβ40, which is considered to be less neurotoxic even though it is present in amyloid plaques. γ-secretase cuts downstream from the transmembrane domain into the ε-site of APP and therefore slightly shortens the AICD cleaving domain [50]. Aβ42 provides the basis for oligomerisation, fibrillation and plaque generation, even with Aβ40 being found with a limited ability to protect neurons in mouse models [51]. The ratio of Aβ42/Aβ40 increases after the AD age of onset but is still relatively low. However, with a binding affinity to Aβ40, fibrils can, as a consequence, bind together, meaning there does not need to be a high concentration to be effective [52].

The Aβ fragments are not always cleaved to the extracellular space either. There are a number of conformations that Aβ fragments can take including monomers, which are found free in neurons as a consequence of APP cleavage. Studies have also shown that fragments can form the shape of α-helices, random coils and even as β-sheets in a neutual pH to add to the complexity [53-56]. These individual fragments maintain the ability to block synaptic neurotransmitter transfer and instigate an apoptotic response via activation of the p53 promoter leading to cell death [57]. Alternatively, soluble Aβ oligomers have been referred to as Aβ-derived diffusible ligands (ADDLs) that have the ability to aggregate into protofibrils, spherical structures of 7-10 nm wide, that can have the ability to interrupt nerve signal transduction leading to cell death [58]. Initial investigations into the Aβ fibrils showed there was a toxic response from the neurons in which they were attached [59].

To target the Aβ fibrils, gene knockout studies of PS1 have found adverse reactions relating to formation of the axial skeleton, neurogenesis and neuronal survival causing effected mice to die late in embryogenesis [60]. These reactions however, can be attributed to a dysfunction of the Notch signalling pathway because of its involvement with cell proliferation, apoptosis and myelin formation, not to mention it is a substrate of γ-secretase [61]. This indicates that there are a number of associated risks with nullifying γ-secretase that with any inhibition, the complex will invariably prevent the cleavage of two regulatory pathways.

3.2. Neuroinflammation

The increase of intra and extracellular Aβ has a direct effect on the complement system and the recruitment of microglia, instigating the activation of inflammatory mechanisms, a trademark of stress on an Alzheimer's brain [62]. The microglia, derived from the mesenchyme and transferred to the CNS where proliferation occurs, are classified as the macrophages of the brain and regulate apoptotic cell abundance [63]. Stress incurred, mainly by amyloid plaque formation, triggers an immune response which leads to the activation of astrocytes and microglia to dismantle the ailing cell. The Aβ fragment has the ability to activate this process via the receptor for advanced glycation end products (RAGE), a multi-ligand member of the immunoglobulin family that is increased in production in an AD brain, and by CD40, an inflammatory signalling receptor [64-66]. The general immune response is aimed at eliminating Aβ, removing disease ridden cells and restoring tissue integrity but does more damage when it becomes of a chronic nature. The activation of reactive oxygen species (ROS), prostaglandins, and pro-inflammatory cytokines are a characteristic of the chronic inflammation and neuronal dysfunction in AD [67].

The onset of AD encourages the migration of microglia to the plaque affected areas. Cultured microglia, from elderly human patients, showed this migration as they coupled with Aβ for the purpose of deconstruction [68]. Similar findings were discovered in sections of cortex tested in vitro for migration but growing evidence suggests that once endocytosed, the microglia struggle to breakdown the Aβ, causing stress and functional changes to the cell [68-70]. Additionally, the APP mRNA translation is upregulated in the event of trauma, nerve damage and brain ischemia, which can be beneficial for the release of more AICD, but can also result in the production of more Aβ [71-73]. BACE1 has also been found to be regulated by Aβ42 via the c-Jun N-terminal kinase (JNK) pathway, otherwise known as the stress-activated signalling pathway which is important for the mediation of pro-inflammatory cytokines [74, 75]. This reiterates the important influence that a variety of stressors have when responding to the amyloidogenic pathway and that there are many different pathways that can be involved in the pathogenesis of amyloid plaques.

All aspects of the amyloid plaque progression relates back to the effectiveness of the BACE1 enzyme. Taking into consideration alternative BACE1 substrates, the proteolytic cleavage of APP can be regulated with an inhibitor. The Aβ concentration increases as the disease gets worse but could be diverted with the use of an effective pharmaceutical intervention. The possibilities and implications will not be recognised until BACE1 is inhibited successfully *in vivo*.

4. BACE1

4.1. BACE1 production and natural degradation

The BACE1 enzyme (also called β-secretase, Asp2 or memapsin2) is developed in the endoplasmic reticulum from a 501 amino acid, 60 kDa, immature precursor protein. The transfer from the endoplasmic reticulum to the Golgi is dependent on the prodomain, which is removed by the proprotein convertase, furin [76]. At this stage the immature BACE1 can already cleave APP so is not a true zymogen but the removal of the prodomain can double the proteolytic effectiveness whilst increasing structural stability [77, 78]. The immature BACE1 is deacetylated and transformed in the golgi by post-translational modification into a type 1 transmembrane protein [79]. A bi-lobal structure is formed with two aspartate motifs (D93TG and D289SG in a D-T/S-G-T/S conformation), which forms the active site that stimulates water molecules to hydrolyse APP peptide bonds, a defining characteristic of aspartic proteases [80, 81]. The proteolytic ability of this motif is only limited by site-directed mutagenesis of the aspartate residues [81]. The active site remains an important structure of this enzyme because of its supposed vulnerability. However, although it has been the focus of inhibition studies since its highly contested discovery in 1999, no effective pharmaceutical options have been elucidated since [34, 82-85]. The distinctiveness surrounding BACE1 is exposed when comparing it to other aspartic proteases and the contrasting characteristics of a C-terminal cytosolic tail and a transmembrane domain.

The transfer from the Golgi to the cell membrane is mediated by transport vesicles because BACE1 is membrane bound. The serine and di-leucine residues of BACE1 act as a signal for the Golgi-localized γ-ear-containing ARF binding protein 1 (GGA1), a sorting protein that aids the link between the transporting endosome and the cell membrane [86]. The endosome provides an optimal transport vesicle because of its internal acidic nature (approximately pH 4.5), a fundamental for the conformational shape and functionality of BACE1, but also because it is much more stable environment for transporting proteins [87, 88]. Changes in pH below 4.0 can have a negative effect on Wat1, a molecule considered to be the nucleophile with the ability to attack the carbonyl carbon of a peptide bond in the active site resulting in the loss of functionality. Changes at the other end of the scale, above that of pH 7.0, render the enzyme inactive and unable to cleave a substrate [87] (Figure 2A,B,C).

The active site placement is also vulnerable as it remains exposed to the extracellular space once it makes the transition to the lipid bi-layer of the membrane where it concludes its intracellular transport. BACE1 becomes susceptible to post-translational modification, protein to protein interactions or even inhibitor attachment because of its availability. It is here, however, that the BACE1 enzyme comes into contact with the membrane bound APP [89]. In some instances, the help of increased cellular cholesterol producing lipid rafts helps improve the availability of APP for BACE1. So what is considered a negative of vulnerability of the enzyme actually serves an important purpose in that a specific environment is created for APP to become more available. The lipid rafts are formed as an essential membrane stabilizer of intermediate space but have also controversially, improved signal transduction and intracellular trafficking ability of the cell [90].

http://dx.doi.org/10.5772/53603

BACE1 is found in a number of tissues throughout the body but majority of expression is found in the brain [91]. The levels of this expression have been of much debate due to conflicting reports separating different tissues in which the samples were taken, animal or human models and the use of controls [92]. The increase in expression could then be argued as a reason for the uncontrollable aggregation of Aβ but reports of little or no increase in expression of BACE1 instigates the influence of another factor is involved [93].

The natural degradation of BACE1 has been found to be involved the ubiquitin proteasome pathway. BACE1 can be transported from endosomes to lysosomes by ubiquitination with help from the sorting proteins, ADP ribosylation factor 6 (ARF6) and GGA3, another member of the GGA family [94-97]. The degradation by lysosomes is still ambiguous with an increase in BACE1 protein available in an AD brain, whilst there is little to no increase in mRNA levels. The failed or impaired lysosome could be a contributing factor to the increase in cellular Aβ or BACE1 could be getting recycled back into endosomes [93] (Figure 2D).

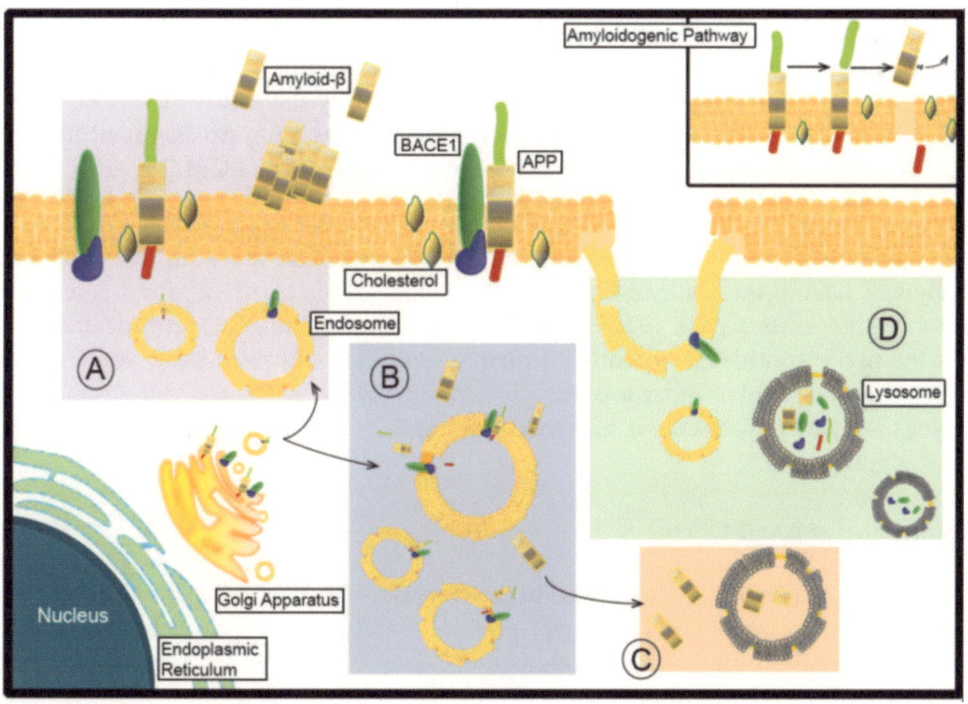

Figure 2. BACE1 Trafficking. BACE1 is constructed in the ER and processed, with the removal of the proBACE1 domain, in the Golgi. A) BACE1 is a membrane bound protease and so is either exocytosed from the Golgi or transported to an endosome with the help of the sorting protein GGA1. From here, the cleavage of APP to produce extracellular Aβ takes place in the lipid raft region of the membrane. The synthesis of Aβ occurs through the amyloidogenic (pathogenic) pathway. B) Processing of APP can otherwise occur whilst present in the endosome and so can release Aβ into the cytosoplasm. C) The Aβ can then either aggregate together or be endocytosed by lysosomes and degraded. D) Once APP proteolysis has occurred, BACE1 is either internalized to endosomes via GGA1 and ARF6 or labelled with ubiquitin and endocytosed. With assistance from the sorting protein, GGA3, the lysosomes will either recycle or degrade BACE1.

Recently, a natural inhibition of BACE1 has been found via the sAPPa fragment produced from the non-amyloidogenic pathway [98]. The sAPPa, once produced from APP, has been found to implicate its own cleavage. The findings showed that sAPPa can bind to BACE1 and interfere with the APP cleavage in a mouse model. This resulted in an overall reduction in Aβ formation under physiological conditions. The consequence of this pathway being impaired in any way, could result in a decrease in BACE1 production thus reducing the cleavage of further units of APP. The sAPPa production or cellular concentration could be a therapeutic intervention strategy in future research.

4.2. BACE2 and closely related proteins

BACE2 is a closely associated β-secretase to BACE1. Sequence analysis show amino acid residue similarities of ~45% and structural comparisons of 75% homology [99]. BACE2 is also classified as an aspartic protease with the ability to cleave APP at the β-site [100]. In vitro studies have also implicated BACE2 as a possible competitor of BACE1 for the cleavage of the APP protein but it is not formally expressed in excess in the brain and does not compensate for the loss of BACE1 in gene knockout models in mice [89, 101]. In fact, over expression of BACE2 has actually been found to reduce Aβ production in primary neuronal cultures derived from APP transgenic mice. This could be caused by the ability of BACE2 to cleave APP before BACE1 or because BACE2 cleaves a longer 79 residue Aβ fragment from APP, which is closer to the cleaved fragment of α-secretase then that of BACE1 [89, 99].

Apart from the sequence homology, BACE2 is not primarily expressed in the brain. It is more commonly expressed in the colon, kidney and pancreas, showing that whilst theoretically still having the ability to increase the pathogenesis of AD it is not considered a threat to Aβ generation [100, 102]. BACE1 is the main amyloidogenic enzyme and still remains the major contributor to amyloid plaque formation but does show some sequence homology with a number other aspartic proteases including renin and cathepsin D. These homologs are generally used for selectivity testing with *in vitro* assays to confirm no unwanted binding occurs.

4.3. Substrates of BACE1

The BACE1 protein is not solely defined to the cleavage of APP and has the ability to cleave other proteins like amyloid like precursor proteins 1 and 2, APPε (which is another closely related *N*-terminal product of APP), neuregulin-1 and -3 involved in axon myelination, β-subunits of voltage gated sodium channels required for neuronal action potentials, P-selectin glycoprotein ligand-1 (PSGL-1), which regulates leukocyte adhesion in the inflammatory process, the interleukin 1 receptor type-II (IL1-R2) and the low density lipoprotein receptor-related protein 1(LLRP1), which is a multifunctional endocytic and signalling receptor [1, 2, 103-106]. With the use of an unbiased, quantitative proteomics method, the identification of 64 new potential substrates were elucidated. The majority of these were type I transmembrane proteins but an added 3 glycophosphatidylinositol anchors and one type II transmembrane protein were also identified, all of which are membrane bound [107]. This suggests that BACE1 has a significant purpose in normal cellular functions but a number of these are

http://dx.doi.org/10.5772/53603

yet to be characterised in vivo and subsequently cannot be verified as a substrate until this time. With the interaction between BACE1 and APP being widely of interest in the prevention of AD, the actual damage by completely inhibiting the enzyme from normal functioning could prove detrimental in its own right. APP may not even be the primary substrate of the enzyme. Therefore, partial inhibition of BACE1 is all that may be required as an intervention therapy to normalize the enhanced BACE1 activity seen in AD patients.

Alternatively, both of the amyloidogenic creating enzymes, BACE1 and γ-secretase, have alternative purposes relating to other substrates. Gene knockout studies in mouse models produced the reaction of hyperactivity, premature death and seizure like behaviours for BACE1 whilst presenilin -/- mice displayed early neurodegenerative behaviours and an increase of Aβ species which could possibly be due to the large number of substrates in which both are effective [108-111]. The γ-secretase complex is essential for the Notch signalling pathway, which is important for the development of the nervous system and this would also be in deficit if inhibited completely [112]. Likewise, the γ-secretase complex is also required for the non-amyloidogenic pathway, suggesting that the complete inhibition or deletion of these proteins will be detrimental to the homeostatic processing related to normal development and function.

5. Challenges

5.1. Past BACE1 inhibitors

Inhibition of BACE1 has been the focus of many studies since it was discovered. The main interest in this enzyme remains with the obvious involvement in plaque formation but also to the positive intervention target for which it provides. Firstly, mouse models have shown that without BACE1, Aβ is no longer produced, which indicates that if a product can reduce the enzymatic ability of BACE1 then plaques will not be formed [109]. The enzyme has been characterised and 3-D structure produced, which will allow for inhibitor modelling [80]. BACE1 also has the ability to bind to a wide variety of peptidic structures, while specific binding is an attribute there is still access to the active site for potential targeting [113]. BACE1 is a part of the large aspartic protease family, which have had the success of at least two members (renin and HIV protease-1(HIV-1) inhibited with success [114]. This shows confidence that BACE1 is a viable option for inhibition and, if successful, could influence the production of Aβ.

Drug intervention of AD is limited between therapeutic relief of symptoms and the prevention of the underlying etiology of the disease [115]. The treatment to minimise symptoms is the only viable option for sufferers of AD. This method slows the decline of cognition, function and behaviour but only masks the underlying neurodegeneration taking place [116]. The drugs currently available to treat AD are divided into two categories of cholinesterase inhibitors and receptor antagonists [115].

Cholinesterase inhibitors attempt to prevent the metabolism of acetylcholine allowing the neurotransmitter to maintain effect in the neuron [117]. Cholinesterase inhibiting drugs like donepezil, galantamine and revastigmine are only effective in the early stages of AD by allowing the retention of acetylcholine [115]. By inhibiting the hydrolysis of acetylcholine by cholinesterase, once the neurotransmitter has crossed the synapse, the cholinergic neuron remains active [117]. This action becomes redundant when inadvertent progression of NFTs interfere with the normal signal transmission of the axon [15]. Cholinesterase inhibitors have shown that they can actually increase the amount of phosphorylated tau which can further the progression of AD, minimising the effectiveness of the drug [118, 119].

The other pharmaceutical option is memantine, an uncompetitive N-methyl-D-aspartate (NMDA) receptor antagonist, which prevents binding of the primary excitatory neurotransmitter in the brain, glutamate [120, 121]. As a result, glutamatergic overstimulation can occur causing neuronal cell damage by increased localized calcium stores or excitotoxicity [122]. Both drug options have important side effects and can only offer therapeutic relief of symptoms and are not useful as a long-term intervention strategy.

Therapeutic relief by drugs like donepezil, galantamine and memantine are required to optimize the productivity of the brain whilst the disease progresses and cannot translate to a definite cure. The production of Aβ is the basis of senile plaques and should be investigated as an important therapeutic target. Theories suggest that by inhibiting BACE1 before it cleaves APP, the formation of the beta amyloid residues would be reduced [123, 124]. To prevent this process, inhibition would be paramount between the translation of BACE1 and its binding to APP, before sAPPβ has been cleaved.

Modern drug discovery for a pharmaceutical intervention aims to hinder the BACE1 enzymatic activity by exactly this process. Notable methods look at high-throughput screening (HTS), fragment-based drug discovery (FBDD) and substrate-based inhibitors [125]. However, none of these methods have been successful in therapeutic trials. The more complex approach, generally taken by larger pharmaceutical companies, relate to either the HTS strategy or a FBDD approach. Both processes use a large library of complex compounds in order to find a suitable hit followed by a long modification process to refine it into a suitable chemical. Initial use of HTS sourced complex, high-molecular weight, compounds that were difficult to manipulate. Potential therapeutic candidates showed strong oral availability and good brain permeability but could not provide the standards of potency and selectivity for therapeutic trials [125, 126]

The HTS method has been substituted by the FBDD approach because it uses smaller and more specific compounds [127]. The screening of a fragment library is more appealing because a higher hit ratio is produced and the options show favourable drug properties. The main problem with the hit compounds is again, the low potency and selectivity. Often, fragments that showed promise were too small to be effective and have not provided any real inhibition with the effectiveness required for therapeutic trials.

A large range of inhibitors are being researched including statins, primary, secondary and tertiary amines, hydroethylamines (HEA) of many different conformations, arylamino compounds and acyclic acylguanidines. Most of these compounds seek to act as transition state mimics with a reduced peptidic structure that preclude them from the same scrutiny as other peptidic structures. To their detriment, hydroxyethylamine derivatives had poor brain exposure, mainly because of p-glycoprotein (PgP) mediated efflux [128-130]. Bristol-Myers Squibb produced a HEA-derivative that contained an indole and a 7-azoindole carboxamide but struggled to maintain brain Aβ levels in vivo [131]. Unfortunately, the inhibitor showed a high potency *in vitro* that had an IC_{50} of 10 nM and a low affinity for BACE2 and cathepsin D.

Another study has looked to hybridize the HEA isotere and replace the sulfonate ester present in one molecule with the sulphonamide of another [132]. The result was a compound that had high potency IC50 of 15 nm to BACE1 that was able to bind to the hydrophobic space of the active site. Unfortunately, this compound was able to bind to BACE2 which minimised the selectivity to BACE1. After problems with HEA structures and brain penetration, Merck decided to use a macrocyclic inhibitor, produced by cross linking the P1 and P3 sidechains of an isophthalamide-based inhibitor. This process helped improve potency but a bolus of 100 mg/kg fed to APP-YAC mouse model could only obtain Aβ decreases of 25% in the first hour and 10% after the third [133].

From another perspective, BACE1 inhibitors have been manufactured from peptide sequences by a substrate-based method. The initial peptide sequences showed promise with high potency and selectivity but did not progress as a viable pharmaceutical target because of the large, unstable products it produced. Branded OM99-2, this peptide was originally used to determine many functions and shapes of BACE1 including the active site. Unfortunately, it was too bulky to cross the BBB but maintained appropriate potency. Revision of this method looked specifically at the structure and function of BACE1 in order to manufacture a peptide sequence that would exploit its weaknesses [134]. It was designed to competitively inhibit the binding regions and shut down the enzymatic properties. The finished product was a long peptide upwards of 18 amino acid residues, which produced a high potency but was not stable enough for use in therapeutic trials.

These studies made it clear that the peptidic structure would fulfil the desired properties required for an inhibitor, the only issue being BBB transport which has motivated the research into small molecules that can freely penetrate the brain. The potential inhibitor needs to be lipophilic enough to permeate the BBB by passive diffusion via the use of a transporter that can maintain entry to the CNS without exiting the same way. Another issue with the peptide inhibitors is the added convolution of ubiquity throughout the body. Since amino acids, peptides and proteins are the building blocks of the human form and function, there is the added complication of anonymity with other proteins and the possibility of unwanted binding causing adverse reactions. If a severe enough reaction to the peptide is apparent, it would be more detrimental then beneficial.

5.2. Crossing the blood brain barrier

The BBB is a network of brain capillaries that regulate the transfer of nutrients and co-factors that are important to the functioning and maintenance of the brain. The conformation begins with the lumen that is lined with a monolayer of capillary endothelial cells, held together with tight gap junctions. This monolayer is complemented by pericytes for the purpose of BBB-specific gene expression and inducing polarisation of the astrocyte end-feet with the surrounding basal lamina [135]. The tight junctions are known to prevent the paracellular diffusion of polar molecules from systemic circulation and brain parenchyma [136]. Complementing the endothelium are a number of compounds that defend against foreign transfer like cytochrome p450 and glutathione S-transferase in conjunction with transporters and the multidrug resistance associated proteins 1 and 2 (Mrp1/2) [137-139].

The defence mechanisms that protect the brain from systemic circulation become a challenging interference when fabricating an inhibitor, especially when it comes to testing the administration of localised drug performance. The molecular weight threshold, which is a relevant property of all membranes, is <450 Da [140]. A molecular model can be used to determine the effect of molecular size on membrane permeability and should be a consideration when investigating an inhibitor [141]. This creates a challenge that goes beyond the production of protein specific intervention strategies. In the case of BACE1, there are a number of different challenges, as previously mentioned, influencing the inhibition of APP cleavage. With the influence of the BBB, the drug will be required to maintain an ability to inhibit BACE1 but also maintain solubility across the tight junctions of vessel epithelium.

The natural functioning of the BBB is to maintain the tight junctions, for which it is idiosyncratic, but in order to transport a required drug, the concept of BBB disruption can be considered. The relaxing of these junctions with hyperosmotic chemicals, for example, could be enough to encourage transport to the brain. The only concern with this method is due to the unfavourable uptake of plasma proteins, like albumin, which is toxic to astrocytes [142]. Consequently, it could also affect drug retention and enhance unwanted migration of otherwise rejected contaminants.

Another drastic, invasive technique involves drilling into the cranium and administering the treatment via intracerebroventricular injection, intracerebral implantation and convection enhanced diffusion. While all are incredibly invasive and risky, the required responses from the drug once applied are generally not that positive [143]. Intracerebroventricular injection specifically has been found to cause haemorrhage after the insertion of a needle into the brain as an adverse reaction but has otherwise has shown good responses [144]. This suggests these invasive techniques are questionable and should be used with extreme caution.

The interesting, non-invasive, concept of lipid carriers has the most potential. The carriers are attached to water soluble inhibitors, that cannot otherwise penetrate the BBB, and turn them lipid soluble [145]. This will allow the transfer into the BBB but once across, the requirement to either shed the carrier or be able to function with it attached in order to maintain functionality, becomes apparent. The naturally occurring, 60 amino acid, galanin-like peptide (GALP) has the ability to cross the BBB where needed with the use of a saturable transport system [146]. The glucose transporter (GLUT1) is another natural carrier system that is used frequently as glucose is the main energy source of the brain [147]. If this method can be transformed for BACE1 inhibitors, the transfer of larger, more potent molecules with an increased selectivity, could be achieved.

5.3. Transporters

The ability to transport potential inhibitors across the blood brain barrier can determine the success or failure of the potential therapeutic intervention. The BBB has motivated the research base to investigate small <450 Da molecules that have the potential to pass the barrier with minimal scrutiny. The issue being a lack of potency and selectivity *in vivo* which indicates that a greater effectiveness could be achieved with a larger style inhibitor. The potential for transporters could revolutionize the future of drug production by providing a medium in which the larger more effective inhibitors can cross this barrier.

The earlier transporters aimed to cross the BBB by utilising the already formed channels and receptors. The idea was to couple an inhibitor with the specific ligand of a surface receptor like that of the H1 histone, insulin, insulin-like growth factors or transferrin [148-151]. These systems can also work by binding the inhibitor to antibodies that identify surface epitopes already present in the BBB. The coupling of an 18mer peptide to transferrin receptor specific antibodies were used to infiltrate the BBB via the transferrin receptor for the inhibition of the rev gene of HIV-1 [152]. This study demonstrated a 15-fold increase in transfer across the BBB. This system can be modified to display a number of different biotinylated peptides specifically but could also be manipulated for other effective compounds.

A more advanced method of targeted liposomes progresses from the inhibitor-ligand structure to a colloidal carrier system. The concept still utilizes BBB receptors and channels but is improved with an increase in the concentration of the inhibitor that it can carry. The liposomal system can hold >10,000 drug molecules [153]. The main question regarding this system is the avoidance of opsonins which are members of the complement system and immunoglobulins that cover the colloidal particle and are able to activate phagocytosis. This method has already been used to transfer monoclonal antibodies across the BBB [153]. The negative of this system however, is the vulnerability to macrophages via opsonisation and the lack of selectivity that liposomes have in regards to the brain and BBB. The targeted liposome system has already been used successfully to transfer sodium borocaptate in defence against malignant glioma, which suggests that further research could provide a neurodegenerative diseases template [154].

Alternatively, fullerenes are an allotropic form of carbon that form an arrangement of 60 atoms into the shape of a hollow sphere that is 1 nanometre in diameter and can be coupled with an inhibitor [155]. These fullerene systems have shown promise in the fight against chronic multiple sclerosis [156]. Whilst still in the early stages of research, recovery has been attributed to a reduction in axon loss and demyelination in the spinal region of the CNS in a mouse model. Another study has shown a reduction of infarct size in gerbils and rats with the use of a hexasulfinonated C60 that was administered intravenously [157, 158]. Further research is required for the use in human studies but there is anticipation for its use against the aggregation of Aβ.

6. Future perspectives

There are a number of exciting directions that future research will take to determine a safe and effective treatment for AD. The regulation of internal pathways for the natural management of BACE1 activity is of key interest as it involves the crossroad from compound based, active site mimics. The recent study identifying the sAPPα as a BACE1 modulator could motivate the investigation of the broader pathway rather than focussing on the enzyme itself [98]. Pathway regulation could reduce side effects and associated pathologies because of the broad spectrum enzymes that envelope amyloidogenesis.

The implication of Aβ signalling in plaque formation is another concept for investigation for the possibility of a feedback system. The promotion of Aβ proliferation could increase the ability for a plaque to form as there is the availability to encourage the process. The application of a potential BACE1 inhibitor is rudimentary to the prevention of this disease because of the potential to bypass the amyloidogenic pathway. With minimal Aβ production the pressure released on the natural inflammatory defences would allow for the metabolism of impeding plaques.

γ-secretase inhibitors have already been progressing to phase III clinical trials which seek to influence the production of Aβ but maintain a number of important consequences that surround this process [159]. The implication of the Notch signalling pathway, important in axon myelination and apoptosis, could be more detrimental than plaque formation because of the regulatory purpose in which it serves [112].

Merck have developed the MK-8931 inhibitor, which is currently undergoing phase II clinical trials [160]. It has already shown an ability to reduce $A\beta_{40}$, $A\beta_{42}$ and sAPPβ levels, is well tolerated *in vivo* and shows minimal adverse reactions, which is encouraging for the <450 Da compounds. Eli Lilly and AstraZeneca are also involved with BACE1 inhibitor clinical trials, which will increase competition once results come to fruition. The opposing mentality behind BACE1 inhibitors, as small <450 Da compounds, could be the answer to years of attempts. The crossing of the barrier is not a major obstacle for this method but show alternative hurdles of selectivity and bioavailability. This has created a race for a pharmaceutically able inhibitor.

Alternatively, the membrane transporters concept for the advantage of allowing the transfer of a range of different inhibitors, in a variety of doses, could produce a platform for a number of different brain based diseases without being overly invasive. The BBB is an ominous obstacle for a number of the earlier peptidic inhibitors, whilst showing a lot of promising pharmaceutical attributes. The combination of the two technologies could provide the difference required for drug penetration and selectivity.

Once an inhibitor has been potentiated, the focus can move into research looking at plaque clearing and neurogenesis that will aid regeneration of the AD brain. One option is the utilization of stem cells to replace lost brain mass by utilizing multi-potent adult neural stem cells found in the subgranular and subventricular zones. The CNS has the ability to regenerate a number of neuronal cell lines with astrocytes, oligodendrocytes, and functional neurons [161]. By utilizing these cell lines the brain could be "rebuilt" to maintain the structures affected by the plaque formation. However, this would be implicated by numerous ethical challenges.

7. Conclusions

The onset of AD is relatively unknown, but early stages of the disease are met with the accumulation of amyloid plaques. The amyloidogenic pathway, mediated by the proteolytic cleavage of APP, is the major focus for the alleviation of AD. BACE1, the defining enzyme of this process, is responsible for the cleavage of the Aβ fragment. The determinant of fragment length, 38-42 amino acids, is coordinated by γ-secretase. The focus is placed specifically on fragments $A\beta_{40}$ and $A\beta_{42}$ because of the influence they maintain over plaque formation and an increased affinity for aggregation.

Whilst there is an indication that γ-secretase maintains the ability to determine the severity of plaque formation, there are a number of reasons to avoid inhibition, mainly because of its involvement in the Notch pathway and the extreme consequences which brings to light the cost outweighing the means. This is a hallmark of plaque formation as the enzymes involved have a number of substrates in different pathways that do not involve AD. This motivates the notion of regulation, as opposed to complete inhibition, to aid the process alleviating majority of the proteolysis.

The recent association between the cleaved product of APP by α-secretase, sAPPα, having an influence on the amyloidogenic pathway adds another perspective to AD and the mechanisms relating to brain homeostasis. It prompts the idea of maintaining normal processing as opposed to initiating inhibition. The BACE1 cleavage of APP is not a response, or trigger, to AD progression but is fundamental in Aβ production, which implies that normal conservation is a natural process and regulation can be achieved with an external stimulus.

A large obstacle with potential BACE1 inhibitors is the ability to maintain the pharmaceutical properties between *in vitro* and *in vivo* testing, namely the BBB. The transfer between the Tight junctions of brain endothelium and the neuronal cells has defined the way BACE1 inhibitors are engaged. The change from basic peptidic structures to that of small <450 Da chemicals has solved one hurdle but has inadvertently created others. The original *in vitro* studies of peptidic inhibitors maintained positive selectivity for BACE1 but were too bulky for transport. The application of a BACE1 inhibitor, whatever structure it is formed from, will be rudimentary in treating and alleviating the devastating prognosis of AD in the years to come.

Author details

Justin Read and Cenk Suphioglu

NeuroAllergy Research Laboratory (NARL), School of Life and Environmental Sciences, Deakin University, Geelong, Victoria, Australia

References

[1] Hu X, Hicks CW, He W, Wong P, Macklin WB, Trapp BD, et al. Bace1 Modulates Myelination in the Central and Peripheral Nervous System. Nature Neuroscience. 2006;9(12):1520-5.

[2] Wong H-K, Sakurai T, Oyama F, Kaneko K, Wada K, Miyazaki H, et al. β Subunits of Voltage-gated Sodium Channels Are Novel Substrates of β-Site Amyloid Precursor Protein-cleaving Enzyme (BACE1) and γ-Secretase. Journal of Biological Chemistry. 2005;280(24):23009-17.

[3] Choi DW. Excitotoxic cell death. Journal of Neurobiology. 1992;23(9):1261-76.

[4] Brun A, Englund E. Regional Pattern of Degeneration in Alzheimer's Disease: Neuronal Loss and Histopathological Grading. Histopathology. 1981;5:549-64.

[5] Brookmeyer R, Johnson E, Ziegler-Graham K, Arrighi HM. Forecasting the Global Burden of Alzheimer's Disease. Alzheimer's and Dementia. 2007;3(3):186-91.

[6] WHO. Dementia: a public health priority. Geneva: World Health Organization and Alzheimer's Disease International. http://www.who.int/mental_health/publications/dementia_report_2012/en/index.html. (accessed 7 July 2012).

[7] Rice DP, Fillit HM, Max W, Knopman DS, Lloyd JR, Duttagupta S. Prevalence, Costs, and Treatment of Alzheimer's Disease and Related Dementia: a Managed Care Perspective. The American Journal of Managed Care. 2001;7(8):809-18.

[8] Malone DC, McLaughlin TP, Wahl PM, Leibman C, Arrighi M, Cziraky MJ, et al. Burden of Alzheimer's Disease and Association With Negative Health Outcomes. The American Journal of Managed Care. 2009;15(8):481-8.

[9] Wenk GL. Neuropathologic Changes in Alzheimer's Disease. The Journal of Clinical Psychiatry. 2003;64 Suppl 9:7-10.

[10] Sultzer DL, Brown CV, Mandelkern MA, Mahler ME, Mendez MF, Chen ST, et al. Delusional Thoughts and Regional Frontal/Temporal Cortex Metabolism in Alzheimer's Disease. American Journal Of Psychiatry. 2003;160:341-9.

[11] Bruen PD, McGeown WJ, Shanks MF, Venneri A. Neuroanatomical Correlates of Neuropsychiatric Symptoms in Alzheimer's Disease. Brain. 2008;131(9):2455-63.

[12] Fountoulakis M, Kossida S. Proteomics-driven Progress in Neurodegeneration Research. Electrophoresis. 2006;27(8):1556-73.

[13] Cai H, Wang Y, McCarthy D, Wen H, Borchelt DR, Price DL, et al. BACE1 is the Major β-secretase for Generation of Aβ Peptides by Neurons. Nature Neuroscience. 2001;4(3):233-4.

[14] Spillantini MG, Goedert M. Tau Protein Pathology in Neurodegenerative Diseases. Trends in Neurosciences. 1998;21(10):428-33.

[15] Lebouvier T, Scales TME, Williamson R, Noble W, Duyckaerts C, Hanger DP, et al. The Microtubule-Associated Protein Tau is Also Phosphorylated on Tyrosine. Journal of Alzheimer's Disease. 2009;18(1):1-9.

[16] Selkoe DJ. Alzheimer Disease: Mechanistic Understanding Predicts Novel Therapies. Annals of Internal Medicine. 2004;140(8):627-38.

[17] Eikelenboom P, Hack C, Rozemuller J, Stam F. Complement Activation in Amyloid Plaques in Alzheimer's Dementia. Virchows Archiv B Cell Pathology Zell-pathologie. 1988;56(1):259-62.

[18] Tuppo EE, Arias HR. The Role of Inflammation in Alzheimer's Disease. The International Journal of Biochemistry & Cell Biology. 2005;37(2):289-305.

[19] Wolfe MS. When Loss is Gain: Reduced Presenilin Proteolytic Function Leads to Increased Aβ42/Aβ40. EMBO Reports. 2007;8(2):136-40.

[20] Arendt T. Synaptic Degeneration in Alzheimer's Disease. Acta Neuropathologica. 2009;118(1):167-79.

[21] Francis PT. Glutamatergic Systems in Alzheimer's Disease. International Journal of Geriatric Psychiatry. 2003;18(S1):S15-S21.

[22] Nixon RA, Wegiel J, Kumar A, Yu WH, Peterhoff C, Cataldo A, et al. Extensive Involvement of Autophagy in Alzheimer Disease: An Immuno-Electron Microscopy Study. Journal of Neuropathology & Experimental Neurology. 2005;64(2):113-22.

[23] Martins IJ, Berger T, Sharman MJ, Verdile G, Fuller SJ, Martins RN. Cholesterol Metabolism and Transport in the Pathogenesis of Alzheimer's Disease. Journal of Neurochemistry. 2009;111(6):1275-308.

[24] Bibel M, Barde Y-A. Neurotrophins: Key Regulators of Cell Fate and Cell Shape in the Vertebrate Nervous System. Genes & Development. 2000;14(23):2919-37.

[25] Morfini GA, Burns M, Binder LI, Kanaan NM, LaPointe N, Bosco DA, et al. Axonal Transport Defects in Neurodegenerative Diseases. The Journal of Neuroscience. 2009;29(41):12776-86.

[26] Hardy J, Duff K, Hardy KG, Perez-Tur J, Hutton M. Genetic Dissection of Alzheimer's Disease and Related Dementias: Amyloid and its Relationship to Tau. Nature Neuroscience. 1998;1(5):355-8.

[27] Varani L, Hasegawa M, Spillantini MG, Smith MJ, Murrell JR, Ghetti B, et al. Structure of Tau Exon 10 Splicing Regulatory Element RNA and Destabilization by Mutations of Frontotemporal Dementia and Parkinsonism Linked to Chromosome 17. Proceedings of the National Academy of Sciences. 1999;96(14):8229-34.

[28] Glenner GG, Wong CW. Alzheimer's Disease: Initial Report of the Purification and Characterization of a Novel Cerebrovascular Amyloid Protein. Biochemical and Biophysical Research Communications. 1984;120(3):885-90.

[29] Tanzi R, Gusella J, Watkins P, Bruns G, St George-Hyslop P, Van Keuren M, et al. Amyloid Beta Protein Gene: cDNA, mRNA Distribution, and Genetic Linkage Near the Alzheimer Locus. Science. 1987;235(4791):880-4.

[30] Kang J, Lemaire H-G, Unterbeck A, Salbaum JM, Masters CL, Grzeschik K-H, et al. The Precursor of Alzheimer's Disease Amyloid Aβ Protein Resembles a Cell-surface Receptor. Nature. 1987;325(6106):733-6.

[31] Lee J, Retamal C, Cuitiño L, Caruano-Yzermans A, Shin J-E, van Kerkhof P, et al. Adaptor Protein Sorting Nexin 17 Regulates Amyloid Precursor Protein Trafficking and Processing in the Early Endosomes. Journal of Biological Chemistry. 2008;283(17):11501-8.

[32] Jorissen E, Prox J, Bernreuther C, Weber S, Schwanbeck R, Serneels L, et al. The Disintegrin/Metalloproteinase ADAM10 Is Essential for the Establishment of the Brain Cortex. The Journal of Neuroscience. 2010;30(14):4833-44.

[33] Selkoe DJ. The Molecular Pathology of Alzheimer's Disease. Neuron. 1991;6(4): 487-98.

[34] Vassar R, Bennett BD, Babu-Khan S, Kahn S, Mendiaz EA, Denis P, et al. β-Secretase Cleavage of Alzheimer's Amyloid Precursor Protein by the Transmembrane Aspartic Protease BACE. Science. 1999;286(5440):735-41.

[35] Kuhn P-H, Wang H, Dislich B, Colombo A, Zeitschel U, Ellwart JW, et al. ADAM10 is the Physiologically Relevant, Constitutive α-secretase of the Amyloid Precursor Protein in Primary Neurons. The EMBO Journal. 2010;29(17):3020-32.

[36] Alves da Costa C, Sunyach C, Pardossi-Piquard R, Sévalle J, Vincent B, Boyer N, et al. Presenilin-Dependent γ-Secretase-Mediated Control of p53-Associated Cell Death in Alzheimer's Disease. The Journal of Neuroscience. 2006;26(23):6377-85.

[37] Madeira A, Pommet J-M, Prochiantz A, Allinquant B. SET Protein (TAF1β, I2PP2A) is Involved in Neuronal Apoptosis Induced by an Amyloid Precursor Protein Cytoplasmic Subdomain. The FASEB Journal. 2005;19(13):1905-07.

[38] Müller T, Concannon CG, Ward MW, Walsh CM, Tirniceriu AL, Tribl F, et al. Modulation of Gene Expression and Cytoskeletal Dynamics by the Amyloid Precursor Protein Intracellular Domain (AICD). Molecular Biology of the Cell. 2007;18(1):201-10.

[39] Dulin F, Léveillé F, Ortega JB, Mornon J-P, Buisson A, Callebaut I, et al. p3 Peptide, a Truncated Form of Aβ Devoid of Synaptotoxic Effect, Does Not Assemble Into Soluble Oligomers. FEBS Letters. 2008;582(13):1865-70.

[40] Walsh DM, Klyubin I, Fadeeva JV, Cullen WK, Anwyl R, Wolfe MS, et al. Naturally Secreted Oligomers of Amyloidβ Protein Potently Inhibit Hippocampal Long-term Potentiation in vivo. Nature. 2002;416(6880):535-9.

[41] De Strooper B. Aph-1, Pen-2, and Nicastrin with Presenilin Generate an Active γ-Secretase Complex. Neuron. 2003;38(1):9-12.

[42] Takasugi N, Tomita T, Hayashi I, Tsuruoka M, Niimura M, Takahashi Y, et al. The Role of Presenilin Cofactors in the γ-secretase Complex. Nature. 2003;422(6930): 438-41.

[43] LaVoie MJ, Fraering PC, Ostaszewski BL, Ye W, Kimberly WT, Wolfe MS, et al. Assembly of the γ-Secretase Complex Involves Early Formation of an Intermediate Subcomplex of Aph-1 and Nicastrin. Journal of Biological Chemistry. 2003;278(39): 37213-22.

[44] Wolfe M, Xia W, Ostaszewski B, Diehl T, Kimberly W, Selkoe D. Two Transmembrane Aspartates in Presenilin-1 Required for Presenilin Endoproteolysis and γ-secretase Activity. Nature. 1999;398(6727):513-7.

[45] Levy-Lahad E, Wasco W, Poorkaj P, Romano D, Oshima J, Pettingell W, et al. Candidate Gene for the Chromosome 1 Familial Alzheimer's Disease Locus. Science. 1995;269(5226):973-7.

[46] Francis R, McGrath G, Zhang J, Ruddy DA, Sym M, Apfeld J, et al. aph-1 and pen-2 Are Required for Notch Pathway Signaling, γ-Secretase Cleavage of βAPP, and Presenilin Protein Accumulation. Developmental Cell. 2002;3(1):85-97.

[47] Tanzi RE, Bertram L. Twenty Years of the Alzheimer's Disease Amyloid Hypothesis: A Genetic Perspective. Cell. 2005;120(4):545-55.

[48] Suzuki N, Cheung T, Cai X, Odaka A, Otvos L, Eckman C, et al. An Increased Percentage of Long Amyloid Beta Protein Secreted by Familial Amyloid Beta Protein Precursor (Beta APP717) Mutants. Science. 1994;264(5163):1336-40.

[49] Burdick D, Soreghan B, Kwon M, Kosmoski J, Knauer M, Henschen A, et al. Assembly and Aggregation Properties of Synthetic Alzheimer's A4/beta Amyloid Peptide Analogs. Journal of Biological Chemistry. 1992;267(1):546-54.

[50] Sato T, Dohmae N, Qi Y, Kakuda N, Misonou H, Mitsumori R, et al. Potential Link between Amyloid β-Protein 42 and C-terminal Fragment γ 49–99 of β-Amyloid Precursor Protein. Journal of Biological Chemistry. 2003;278(27):24294-301.

[51] Zou K, Kim D, Kakio A, Byun K, Gong J-S, Kim J, et al. Amyloid β-protein (Aβ)1–40 Protects Neurons from Damage Induced by Aβ1–42 in Culture and in Rat Brain. Journal of Neurochemistry. 2003;87(3):609-19.

[52] Duering M, Grimm MOW, Grimm HS, Schröder J, Hartmann T. Mean Age of Onset in Familial Alzheimer's Disease is Determined by Amyloid Beta 42. Neurobiology of Aging. 2005;26(6):785-8.

[53] Coles M, Bicknell W, Watson AA, Fairlie DP, Craik DJ. Solution Structure of Amyloid β-Peptide(1−40) in a Water−Micelle Environment. Is the Membrane-Spanning Domain Where We Think It Is? Biochemistry. 1998;37(31):11064-77.

[54] Crescenzi O, Tomaselli S, Guerrini R, Salvadori S, D'Ursi AM, Temussi PA, et al. Solution Structure of the Alzheimer Amyloid β-peptide (1–42) in an Apolar Microenvironment. European Journal of Biochemistry. 2002;269(22):5642-8.

[55] Zhang S, Iwata K, Lachenmann MJ, Peng JW, Li S, Stimson ER, et al. The Alzheimer's Peptide Aβ Adopts a Collapsed Coil Structure in Water. Journal of Structural Biology. 2000;130(2–3):130-41.

[56] Barrow C, Zagorski M. Solution Structures of Beta Peptide and its Constituent Fragments: Relation to Amyloid Deposition. Science. 1991;253(5016):179-82.

[57] Ohyagi Y, Asahara H, Chui D-H, Tsuruta Y, Sakae N, Miyoshi K, et al. Intracellular Aβ42 Activates p53 Promoter: a Pathway to Neurodegeneration in Alzheimer's Disease. The FASEB Journal. 2004;19(2):255-57.

[58] Hartley DM, Walsh DM, Ye CP, Diehl T, Vasquez S, Vassilev PM, et al. Protofibrillar Intermediates of Amyloid β-Protein Induce Acute Electrophysiological Changes and Progressive Neurotoxicity in Cortical Neurons. The Journal of Neuroscience. 1999;19(20):8876-84.

[59] Yankner B, Dawes L, Fisher S, Villa-Komaroff L, Oster-Granite M, Neve R. Neurotoxicity of a Fragment of the Amyloid Precursor Associated with Alzheimer's Disease. Science. 1989;245(4916):417-20.

[60] Shen J, Bronson RT, Chen DF, Xia W, Selkoe DJ, Tonegawa S. Skeletal and CNS Defects in Presenilin-1-Deficient Mice. Cell. 1997;89(4):629-39.

[61] De Strooper B, Saftig P, Craessaerts K, Vanderstichele H, Guhde G, Annaert W, et al. Deficiency of Presenilin-1 Inhibits the Normal Cleavage of Amyloid Precursor Protein. Nature. 1998;391(6665):387-90.

[62] Wyss-Coray T, Mucke L. Inflammation in Neurodegenerative Disease—A Double-Edged Sword. Neuron. 2002;35(3):419-32.

[63] Rezaie P, Male D. Mesoglia & Microglia-A Historical Review of the Concept of Mononuclear Phagocytes Within the Central Nervous System. Journal of the History of the Neurosciences. 2002;11(4):325.

[64] Yan SD, Roher A, Schmidt AM, Stern DM. Cellular Cofactors for Amyloid β-Peptide-Induced Cell Stress: Moving from Cell Culture to in vivo. The American Journal of Pathology. 1999;155(5):1403-11.

[65] Yan SD, Chen X, Fu J, Chen M, Zhu H, Roher A, et al. RAGE and Amyloid-β Peptide Neurotoxicity in Alzheimer's Disease. Nature. 1996;382(6593):685-91.

[66] Tan J, Town T, Paris D, Mori T, Suo Z, Crawford F, et al. Microglial Activation Resulting from CD40-CD40L Interaction After β-Amyloid Stimulation. Science. 1999;286(5448):2352-5.

[67] Mrak RE, Griffin WST. Glia and Their Cytokines in Progression of Neurodegeneration. Neurobiology of Aging. 2005;26(3):349-54.

[68] Walker DG, Lue LF. Investigations with Cultured Human Microglia on Pathogenic Mechanisms of Alzheimer's Disease and Other Neurodegenerative Diseases. Journal of Neuroscience Research. 2005;81(3):412-25.

[69] Bard F, Cannon C, Barbour R, Burke R-L, Games D, Grajeda H, et al. Peripherally Administered Antibodies Against Amyloid β-peptide Enter the Central Nervous System and Reduce Pathology in a Mouse Model of Alzheimer Disease. Nature Medicine. 2000;6(8):916-9.

[70] Majumdar A, Chung H, Dolios G, Wang R, Asamoah N, Lobel P, et al. Degradation of Fibrillar Forms of Alzheimer's Amyloid β-peptide by Macrophages. Neurobiology of Aging. 2008;29(5):707-15.

[71] Banati RB, Gehrmann J, Czech C, Mönning U, Jones LL, König G, et al. Early and Rapid de novo Synthesis of Alzheimer βA4-Amyloid Precursor Protein (APP) in Activated Microglia. Glia. 1993;9(3):199-210.

[72] Shi J, Yang SH, Stubley L, Day AL, Simpkins JW. Hypoperfusion Induces Overexpression of β-amyloid Precursor Protein mRNA in a Focal Ischemic Rodent Model. Brain Research. 2000;853(1):1-4.

[73] Ciallella JR, Ikonomovic MD, Paljug WR, Wilbur YI, Dixon CE, Kochanek PM, et al. Changes in Expression of Amyloid Precursor Protein and Interleukin-1beta After Experimental Traumatic Brain Injury in Rats. Journal of Neurotrauma. 2002;19(12): 1555-67.

[74] Guglielmotto M, Monteleone D, Giliberto L, Fornaro M, Borghi R, Tamagno E, et al. Amyloid-β_{42} Activates the Expression of BACE1 Through the JNK Pathway. Journal of Alzheimer's Disease. 2011;27(4):871-83.

[75] Davies C, Tournier C. Exploring the Function of the JNK (c-Jun N-terminal Kinase) Signalling Pathway in Physiological and Pathological Processes to Design Novel Therapeutic Strategies. Biochemical Society Transactions 2012;40(1):85-9.

[76] Benjannet S, Elagoz A, Wickham L, Mamarbachi M, Munzer JS, Basak A, et al. Post-translational Processing of β-Secretase (β-Amyloid-converting Enzyme) and its Ectodomain Shedding. Journal of Biological Chemistry. 2001;276(14):10879-87.

[77] Creemers JWM, Ines Dominguez D, Plets E, Serneels L, Taylor NA, Multhaup G, et al. Processing of β-Secretase by Furin and Other Members of the Proprotein Convertase Family. Journal of Biological Chemistry. 2001;276(6):4211-7.

[78] Shi X-P, Chen E, Yin K-C, Na S, Garsky VM, Lai M-T, et al. The Pro Domain of β-Secretase Does Not Confer Strict Zymogen-like Properties but Does Assist Proper Folding of the Protease Domain. Journal of Biological Chemistry. 2001;276(13): 10366-73.

[79] Haniu M, Denis P, Young Y, Mendiaz EA, Fuller J, Hui JO, et al. Characterization of Alzheimer's β-Secretase Protein BACE. Journal of Biological Chemistry. 2000;275(28): 21099-106.

[80] Hong L, Koelsch G, Lin X, Wu S, Terzyan S, Ghosh AK, et al. Structure of the Protease Domain of Memapsin 2 (β-Secretase) Complexed with Inhibitor. Science. 2000;290(5489):150-3.

[81] Charlwood J, Dingwall C, Matico R, Hussain I, Johanson K, Moore S, et al. Characterization of the Glycosylation Profiles of Alzheimer's β-Secretase Protein Asp-2 Expressed in a Variety of Cell Lines. Journal of Biological Chemistry. 2001;276(20): 16739-48.

[82] Hussain I, Powell D, Howlett DR, Tew DG, Meek TD, Chapman C, et al. Identification of a Novel Aspartic Protease (Asp 2) as β-secretase. Molecular and Cellular Neurosciences. 1999;14(6):419-27.

[83] Sinha S, Anderson JP, Barbour R, Basi GS, Caccaveffo R, Davis D, et al. Purification and Cloning of Amyloid Precursor Protein β-secretase from Human Brain. Nature. 1999;402(6761):537-40.

[84] Yan R, Blenkowski MJ, Shuck ME, Miao H, Tory MC, Pauley AM, et al. Membrane-anchored Aspartyl Protease with Alzheimer's Disease β-secretase Activity. Nature. 1999;402(6761):533-7.

[85] Lin X, Koelsch G, Wu S, Downs D, Dashti A, Tang J. Human Aspartic Protease Memapsin 2 Cleaves the β-secretase Site of β-amyloid Precursor Protein. Proceedings of the National Academy of Sciences of the United States of America. 2000;97(4): 1456-60.

[86] Walter J, Fluhrer R, Hartung B, Willem M, Kaether C, Capell A, et al. Phosphorylation Regulates Intracellular Trafficking of β-Secretase. Journal of Biological Chemistry. 2001;276(18):14634-41.

[87] Shimizu H, Tosaki A, Kaneko K, Hisano T, Sakurai T, Nukina N. Crystal Structure of an Active Form of BACE1, an Enzyme Responsible for Amyloid β Protein Production. Molecular and Cellular Biology. 2008;28(11):3663-71.

[88] Pasternak SH, Bagshaw RD, Guiral M, Zhang S, Ackerley CA, Pak BJ, et al. Presenilin-1, Nicastrin, Amyloid Precursor Protein, and γ-Secretase Activity are Co-localized in the Lysosomal Membrane. Journal of Biological Chemistry. 2003;278(29):26687-94.

[89] Yan R, Munzner JB, Shuck ME, Bienkowski MJ. BACE2 Functions as an Alternative α-Secretase in Cells. Journal of Biological Chemistry. 2001;276(36):34019-27.

[90] Lingwood D, Simons K. Lipid Rafts As a Membrane-Organizing Principle. Science. 2010;327(5961):46-50.

[91] Lin X, Koelsch G, Wu S, Downs D, Dashti A, Tang J. Human Aspartic Protease Memapsin 2 Cleaves the β-secretase Site of β-amyloid Precursor Protein. Proceedings of the National Academy of Sciences. 2000;97(4):1456-60.

[92] Zhao J, Fu Y, Yasvoina M, Shao P, Hitt B, O'Connor T, et al. β-Site Amyloid Precursor Protein Cleaving Enzyme 1 Levels Become Elevated in Neurons around Amyloid Plaques: Implications for Alzheimer's Disease Pathogenesis. The Journal of Neuroscience. 2007;27(14):3639-49.

[93] Coulson DTR, Beyer N, Quinn JG, Brockbank S, Hellemans J, Irvine GB, et al. BACE1 mRNA Expression in Alzheimer's Disease Postmortem Brain Tissue. Journal Of Alzheimer's Disease: JAD. 2010;22(4):1111-22.

[94] Davies BA, Lee JRE, Oestreich AJ, Katzmann DJ. Membrane Protein Targeting to the MVB/Lysosome. Chemical Reviews. 2009;109(4):1575-86.

[95] Kang EL, Cameron AN, Piazza F, Walker KR, Tesco G. Ubiquitin Regulates GGA3-mediated Degradation of BACE1. Journal of Biological Chemistry. 2010;285(31): 24108-19.

[96] Koh YH, von Arnim CAF, Hyman BT, Tanzi RE, Tesco G. BACE Is Degraded via the Lysosomal Pathway. Journal of Biological Chemistry. 2005;280(37):32499-504.

[97] Sannerud R, Declerck I, Peric A, Raemaekers T, Menendez G, Zhou L, et al. ADP Ribosylation Factor 6 (ARF6) Controls Amyloid Precursor Protein (APP) Processing by Mediating the Endosomal Sorting of BACE1. Proceedings of the National Academy of Sciences. 2011;108(34):E559–E68.

[98] Obregon D, Hou H, Deng J, Giunta B, Tian J, Darlington D, et al. Soluble Amyloid Precursor Protein-α Modulates β-secretase Activity and Amyloid-β Generation. Nature Communicationa. 2012;3:777.

[99] Sun X, Wang Y, Qing H, Christensen MA, Liu Y, Zhou W, et al. Distinct Transcriptional Regulation and Function of the Human BACE2 and BACE1 Genes. The FASEB Journal. 2005;19(7):739-49.

[100] Farzan M, Schnitzler CE, Vasilieva N, Leung D, Choe H. BACE2, a β-secretase Homolog, Cleaves at the β Site and Within the Amyloid-β Region of the Amyloid-β Precursor Protein. Proceedings of the National Academy of Sciences.2000;97(17):9712-7.

[101] Luo Y, Bolon B, Damore MA, Fitzpatrick D, Liu H, Zhang J, et al. BACE1 (β-secretase) Knockout Mice do not Acquire Compensatory Gene Expression Changes or Develop Neural Lesions Over Time. Neurobiology of Disease. 2003;14(1):81-8.

[102] Bennett BD, Babu-Khan S, Loeloff R, Louis J-C, Curran E, Citron M, et al. Expression Analysis of BACE2 in Brain and Peripheral Tissues. Journal of Biological Chemistry. 2000;275(27):20647-51.

[103] von Arnim CAF, Kinoshita A, Peltan ID, Tangredi MM, Herl L, Lee BM, et al. The Low Density Lipoprotein Receptor-related Protein (LRP) is a Novel β-Secretase (BACE1) Substrate. Journal of Biological Chemistry. 2005;280(18):17777-85.

[104] Li Q, Südhof TC. Cleavage of Amyloid-β Precursor Protein and Amyloid-β Precursor-like Protein by BACE 1. Journal of Biological Chemistry. 2004;279(11):10542-50.

[105] Lichtenthaler SF, Dominguez D-i, Westmeyer GG, Reiss K, Haass C, Saftig P, et al. The Cell Adhesion Protein P-selectin Glycoprotein Ligand-1 is a Substrate for the Aspartyl Protease BACE1. Journal of Biological Chemistry. 2003;278(49):48713-9.

[106] Kuhn P-H, Marjaux E, Imhof A, De Strooper B, Haass C, Lichtenthaler SF. Regulated Intramembrane Proteolysis of the Interleukin-1 Receptor II by α-, β-, and γ-secretase. Journal of Biological Chemistry. 2007;282(16):11982-95.

[107] Hemming ML, Elias JE, Gygi SP, Selkoe DJ. Identification of β-Secretase (BACE1) Substrates Using Quantitative Proteomics. PLoS ONE. 2009;4(12):e8477.

[108] Dominguez D, Tournoy J, Hartmann D, Huth T, Cryns K, Deforce S, et al. Phenotypic and Biochemical Analyses of BACE1- and BACE2-deficient Mice. Journal of Biological Chemistry. 2005;280(35):30797-806.

[109] Hitt B, Jaramillo T, Chetkovich D, Vassar R. BACE1-/- Mice Exhibit Seizure Activity that does not Correlate with Sodium Channel Level or Axonal Localization. Molecular Neurodegeneration. 2010;5(1):31.

[110] Siman R, Reaume AG, Savage MJ, Trusko S, Lin Y-G, Scott RW, et al. Presenilin-1 P264L Knock-In Mutation: Differential Effects on Aβ Production, Amyloid Deposition, and Neuronal Vulnerability. The Journal of Neuroscience. 2000;20(23):8717-26.

[111] Flood DG, Reaume AG, Dorfman KS, Lin Y-G, Lang DM, Trusko SP, et al. FAD Mutant PS-1 Gene-Targeted Mice: Increased Aβ42 and Aβ Deposition Without APP Overproduction. Neurobiology of Aging. 2002;23(3):335-48.

[112] Louvi A, Artavanis-Tsakonas S. Notch Signalling in Vertebrate Neural Development. Nature Reviews Neuroscience. 2006;7(2):93-102.

[113] Grüninger-Leitch F, Schlatter D, Küng E, Nelböck P, Döbeli H. Substrate and Inhibitor Profile of BACE (β-Secretase) and Comparison with Other Mammalian Aspartic Proteases. Journal of Biological Chemistry. 2002;277(7):4687-93.

[114] Nguyen J-T, Hamada Y, Kimura T, Kiso Y. Design of Potent Aspartic Protease Inhibitors to Treat Various Diseases. Archiv der Pharmazie. 2008;341(9):523-35.

[115] Hansen RA, Gartlehner G, Webb AP, Morgan LC, Moore CG, Jonas DE. Efficacy and Safety of Donepezil, Galantamine, and Rivastigmine for the Treatment of Alzheimer's Disease: A Systematic Review and Meta-analysis. Dove Medical Press. 2008;3(2): 211-25.

[116] Ghosh AK, Kumaragurubaran N, Hong L, Koelsh G, Tang J. Memapsin 2 (Beta-Secretase) Inhibitors: Drug Development. Current Alzheimer Research. 2008;5(2):121-31.

[117] Román GC, Kalaria RN. Vascular Determinants of Cholinergic Deficits in Alzheimer Disease and Vascular Dementia. Neurobiology of Aging. 2006;27(12):1769-85.

[118] Hellström-Lindahl E, Moore H, Nordberg A. Increased Levels of Tau Protein in SH-SY5Y Cells After Treatment with Cholinesterase Inhibitors and Nicotinic Agonists. Journal of Neurochemistry. 2000;74(2):777-84.

[119] Chalmers K, Wilcock G, Vinters H, Perry E, Perry R, Ballard C, et al. Cholinesterase Inhibitors may Increase Phosphorylated Tau in Alzheimer's Disease. Journal of Neurology. 2009;256(5):717-20.

[120] Danysz W, Parsons C, MÖbius H-J, StÖffler A, Quack G. Neuroprotective and Symptomatological Action of Memantine Relevant for Alzheimer's Disease — a Unified Glutamatergic Hypothesis on the Mechanism of Action. Neurotoxicity Research. 2000;2(2):85-97.

[121] Orrego F, Villanueva S. The Chemical Nature of the Main Central Excitatory Transmitter: A Critical Appraisal Based Upon Release Studies and Synaptic Vesicle Localization. Neuroscience. 1993;56(3):539-55.

[122] Lipton SA, Rosenberg PA. Excitatory Amino Acids as a Final Common Pathway for Neurologic Disorders. New England Journal of Medicine. 1994;330(9):613-22.

[123] Luo X, Yan R. Inhibition of BACE1 for Therapeutic use in Alzheimer's Disease. International Journal of Clinical and Experimental Pathology. 2010;3(6):618-28.

[124] Guo T, Hobbs DW. Development of BACE1 Inhibitors for Alzheimer's Disease. Current Medicinal Chemistry. 2006;13(15):1811-29.

[125] Baxter EW, Conway KA, Kennis L, Bischoff F, Mercken MH, De Winter HL, et al. 2-Amino-3,4-dihydroquinazolines as Inhibitors of BACE-1 (β-Site APP Cleaving En-

zyme): Use of Structure Based Design to Convert a Micromolar Hit into a Nanomolar Lead. Journal of Medicinal Chemistry. 2007;50(18):4261-4.

[126] Cole DC, Manas ES, Stock JR, Condon JS, Jennings LD, Aulabaugh A, et al. Acylguanidines as Small-Molecule β-Secretase Inhibitors. Journal of Medicinal Chemistry. 2006;49(21):6158-61.

[127] Edwards PD, Albert JS, Sylvester M, Aharony D, Andisik D, Callaghan O, et al. Application of Fragment-Based Lead Generation to the Discovery of Novel, Cyclic Amidine β-Secretase Inhibitors with Nanomolar Potency, Cellular Activity, and High Ligand Efficiency. Journal of Medicinal Chemistry. 2007;50(24):5912-25.

[128] Hussain I, Hawkins J, Harrison D, Hille C, Wayne G, Cutler L, et al. Oral Administration of a Potent and Selective Non-peptidic BACE-1 Inhibitor Decreases β-cleavage of Amyloid Precursor Protein and Amyloid-β Production in vivo. Journal of Neurochemistry. 2007;100(3):802-9.

[129] Iserloh U, Pan J, Stamford AW, Kennedy ME, Zhang Q, Zhang L, et al. Discovery of an Orally Efficaceous 4-phenoxypyrrolidine-based BACE-1 Inhibitor. Bioorganic and Medicinal Chemistry Letters. 2008;18(1):418-22.

[130] Kortum SW, Benson TE, Bienkowski MJ, Emmons TL, Prince DB, Paddock DJ, et al. Potent and Selective Isophthalamide S2 Hydroxyethylamine Inhibitors of BACE1. Bioorganic and Medicinal Chemistry Letters. 2007;17(12):3378-83.

[131] Marcin LR, Higgins MA, Zusi FC, Zhang Y, Dee MF, Parker MF, et al. Synthesis and SAR of Indole-and 7-azaindole-1,3-dicarboxamide Hydroxyethylamine Inhibitors of BACE-1. Bioorganic & Medicinal Chemistry Letters. 2011;21(1):537-41.

[132] Stachel SJ, Coburn CA, Steele TG, Jones KG, Loutzenhiser EF, Gregro AR, et al. Structure-Based Design of Potent and Selective Cell-Permeable Inhibitors of Human β-Secretase (BACE-1). Journal of Medicinal Chemistry. 2004;47(26):6447-50.

[133] Stachel SJ, Coburn CA, Sankaranarayanan S, Price EA, Pietrak BL, Huang Q, et al. Macrocyclic Inhibitors of β-Secretase: Functional Activity in an Animal Model. Journal of Medicinal Chemistry. 2006;49(21):6147-50.

[134] Tung JS, Davis DL, Anderson JP, Walker DE, Mamo S, Jewett N, et al. Design of Substrate-Based Inhibitors of Human β-Secretase. Journal of Medicinal Chemistry. 2001;45(2):259-62.

[135] Armulik A, Genove G, Mae M, Nisancioglu MH, Wallgard E, Niaudet C, et al. Pericytes Regulate the Blood-brain Barrier. Nature. 2010;468(7323):557-61.

[136] Brightman MW, Reese TS. Junctions Between Intinately Apposed Cell Membranes in the Verterbrate Brain. The Journal of Cell Biology. 1969;40(3):648-77.

[137] Ghersi-Egea JF, Leninger-Muller B, Suleman G, Siest G, Minn A. Localization of Drug-metabolizing Enzyme Activities to Blood-Brain Interfaces and Circumventricular Organs. Journal of Neurochemistry. 1994;62(3):1089-96.

[138] Meyer RP, Gehlhaus M, Knoth R, Volk B. Expression and Function of Cytochrome p450 in Brain Drug Metabolism. Current Drug Metabolism. 2007;8(4):297-306.

[139] Bauer B, Hartz AMS, Lucking JR, Yang X, Pollack GM, Miller DS. Coordinated Nuclear Receptor Regulation of the Efflux Transporter, Mrp2, and the Phase-II Metabolizing Enzyme, GST[pi], at the Blood-brain Barrier. Journal of Cerebral Blood Flow Metabolism. 2008;28(6):1222-34.

[140] Fischer H, Gottschlich R, Seelig A. Blood-Brain Barrier Permeation: Molecular Parameters Governing Passive Diffusion. Journal of Membrane Biology. 1998;165(3): 201-11.

[141] Träuble H. The Movement of Molecules Across Lipid Membranes: A Molecular Theory. Journal of Membrane Biology. 1971;4(1):193-208.

[142] Nadal A, Fuentes E, Pastor J, McNaughton PA. Plasma Albumin is a Potent Trigger of Calcium Signals and DNA Synthesis in Astrocytes. Proceedings of the National Academy of Sciences of the United States of America. 1995;92(5):1426-30.

[143] Pardridge WM. Blood–brain Barrier Delivery. Drug Discovery Today. 2007;12(1–2): 54-61.

[144] Tuszynski MH, Thal L, Pay M, Salmon DP, U HS, Bakay R, et al. A Phase 1 Clinical Trial of Nerve Growth Factor Gene Therapy for Alzheimer Disease. Nature Medicine. 2005;11(5):551-5.

[145] Bodor N, Prokai L, Wu W, Farag H, Jonalagadda S, Kawamura M, et al. A Strategy for Delivering Peptides into the Central Nervous System by Sequential Metabolism. Science. 1992;257(5077):1698-700.

[146] Kastin AJ, Akerstrom V, Hackler L. Food Deprivation Decreases Blood Galanin-like Peptide and its Rapid Entry into the Brain. Neuroendocrinology. 2001;74(6):423-32.

[147] Simpson IA, Carruthers A, Vannucci SJ. Supply and Demand in Cerebral Energy Metabolism: the Role of Nutrient Transporters. Journal of Cerebral Blood Flow Metabolism. 2007;27(11):1766-91.

[148] Duffy KR, Pardridge WM. Blood-brain Barrier Transcytosis of Insulin in Developing Rabbits. Brain Research. 1987;420(1):32-8.

[149] Fishman JB, Rubin JB, Handrahan JV, Connor JR, Fine RE. Receptor-mediated Transcytosis of Transferrin Across the Blood-brain Barrier. Journal of Neuroscience Research. 1987;18(2):299-304.

[150] Reinhardt RR, Bondy CA. Insulin-like Growth Factors Cross the Blood-brain Barrier. Endocrinology. 1994;135(5):1753-61.

[151] Tadayoni BM, Friden PM, Walus LR, Musso GF. Synthesis, in vitro Kinetics and in vivo Studies on Protein Conjugates of AZT: Evaluation as a Transport System to Increase Brain Delivery. Bioconjugate Chemistry. 1993;4(2):139-45.

[152] Penichet ML, Kang Y-S, Pardridge WM, Morrison SL, Shin S-U. An Antibody-Avidin Fusion Protein Specific for the Transferrin Receptor Serves as a Delivery Vehicle for Effective Brain Targeting: Initial Applications in Anti-HIV Antisense Drug Delivery to the Brain. The Journal of Immunology. 1999;163(8):4421-6.

[153] Huwyler J, Wu D, Pardridge WM. Brain Drug Delivery of Small Molecules Using Immunoliposomes. Proceedings of the National Academy of Sciences. 1996;93(24): 14164-9.

[154] Doi A, Kawabata S, Iida K, Yokoyama K, Kajimoto Y, Kuroiwa T, et al. Tumor-specific Targeting of Sodium Borocaptate (BSH) to Malignant Glioma by Transferrin-PEG Liposomes: a Modality for Boron Neutron Capture Therapy. Journal of Neuro-Oncology. 2008;87(3):287-94.

[155] Bosi S, Da Ros T, Spalluto G, Prato M. Fullerene Derivatives: an Attractive Tool for Biological Applications. European Journal of Medicinal Chemistry. 2003;38(11–12): 913-23.

[156] Basso AS, Frenkel D, Quintana FJ, Costa-Pinto FA, Petrovic-Stojkovic S, Puckett L, et al. Reversal of Axonal Loss and Disability in a Mouse Model of Progressive Multiple Sclerosis. The Journal of Clinical Investigation. 2008;118(4):1532-43.

[157] Huang SS, Tsai SK, Chih CL, Chiang L-Y, Hsieh HM, Teng CM, et al. Neuroprotective Effect of Hexasulfobutylated C60 on Rats Subjected to Focal Cerebral Ischemia. Free Radical Biology and Medicine. 2001;30(6):643-9.

[158] Yang DY, Wang MF, Chen IL, Chan YC, Lee MS, Cheng FC. Systemic Administration of a Water-soluble Hexasulfonated C60 (FC4S) Reduces Cerebral Ischemia-induced Infarct Volume in Gerbils. Neuroscience Letters. 2001;311(2):121-4.

[159] Henley DB, May PC, Dean RA, Siemers ER. Development of Semagacestat (LY450139), a Functional γ-secretase Inhibitor, for the Treatment of Alzheimer's Disease. Expert Opinion on Pharmacotherapy. 2009;10(10):1657-64.

[160] Forman M, Tseng J, Palcza J, Leempoels J, Ramael S, Krishna G, et al. The Novel BACE Inhibitor MK-8931 Dramatically Lowers CSF Aβ Peptides in Healthy Subjects: Results from a Rising Single Dose Study (PL02.004) 64th American Academy of Neurology Annual Meeting; 2012; New Orleans: Neurology.

[161] Ming GL, Song H. Adult Neurogenesis in the Mammalian Central Nervous System. Annual Review of Neuroscience. 2005;28:223-50.

Chapter 11

QSAR Analysis of Purine-Type and Propafenone-Type Substrates of P-Glycoprotein Targeting β-Amyloid Clearance

Jie Yang and Jie Chen

Additional information is available at the end of the chapter

http://dx.doi.org/10.5772/54975

1. Introduction

Therapy for central nervous system (CNS) diseases requires drugs that can cross the blood-brain barrier (BBB) (Cheng et al, 2010). BBB not only maintains the homeostasis of the CNS, but also refuses many potentially important diagnostic and therapeutic agents from entering into the brain (Chen et al, 2009). The pathogenesis of Alzheimer's disease (AD) senile plaque and neurofibrillary tangle lesions putatively involves a compromised BBB (Jevnes & Provias, 2011), which protects the brain against endogenous and exogenous compounds and plays an important part in the maintenance of the microenvironment of the brain (Vogelgesang et al, 2011). The ability of drug permeating across BBB becomes critical in the development of new medicines, especially in the design of new drugs which are active in brain tissue. In particular, the importance of brain-to-blood transport of brain-derived metabolites across the BBB has gained increasing attention as a potential mechanism in the pathogenesis of neurodegenerative disorders such as Parkinson's disease (Bartels, 2011) and AD characterized by the aberrant polymerization and accumulation of specific misfolded proteins, particularly β-amyloid (Aβ), a neuropathological hallmark of AD. P-glycoprotein (P-gp or MDR1/ABCB1) is a 170-kDa transmembrane protein widely expressed from the epithelial cells of the intestine, liver, kidney, placenta, uterus, and testis to endothelial cells of the BBB (Gottesman & Pastan, 1993). It belongs to the ABC (ATP-binding cassette) transporter family and serves to pump exogenous substances out of the cells (Suresh et al, 1999). The domain topology of P-gp consist of two homologous halves each consist a transmembrane domain preceding a cytosolic nucleotide binding domain. Each transmembrane domain is composed of six transmembrane α-helix segments involved in efflux as well as in drug binding (Kast et al, 1996). The ABC transport protein P-gp, a major component of the BBB, mediates the efflux of Aβ from the brain as well as a major factor in mediating resistance to brain entry by numerous exogenous chemicals, including therapeutic pharmaceuticals (Bendayan et al, 2002). P-gp plays a role in the etiology of AD through the clearance of Aβ from the brain. Some drugs, such as rifampicin, dexamethasone, caffeine, verapamil, hyperforin, β-estradiol and pentylenetetrazole, were able to improve the efflux of Aβ from the cells via P-gp up-regulation (Abuznait et al, 2011). Meanwhile, some compounds have been shown to reverse the P-gp mediated multidrug resistance (MDR), including verapamil, adriamycin, cyclosporin, and dexverapamil (Kothandan et al, 2011). Harta et al (2010) have shown that up-regulate P-gp in the early stages of AD has the potential to increase Aβ clearance from the brain and reduce Aβ brain accumulation by a transgenic mouse model of AD (human amyloid precursor protein-overexpressing mice). Abuznait et al (2011) have also elucidated the impact of P-gp up-regulation on the clearance of Aβ, which indicated targeting Aβ clearance via P-gp up-regulation effective in slowing or halting the progression of AD and the possibility of P-gp as a potential therapeutic target for AD.

P-gp at the BBB functions as an active efflux pump by extruding a substrate from the brain, which is important for maintaining loco-regional homeostasis in the brain and protection against toxic compounds (Bartels, 2011). P-gp is also discovered in various resistant tumor cells and expressed widely in many normal tissues and plays a very important role in drug ADME-Tox (absorption, distribution, metabolism, excretion, and toxicity). MDR is a matter of growing concern in chemotherapy. Cells which express the multidrug resistance phenotype can over-express efflux transporters after exposure to a single agent. As a result, these cells become resistant to the selective agent and cross-resistant to a broad spectrum of structurally and functionally dissimilar drugs. The drug efflux pump P-gp has been shown to promote MDR in tumors as well as to influence ADME properties of drug candidates (Jabben et al, 2012). P-gp is expressed at the BBB, the blood-cerebrospinal fluid barrier, and the intestinal barrier, thus modulating the absorption and excretion of xenobiotics across these barriers. P-gp and its ligands (substrates and inhibitors) are therefore extensively studied both with respect to reversing MDR in tumors and for modifying ADME-Tox properties of drug candidates, such as CNS active agents (Jabben et al, 2012). P-gp possesses broad substrate specificity and substrates include members of many clinically important therapeutic drug classes, including anti-HIV protease inhibitors, calcium channel blockers used in the treatment of angina, hypertension, antibiotics and cancer chemotherapeutics (Stouch & Gudmundsson, 2002). In this active efflux process, energy originating from ATP hydrolysis is directly consumed. Because of such a wide distribution of P-gp, so if a drug such as quinidine or verapamil inhibits the function of P-gp, it will also inhibit the excretion of digoxin by P-gp leading to increased plasma levels and toxicity due to digoxin. It is believed to be an important protective mechanism against environmental toxins (Martin, 2004). Since the function of P-gp always results in lack of intracellular levels of the drug necessary for effective therapy, the overexpression of P-gp in certain malignant cells is always associated with MDR phenotype (Sharom, 1997). Although recently low resolution structure of P-gp is obtained, its physiological function and mechanisms of MDR modulation are still not very clear (Li et al, 2005). It is well known that a large number of structurally and functionally diverse compounds act as substrates or modulators of P-gp, including calcium and sodium channel blockers, calmodulin antagonists and structural analogues, protein kinase C inhibitors, steroidal and structurally related com-

http://dx.doi.org/10.5772/54975

pounds, indole alkaloids, cyclic peptides and macrolide compounds, flayanoids and miscellaneous compounds (Wang et al, 2003), which mostly share common structural features, such as aromatic ring structures and high lipophilicity. Some of them possess MDR reversing activity. But only a small number of them have entered clinical study and classification of candidate drugs as substrates or inhibitors of the carrier protein is of crucial importance in drug development (Wang et al, 2005).

On the other hand, the prerequisite to cure neurological disorders is that the drug distribution in CNS can reach effectively therapeutic concentrations (Chen et al, 2009). Usually, the high BBB penetration is needed for drugs that activate in brain. The molecule negotiating the BBB must go through cellular membranes comprising of a lipid bilayer. Until now, it is widely accepted that interaction of compounds with P-gp is a complex process and at this time the details of its mechanism of action are still the subject on hot debate. Although the experimental analysis of drug permeability is essential but the procedure of experiment is time consuming and complicated, a theoretical model of drug permeability is effective to give predictions. Membrane-interaction (MI)-QSAR (quantitative structure-activity relationship) method is a structure-based design methodology combined with classic intramolecular QSAR analysis to model chemically and structurally diverse compounds interacting with cellular membranes. Our modified MI-QSAR method that combines QSAR with solute-membrane-water complex simulating the BBB environment is more close to the body condition than MI-QSAR and possesses higher ability to predict organic compounds across BBB (Chen & Yang, 2006). Before we construct any QSAR models, several things should be consider seriously first. There are several critical assumptions that can influence validity and correctness of any QSAR study as follows: the same mechanism of action of all studied analogs; a comparable manner of their binding to the receptor; correlation of binding to the interaction energies; correlation of measured biological activities to the binding affinities (Kubinyi, 1995). All the accuracy answer and research based on the questions above may guarantee that proper and reliable relationships are obtained. However, in case of MDR modulators different mechanisms and different binding sites may be involved. Several screening assays can help in the identification of substrates and inhibitors although they have both advantages and drawbacks, such as cytotoxity assays (Wiese & Pajeva, 2001), inhibition of efflux assays (Stouch & Gudrmundsson, 2001), P-gp-ATPase activation assays, and drug transport assays (Taub et al, 2005).

The goal of a QSAR study is to find a means of predicting the activity of a new compound. If possible, a desirable goal is the understanding of the biology and chemistry that give rise to that activity and the consequential possibility of reengineering the compound to remove or enhance that activity. One successful example is the transformation of nalidixic acid with the help of QSAR into an important family of drug: the quinolone carboxylates, such as norfloxacin, fleroxacin, ciprofloxacin, and levofloxacin (Alka, 2003). Since the method was established in the 1960s, QSAR equations have been used to describe the biological activities of thousands of different drugs and drug candidates (Kuo et al, 2004). The method definitely provides a more accurate way to synthesize or filtrate the new chemical compounds. At last, the final destination is to degrade the cost of research and manufacture. To date, so many methods have been used in QSAR study and some of them have got successful results. There are general methods used in the literatures these years, such as multiple linear regression (MLR) method, partial least square regression (PLSR) (Li et al, 2005), MI-QSAR analysis (Chen & Yang, 2006), and three-dimension (3D) QSAR (Cramer et al, 1988), and artificial neural network (ANN) (Chen et al, 2006). In order to get more accurate results and QSAR models, we have used two different analyses: MLR and PLSR. Moreover, we focus on constructing theoretical models of the interaction between organic compounds and P-gp as well as the predictive models of blood-brain barrier partitioning of organic compounds on the basis of QSAR analysis and MI-QSAR analysis.

2. Materials and methods

2.1. P-glycoprotein ligands

Building of some compounds 36 purine derivatives were selected and used in QSAR analysis (table 1) (Dhainaut et al, 1996). These compounds were divided into two sets: the training set and the test set. The study of the MDR-reversing properties of these derivatives was carried out in vitro on P388/VCR-20 cells, a murine leukemia cell line whose resistance was induced by vincristine (VCR), and KB-A1 cells, a human epidermoid carcinoma cell line whose resistance was induced by adriamycin (ADR). The compounds were tested at four concentrations (0.5–5 μM) in association with VCR (P388/VCR-20 cells) or ADR (KB-A1 cells). In this test, MDR ratio in P388/VDR-20 and KB-A1 in vitro was used as biological activity for the whole dataset, namely $MDR_{ratio} = \frac{IC_{50}(CD)}{IC_{50}(CD + \text{mod})}$. Here "CD" is the abbreviation for cytotoxic drug (such as VCR and ADR) in cytotoxity assays, and "mod" means modulators. It is defined as ratio between the IC_{50} values (concentration that inhibits the growth of MDR cells by 50%) of the cytotoxic agent in absence and presence of relatively nontoxic concentration of the modifier (Wiese & Pajeva, 2001). Most often the IC_{50} for several concentration of a cytotoxic drug is evaluated in the presence and absence of a nontoxic concentration of a P-gp modifier. In this assay modulators that interact with P-gp and thus, reduce the efflux of the cytotoxic compounds, will increase the apparent toxicity of the cytotoxic compound. It is important to keep in mind that it is based on a general assessment of cytotoxicity and thus may account for more then one acting mechanism in the resistant cells used (Stouch & Gudmundsso,. 2001). Furthermore, it is well known that the MDR ratio for any given compound can vary greatly depending on the cell type used for the assay as well as the intrinsic cytotoxicity of the compounds used. The data is also dependent on the concentration of the P-gp substrates or modulators used in the studies (Ford et al, 1990).

Similarly, another 21 propafenone analogs were selected from the literature of Diethart Schmid et al (1999) and used in QSAR analysis (table 2). In this test Ka of P-gp ATPase in the adriamycin-resistant subline CCRF ADR5000 was used as biological activity for the whole dataset (Schmid et al, 1999). The assays were performed based on the colorimetric determination of inorganic phosphate released by the hydrolysis of ATP. Table 2 shows all the structures and the experimental biological activity value.

No.	Structure	in vitro reversal fold reversion (MDR ratio)		No.	Structure	in vitro reversal fold reversion (MDR ratio)	
		P388/ VCR-20	KB-A1			P388/VCR-20	KB-A1
A1	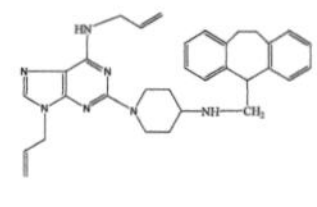	50	171	A19	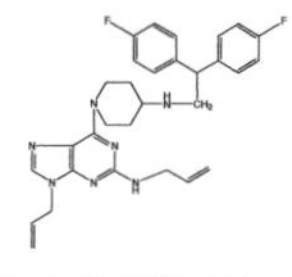	36	49
A2	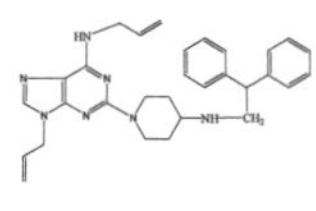	78	278	A20	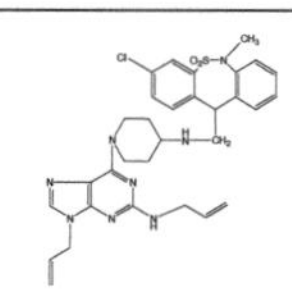	70	214
A3	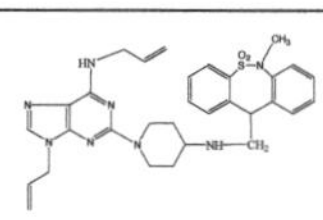	75	238	A21	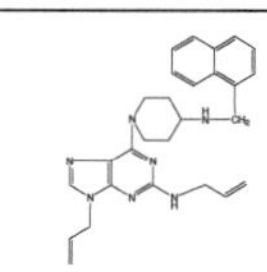	35	113
A4	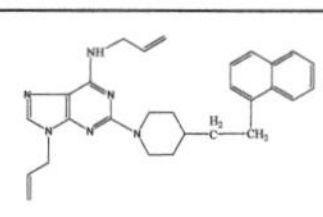	53	236	A22	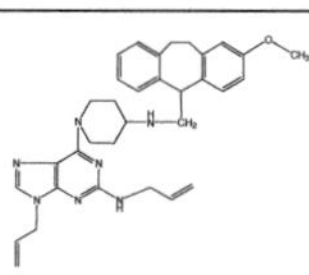	133	200
A5	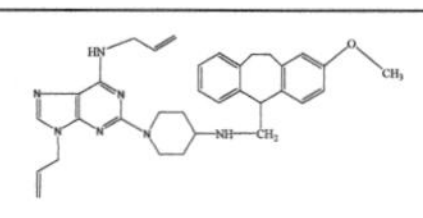	236	160	A23	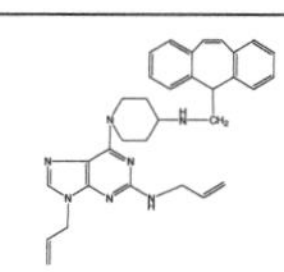	193	189
A6	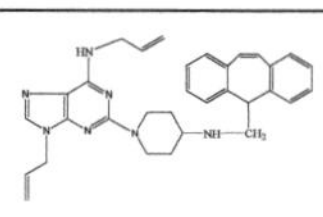	93	208	A24	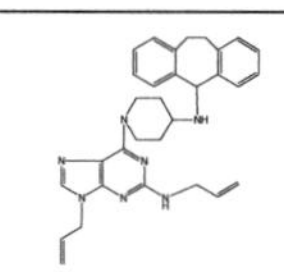	24	142
A7	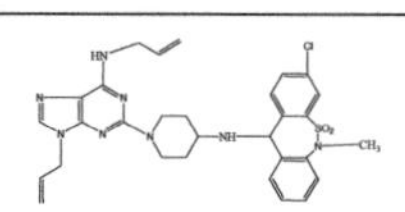	124	102	A25	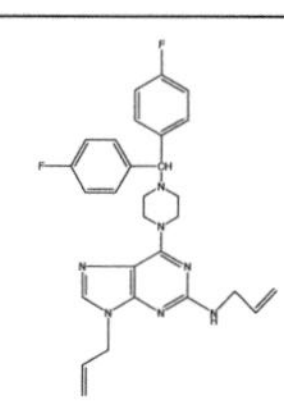	13	6
A8	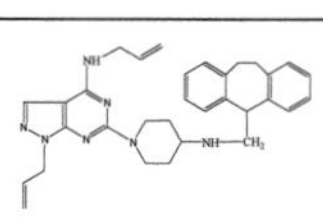	30	120	A26	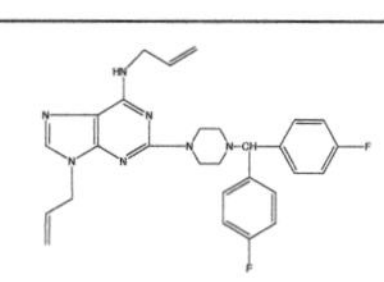	24	9
A9	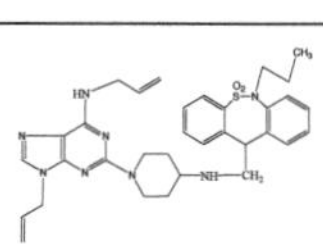	57	75	A27	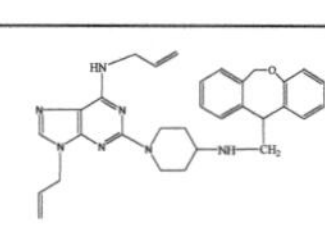	84	406

No.	Structure	in vitro reversal fold reversion (MDR ratio)		No.	Structure	in vitro reversal fold reversion (MDR ratio)	
		P388/ VCR-20	KB-A1			P388/VCR-20	KB-A1
A10	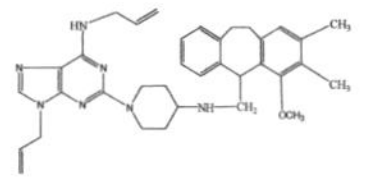	108	136	A28	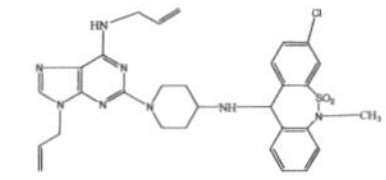	57	68
A11	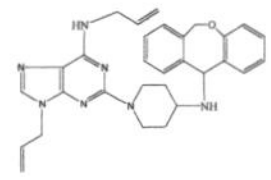	37	44	A29	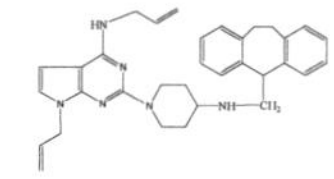	108	723
A12	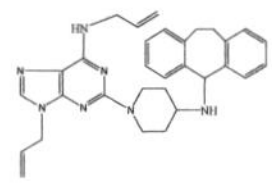	15	83	A30	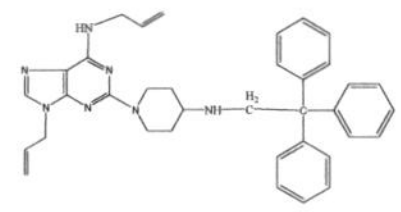	27	370
A13	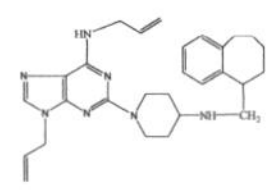	78	272	A31	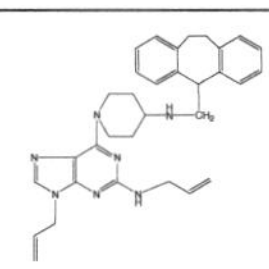	288	210
A14	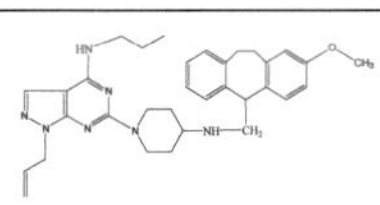	56	147	A32	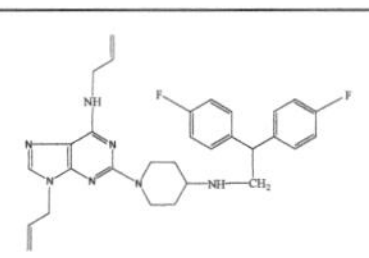	59	121
A15	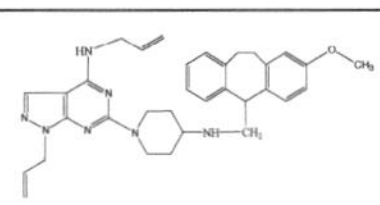	75	152	A33	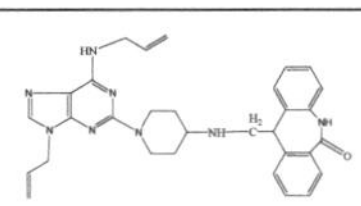	71	499
A16	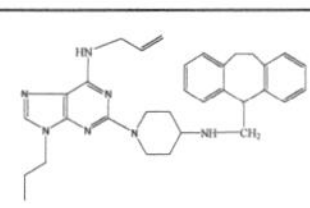	51	209	A34	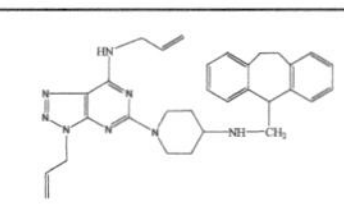	13	264
A17	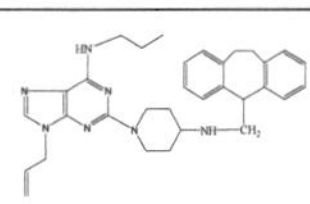	70	171	A35	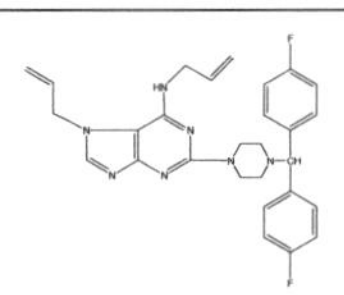	3	5
A18	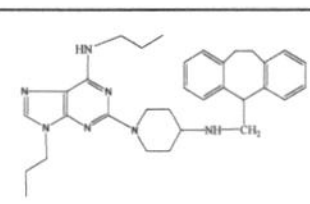	129	156				

Note: Ratio of IC_{50} (cytotoxic alone (VCR for P388/VCR-20, ADR for KB-A1 cells))/IC_{50} (cytotoxic + modulator) (1μM in association with VCR or 2.5 μM in association with ADR) (Dhainaut et al, 1996).

Table 1. The structures and MDR ratios of 35 purine derivatives in the training/test sets.

No.	Structure	Ka(μM/L)	LogP	No.	Structure	Ka(μM/L)	LogP
A36	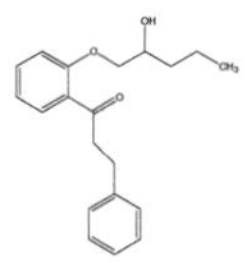	3.34	3.39	A45	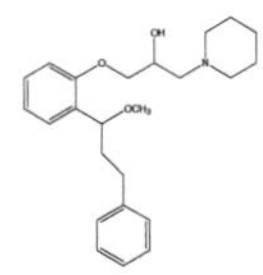	1.53	4.3
A37	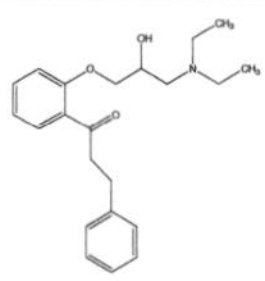	5.3	3.62	A46	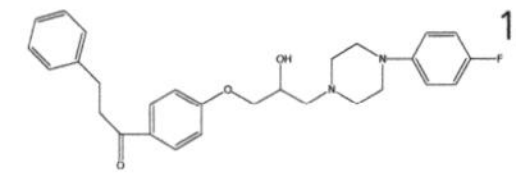	1.47	4.93
A38	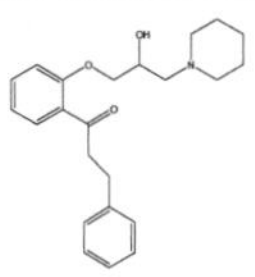	2.59	3.67	A47	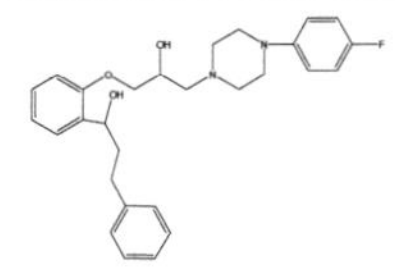	0.55	5.2
A39	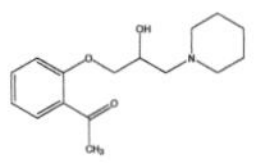	122	1.42	A48	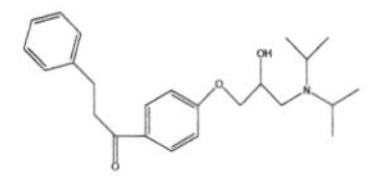	7.64	4.25
A40	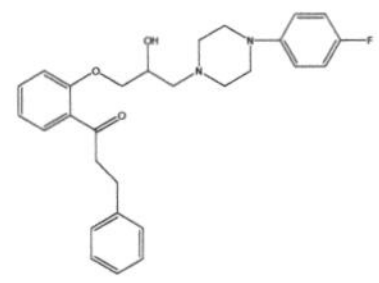	0.36	4.93	A49	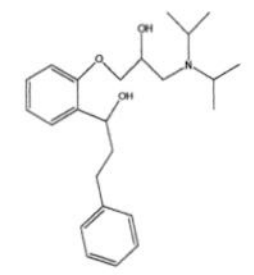	12.2	4.52
A41	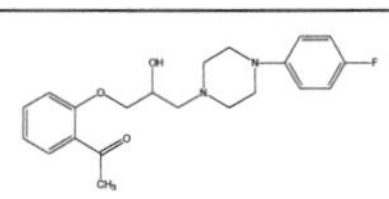	6.13	2.67	A50	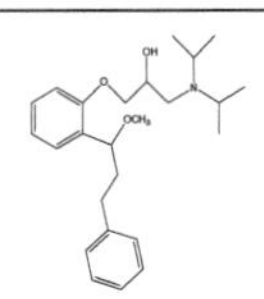	2.26	4.88
A42	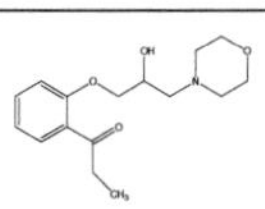	120	0.94	A51	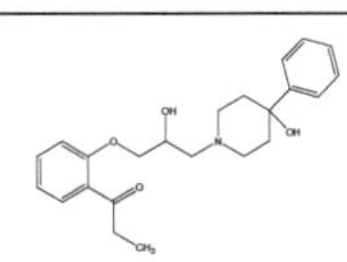	10.5	2.38
A43	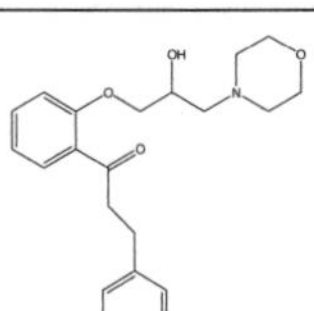	18.5	2.54	A52	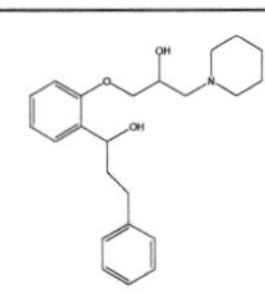	12.8	3.94
A44	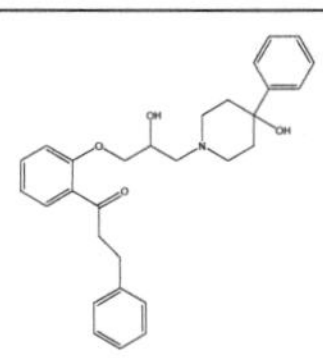	1.01	3.98	A53	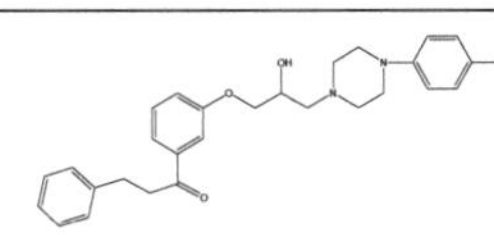	4.15	4.93

Table 2. The structures and Ka values and LogP of 18 propafenone analogs in the training/test sets.

Finally, all two-dimensional structures of these compounds mentioned above were constructed using the chemical drawing software ChemDraw 8.0 and prepared for the next calculation.

Calculation of some descriptors Molecular descriptors are "numbers that characterize a specific aspect of the molecular structure" (Karelson, 2000). There are a great number of molecular descriptors that can be used in QSAR studies in the structure parameterization form, which include physicochemical properties (such as hydrophobicity, aqueous solubility, molecular electronegativity, and molecular refractivity), quantum chemical parameters (i.g. atomic charges, energies of HOMO (highest occupied molecular orbital) and LUMO (lowest unoccupied molecular orbital)) (Karelson & Lobanov, 1996), topological indexes (i.e. molecular connectivity indexes) (Ponce et al, 2004), and other three-dimentional (3D) descriptors. Molecular descriptors were mostly calculated by the commercial software packages Chemoffice Chem3D Ultra 8.0, which included molecular mechanism parameters (Bending Energy (E_{bend}), Stretch-Bend Energy ($E_{stretch}$), Torsion Energy ($E_{torsion}$), Total Energy (E_{total}), van der Waals Energy (E_{VDW}), etc), quantum chemistry parameters (i.e. Electronic Energy ($E_{electronic}$), HOMO Energy (E_{HOMO}) and LUMO Energy (E_{LUMO})), hydrophobic parameters (such as Clog P), stereo parameters (eg. Es, Balaban Index (BI), Connolly Accessible Area (CAA), Molecular Weight (MW), Shape Attribute (ShA), Total Connectivity (T_{con}), and Wiener Index (WI)), thermodynamic parameters, including Henry's Law Constant (H), Hydration Energy (E_{hyd}), Logarithm of partition coefficient in n-octanol/water (LogP), Molar Refractivity (MR), and molecular polar surface area (PSA). PSA is defined as the surface area ($Å^2$) occupied by polar atoms, usually oxygen, nitrogen and hydrogen attached to them, which will restrict molecule penetration into the membranes (Chen et al, 2009). The other properties involved in number of hydrogen bond acceptor (NBA) and number of hydrogen bond donor (NBD).

The energy parameters root in the results of molecular mechanism and molecular dynamics. The total energy of a system expressed as follows (Iyer et al 2002): $E_{total} = E_{valence} + E_{crossterm} + E_{nonbone}$.

Here, the valence interactions includes bond stretching (bond), valence angle bending (angle), dihedral angle torsion (torsion), and inversion, also called out-of-plane interactions (oop) terms, which are part of nearly all forcefields for covalent systems. A Urey-Bradley term (UB) may be used to account for interactions between atom pairs involved in 1-3 configurations (i.e., atoms bound to a common atom): $E_{valence} = E_{bond} + E_{angle} + E_{torsion} + E_{oop} + E_{UP}$. Modern (second-generation) forcefields generally achieve higher accuracy by including cross terms to account for such factors as bond or angle distortions caused by nearby atoms. Crossterms can include the following terms: stretch-stretch, stretch-bend-stretch, bend-bend, torsion-stretch, torsion-bend-bend, bend-torsion-bend, stretch-torsion-stretch. The interaction energy between non-bonded atoms is accounted by van der Waals (VDW), electrostatic (Coulomb), and hydrogen bond (hbond) terms in some older forcefields. $E_{non-bond} = E_{VDW} + E_{Coulomb} + E_{hbond}$. Restraints that can be added to an energy expression include distance, angle, torsion, and inversion restraints. Restraints are useful if you, for example, are interested in only part of a structure for information on restraints and their implementation and use, and also the documentation for the particular simulation engine.

With the aid of Chemoffice Chem3D Ultra 8.0 and Hyperchem 7.5, we calculated the following descriptors by the procedure in detail below: (1) Draw the structures in ChemDraw 8.0; (2) Change structures to 3D by Chem3D; (3) Considering our chosen compounds, minimize the energy of the molecule based on molecular mechanism MM2 Force Field (Because under the MM2 force field, the time required for performing computations increases as N^2, where N is the number of atoms.). We have chosen the job type as minimize energy to minimum RMS (root mean square) Gradient of 0.100 (the default value of 0.100 is a reasonable compromise between accuracy and speed). (4) Under the menu of Analyze-compute properties, select the properties to calculate and get every descriptor value of each compound.

QSAR models QSAR model of some purine derivatives (table 1) are achieved by partial sum of squares for regression with software SPSS 10.0. Some biological activity data are so large or small that the group of data cannot form a normal school, which is very important in lineal regression, and will surely degrade the accuracy of QSAR equations. So we discarded several data out of the normal school and some without necessary descriptors value. A training set of 26 structurally diverse purine derivatives are measured is used to construct QSAR models. The QSAR models are optimized using MLR fitting and stepwise method (Eq.1-Eq.5). A test set of five compounds is evaluated using the QSAR models as part of a validation process. Take MDR ratio in vitro in P388/VDR cell lines as dependent variable and molecule descriptors as independent variable. With the aid of Virtual Computational Chemistry Laboratory software (Wang et al, 2005), QSAR modeling was constructed by PLSR (Eg. 6).

Similarly, a training set of 18 structurally diverse propafenone analogs (table 2) are measured is used to construct QSAR models. The QSAR models are optimized using MLR fitting and stepwise method (Eq.7-Eq.11). Another QSAR modeling was constructed by PLSR (Eg. 12). A test set of five compounds is evaluated using the QSAR models as part of a validation process.

2.2. Blood-brain-barrier

Building of some compounds 37 organic compounds (Abraham et al, 1995; Abraham et al, 1997) were elected, composed a train set, and another 8 organic compounds were acted as a test set (table 3). The dependent variable used in this predictive model is the logarithm of the BBB partition coefficient, log BB = log (C_{brain} / C_{blood}), where C_{brain} is the concentration of the test compound in the brain, and C_{blood} is the concentration of the test compound in blood. Experimental values of log BB published to date lie approximately between -2.00 to +1.04. Compounds with log BB values of > 0.30 are readily distributed to the brain whereas compounds with values < -1.00 are poorly distributed to the brain. Building of all these compounds was performed on a PC computer using the Build modules of the commercial software packages Hyperchem 7.5. First, the geometry of these compounds was opitimized using the Amber 94 force field in gas state. Second, they were placed at a periodic solvent box whose volume was X=16Å, Y=10Å, Z=18Å, which included 96 water molecules. Here, temperature is 300ºK and pressure is 1 standard atmosphere. Then, the compounds in water were minimized by the above method. Third, the compounds in water were simulated by Monte Carlo method and minimized by the above method.

No	Structure	LogBB	No	Structure	LogBB
		Training set			
B1	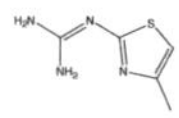	-0.04	B20	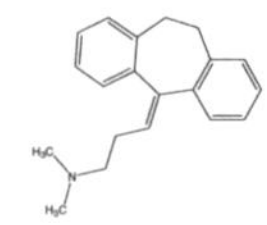	0.85
B2	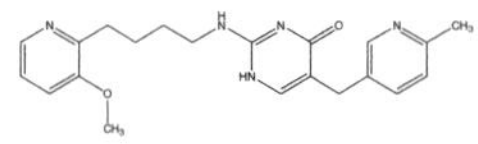	-2.00	B21		0.03
B3	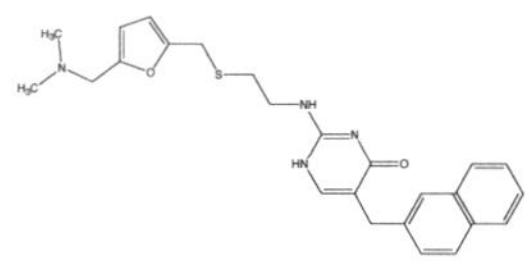	-1.30	B22	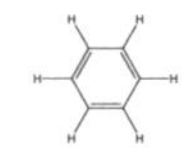	0.37
B4	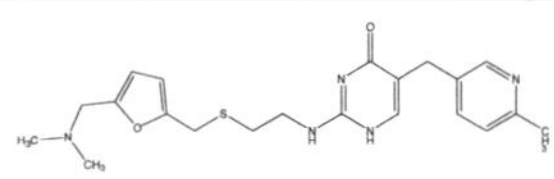	-1.06	B23	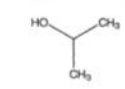	-0.15
B5	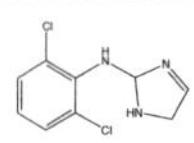	0.11	B24	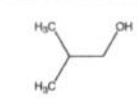	-0.17
B6	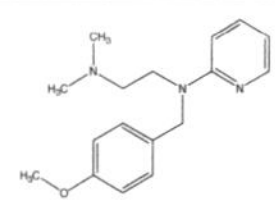	0.49	B25	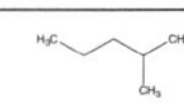	0.97
B7	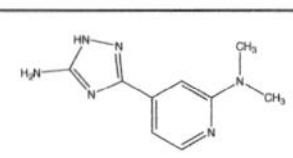	-1.17	B26	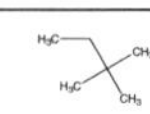	1.04
B8	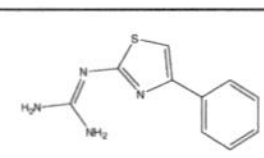	-0.18	B27	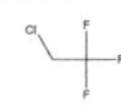	0.08
B9	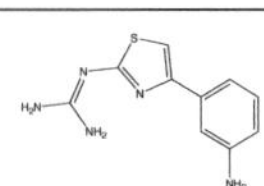	-1.15	B28	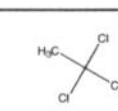	0.40
B10	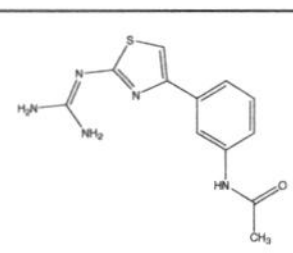	-1.57	B29	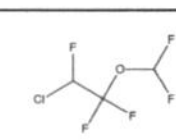	0.24
B11	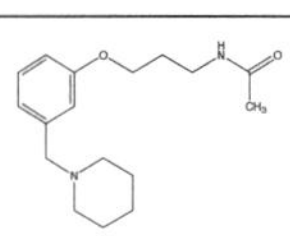	-0.46	B30	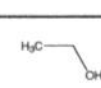	-0.16
B12	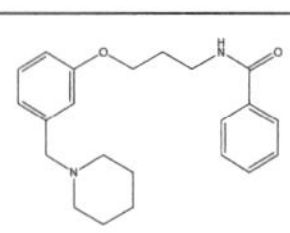	-0.24	B31	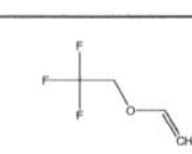	0.13

No	Structure	LogBB	No	Structure	LogBB
B13	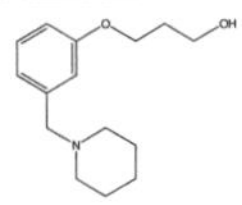	-0.02	B32	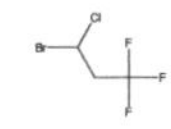	0.35
B14	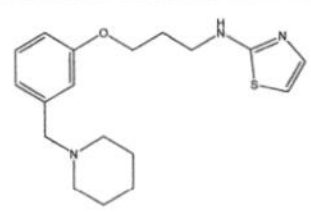	0.44	B33	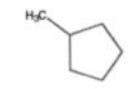	0.93
B15	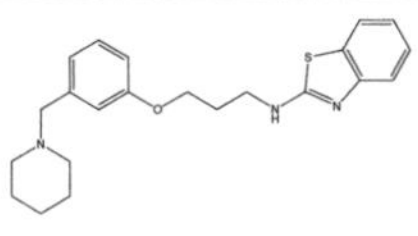	0.14	B34	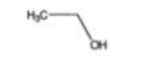	-0.16
B16	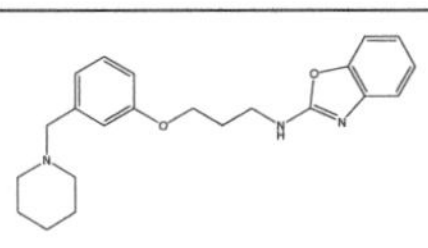	0.22	B35	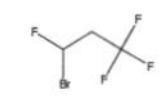	0.27
B17	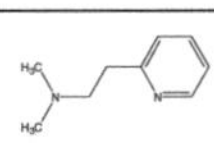	-0.06	B36	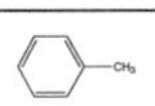	0.37
B18	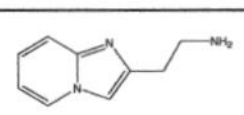	-1.40	B37	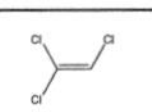	0.34
B19	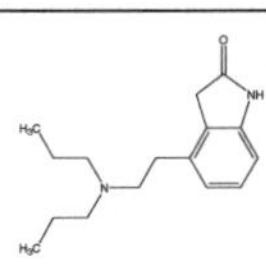	0.25			
		Test set			
T1	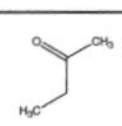	-0.08	T5	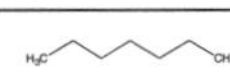	0.81
T2	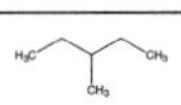	1.01	T6	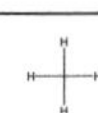	0.04
T3	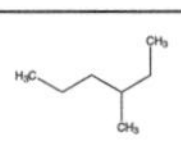	0.90	T7	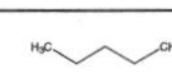	0.76
T4	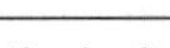	0.00	T8	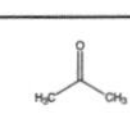	-0.15

Table 3. The structures and LogBB values of some compounds in the training/test sets.

Molecular modeling of a DMPC monolayer membrane complex with a layer of water. A model of dimyristoylphosphatidylcholine (DMPC) monolayer membrane was constructed using the software Material Studio, and minimized for 200 steps with the smart minimizer. The DMPC monolayer membrane was composed of 25 DMPC molecules ($5\times5\times1$). Here, the parameter of the single crystal of DMPC was a=8Å, b=8Å, and $\gamma=96.0$, which resulted average area of each lipid molecule 64Å^2 similar to Stouch's research results (Bassolino-Klimas et al, 1993). Moreover, we add a layer of water ($40\times40\times10$) including 529 water molecules to the polar side of the DMPC monolayer membrane. Figure 1 showed the dominant conformation of B1 compound colored by atom-type in water. The red box denotes the water solvent box defined in Monte Carlo simulation.

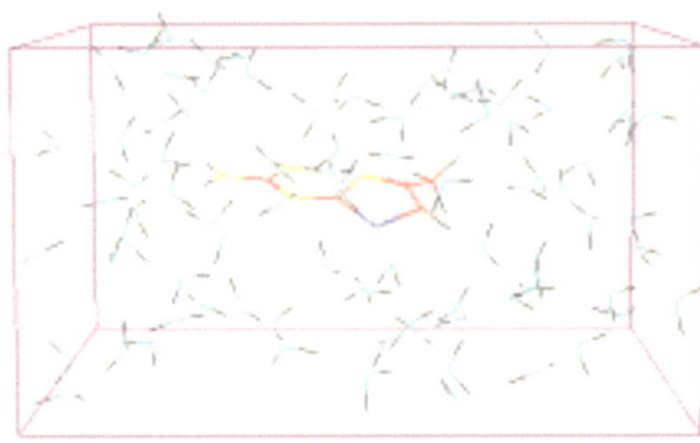

Figure 1. The dominant conformation of B1 compound colored by atom-type in water. The red box denotes the water solvent box defined in Monte Carlo simulation.

Molecular dynamic simulation of a small molecule complex with DMPC-water model. A DMPC molecule at the center of the above DMPC monolayer membrane complex with a layer of water was replaced with an organic compound to form a solute-membrane-water complex. The center organic compound was inserted at three different positions in the DMPC-water model before the start of each of the three corresponding molecular dynamics simulation. Molecular dynamic simulation of the complex was performed for 1000 steps by Discover module with Materials Studios, using Compass force field. Here, the three-dimensional volume was restricted to a border of X=40Å, Y=40Å, Z=91.76Å, and γ=96.0 .

QSAR model of BBB partitioning of some compounds. MI-QSAR model of some organic compounds through BBB are achieved by partial sum of squares for regression with software SPSS. A training set of 37 structurally diverse compounds whose BBB partition coefficients are measured is used to construct QSAR models. Molecular dynamics simulations are used to determine the explicit interaction of each test compound with a model of DMPC monolayer membrane complex with a layer of water. An additional set of intramolecular solute descriptors are computed and considered in the trial pool of descriptors for building MI-QSAR models. The QSAR models are optimized using multidimensional linear regression fitting and stepwise method. A test set of eight compounds is evaluated using the MI-QSAR models as part of a validation process.

3. Results

3.1. QSAR analysis based on MDR ratio in P388/VDR-20 and KB-A1 in vitro

Take MDR ratio in vitro in KB-A1/ADR cell lines as dependent variable and molecule descriptors as independent variable. A training set of 26 structurally diverse compounds (Table 4) was

http://dx.doi.org/10.5772/54975

used to construct QSAR models. The QSAR models were optimized using MLR fitting and stepwise method by the SPSS software (Eq.1-Eq.5). A test set of 5 compounds (compound A27-A31) was evaluated using the models as part of a validation process (figure 2 upper, Table 5).

Meanwhile, take MDR ratio in vitro in P388/VDR cell lines as dependent variable and molecule descriptors as independent variable. With the aid of Virtual Computational Chemistry Laboratory software (http://vcclab.org) (Wang et al, 2005), construct QSAR modeling by PLSR (Eg.6, figure 2 down). Table 6 shows the calculated descriptors mentioned above and the result of predicted value was in Table 5.

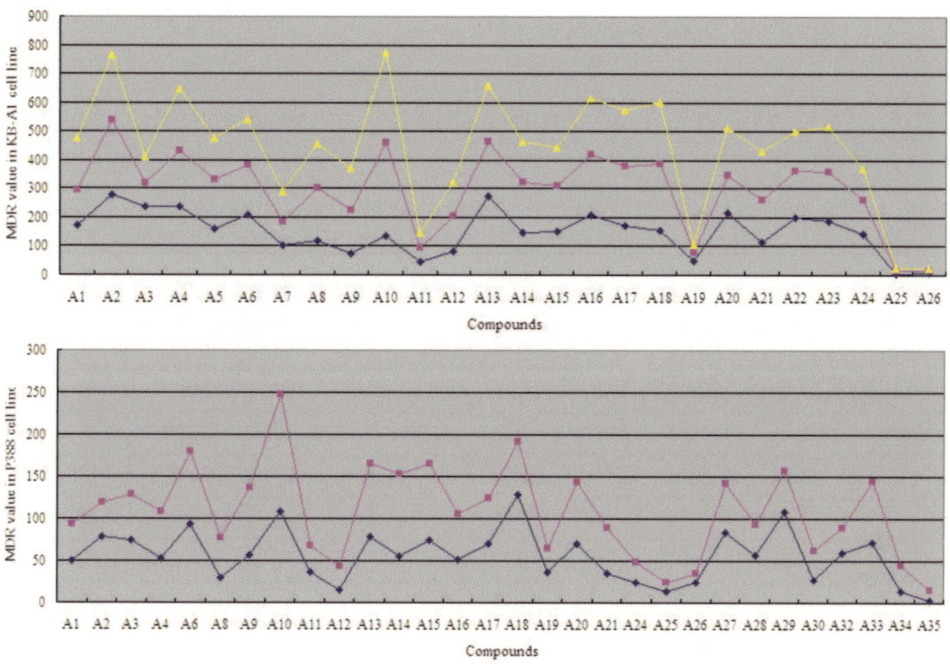

Figure 2. Comparison of the experimental MDR values with the corresponding predicted MDR values. Upper: MDR value in KB-A1/ADR cell lines (blue rhombic dots); MDR as predicted by Eg.4 MLR model (red square dots) and by Eg.5 MLR model (yellow triangle dots) for all the molecules of the training and test set. Down: MDR value in P388/VDR cell lines (blue rhombic dots); MDR as predicted by the method of PLSR (Eg. 6) (red square dots) for all the molecules of the training and test set. The rhombic dots represented the experimental values (P388) and the predicted values of MDR, respectively.

$$LogMDR = -6.537 + 7.162LogMR$$
$$N= 27; R= 0.445; F=6.187 \tag{1}$$

$$LogMDR = -37.830 + 48.862LogMR - 0.499ShA$$
$$N= 27; R= 0.889; F=45.415 \tag{2}$$

$$LogMDR = -35.816 + 52.416 LogMR - 0.717 \times ShA + 6.612 \times 10^{-7} BI$$
$$N= 27;\ R= 0.919;\ F=41.442 \quad (3)$$

$$LogMDR = -38.791 + 56.923 LogMR - 0.769 ShA + 5.897 \times 10^{-7} BI - 0.159 LogP$$
$$N = 27;\ R = 0.927;\ F = 33.504 \quad (4)$$

$$LogMDR = -42.192 + 61.818 LogMR -$$
$$-0.801 ShA + 4.791 \times 10^{-7} BI - 0.369 LogP + 3.595 \times 10^{-2} E_{hyd} \quad (5)$$
$$N= 27;\ R= 0.936;\ F=29.749$$

$$LogMDR = 7.611 + 3.138 \times 10^{-2} LogP - 0.245 MR + 0.495 E_{VDW} - 0.509 ShA + 8.802 \times 10^{-4} WI$$
$$N=30;\ Q^2=0.4650 \quad (6)$$

No.	Log MR	ShA	BI	LogP	E_{hyd} (kcal/mol)	No.	Log MR	ShA	BI	LogP	E_{hyd} (kcal/mol)
Training set											
A1	1.20	37.03	2662570	3.33	-3.56	A14	1.22	39.02	3358755	1.48	-19.64
A2	1.18	35.03	2440928	2.59	-13.71	A15	1.22	39.02	3358755	1.48	-19.71
A3	1.22	40.02	3649082	1.14	-16.23	A16	1.20	37.03	2662570	2.13	-15.99
A4	1.14	32.03	1669953	2.21	-13.54	A17	1.202	37.03	2662570	2.13	-16.23
A5	1.22	39.02	3358755	1.33	-19.71	A18	1.202	37.03	2662570	2.13	-15.95
A6	1.20	37.03	2662570	2.13	-16.22	A19	1.18	37.03	3091919	1.61	-15.9
A7	1.22	40.02	3491392	0.76	-17.67	A20	1.23	41.02	4008723	0.76	-17.36
A8	1.20	37.03	2662570	2.28	-16.3	A21	1.14	32.03	1651352	1.9	-13.79
A9	1.24	42.02	4491514	1.29	-16.34	A22	1.22	39.02	3324212	1.33	-20.06
A10	1.24	41.02	4055919	0.99	-19.77	A23	1.20	37.03	2634052	2.13	-15.77
A11	1.18	36.03	2271976	1.41	-17.73	A24	1.19	36.03	2246188	2.13	-16.15
A12	1.19	36.03	2271976	2.13	-16.17	A25	1.15	35.03	2244801	1.71	-14.88
A13	1.15	33.03	1900460	2.28	-13.57	A26	1.15	35.03	2271261	1.71	-15.03
Test set											
A27	1.19	37.03	2662570	1.41	-18.09	A30	1.25	41.02	3977672	2.98	-13.52
A28	1.22	40.02	3491392	0.76	-17.61	A31	1.20	37.03	2634052	2.13	-15.95
A29	1.21	37.03	2662570	2.75	-15.55						

Table 4. The molecular descriptors of some compounds related to MDR ratios in the training/test sets

No.	MDR ratio (KB-A1)	Predictive values of MDR ratio					No.	MDR ratio (KB-A1)	Predictive values of MDR ratio				
		Eq.1	Eq.2	Eq.3	Eq.4	Eq.5			Eq.1	Eq.2	Eq.3	Eq.4	Eq.5
Training set													
A1	171	114.32	215.61	200.33	123.15	180.87	A14	147	151.94	151.04	171.02	173.75	144.79
A2	278	80.79	200.54	305.22	260.52	228.39	A15	152	150.27	140.09	157.75	159.16	130.87
A3	238	161.08	71.37	78.37	79.12	92.55	A16	209	115.64	233.15	217.87	209.32	197.83
A4	236	44.84	113.11	178.94	196.99	213.61	A17	171	115.64	233.15	217.87	209.32	193.94
A5	160	150.27	140.09	157.75	168.14	148.66	A18	156	116.97	252.09	236.91	229.26	219.10
A6	208	113.02	199.36	184.18	174.42	159.21	A19	49	81.98	22.31	33.79	29.47	25.56
A7	102	163.01	77.39	67.24	80.67	105.63	A20	214	198.44	93.91	119.73	132.46	165.76
A8	120	114.32	215.61	200.33	180.88	153.75	A21	113	42.69	80.90	121.41	145.60	174.56
A9	75	237.62	101.82	179.28	149.94	146.81	A22	200	150.27	140.09	149.67	160.44	139.02
A10	136	222.49	204.96	297.19	322.30	315.82	A23	189	113.02	199.36	176.36	167.80	160.14
A11	44	79.86	58.80	41.66	49.61	53.08	A24	142	92.42	159.30	116.68	117.52	112.54
A12	83	92.42	159.30	121.35	121.70	115.60	A25	6	52.12	10.08	9.16	8.45	8.02
A13	272	53.80	124.41	185.32	190.50	197.66	A26	9	52.12	10.08	9.53	8.76	8.16
Testset													
A27	406	99.21	81.97	70.98	80.61	81.67	A30	370	243.10	375.08	504.47	282.78	192.47
A28	68	163.01	77.39	67.24	80.67	106.16	A31	210	114.32	215.61	191.82	183.83	174.21
A29	723	125.69	411.51	400.76	323.36	248.59							

Table 5. The experimental values and the predictive values of MDR ratio of these compounds.

No.	MDR (P388)	Pred MDR	LogP	MR	E_{VDW}	ShA	WI	No.	MDR (P388)	Pred MDR	LogP	MR	E_{VDW}	ShA	WI
A1	50	43.66	3.33	15.85	32.21	37.03	5476	A18	129	62.87	2.13	15.90	27.08	37.03	5476
A2	78	40.71	2.59	15.10	21.84	35.08	4872	A19	36	29.48	1.61	15.13	21.63	37.03	5585
A3	75	53.15	1.14	16.63	24.83	40.02	6522	A20	70	73.87	0.76	17.12	25.52	41.02	6855
A4	53	55.39	2.21	13.91	20.16	32.03	3916	A21	35	54.41	1.9	13.82	20.17	32.03	3874
A6	93	86.84	2.13	15.83	32.75	37.03	5476	A24	24	24.57	2.13	15.39	23.42	36.03	4855
A8	30	47.64	2.28	15.85	25.21	37.03	5476	A25	13	11.32	1.71	14.21	22.20	35.03	4487
A9	57	79.51	1.29	17.56	26.03	42.02	7353	A26	24	11.44	1.71	14.21	20.92	35.03	4538
A10	108	138.69	0.99	17.40	29.44	41.02	6935	A27	84	58.01	1.41	15.54	26.05	37.03	5476

No.	MDR (P388)	Pred MDR	LogP	MR	E_{VDW}	ShA	WI	No.	MDR (P388)	Pred MDR	LogP	MR	E_{VDW}	ShA	WI
A11	37	30.21	1.41	15.08	24.04	36.03	4909	A28	57	35.88	0.76	16.66	23.78	40.02	6244
A12	15	27.61	2.13	15.39	23.512	36.03	4909	A29	108	49.03	2.75	16.06	25.95	37.03	5476
A13	78	87.23	2.28	14.27	29.12	33.03	4216	A30	27	35.79	2.98	17.61	26.49	41.02	6804
A14	56	96.24	1.48	16.50	28.19	39.02	6288	A32	59	30.18	1.83	15.13	22.08	37.03	5642
A15	75	89.20	1.48	16.47	27.54	39.02	6288	A33	71	73.84	0.86	15.79	27.62	38.03	5822
A16	51	54.90	2.13	15.88	25.61	37.03	5476	A34	13	31.95	2.58	15.64	25.36	37.03	5476
A17	70	54.43	2.13	15.88	25.49	37.03	5476	A35	3	12.22	1.71	14.21	20.40	35.03	4589

Table 6. Comparison of experimental value of MDR ratio with predicted value of MDR ratio by PLSR.

3.2. QSAR analysis based on Ka of ATPase in CCRF ADR5000 cell lines

Similarly, take Ka of ATPase in CCRF ADR5000 cell lines as dependent variable and molecule descriptors as independent variable. We construct QSAR models using two methods, MLD method (Eq.7-Eq.11) and PLSR method (Eg.12) (see figure 3).

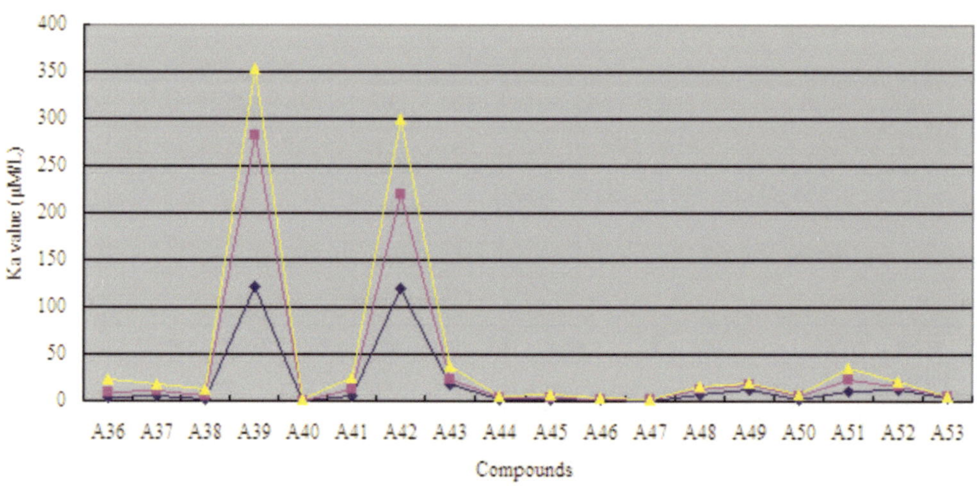

Figure 3. Comparison of the experimental Ka value (blue rhombic dots) with the corresponding predicted Ka as predicted by Eg.11 MLR model (red square dats) and by Eg.12 PLSR model (yellow triangle dots) for all the molecules of the training and test.

A training set of 16 structurally diverse compounds was used to construct QSAR models. All the molecular descriptors were calculated as Table 7. The QSAR models were optimized using MLR fitting and stepwise method. A test set of 2 compounds was evaluated using the models as part of a validation process. Table 8 displays the comparison of the experiment and prediction value.

http://dx.doi.org/10.5772/54975

$$LogKa = 2.424 - 0.484LogP$$
N= 16; R= 0.860; F=39.748 (7)

$$LogKa = 3.612 - 0.285LogP - 0.0732ShA$$
N= 16; R= 0.900; F=27.676 (8)

$$LogKa = 2.573 - 0.480LogP - 0.285ShA + 0.651MR$$
N= 16; R= 0.914; F=20.251 (9)

$$LogKa = 7.313 - 0.752LogP - 0.647ShA + 1.642MR + 0.605E_{HOMO}$$
N= 16; R= 0.928; F=17.111 (10)

$$LogKa = 10.021 - 0.875LogP - 1.044ShA + 2.263MR + 0.673E_{HOMO} + 6.734 \times 10^{-4} WI$$
N= 16; R=0.945; F=16.832 (11)

$$LogKa = 3.662 - 0.279LogP - 4.71 \times 10^{-3} MW + 1.223 \times 10^{-2} E_{HOMO}$$
N=18, Q^2=0.7100 (12)

No.	LogP	ShA	MR	E_{HOMO} (eV)	WI	MW	No.	LogP	ShA	MR	E_{HOMO} (eV)	WI	MW
A36	3.39	21.04	9.254	-9.14	1366	312.41	A45	4.3	26.04	11.42	-9.17	2345	383.53
A37	3.62	24.04	10.55	-9.20	1949	355.48	A46	4.93	32.03	13.27	-8.24	4689	462.57
A38	3.67	25.04	10.84	-9.16	2172	367.49	A47	5.2	32.03	13.38	-8.19	4329	464.58
A39	1.42	18.05	7.86	-9.12	920	277.37	A48	4.25	26.04	11.45	-9.24	2607	383.53
A40	4.93	32.03	13.27	-8.16	4329	462.57	A49	4.52	26.04	11.59	-8.94	2367	385.55
A41	2.67	25.04	10.29	-8.15	2244	372.44	A50	4.88	27.03	12.06	-8.94	2550	399.58
A42	0.94	19.05	8.01	-9.15	1050	293.37	A51	2.38	26.04	10.99	-9.09	2400	383.49
A43	2.54	25.04	10.52	-9.20	2172	369.46	A52	3.94	25.04	10.95	-9.05	2172	369.51
A44	3.98	32.03	13.50	-9.16	4227	459.59	A53	4.93	32.03	13.27	-8.19	4509	462.57

Table 7. The molecular descriptors of some compounds related to ATPase in the training/test sets.

No.	Ka (μM/L)	Predictive values of Ka						No.	Ka (μM/L)	Predictive values of Ka					
Eg.7	Eg.8	Eg.9	Eg.10	Eg.11	Eg.12	Eg.7	Eg.8	Eg.9	Eg.10	Eg.11	Eg.12				
A36	3.34	6.07	12.75	9.37	6.43	6.14	13.57	A45	1.53	2.20	3.02	3.32	2.69	2.08	3.50
A37	5.30	4.70	6.62	7.10	6.19	5.60	7.33	A46	1.47	1.09	0.73	0.52	0.48	0.81	1.02
A38	2.59	4.44	5.41	5.36	3.98	3.06	6.24	A47	0.55	0.81	0.61	0.46	0.50	0.53	0.84
A39	122	54.54	76.92	73.09	90.64	160.46	70.37	A48	7.64	2.33	3.13	3.83	3.33	4.22	3.60
A40	0.36	1.09	0.73	0.52	0.53	0.51	1.02	A49	12.20	1.72	2.62	3.39	4.98	5.00	2.99
A41	6.13	13.54	10.43	7.17	11.79	7.23	11.56	A50	2.26	1.15	1.75	2.37	3.50	3.28	2.04
A42	120.00	93.12	89.09	81.21	80.47	99.37	80.44	A51	10.50	18.71	10.66	14.57	16.6	13.20	12.02
A43	18.50	15.65	11.36	11.73	8.26	5.56	12.59	A52	12.80	3.29	4.53	4.74	4.57	3.91	5.15
A44	1.01	3.15	1.36	2.10	1.66	2.13	1.88	A53	4.15	1.09	0.73	0.52	0.51	0.65	1.02

Table 8. Comparison the experimental values with the predictive values of Ka of these compounds.

3.3. QSAR analysis based on blood-brain barrier partitioning of organic compounds

37 organic compounds of training set and 8 compounds of test set are built and minimized, dissolved in liquid, and are optimized by Monte Carlo method and molecular mechanism, finally the dominant conformation of these compounds are obtained. Molecular modeling of a small molecule complex with the membrane-water model reveals that the energy of an organic compound inserted at the middle position in the DMPC model with a layer of water is lower than that of the other two positions. MI-QSAR analysis has been used to develop predictive models of some organic compounds through BBB, in part, simulating the interaction of an organic compound with the phospholipide-rich regions of cellular membranes surrounding by a layer of water. Molecular descriptors of compounds in a training set and a test set are listed in Table 9. Six QSAR equations were constructed based on Table 9 and were listed as follows.

$$\log BB = 0.552 - 1.73 \times 10^{-2} PSA \qquad (13)$$
$$n = 37 \quad R = 0.835 \quad S = 0.398$$

$$\log BB = 0.229 - 1.70 \times 10^{-2} PSA + 0.131 C\log P \qquad (14)$$
$$n = 37 \quad R = 0.878 \quad S = 0.352$$

$$\log BB = 4.965 \times 10^{-2} - 1.28 \times 10^{-2} PSA + 0.211 C\log P - 6.40 \times 10^{-7} BI \qquad (15)$$
$$n = 37 \quad R = 0.924 \quad S = 0.285$$

$$\log BB = 6.262\times10^{-2} - 1.36\times10^{-2} PSA + 0.205C\log P - 7.11\times10^{-7} BI - 0.185E_{stretch}$$
$$n = 37 \quad R = 0.938 \quad S = 0.264 \tag{16}$$

$$\log BB = 6.580\times10^{-2} - 1.21\times10^{-2} PSA + 0.206C\log P - 7.77\times10^{-7} BI - 0.197E_{stretch} +$$
$$+1.330\times10^{-3}\Delta E_{total} \tag{17}$$
$$n = 37 \quad R = 0.947 \quad S = 0.248$$

$$\log BB = 8.730\times10^{-2} - 1.04\times10^{-2} PSA + 0.222C\log P - 9.60\times10^{-7} BI - 0.183E_{stretch} +$$
$$+1.364\times10^{-3}\Delta E_{total} - 2.68\times10^{-3}\Delta E_{torsion} \tag{18}$$
$$n = 37 \quad R = 0.955 \quad S^2 = 0.232$$

Here, n means the number of compounds in a training set, R means the correlative coefficient, and S means the standard residual error. Log BB = log (C_{brain}/C_{blood}). PSA means the total polar surface area of a molecule. CLogP and BI display calculated LogP and connective index of molecular average total distance (relative covalent radius), respectively. They come from CS calculation. ΔE_{total} and $\Delta E_{torsion}$ are related to interaction between an organic compound and membrane-water model. The total energy and the torsion energy of the DMPC monolayer membrane complex with a layer of water are -340.7589 and -1724.4164 (Kcal/mol), respectively. ΔE_{total} is the change in the total potential energy of the solute-membrane-water complex comparing with that of the membrane-water model and so is $\Delta E_{torsion}$.

No	PSA (Å²)	ClogP	BI(Å)	$E_{stretch}$ (Kcal/mol)	E_{total} [a] (Kcal/mol)	$E_{torsion}$ [a] (Kcal/mol)	ΔE_{total} [b] (Kcal/mol)	$\Delta E_{torsion}$ [b] (Kcal/mol)
				Training set				
B1	78.90	1.20	12378	-1.35503	-298.2972	-1713.1146	42.46	11.30
B2	94.00	1.99	1101758	-0.15595	-406.0803	-1789.8084	-65.32	-65.39
B3	73.00	3.80	1738650	-1.48472	-256.3021	-1703.1425	84.46	21.27
B4	87.00	1.63	1346396	-1.39112	-302.7543	-1841.5635	38.00	-117.15
B5	39.00	1.02	41807	0.58131	-226.3773	-1734.7452	114.38	-10.33
B6	26.80	3.23	305770	-0.09264	-228.2923	-1679.4604	112.47	44.96
B7	88.80	1.01	58510	0.71038	-279.0781	-1671.3414	61.68	53.07
B8	76.60	2.80	62216	-0.38334	-309.2981	-1654.6730	31.46	69.74

No	PSA (Å²)	ClogP	BI(Å)	$E_{stretch}$ (Kcal/mol)	E_{total} [a] (Kcal/mol)	$E_{torsion}$ [a] (Kcal/mol)	ΔE_{total} [b] (Kcal/mol)	$\Delta E_{torsion}$ [b] (Kcal/mol)
				Training set				
B9	104.40	1.77	83798	-0.35599	-313.4237	-1639.9898	27.34	84.43
B10	108.80	2.00	193593	-0.52172	-548.5593	-1640.9214	-207.80	83.49
B11	47.90	2.51	352512	-0.09496	-312.1226	-1656.7465	28.64	67.67
B12	45.20	4.27	779210	0.00479	-163.8011	-1716.3101	176.96	8.11
B13	38.50	2.61	158640	-0.09491	-170.3338	-1716.7159	170.43	7.70
B14	40.00	4.28	431722	-1.30506	-247.0951	-1748.0241	93.66	-23.61
B15	39.20	5.88	766256	0.09911	-289.2825	-1735.4004	51.48	-10.98
B16	54.90	5.14	766256	-0.14215	-181.0636	-1743.6068	159.70	-19.19
B17	18.80	0.62	20863	0.18071	-331.7044	-1695.6999	9.05	28.72
B18	46.70	0.27	20264	-1.36843	-209.4697	-1644.6752	131.29	79.74
B19	44.10	2.80	190375	-2.97778	-311.9182	-1713.8942	28.84	10.52
B20	5.40	4.85	210631	-0.06079	-235.7250	-1704.3399	105.03	20.08
B21	0.00	-0.47	4	0.00000	-407.3194	-1729.3793	-66.56	-4.96
B22	0.00	2.14	972	-0.00009	-239.8807	-1675.1827	100.88	49.23
B23	23.40	0.07	213	0.00000	-160.1278	-1672.3898	180.63	52.03
B24	22.60	0.69	712	0.00000	-319.0674	-1742.6968	21.69	-18.28
B25	0.00	3.74	1899	0.00067	-282.3721	-1751.6193	58.39	-27.20
B26	0.00	3.61	1661	0.00000	-285.7132	-1731.9518	55.05	-7.54
B27	0.00	1.43	1661	-0.00008	-238.7249	-1731.3090	102.03	-6.89
B28	0.00	2.48	633	0.00003	-291.5583	-1725.7370	49.20	-1.32
B29	11.60	2.46	21380	-0.00005	-418.0323	-1682.7138	-77.27	41.70
B30	24.40	-0.24	47	0.00000	-329.3150	-1704.6187	11.44	19.80
B31	10.70	1.27	7864	-0.00002	-253.3453	-1747.7044	87.41	-23.29
B32	0.00	2.37	7322	-0.00003	-268.8335	-1714.2486	71.93	10.17
B33	0.00	3.31	931	0.02567	-353.8395	-1739.7672	-13.08	-15.35
B34	24.40	-0.24	47	0.00000	-187.4520	-1720.5500	153.31	3.87
B35	0.00	1.93	7322	-0.00003	-177.4875	-1728.8621	163.27	-4.45

http://dx.doi.org/10.5772/54975

No	PSA (Å²)	ClogP	BI(Å)	$E_{stretch}$ (Kcal/mol)	E_{total} [a] (Kcal/mol)	$E_{torsion}$ [a] (Kcal/mol)	ΔE_{total} [b] (Kcal/mol)	$\Delta E_{torsion}$ [b] (Kcal/mol)
				Training set				
B36	0.00	2.64	2050	-0.02344	-220.3940	-1681.1548	120.36	43.26
B37	0.00	2.63	712	-0.00002	-231.5752	-1722.2582	109.18	2.16
				Test set				
T1	22.70	0.321	712	0.00000	-274.7201	-1713.7409	66.04	10.68
T2	0.00	3.738	1838	0.00000	-225.6308	-1716.6234	115.13	7.79
T3	0.00	4.267	4150	0.00000	-331.3754	-1700.6397	9.38	23.78
T4	11.30	0.870	791	0.00000	-181.5954	-1700.8447	159.16	23.57
T5	0.00	4.397	4650	0.00000	-404.2903	-1741.2420	-63.53	-16.83
T6	0.00	1.103	0	0.00000	-282.9386	-1746.1889	57.82	-21.77
T7	0.00	3.339	791	0.00063	-271.9174	-1681.9440	68.84	42.47
T8	22.70	-0.208	213	0.00000	-364.8884	-1695.3605	-24.13	29.06

Note: [a] E_{total} and $E_{torsion}$ mean the total energy and the torsion energy of the complex with an organic compound and DMPC monolayer membrane. [b] The total energy and the torsion energy of the DMPC monolayer membrane are -340.758901 and -1724.416387 (Kcal/mol). ΔE_{total} and $\Delta E_{torsion}$ are the residues between a complex of an organic compound with DMPC monolayer membrane and the DMPC monolayer membrane.

Table 9. The molecular descriptors of the compounds related to BBB in the training/test sets

With the increase of the variable from one to six, the relativity of QSAR equation is also improved, and the predictive ability of the model is enhanced. Eq.18 is most significant, which means that the capability of an organic compound through BBB depends upon PSA, ClogP, BI, $E_{stretch}$, ΔE_{total}, and $\Delta E_{torsion}$. Moreover, the potential of an organic compound through BBB is directly proportional to ClogP and ΔE_{total}, but inversely proportional to PSA, BI, $E_{stretch}$, and $\Delta E_{torsion}$. The observed and predicted log BB values of the training set compounds are listed in Table 10. Figure 4 shows the comparison of the experimental log BB values for all the molecules of the training set with the corresponding predicted log BB as predicted by Eg.17 and -18 MI-QSAR models. Compound B18 in the training set is predicted to have a much higher log BB than observed, and this molecule has also been identified as an outlier in other studies (Iyer et al, 2002). Protonation of the molecule could account for its low log BB value.

A test set of eight solute compounds was constructed as one way to attempt to validate the QSAR models given by six equations mentioned. The test set compounds were selected so as to span almost the entire range in BBB partitioning. The observed and predicted log BB values for this test set are given in Table 10 and plotted in Figure 4 (right). It seems to suggest that Eg. 17and -18 QSAR models could predict log BB for other compounds in drug design.

No	LogBB	Predictive Value of logBB						No	LogBB	Predictive Value of logBB					
		Eg.13	Eg.14	Eg.15	Eg.16	Eg.17	Eg.18			Eg.13	Eg.14	Eg.15	Eg.16	Eg.17	Eg.18
Training set															
B1	-0.04	-0.81	-0.95	-0.71	-0.52	-0.33	-0.20	B20	0.85	0.46	0.77	0.87	0.85	0.99	1.01
B2	-2.00	-1.07	-1.11	-1.44	-1.56	-1.57	-1.39	B21	0.03	0.55	0.17	-0.05	-0.03	-0.12	-0.10
B3	-1.30	-0.71	-0.51	-1.20	-1.11	-0.98	-1.17	B22	0.37	0.55	0.51	0.50	0.50	0.64	0.57
B4	-1.06	-0.95	-1.04	-1.58	-1.49	-1.37	-1.13	B23	-0.15	0.15	-0.16	-0.23	-0.24	0.04	-0.03
B5	0.11	-0.12	-0.30	-0.26	-0.40	-0.19	-0.06	B24	-0.17	0.16	-0.06	-0.09	-0.10	-0.04	0.08
B6	0.49	0.09	0.20	0.19	0.16	0.34	0.28	B25	0.97	0.55	0.72	0.84	0.83	0.91	1.07
B7	-1.17	-0.98	-1.15	-0.91	-1.11	-0.90	-0.86	B26	1.04	0.55	0.70	0.81	0.80	0.88	0.98
B8	-0.18	-0.77	-0.71	-0.38	-0.38	-0.22	-0.22	B27	0.08	0.55	0.42	0.35	0.35	0.49	0.56
B9	-1.15	-1.25	-1.31	-0.97	-0.99	-0.79	-0.81	B28	0.40	0.55	0.55	0.57	0.57	0.64	0.71
B10	-1.57	-1.33	-1.36	-1.05	-1.05	-1.16	-1.20	B29	0.24	0.35	0.35	0.41	0.39	0.31	0.27
B11	-0.46	-0.28	-0.26	-0.26	-0.31	-0.21	-0.32	B30	-0.16	0.13	-0.22	-0.31	-0.32	-0.26	-0.26
B12	-0.24	-0.23	0.02	-0.13	-0.23	0.03	0.04	B31	0.13	0.37	0.21	0.18	0.17	0.31	0.43
B13	-0.02	-0.11	-0.08	0.01	-0.02	0.26	0.34	B32	0.35	0.55	0.54	0.55	0.54	0.64	0.68
B14	0.44	-0.14	0.11	0.17	0.33	0.51	0.64	B33	0.93	0.55	0.66	0.75	0.74	0.73	0.84
B15	0.14	-0.13	0.33	0.30	0.17	0.26	0.33	B34	-0.16	0.13	-0.22	-0.31	-0.32	-0.07	-0.02
B16	0.22	-0.40	-0.03	-0.06	-0.15	0.10	0.22	B35	0.27	0.55	0.48	0.45	0.45	0.68	0.74
B17	-0.06	0.23	-0.01	-0.07	-0.11	-0.07	-0.09	B36	0.37	0.55	0.57	0.61	0.61	0.77	0.72
B18	-1.40	-0.26	-0.53	-0.50	-0.28	-0.02	-0.14	B37	0.34	0.55	0.57	0.60	0.60	0.75	0.81
B19	0.25	-0.21	-0.15	-0.05	0.45	0.59	0.62								
Test set															
T1	-0.08	0.16	-0.11	-0.17	-0.18	-0.06	-0.02	T5	0.81	0.55	0.81	0.97	0.96	0.88	1.02
T2	1.01	0.55	0.72	0.84	0.83	0.99	1.05	T6	0.04	0.55	0.37	0.28	0.29	0.37	0.47
T3	0.90	0.55	0.79	0.95	0.93	0.95	0.98	T7	0.76	0.55	0.67	0.75	0.75	0.84	0.81
T4	0.00	0.36	0.15	0.09	0.09	0.32	0.32	T8	-0.15	0.16	-0.18	-0.28	-0.29	-0.28	-0.31

Table 10. The experimental values and the predictive values of LogBB of these compounds.

http://dx.doi.org/10.5772/54975

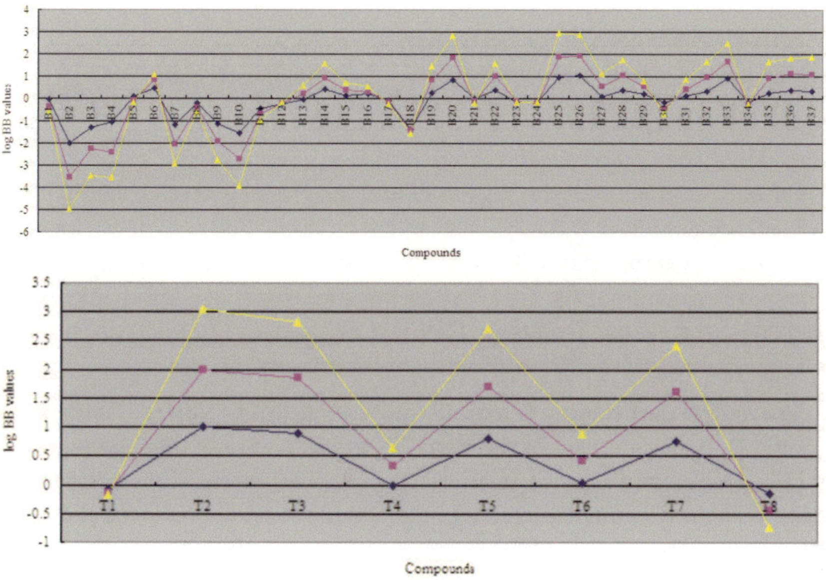

Figure 4. Comparison of the experimental log BB values (blue rhombic dots) for all the molecules of the training sets (upper) or the test set (down) to the corresponding predicted log BB as predicted by Eg.17 MI-QSAR model (red square dots) and by Eg.18 MI-QSAR model (yellow triangle dots).

4. Discussion

We have built some predictive models of MDR, Ka and BBB partitioning of organic compounds by simulating the interaction of modulators or drugs interact with P-gp and/or of an organic compound with the phospholipide-rich regions of cellular membranes. As we know in the introduction part, modulators or drugs interact with P-gp and thus reduce the efflux of the cytotoxic compounds will increase the apparent toxicity of the cytotoxic compounds. It is very important to keep in mind that it is based on a general assessment of cytotoxicity and thus may account for more than one acting mechanism in the resistant cells used. So there are many uncertainty factors in the MDR ratio assay method and it is also convinced by our linear regression models. Our research results using two different statistic methods, MLR and PLSR, have revealed that the QSAR equation was also improved and the predictive ability of the models was enhanced with the increase of the variable. Eg.5 is built on KB-A1 cell line with a cytotoxic compound of 2.5μM ADR while Eg.6 is based on P388/VDR-20 cell line with 1.5μM VCR. Here, most of the models gave satisfactory cross-validated Q^2 above 0.500, conventional R above 0.800 and less SE values indicating their proper predictive ability. Significant differences between values were examined using two-tailed paired T test provided by SPSS. All the results were considered not significant if $P<0.05$. Eg.5 model is the most significant and indicated that the capability of P-gp modulators interacted with P-gp depends upon MR, BI, E_{hyd}, ShA, and LogP. The former three display positive contributions to the MDR activity of P-gp, suggesting that the MDR activity increase accordingly with MR increase. The latter two displays negative contribution to the MDR activity of P-gp.

On the other hand, we have built the predicted models for Ka of ATPase of some compounds using the same statistic methods in order to get a more accurate model. Both models, Eg.11 by MLR and Eg.12 by PLSR, point out that LogP and E_{HOMO} are both important parameters with the affinity for and simulation of the P-gp ATPase. LogP is negative related with the activity of P-gp ATPase, suggesting that the ATPase activity also decrease with the increase of LogP. Figure 3 showed that molecular A39 and A42 have higher Ka value of ATPase and is a departure from other compounds. This may be because they have lower lipophilicity, which is supported by the research results of Diethart Schmid et al (1999). Another significant descriptor E_{HOMO} is positive related with the activity of P-gp ATPase.

In another aspect, BBB partitioning is mainly found to depend upon two parameters, namely PSA and ClogP. With the increase of the variable, the relativity of QSAR equation is also improved, and the predictive ability of the model is enhanced, especially Eq.18 most significant. Moreover, the BBB partitioning measures of the test set compounds were predicted with the same accuracy as the compounds of the training set. The family of these QSAR models reveal that the capability of BBB partitioning of an organic compound focus on six significant features, which are PSA, ClogP, BI, $E_{stretch}$, ΔE_{total}, and $\Delta E_{torsion}$ (Eg. 18). Obviously, two of the six descriptors of the QSAR models have positive regression coefficients and the other four descriptors have negative regression coefficients. The potential of an organic compound through BBB is directly proportional to ClogP and ΔE_{total}, but inversely proportional to PSA, BI, $E_{stretch}$, and $\Delta E_{torsion}$. Moreover, PSA descriptor is found as a dominant descriptor in these QSAR models, which related to the aqueous solubility of the solute compound along with a direct lipophilicity descriptor (Clark et al, 1999). When the value of PSA of a molecule lessens within the range from 0 to 108.80 Å^2, its value of LogBB will increase. This is consistent with the experimental results that the more polarity it possesses, the more difficultly a molecule enters the hydrophobic environment of BBB (Stouch, 1993). BI is the connective index of molecular average total distance, which pertains to the volume parameter. Our research result points it out that with the accretion of its bulk, a molecule more and more difficultly across through BBB by diffusion. However, the value of LogBB of a molecule increases with the increase of ClogP. It means that the hydrophobic molecule can pass through BBB more easily than the hydrophilic molecule does, which is supported by the experimental results (Kaliszan & Markuszewski, 1996). The presence of $E_{stretch}$ descriptor suggests that with the decrease of the stretch-bend energy of a molecule, its value of LogBB increases. Two of the descriptors, found in the log BB QSAR models (Eg.17 and Eq.18), reflect the behavior of the solute in the membrane and the entire membrane-solute complex. Along with the meaning mentioned, ΔE_{total} is equivalent to the change in average total potential energy between the triple member complex and the double member complex. Similarly, $\Delta E_{torsion}$ is the difference between the dihedral torsion energy of the triple complex and that of the double complex. Here, the more the change value of ΔE_{total} is, the more its value of LogBB increases. This is because small molecule across BBB membrane leads to the change of the structure of the complex. The more changeability of the structure results in greater change of total potential energy, while the accretion of the energy change is the important cause of the increase of the capability of a small molecule through BBB. On the contrary, the less the difference of the torsion energy is, the

http://dx.doi.org/10.5772/54975

larger its value of LogBB is. It displays that a small molecule tight combining with the membrane-water complex leads to increase its value of LogBB. And the relationship would suggest that as the solute becomes more flexible within the membrane-water complex, the greater would be its log BB value, which is in agreement with the research results of Iyer M et al (2002).

Several non-MI-QSAR computational models to describe and predict BBB partitioning have been reported that includes other descriptors besides PSA and ClogP (Lombardo et al, 1996; Keseru & Molnar, 2001; Crivori et al, 2000). An alternative, complementary approach to BBB partitioning prediction uses MI-QSAR analysis developed by Iyer M et al (2002). Their research results show that BBB partitioning of an organic compound depend upon PSA, CLogP, and the conformational flexibility of the compounds as well as the strength of their "binding" to the model biologic membrane. The MI-QSAR models indicate that BBB partitioning process can be reliably described for structurally diverse molecules provided interactions of the molecule with the phospholipide-rich regions of cellular membranes are explicitly considered. An extension of these approaches that combines QSAR with solute-membrane-water complex has been developed by us, which is addition of a layer of water on the hydrophilic side of DMPC monolayer membrane in our research. And so, it is more analogous to the truth BBB environment. Our results reveal that the distribution of organic molecules through BBB was not only influenced by the properties of organic solutes, but also related to the property of the solute-membrane-water complex. The former involves the polarity, hydrophobic, size, and conformational freedom degree of organic molecules. The latter deals with the strength of an organic molecule combined with BBB membrane and the structural changeability of a solute-membrane-water complex. Furthermore, the capability of a small molecule across BBB is mainly related to four physicochemical factors, which depend on the relative polarity of a small molecule, the molecular volume, the strength of a small molecule combined with DMPC-water model, and the changeability of the structure of a solute-membrane-water complex. The relative polarity of a small molecule includes two parameters, namely PSA and ClogP. The QSAR model shows that less polarity and more hydrophobic molecules relatively easily pass through BBB and enter brain to cure. The molecular volume involves one parameter, namely BI. The strength of a small molecule combined with DMPC monolayer membrane complex with a layer of water involves one parameter, namely $\Delta E_{torsion}$. The changeability of the structure of a complex between a small molecule and the membrane-water complex includes one parameter, namely ΔE_{total}. The reason for the change of total energy is that small molecule across BBB membrane leads to the change of the structure of the solute-membrane-water complex. The more the changeability of the complex structure is, the more the change value of total energy is, and the more easily a small molecule penetrates BBB.

Cerebral clearance of Aβ is considered to occur via elimination across BBB, as well as proteolytic degradation. Attenuation of its elimination is likely to result in increased cerebral Aβ deposition, which may facilitate progression of AD (Ohtsuki et al, 2010). P-gp detoxifies cells by exporting hundreds of chemically unrelated toxins but has been implicated in MDR in the treatment of cancers. Substrate promiscuity is a hallmark of P-gp activity, thus a structural description of poly-specific drug-binding is important for the rational design of anti-amyloid accumulation drugs, anticancer drugs and MDR inhibitors. The x-ray structure of apo P-gp at

3.8 angstroms reveals an internal cavity of approximately 6000 angstroms cubed with a 30 angstrom separation of the two nucleotide-binding domains. Two additional P-gp structures with cyclic peptide inhibitors demonstrate distinct drug-binding sites in the internal cavity capable of stereoselectivity that is based on hydrophobic and aromatic interactions. Apo and drug-bound P-gp structures have portals open to the cytoplasm and the inner leaflet of the lipid bilayer for drug entry. The inward-facing conformation represents an initial stage of the transport cycle that is competent for drug binding (Aller et al, 2009). Currently, P-gp is identificated as an energy-dependent pump, ATPase activity as an assay in itself is possibly problematical cause it is based upon one assumption that drug-induced ATP hydrolysis reflects transport by the transporter (Stouch & Gudmundsson, 2001). There may be many ways in which this activity could be altered, including direct action on the ATP binding domain. Scientists once observed some compounds such as daunomycin and vinblastine inhibit ATPase activity, but increase in others, suggesting that modulation of ATPase activity is highly dependent on experimental conditions and may not correlate well with the ability of P-gp to transport the drug (Ambudkar et al, 1992; Shapiro & Ling, 1994; Doige et al, 1993). The work of Litman et al was one of the few studies suggesting that affinity between drugs and ATPase activity has no correlation to LogP, but Surface Area (Litman et al, 1997). Because of the less comparability of molecular structures in a training set, our QSAR equation possesses universal significance. However, the precision of QSAR equation is so low that there is still a distance to its application. So a series of organic compounds with similar structures are chosen and consist of a training set, thus the precision of QSAR simulation is largely increased, while the prediction of the analogues through BBB is greatly improved.

5. Conclusion

P-gp is involved in MDR and in neurodegenerative disorders such as Parkinson disease, AD and epilepsy. The xenobiotic efflux pump P-gp limits intracellular drug accumulation by active extrusion of compounds out of cells. P-gp mediates the efflux of Aβ from the brain together with mediating MDR, while P-gp transports neutral or positively-charged hydrophobic substrates with consuming energy from ATP hydrolysis. We have built up theoretical models of the interaction between organic compounds and P-gp and compounds with the affinity for and simulation of the P-gp ATPase. The interaction between compounds and p-gp (P-gp binding or MDR-reversal activity of compounds) is found to depend on LogP, LogMR, and ShA of compounds it transports, which proportional to LogMR while inversely proportional to LogP and ShA (see Eg.1 to Eg.5). Until now we have not convinced that ATPase activity of P-gp is well correlated with the ability of P-gp to transport the drugs. However, our constructed model based on the analogies of purine and propafenone analogs suggests that the enzyme hydrolysis of these compounds largely depends on LogP, MR, ShA, MW and E_{HOMO}, especially positive related to MR but negative to LogP and ShA (see Eg.7 to Eq.11). This shows that the P-gp binding capacity of these compounds shares common characteristics with their ATPase hydrolysis, namely their hydrophobic parameters (such as log P) and steric parameters (eg. MW, ShA, MR, and WI).

Additionally, our constructed MI-QSAR model indicates that the distribution of organic molecules through BBB was not only influenced by organic solutes themselves, but also related to the properties of the solute-membrane water complex, namely interactions of the molecule with the phospholipide-rich regions of cellular membranes. Moreover, our results reveal that the ability of organic molecules permeating across BBB is proportional to LogP but inversely proportional to PSA (see Eg.13 to 18), which is consistent with the research results of Chen and co-worker (2009), namely the increasing PSA decreased LogBB rapidly while LogP positively related to LogBB. It indicates that molecules with higher lipophilic will be partitioned into the lipid bilayer more easily with more chances to penetrate BBB, supported by the research result of Wang et al (2003), namely a large number of structurally and functionally diverse compounds as substrates or modulators of P-gp mostly sharing common structural features, such as aromatic ring structures and high lipophilicity. PSA of CNS active drug should be lower than 90 Å^2 (Chen et al, 2009), while the penetration through the BBB is optimal for LogP value in the range 1.5–2.7 (Norinder & Haeberlein, 2002).

In comparison with the ability of organic molecules permeating across BBB, P-gp binding or MDR-reversal activity of compounds has a negative correlation with LogP. There are two reasons for this phenomenon. Firstly, the compounds with higher liposolubility are more vulnerable to cytochrome P450 metabolism, leading to faster clearance (Waterhouse, 2003). P450 enzymes (CYP450s) catalyze the metabolism of a wide variety of endogenous and

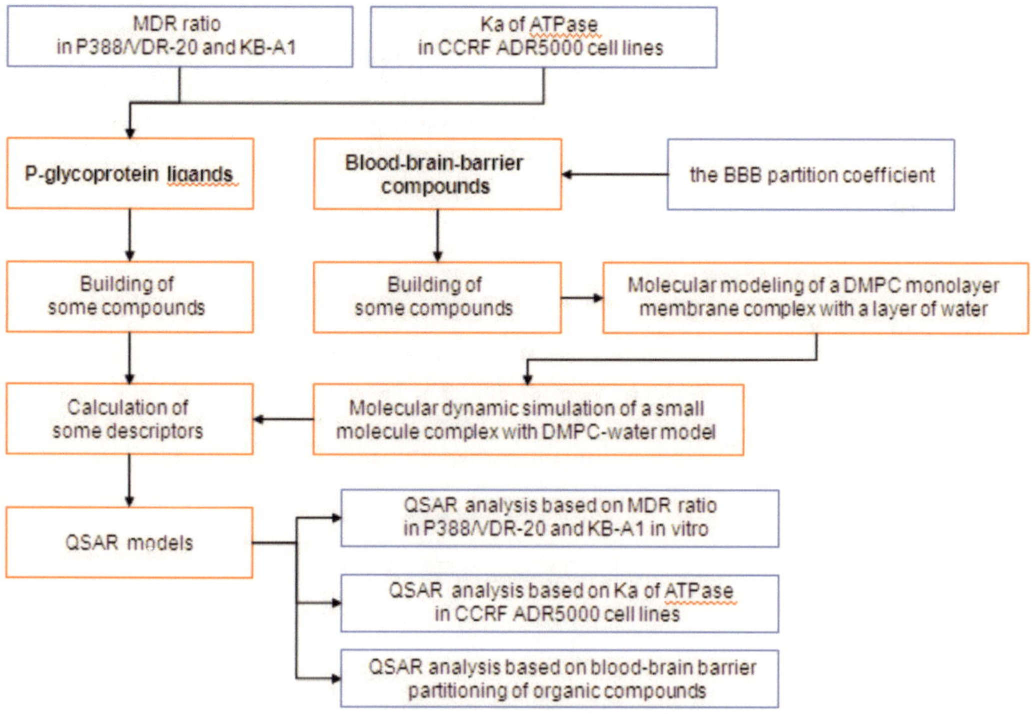

Scheme 1. Flowchart for QSAR analysis of some substrates of P-glycoprotein targeting β-amyloid clearance.

exogenous compounds including xenobiotics, drugs, environmental toxins, steroids, and fatty acids. Aminated thioxanthones have recently been reported as P-gp inhibitors as well as its interaction with cytochrome P450 3A4 (CYP3A4), as many substrates of P-glycoprotein and CYP3A4 are common (Palmeira et al, 2012). The second reason is related to the mechanism of P-gp action. According to model proposed by Higgins and Gottesman (1992), after entering into the phospholipid bilayer, compound may interact with P-gp in the inner leaflet of the lipid bilayer. Upon interaction with P-gp, the compound is flipped from the inner leaflet to the outer leaflet of the lipid bilayer. The lipophilic compounds with high LogP enter into cellular membrane easily and intend to retain there, so its opportunity to interact with P-gp increases. The LogP not only offers opportunity to penetrate the lipid bilayer, but also gives favorable contribution to binding with protein, such as P450, P-gp.

In conclusion, the predictive model of BBB partitioning of organic compounds contributes to discovery of some molecules through BBB as potential AD therapeutic drugs. Moreover, the interaction model of P-gp and modulators for treatment of multidrug resistance indicates discovery of some molecules to increase Aβ clearance from the brain and reduce Aβ brain accumulation by regulate BBB P-gp in the early stages of AD. The mechanism suggests new therapeutic strategy in AD.

Acknowledgements

This work was supported by a grant from Basic Scientific Research Expenses of Central University (020814360012), National Key Technology R&D Program (2008BAI51B01) and Specialized Research Fund for the Doctoral Program of Higher Education (20120091110038).

Author details

Jie Yang* and Jie Chen

*Address all correspondence to: luckyjyj@sina.com.cn

State Key Laboratory of Pharmaceutical Biotechnology, Life College, Nanjing University, Nanjing, China

References

[1] Abraham, M. H, Chadha, H. S, & Mitchell, R. C. (1995). Hydrogen bonding. 36. Determination of blood-brain barrier distribution using octanol-water partition coefficients. *Drug Des Discov* (Nov 1995), 1055-9612, 13(2), 123-131.

[2] Abraham, M. H, Takacs-novak, K, & Mitchell, R. C. (1997). On the partition of ampholytes: Application to blood-brain distribution. *J Pharm Sci* (Mar 1997), 0022-3549, 86(3), 310-315.

[3] Abuznait, A. H, Cain, C, Ingram, D, Burk, D, & Kaddoumi, A. (2011). Up-regulation of P-glycoprotein reduces intracellular accumulation of beta amyloid: investigation of P-glycoprotein as a novel therapeutic target for Alzheimer's disease. J Pharm Pharmacol. (Aug 2011), 0022-3573, 63(8), 1111-1118.

[4] Alka, K. (2003). C-QSAR: a database of 18000 QSARs and associated biological and physical data. *J Comput Aided Mol Des* (Feb-Apr 2003), 1573-4951, 17(2-4), 187-196.

[5] Aller, S. G, Yu, J, Ward, A, Weng, Y, Chittaboina, S, Zhuo, R, Harrell, P. M, Trinh, Y. T, Zhang, Q, Urbatsch, I. L, & Chang, G. (2009). Structure of P-glycoprotein reveals a molecular basis for poly-specific drug binding. *Science.* (Mar 2009), 0036-8075, 323(5922), 1718-1722.

[6] Ambudkar, S. V, Dey, S, Hrycyna, C. A, Ramachandra, M, Pastan, I, & Gottesman, M. M. (1999). Biochemical, cellular, and pharmacological aspects of the multidrug transporter. *Annu. Rev. Pharmacol. Toxicol.* (Apr 1999), 0362-1642, 39, 361-398.

[7] Ambudkar, S. V, Lelong, I. H, Zhang, J, Cardarelli, C. O, Gottesman, M. M, & Pastan, I. (1992). Partial purification and reconstitution of the human multidrug-resistance pump: characterization of the drug-stimulatable ATP hydrolysis. *Proc. Natl. Acad. Sci. USA* (Sep 1992), 0027-8424, 89(18), 8472-8476.

[8] Bartels, A. L. (2011). Blood-brain barrier P-glycoprotein function in neurodegenerative disease. *Curr Pharm Des.* 1381-6128, 17(26), 2771-2777.

[9] Bassolino-klimas, D, Alper, H. E, & Stouch, T. R. (1993). Solute diffusion in lipid bilayer membranes: an atomic level study by molecular dynamics simulation. *Biochemistry.* (Nov 1993), 0006-2960, 32(47), 12624-12637.

[10] Bendayan, R, Lee, G, & Bendayan, M. (2002). Functional expression and localization of p-glycoprotein at the blood brain barrier. Microsc. Res. Tech., (Jun 2002), 0105-9910X., 57(5), 365-380.

[11] Chen, C, & Yang, J. (2006). MI-QSAR models for prediction of corneal permeability of organic compounds. *Acta Pharmacologica Sinica.* (Feb 2006), 1745-7254, 27(2), 193-204.

[12] Chen, L. J, Lian, G. P, & Han, L. J. (2007). Prediction of human skin permeability using artificial neural network (ANN) modeling. *Acta Pharmacologica Sinica,* (Apr 2007), 1745-7254, 28(4), 591-600.

[13] Chen, Y, Zhu, Q. J, Pan, J, Yang, Y, & Wu, X. P. (2009). A prediction model for blood-brain barrier permeation and analysis on its parameter biologically. *Comput Methods Programs Biomed.,* (Sep 2009), 0169-2607, 95(3), 280-287.

[14] Cheng, Z, Zhang, J, Liu, H, Li, Y, Zhao, Y, & Yang, E. (2010). Central nervous system penetration for small molecule therapeutic agents does not increase in multiple scle-

rosis- and Alzheimer's disease-related animal models despite reported blood-brain barrier disruption. *Drug Metab Dispos.* (Aug 2010), 0090-9556, 38(8), 1355-1361.

[15] Cramer, R. D, Patterson, D. E, & Bunce, J. D. (1988). Comparative molecular field analysis (CoMFA). 1. Effect of shape on binding of steroids to carrier proteins. *J. Am. Chem. Sci.* (Aug 1988), 0002-7863, 110(18), 5959-5967.

[16] Dhainaut, A, Regnier, G, Tizot, A, Pierre, A, Leonce, S, Guilbaud, N, Kraus-berthier, L, & Atassi, G. (1996). New purines and purine analogs as modulators of multidrug resistance. *J. Med. Chem.* (Sep 1996), 0223-5234, 39(20), 4099-4108.

[17] Doige, C. A, Yu, X, & Sharom, F. J. (1993). The effects of lipids and detergents on ATPase-active P-glycoprotein. *Biochim. Biophys. Acta* (Feb 1993), 0006-3002, 1146(1), 65-72.

[18] Ford, J. M, Bruggemann, E. P, Pastan, I, Gottesman, M. M, & Hait, W. N. (1990). Cellular and biochemical characterization of thioxanthenes for revesal of multidrug resistance in human and murine cell lines. *Cancer Res.* (Mar 1990), 0008-5472, 50(6), 1748-1756.

[19] Fromm, M. F. (2004). Importance of P-glycoprotein at blood-tissue barriers. *Trends Pharmacol Sci.* (August 2004), 0165-6147, 25(8), 423-429.

[20] Gottesman, M. M, & Pastan, I. (1993). Biochemistry of Multidrug Resistance Mediated by the Multidrug Transporter, *Annu Rev Biochem* No. (July 1993), 0066-4154, 62, 385-427.

[21] Hartz, A. M, Miller, D. S, & Bauer, B. (2010). Restoring blood-brain barrier P-glycoprotein reduces brain amyloid-beta in a mouse model of Alzheimer's disease. *Mol Pharmacol.* (May 2010), 0002-6895X., 77(5), 715-723.

[22] Higgins, C. F, & Gottesman, M. M. (1992). Is the multidrug transporter a flippase? *Trends. Biol. Sci.*, 0962-8924, 17, 18-21.

[23] Iyer, M, Mishra, R, Han, Y, & Hopfinger, A. J. (2002). Predicting Blood-Brain Barrier Partitioning of Organic Molecules Using Membrane-Interaction QSAR Analysis. *Pharmaceutical Res* Nov 2002), 0724-8741, 19(11), 1611-1621.

[24] Jabeen, I, Pleban, K, Rinner, U, Chiba, P, & Ecker, G. F. (2012). Structure-activity relationships, ligand efficiency, and lipophilic efficiency profiles of benzophenone-type inhibitors of the multidrug transporter p-glycoprotein. J. Med. Chem. Apr 2012), 0223-5234, 55(7), 3261-3273.

[25] Jeynes, B, & Provias, J. (2011). An investigation into the role of P-glycoprotein in Alzheimer's disease lesion pathogenesis. Neurosci Lett. Jan 2011), 0168-0102, 487(3), 389-393.

[26] Kast, C, Canfield, V, Levenson, R, & Gros, P. (1996). Transmembrane organization of mouse P-glycoprotein determined by epitope insertion and immunofluorescence. J Biol Chem. Apr 1996), 0021-9258, 271(16), 9240-9248.

[27] Karelson, M. (2000). Molecular Descriptors in QSAR/ QSPR; John Wiley & Sons: New York. 0-47135-168-7

[28] Karelson, M, Lobanov, V. S, & Katritzky, A. R. (1996). Quantum-chemical descriptors in QSAR/QSPR studies. Chem. Rev. May 9), 0003-6021X., 96(3), 1027-1044.

[29] Kothandan, G, Gadhe, C. G, Madhavan, T, Choi, C. H, & Cho, S. J. (2011). Docking and 3D-QSAR (quantitative structure activity relationship) studies of flavones, the potent inhibitors of p-glycoprotein targeting the nucleotide binding domain. Eur J Med Chem. Sep 2011), 0223-5234, 46(9), 4078-4088.

[30] Kubinyi, H. (1995). Strategies and recent technologies in drug discovery. Pharmazie. Oct 1995), 0031-7144, 50(10), 647-662.

[31] Kuo, C. L, Assefa, H, Kamath, S, Brzozowski, Z, Slawinski, J, Saczewski, F, Buolamwini, J. K, & Neamati, N. (2004). Application of CoMFA and CoMSIA 3D-QSAR and docking studies in optimization of mercaptobenzenesulfonamides as HIV-1 integrase inhibitors. J Med Chem. Jan 2004), 0223-5234, 47(2), 385-399.

[32] Li, Y, Wang, Y. H, Yang, L, Zhang, S. W, Liu, C. H, & Yang, S. L. (2005). Comparison of steroid substrates and inhibitors of P-glycoprotein by 3D-QSAR analysis. J. Mol. Struct. Sep 2005), 0166-1280, 733(1-3), 111-118.

[33] Litman, T, Zeuthen, T, Skovsgaard, T, & Stein, W. D. (1997). Structure-activity relationships of P-glycoprotein interacting drugs: kinetic characterization of their effects on ATPase activity, Biochem. Biophys. Acta Aug 1997), 0006-3002, 1361(2), 159-168.

[34] Ma, X. L, Chen, C, & Yang, J. (2005). Predictive model of blood-brain barrier penetration of organic compounds. Acta Pharmacologica Sinica. Apr 2005), 1745-7254, 26(4), 500-512.

[35] Norinder, U, & Haeberlein, M. (2002). Computational approaches to the prediction of the blood-brain distribution. Adv Drug Deliv Rev., (Mar 2002):291-313, 0016-9409X., 54(3)

[36] Ohtsuki, S, Ito, S, & Terasaki, T. (2010). Is P-glycoprotein involved in amyloid-β elimination across the blood-brain barrier in Alzheimer's disease? *Clin Pharmacol Ther.* (Oct 2010), 0009-9236, 88(4), 443-445.

[37] Ooms, F, Wouters, J, Collin, S, Durant, F, Jegham, S, & George, P. (1998). Molecular lipophilicity potential by CLIP, a reliable tool for the description of the 3D distribution of lipophilicity: application to 3-phenyloxazolidin-2-one, a prototype series of reversible MAOA inhibitors. *Bioorg. Med. Chem. Lett.* (Jun 1998), 0096-0894X., 8(11), 1425-1430.

[38] Palmeira, A, Sousa, E, Fernandes, M. X, Pinto, M. M, & Vasconcelos, M. H. (2012). Multidrug resistance reversal effects of aminated thioxanthones and interaction with cytochrome P450 3A4. J Pharm Pharm Sci., (Jan 2012), 1482-1826, 15(1), 31-45.

[39] Ponce, Y. M, Garit, J. A, Torrens, F, Zaldivar, V. R, & Castro, E. A. (2004). Atom, atom-type, and total linear indices of the "molecular pseudograph's atom adjacency matrix": application to QSPR/QSAR studies of organic compounds. Molecules (Dec. 31), 1420-3049, 9(12), 1100-1123.

[40] Schmid, D, Ecker, G, Kopp, S, Hitzler, M, & Chiba, P. (1999). Structure-activity relationship studies of propafenone analogs cased on P-glycoprotein ATPase activity measurements. *Biochem Pharmacol.* (Nov 1999), 0300-5127, 58(9), 1447-1456.

[41] Shapiro, A. B, & Ling, V. (1994). ATPase activity of purified and reconstituted P-glycoprotein from Chinese hamster ovary cells. *J. Biol. Chem.* (Feb 1994), 0021-9258, 269(5), 3745-3754.

[42] Sharom, F. J. (1997). The P-Glycoprotein Efflux Pump: How Does it Transport Drugs? *J. Membr. Biol.* (Dec 1997), 0022-2631, 160(3), 161-175.

[43] Stouch, T. R, & Gudmundsson, O. (2002). Progress in understanding the structure-activity relationships of P-glycoprotein. *Adv Drug Deliv Rev.* (Mar 2002), 0016-9409X., 54(3), 315-328.

[44] Taub, M. E, Podila, L, Ely, D, & Almeida, I. (2005). Functional assessment of multiple P-glycoprotein (P-gp) probe substrates: influence of cell line and modulator concentration on P-gp activity. *Drug Metab Dispos.* (Nov 2005), 0090-9556, 33(11), 1679-1687.

[45] Vogelgesang, S, Jedlitschky, G, Brenn, A, & Walker, L. C. (2011). The role of the ATP-binding cassette transporter P-glycoprotein in the transport of β-amyloid across the blood-brain barrier. *Curr Pharm Des.*171381-6128(26), 2778-2786.

[46] Wang, R. B, Kuo, C. L, Lien, L. L, & Lien, E. J. (2003). Structure-activity relationship: analyses of p-glycoprotein substrates and inhibitors. *J Clin Pharm Ther.* (Jun 2003), 0269-4727, 28(3), 203-228.

[47] Wang, Y. H, Li, Y, Yang, S. L, & Yang, L. (2005). An in silico approach for screening flavonoids as P-glycoprotein inhibitors based on a Bayesian-regularized neural network. *J Comput Aided Mol Des.* (Mar 2005), 0092-0654X., 19(3), 137-147.

[48] Wang, Y. H, Li, Y, Yang, S. L, & Yang, L. (2005). Classification of Substrates and Inhibitors of P-Glycoprotein Using Unsupervised Machine Learning Approach. *J. Chem. Inf. Model.* (May 2005), 1549-9596, 45(3), 750-757.

[49] Waterhouse, R. N. (2003). Determination of lipophilicity and its use as a predictor of blood-brain barrier penetration of molecular imaging agents. *Mol Imaging Biol.*, (Nov-Dec 2003), 1536-1632, 5(6), 376-389.

[50] Wiese, M, & Pajeva, I. K. (2001). Structure-Activity Relationships of Multidrug Resistance Reversers. *Curr. Med. Chem.* (May 2001), 0929-8673, 8(6), 685-713.

Chapter 12

Therapeutic Interventions in Alzheimer Disease

Analava Mitra and Baishakhi Dey

Additional information is available at the end of the chapter

http://dx.doi.org/10.5772/54915

1. Introduction

Alzheimer disease (AD), was first recognized in the early 1900's by Alois Alzheimer, a German psychiatrist and neuro pathologist and named after him (Fig.1). Auguste Deter, in 1902 is a reported patient of Dr. Alois (Fig.2). AD is the most common form of dementia affecting millions of the geriatric population worldwide, mostly those above 65-85 yrs of age. Women are more commonly affected than man [1]. Alzheimer currently afflicts about 5.2 million Americans and with the rapid escalation of the prevalence of the disease, the figure is expected to double by 2020. According to WHO, there are about 18 million people worldwide with AD, the figure will be projected to nearly double by 2025 to 34 million. Developing countries like India and China will be among the countries worst hit by AD due to ageing of the population and likely some genetic factors. In 2000, India had 3.5 million Alzheimer patients, however with the fast graying of population and growth rate being fastest in the 80+ segment of the society, the number of Alzheimer patients have been growing at a phenomenal rate [2]. This neurodegenerative fatal brain disorder generally begins in late life and disease progression is gradual and continuous, the longevity of a patient is about 8-10 yrs after symptoms appear. The disease conditions range from mild, moderate to severe; in mild conditions patients have some functional impairments, in moderate conditions there's a dependence on care givers for some important daily activities, in severe conditions there is complete neuronal and memory loss, motor impairment making the patient absolutely dependent on care givers. Age related behavioral changes and symptoms of Alzheimer should not be confused.

Typical clinical symptoms of Alzheimer include: signs of progressive memory loss disturbing daily activities, difficulty in completing daily activities, poor judgment, vision problems, sudden changes in mood and personality, self withdrawal from hobbies or social contacts, loss of cognition, loss of coordination, etc. Ageing is the greatest risk factor of AD though Alzheimer is not a normal part of aging since people below 65yrs of age can also develop AD referred to as 'younger or early onset' [1,2]. The differences between a normal aged brain and the brain of an

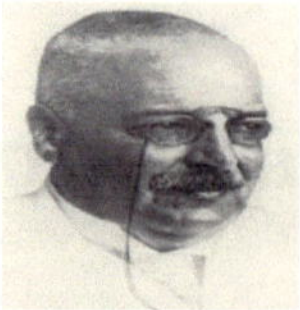

Figure 1. Dr. Alois Alzheimer(1864-1915)

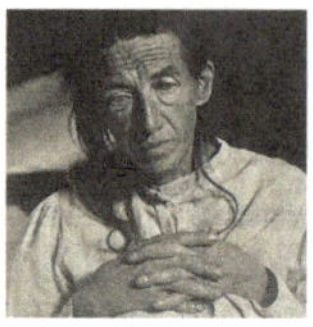

Figure 2. Auguste Deter (1902), patient of Dr. Alois

Alzheimer patient have been depicted in Fig.3. Other prominent risk factors in AD include family history, heredity (genetics), environmental factors. A genetic factor in late onset AD is ApoE ε4. The gene for apolipoprotein E (ApoE) on chromosome 19 has gained much recent attention in the pathogenesis of AD. ApoE is a protein modulator of phospholipid transport that might have a role in synaptic remodeling. ApoE has three common alleles, ApoE ε2, ε3, and ε4, which are expressed in varying amounts in the normal person. It is the ApoE ε4 genotype that is associated with the risk of AD. Everyone inherits one form of APoE gene from each parent; those who receive ApoE ε4 gene are at the risk of developing AD than those who receive ApoE ε2, ApoE ε3. Individuals who inherit two ApoE ε4 genes are at even higher risk; however inheriting one or two copies of genes does not gurantee that the individual will develop Alzheimer [3,4,5]. Moderate and severe head trauma, traumatic brain injuries are associated with increased risk of AD. Head injury resulting in loss of consciousness or post traumatic amnesia lasting about 30mins is associated with twice the risk of developing AD; severe head injuries have about 4.5 fold risks. Mild cognitive impairment (MCI) has an established link with AD in which a person has problems with memory, language, and some essential cognitive ability severe enough to be noticeable to others and shown upon cognitive tests but not severe enough to interfere with the daily life. However there is no clear explanation on the fact that why some people with MCI develops dementia and in some cases it is not. The overall health of the heart and blood vessels shows a close linkage with the brain health since a brain is nourished by the rich network of blood vessels and a healthy heart pumps nutrient and oxygen rich blood to these vessels. Cardiovascular diseases, high blood pressure, hypertensions, type 2 diabetes, cholesterolemia, obesity, smoking habits, and physical inactivity potentially increases the risk of AD [6-9].

2. Patho physiology of Alzheimer

The human brain consists of 100 millions of neurons connected to each other through synapses forming communication network; each cells entitled to perform their own duties relating to

http://dx.doi.org/10.5772/54915

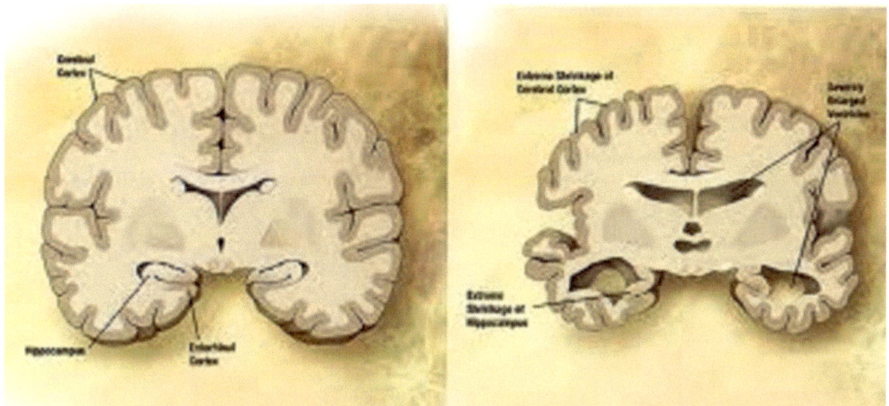

Figure 3. Alzheimer disease diagram, normal aged brain (left), Alzheimer brain (right)

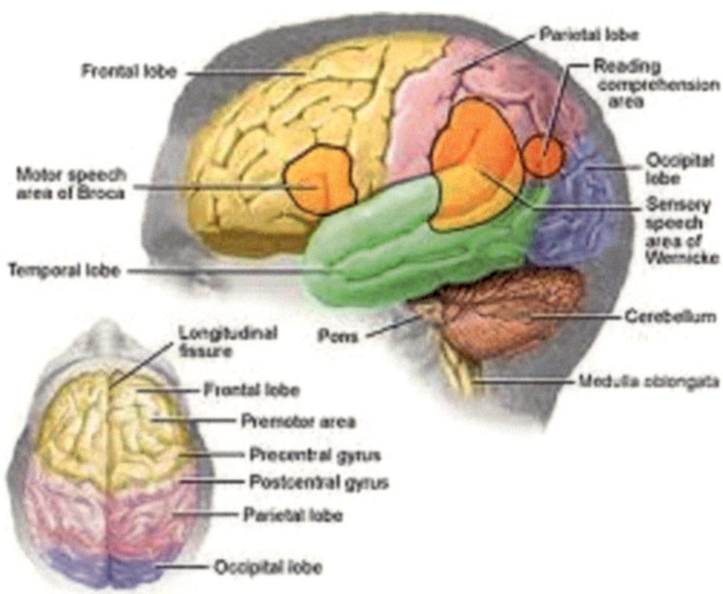

Figure 4. Shrinkage of Brain tissue in Alzheimer disease

memory, thinking, smell, taste, emotions etc. In case of AD these brain cells can't perform their duties. Patho physiology of Alzheimer disease being complex and multi factorial shows important pathological changes in brain like accumulation of amyloid cerebral plaques and neurofibrillary tangles of abnormal insoluble 'tau' protein (Fig.6,8,9). AD is also considered a 'tauopathy' due to abnormal aggregation of the tau protein. Every neuron has a cytoskeleton, an internal support structure partly made up of structures called microtubules. These micro-tubules act like tracks, guiding nutrients and molecules from the body of the cell to the ends of the axon and back. A protein called *tau* stabilizes the microtubules when phosphorylated, and is therefore called a microtubule-associated protein. In AD, tau undergoes chemical

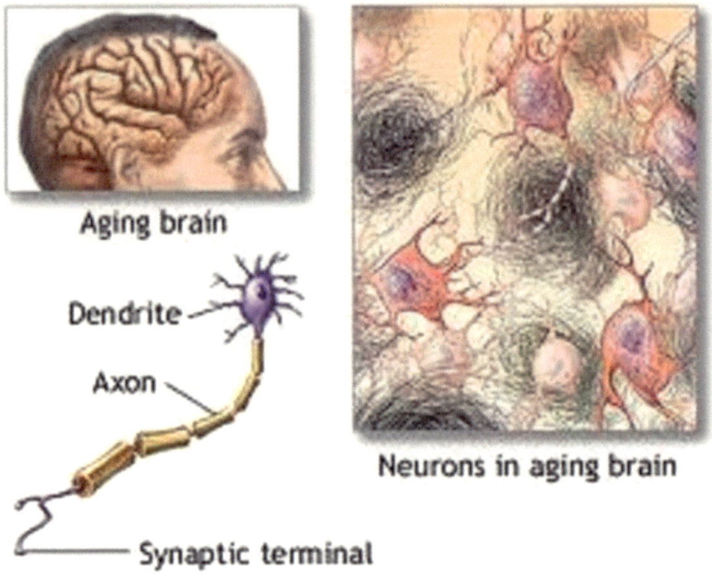

Figure 5. Normal homeostasis of Alzheimer Disease

changes, becoming hyperphosphorylated; it then begins to pair with other threads, creating neurofibrillary tangles and disintegrating the neuron's transport system [10,11].

As per the amyloid hypothesis, the neuropathologic hallmarks of AD are neuritic plaques and neurofibrillary tangles, consisting of hyper-phosphorylated microtubule-associated protein called 'tau' and extracellular amyloid plaques. The main component of amyloid plaques in AD is amyloid β (Aβ) peptide (38–43 amino acids) which is a proteolytic by-product from the amyloid precursor protein (APP) generated by the sequential β-secretase and γ-secretase cleavage (Fig.7). Research data have been shown that oligomeric Aβ species (smallest of which are dimers) isolated from AD brains are the most synaptotoxic forms. Aggregated amyloid fibrils, which are believed to be the toxic form of the protein disrupts the cell's calcium ion homeostasis, induces programmed cell death or apoptosis (Fig.7). It is also known that Aβ selectively builds up in the mitochondria in the cells of Alzheimer's-affected brains, and it also inhibits certain enzyme functions and the utilization of glucose by neurons [3,11-13].

The brain of a Alzheimer patient shows marked histo-pathophysiological changes like, widened sulci and shrinkage of the gyri (Fig.10). In the great majority of cases, every part of the cerebral cortex is involved; however, the occipital pole is often relatively spared. The cortical ribbon may be thinned and ventricular dilatation apparent, especially in the temporal horn, due to atrophy of the amygdala and hippocampus. Microscopically, there is significant loss of neurons, in addition to shrinkage of large cortical neurons, synapses, in association with shrinkage of the dendritic arbor of large neurons, is thought to be the critical pathological substrate (Fig.4). Neurofibrillary tangles are the other characteristic neurohistopathologic hallmarks seen in AD. These tangles found inside the neurons, concentrated in vulnerable

http://dx.doi.org/10.5772/54915

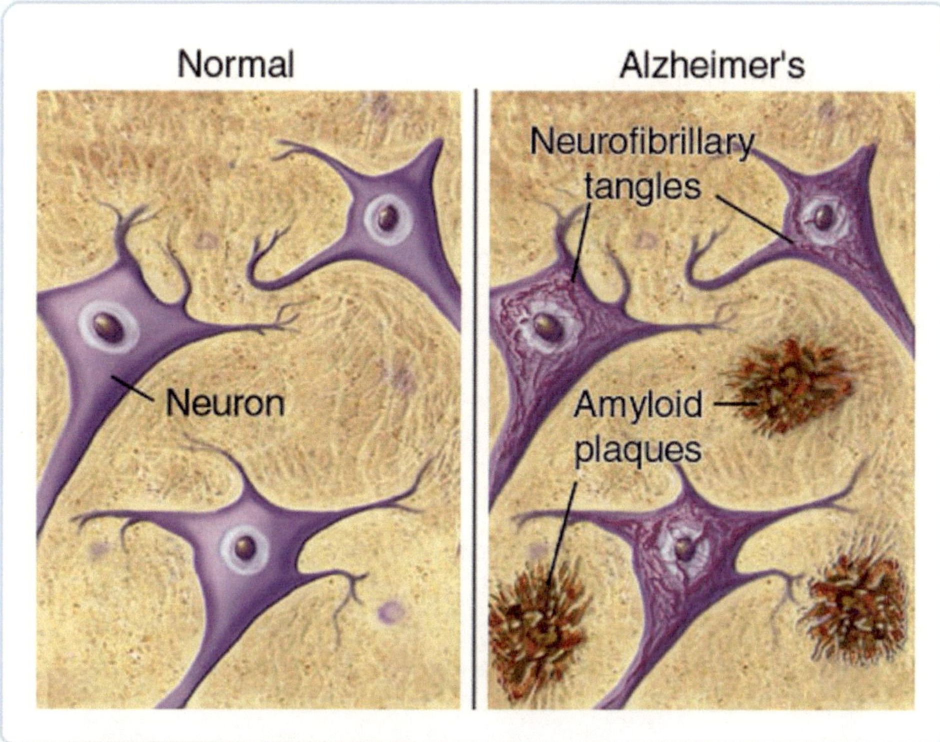

Figure 6. Normal Neuron (left), Neurofibrillary tangles, Amyloid plaques in Alzheimer (right)

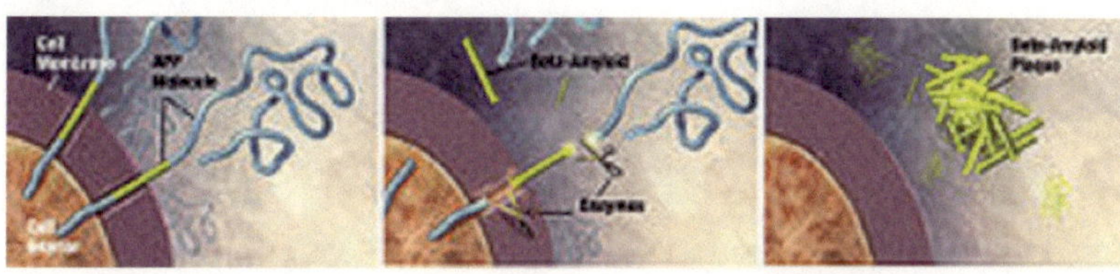

Figure 7. Enzyme action on APP (Amyloid precursor protein) and its fragmentation

neural systems and composed of paired helical filaments of hyperphosphorylated microtubule-associated tau protein that may cause disruption of normal cytoskeletal architecture with subsequent neuronal cell death. Other pathological alterations commonly seen in the brains of AD patients include neuropil threads, granulovacuolar degeneration, and amyloid angiopathy. Amyloid angiopathy is a distinct vascular lesion found in many AD brains, consisting of amyloid deposition in the walls of small-to medium-sized cortical and leptomeningeal arteries. As a result of the deposits, the involved vessels may become compromised with resultant hemorrhage [14-17].

Inflammatory processes and cytokines play a controversial role in the pathology of Alzheimer's disease. Inflammation is a general marker of tissue damage in any disease, and may be either secondary to tissue damage in AD or a marker of an immunological response. Some studies have demonstrated the presence of activated microglia, a marker of the brain's immune response. Alterations in the distribution of different neurotrophic factors and in the expression of their receptors such as the brain derived neurotrophic factor (BDNF) have been found in AD. Microglia have been shown to be significantly activated in AD brains and localized at sites of amyloid deposition. Early activation of microglia in early AD pathogenesis has been shown to be beneficial in scavenging and clearing toxic Aβ from the brain. Peri vascular macrophages like CD163 (hemoglobin-haptoglobin scavenger receptor) and CD206 (mannose receptor) are antigen-presenting phagocytic cells located in outer aspects of blood vessels within the brain, have shown to respond to CNS inflammation. Results of clinical trials have shown that, blood-derived macrophages from AD patients were shown to be less effective at phagocytosing Aβ compared with cells derived from non-demented control patients. Microglial and peri vascular macrophages may play role in clearing Aβ from the brain and in enhancing AD-related inflammation [18-20].

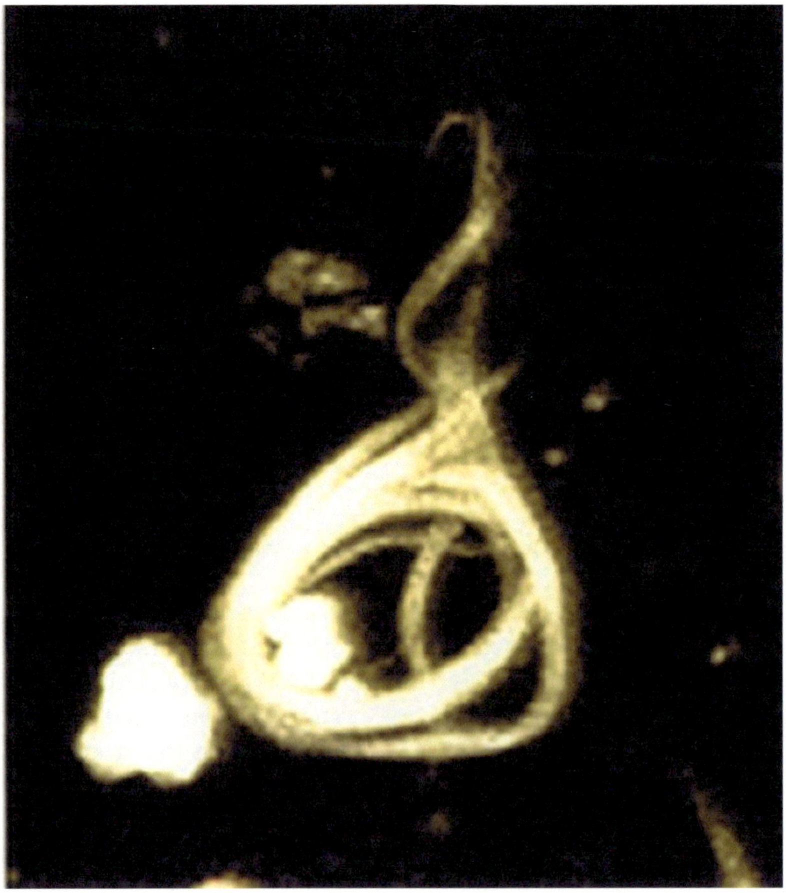

Figure 8. Neuro-fibrillary tangle with hyperphosphorylated Tau Protein(high resolution)

http://dx.doi.org/10.5772/54915

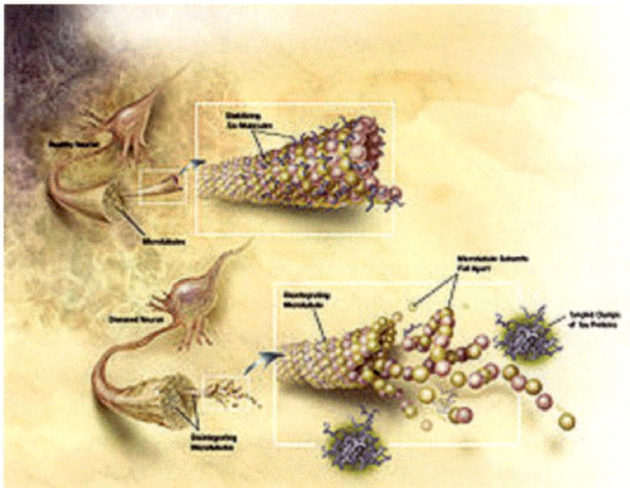

Figure 9. Changes in Tau protein & disintegration of microtubules in brain cells

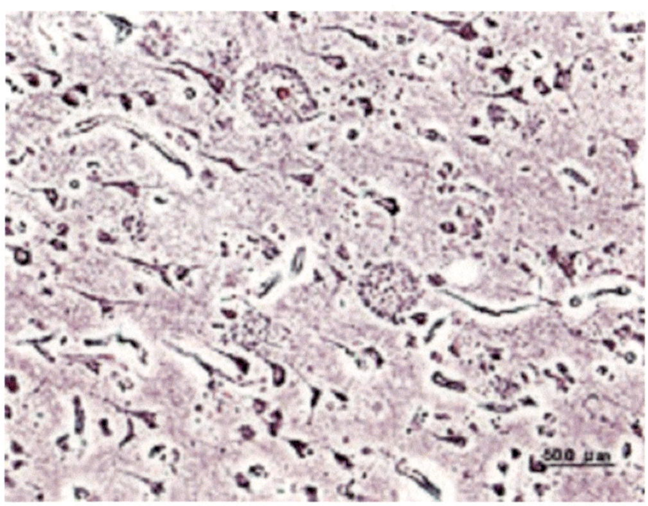

Figure 10. Histopathologic image of senile plaques in Alzheimer Brain

Vascular dysfunction has a critical role in AD. Results of epidemiological and pathological studies have demonstrated positive links between cerebro vascular disorders and AD. For example a person with severe atherosclerosis is at a threefold increased risk of developing AD or vascular dementia. Due to reduced cerebral blood flow in AD there are abnormal cholinergic innervations of intra cerebral blood vessels leading to brain hypo perfusion. Results of recent investigations have shown that, the upregulation of two transcription factors myocardin (MYOCD) and serum response factor (SRF) in AD lead to arterial hypercontractility potentiating reduced cerebral blood flow. Other vascular anatomical defects observed in AD include atrophy and irregularities of arterioles and capillaries, increase in collagen IV, heparin sulfate proteoglycans and laminin deposition in the basement membrane, disruption of the basement membrane, reduced total micro vascular density, occasional swelling of astrocytic endfeets, and extensive degeneration of the endothelium during the disease progression [21-24].

Decreased cerebral blood flow (CBF) has a negative impact on the protein synthesis necessary for memory and learning, and may eventually lead to neuritic injury and neuronal death. Moreover due to cerebral hypo perfusion amyloid β-peptide (Aβ) clearance across the blood–brain barrier (BBB) will be impaired leading to accumulation of Aβ on cerebral blood vessels and brain parenchyma causing cerebral amyloid angiopathy (CAA), which is associated with cognitive decline and is another significant factor in the pathogenesis of AD. CAA can severely disrupt the integrity of the blood vessel wall resulting in micro or macro intra cerebral bleedings that exacerbates neurodegenerative process and inflammatory response and may lead to hemorrhagic stroke. Cerebral amyloid angiopathy (CAA) with Aβ deposits in the vascular smooth muscle cell layer is a major pathological threat to the neurovascular unit in AD [13,17,20,21].

Research evidences have suggested that imbalances between Aβ production and clearance from the brain cause accumulation of Aβ in the wall of cerebral vessels and in the brains of AD individuals. Aβ that is produced both in the brain and periphery by a number of different cell types is transported across the BBB via receptor-mediated transcytosis; the key receptors being involved are: RAGE (Receptor for Advanced Glycation End products) that transports Aβ from the blood into the brain and LRP (low-density lipoprotein receptor related protein-1) that is the major cell surface Aβ clearance receptor that transports Aβ out of the brain across the BBB and promotes Aβ clearance on VSMC. Aβ is not only cleared from the brain interstitial fluid (ISF) as a soluble peptide, but can also be transported by its chaperone proteins in the ISF, such as apolipoprotein E (apoE), apolipoprotein J, and α2-macroglobulin. Apart from direct Aβ clearance into the blood, alternative perivascular route for the clearance of Aβ in the human brain also exists. The pulsation force of cerebral blood vessels has been proposed to drive an Aβ drainage route along the perivascular spaces. Vessel constriction or stiffening reduces the pulsatile blood flow which in turn reduces Aβ clearance along the perivascular spaces leading to increase in Aβ deposition in the arterial wall of AD patients [20-24].

ApoE is a reactive apolipoprotein that exists in 3 iso forms (apoE2, apoE3, and apoE4) in humans has a major function in the transport of lipids and cholesterol in our body. Individuals who carry at least one apoE4 allele have great chances to develop AD. ApoE, an Aβ chaperone protein is found to be associated with impaired transport of Aβ across the BBB. Free Aβ can be rapidly cleared from the brain mainly via LRP or RAGE receptor mediated transcytosis, but Aβ-ApoE complexes (mostly apoE4-Aβ complexes in contrast to apoE2-Aβ and apoE3-Aβ complexes) are cleared by the very low-density lipoprotein receptor at a much slower rate, causing Aβ retention in the brain. Transport of Aβ via the receptor for advanced glycation endproducts (RAGE) across the BBB provides a major source of Aβ that can deposit in the brain and can directly lead to neuroinflammation by activating nuclear factor-κB mediated secretion of pro-inflammatory cytokines, such as tumor necrosis factor-α and interleukin 6 that may reduce the BBB potency [13,17,24-29].

http://dx.doi.org/10.5772/54915

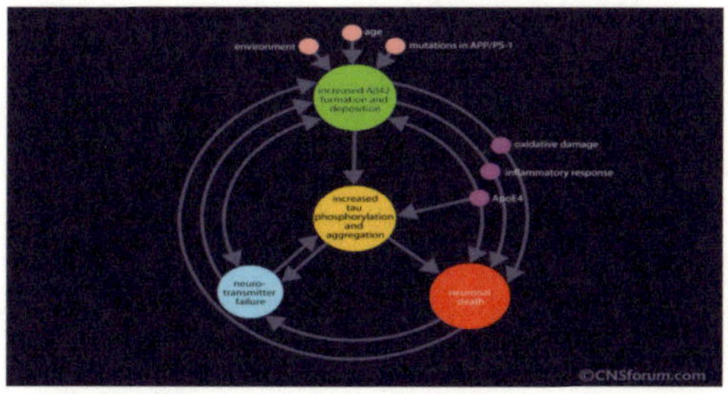

Figure 11. Cascade of events in Alzheimer Disease

From the genetic point of view it has been found that the distribution of cerebrovascular amyloid in AD varies with apoE genotype and specifically the increasing dose of apoE4 alleles has been associated with increased CAA. Understanding the cellular and molecular mechanism by which apoE genotype influences the pathogenicity of the disease process in AD individuals can act as important targets in developing new therapeutic interventions and diagnostic aids for AD.

Interactions of Aβ with human Vascular Smooth Muscle Cells has been found to significantly increase the activation of matrix metalloproteinase 2 (MMP2) via increasing the mRNA expression of membrane type 1 (MT1)-MMP, the primary MMP2 activator at the cell surface. MMP9 specifically has been found in postmortem AD tissue in significant amounts. Activated MMP9 can degrade basement membranes, extracellular matrix proteins and tight junction proteins subsequently damaging the integrity of the BBB and potentially leading to spontaneous cerebral hemorrhages. Similarly high levels of ROS in AD may damage proteins essentials for important neurovascular mechanisms. The breakdown of the BBB may in turn disrupt the normal transport of nutrients, vitamins and electrolytes across the BBB, which are essential for proper neuronal functioning. Therefore, therapies that reduce ROS, MMP2, and MMP9, or that block RAGE-Aβ interaction may offer potentially useful strategies to correct BBB dysfunction in AD [12,25,27-30].

Research data of epidemiological studies have shown controversial results as regards the association between APOE polymorphism and the rate of progression of cognitive decline in AD after onset. Some reports have suggested that homozygous APOE ε4 patients have more rapid cognitive and functional decline following clinical disease onset, but an MRI study on a large cognitively normal population showed rate of volume decrease of entorhinal cortex and hippocampus suggesting potential development. Thus though the role of APOE in the predisposition of AD is well established, still further studies are needed to understand the possible association of APOE with rate of AD progression. The cascade of events in Alzheimer disease is depicted in Fig.11.

3. Diagnosis of Alzheimer

Alzheimer's disease is usually diagnosed clinically from the patient history, collateral history from relatives, and clinical observations, based on the presence of characteristic neurological and neuropsychological features and the absence of alternative conditions. Advanced medical imaging technologies like computed tomography (CT) or magnetic resonance imaging (MRI), single photon emission computed tomography (SPECT) or positron emission tomography (PET) can be used to study the cerebral histo pathophysiological conditions of Alzheimer's disease. The Alzheimer's Disease and Related Disorders Association (now known as the Alzheimer's Association) have set up certain criteria for AD diagnosis which points to eight cognitive domains that are most commonly impaired in AD—memory, language, perceptual skills, attention, constructive abilities, orientation, problem solving and functional abilities. The presence of such symptoms should be confirmed by neuropsychological testing for a clinical diagnosis of possible or probable AD. A histopathologic confirmation including a microscopic examination of brain tissue is required for a definitive diagnosis. In addition to histopathologic confirmation, definite AD requires the clinical finding of dementia as determined by the Mini-Mental State Examination (MMSE) or other standardized neuropsychological testing; the examination must demonstrate deficits in two or more areas of cognition, with progressive memory loss in the absence of delirium. Assessment of intellectual functioning including memory testing can further characterize the state of the disease. The diagnosis can be confirmed with very high accuracy post-mortem when brain material is available and can be examined histologically. Neuropsychological screening tests can help in the diagnosis of AD. In the tests, people are instructed to copy drawings similar to the one shown in the picture, remember words, read, and subtract serial numbers. Neuropsychological tests such as the mini-mental state examination (MMSE), are widely used to evaluate the cognitive impairments needed for diagnosis. More comprehensive test arrays are necessary for high reliability of results, particularly in the earliest stages of the disease. Neurological examination in early AD will usually provide normal results, except for obvious cognitive impairment, which may not differ from that resulting from other diseases processes, including other causes of dementia. Interviews of family members and informations from caregivers about the patient's daily living abilities, the person's mental function are very important in this regard. Psychological tests for depression are also employed, since depression can either be concurrent with AD, an early sign of cognitive impairment, or even the cause [3,4,22].

With the advancements in imaging technology, computed tomography (CT) and magnetic resonance imaging (MRI) can be used to study the cortical atrophy, disproportionate volume loss in the medial temporal lobe structures and also normal age related changes that may be present at the early onset of disease. Functional imaging studies like the positron emission tomography (PET) and single-photon emission computed tomography (SPECT) scans, can be used as a diagnostic tool, which demonstrate hypometabolism and hypoperfusion, respectively, in the temporal-parietal regions bilaterally; for neuro imaging to confirm a diagnosis of Alzheimer's in conjunction with evaluations involving mental status examination (Fig.12). In a person already having dementia, SPECT appears to be superior in differentiating Alzheimer's disease from other possible causes, compared with the usual attempts employing mental testing and medical history analysis. Amyloid burden imaging compounds are under development. A new technique known as PiB PET has been developed that uses carbon-11 PET scanning for directly and clearly imaging beta-amyloid deposits in vivo using a tracer that binds selectively to the A-beta deposits with high levels of accuracy in predicting which people with mild cognitive impairment will develop Alzheimer's disease within two years. Volumetric MRI can detect changes in the size of brain regions and measure the atropy in those regions in order to study the progress of AD. Amyloid imaging used in conjunction with other markers can serve as an important diagnostic tool [3,4].

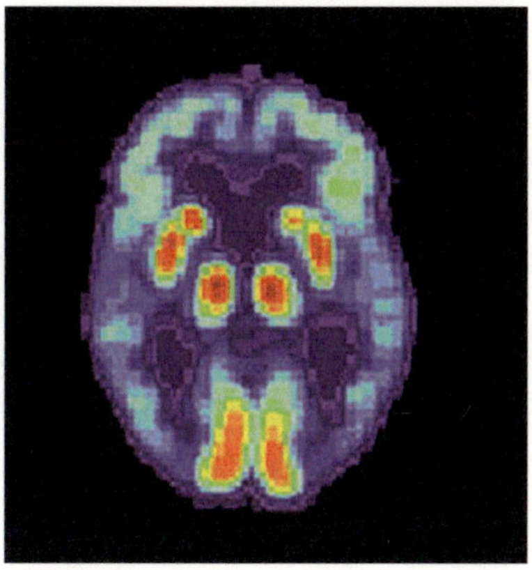

Figure 12. PET scan in the brain of Alzheimer patient (loss of function in temporal lobe)

Results of routine laboratory tests on chemistry panels, blood counts, metabolic panels (e.g., TSH) spinal fluid analyses, and inflammatory markers are all found to be within normal limits in patients with AD. Electroencephalographic (EEG) recordings are usually normal or show diffuse slowing in later stages of the disease. However it has been found that in AD patients it have been found that the levels of glutamate, creatinine, myo-inositol, N-acetyl aspartate are decreased as compared to normal people. Both decrease in N-acetyl aspartate/Creatinine ratio and decrease in hippocampal glutamate may be an early indicator of AD. Monitoring the level of blood dehydroepiandrosterone (DHEA) variations in response to an oxidative stress could be a useful proxy test for AD since experimental research data have shown that the subjects with Mild Cognitive Impairment did not have a DHEA variation, while the healthy controls did [3,4,8].

Another important marker of the disease is the analysis of cerebrospinal fluid for amyloid beta or tau proteins, both total tau protein and phosphorylated tau_{181P} protein concentrations which predicts the onset of AD with a sensitivity of 94-100%. When used in conjunction with existing neuro imaging techniques, doctors can identify people with significant memory loss who are already developing the disease. Spinal fluid tests are commercially available, unlike the latest neuro imaging technology.

The differential diagnosis for AD is extensive and includes a multitude of neurodegenerative diseases that are associated with the development of dementia including Pick's disease, Lewy body disease, and other diseases such as vascular dementia and Creutzfeldt-Jakob disease. Most of these entities can be differentiated from AD by the clinical history and a careful examination. However, the challenge lies to test new hypotheses and not just to continue descriptive studies using better tools, technologies, increased parameters in CSF analysis and routine lab testing's, and more descriptions about the amount of amyloid in the brain [3,4].

4. Therapeutic interventions in Alzheimer

Virtually there are no proven modalities for cure of Alzheimer's disease; however there are treatment regimens that may improve symptoms and may even delay their progression in the early and middle stages of the disease, allowing patients to maintain certain daily functions for longer. Various country- or region-specific, evidence-based guidelines have been developed for the treatment of Alzheimer's disease. These make recommendations that vary according to available resources, funding practices, and local practice. In general, however, the guidelines provide recommendations regarding psychiatric management, psychosocial treatments, and the treatment of specific target symptoms. There are relatively few diseases that have been successfully prevented or even controlled without an understanding of specific etiology of the disease. Apart from the first line and second line FDA recommended synthetic drugs of choice in treating AD, some of the preventive strategies proved to be beneficial in AD include treatment of hypertension, omega fatty acid supplementation, physical activity and cognitive engagement.

5. Conventional therapeutic regimen in Alzheimer

From the point of conventional approach, major six classes of drugs are included in the treatment of AD: Acetylcholinesterase inhibitors (AChE-I), N-methyl-D-aspartate (NMDA) receptor antagonists, monoamine oxidase (MAO) inhibitors, antioxidants, metal chelators, anti-inflammatory drugs. AChE inhibitors are the first line agents for the treatment of mild to moderate AD. FDA approved five prescription drugs to control the symptoms of AD include: Donepezil, Galantamine, Rivastigmine, Tacrine among the AChE inhibitors and Memantine coming under NMDA receptor antagonists. However tacrine have been withdrawn due to the hepato toxicity effects. AChE inhibitors are prescribed to treat symptoms relating to memory, thinking, language, judgment and other thought processes. Cholinesterase inhibitors primarily act by increasing the levels of acetylcholine, the chemical messenger involved in memory, judgment and other thought processes. In AD the cells producing or using ACh are destroyed and thus less amount of ACh is available to carry messages. ACh is produced from acetyl-CoA and choline by cholineacetyltransferase which is released into the synaptic cleft and hydrolyzed by the actions of AChE to choline and acetic acid. This choline is reutilized in ACh synthesis. In the early stages of AD, the activity of AChE is found to be increased in the neuritic plaques and neurofibrillary tangles that accelerate aggregations of beta-amyloid. AChE inhibitors reversibly bind and block the activity of the enzyme acetyl cholinesterase that degrades ACh. AChE inhibitors block the actions of AChE thereby facilitating ACh neurotransmission and reducing beta-amyloid burden [31-34].

Basing on the cholinergic theory, different classes of drugs have been developed to enhance cholinergic deficit in AD patients. Amongst them, AChE inhibitors block the activity of AChE enzyme to improve cognitive function, choline precursors like phosphatidylcholine improves the bioavailability of choline, ACh releasers enhance the release of ACh, M1 and M3 receptor agonists mimic ACh on postsynaptic end terminal receptors, M2 and M3 receptor antagonists regulate ACh release via negative feedback, nicotinic agonists which would enhance ACh release.

AChE inhibitors are mostly well tolerated by the patients; however common side effects include nausea, vomiting, loss of appetite, increased frequency of bowel movements etc. Tacrine, the first FDA approved AD-drug, which inhibits AChE reversibly in a non-competitive manner is no longer in use due to severe side effects (hepatotoxicity) and short biological half life. Donepezil hydrochloride is the second drug of choice approved by USFDA for treatment of mild to moderate AD. This drug is a centrally acting, reversible and non-competitive AChE inhibitor having an N-benzylpiperidine and an indanone moiety which shows longer and more selective action. However it also suffers from the side effects of GI disturbances, nausea, vomiting, headache etc [31,33].

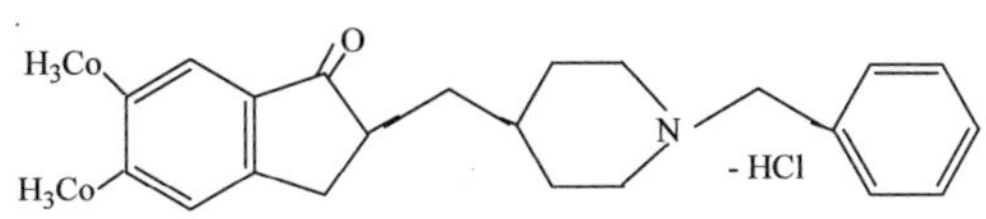

Figure 13. Donepezil hydrochloride

Galantamine reversibly inhibits AChE in a competitive manner and also acts on nicotinic acetylcholine receptors, beneficial for cognitive and non-cognitive AD symptoms. Results of clinical trials have reported this drug to be 50 times more potent against human AChE than butyrylcholinesterase at therapeutic doses. With escalations in drug doses some of the notable adverse effects include vomiting, nausea, diarrhoea etc. Rivastigmine is a reversible carbamate AChE inhibitor that interacts preferentially with acetylcholinesterase G1 with high brain selectivity; this drug has been approved in at least 40 countries around the world. Rivastigmine has the ability to inhibit the activity of butyrylcholinesterase. It binds to both the esteratic and ionic locations of AChE but dissociates at a much slower rate than AChE. Metrifonate, a precursor to the active pseudo irreversible AChE inhibitor DDVP (2,2-dichlorovinyl dimethyl phosphate) rapidly enters the brain with a longer plasma half life than donepezil but shows side effects of diarrhea and muscular cramps and hence could not achieve the market due to muscular weakness. There are certain AChE inhibitors of natural origin finding its use in AD. Physostigmine, a parasympathomimetic plant alkaloid isolated from the seeds of *Physostigma venenosum* have the ability to cross the BBB, having role in cholinergic transmission, can stimulate indirectly both nicotinic and muscarinic receptors. However physostigmine also inhibits another enzyme butyrylcholinesterase which has a role in AD and some of the adverse effects of this drug like nausea, vomiting, headache, diarrhea are attributed to its inhibitory actions on butyrylcholinesterase. Despite of the advantage to cross the BBB, the short half life, narrow margin of therapeutic index has restricted its potentiality. Galanthamine is an alkaloid isolated from *Galanthus nivalis* with competitive reversible AChE inhibitory activity. Galanthamine shows dual mechanism of action, AChE inhibition and allosteric modulation of nicotinic acetyl choline receptors. This drug has 10 fold selectivity for AChE than butyrylcholinesterase. Alpha-7 nicotinic acetylcholine receptors have a role in beta-amyloid mediated neurotoxiciy and since galanthamine can modulate nicotinic acetylcholine receptors it is suggested to prevent beta-amyloid mediated neurotoxicity. Huperzine A, an alkaloid drug isolated from club moss (*Huperzia serrata*) is claimed to show neuroprotective properties with significant improvements in cognitive function and results of clinical trials have shown this drug to be free from unexpected toxicities. This drug has attracted the attention of the scientists due to its strong AChE activities; (-)-huperzine A, a natural isomer have shown strongest dose dependent inhibitory activity against AChE, in comparison to commercially available synthetic drugs like donepezil, tacrine etc [31-33].

Memantine is an uncompetitive low-to-moderate affinity *N*-methyl-D-aspartate (NMDA) receptor antagonist that regulates glutamate activity. Glutamate plays an essential role in learning and memory by triggering NMDA receptors to let a controlled amount of calcium into the nerve cell. This calcium creates the chemical environment required for information storage. Excess glutamate on the other hand, over stimulates NMDA receptors so that they allow too much calcium into nerve cells leading to disruption and death of these cells. Memantine protects cells against excess glutamate by partially blocking NMDA receptors. It's a recently FDA approved NMDA antagonist for the treatment of cognition in moderate to severe Alzheimer's disease, having a half life period between 3-7 h and free from harsh adverse side effects. Memantine can be administered with AChE inhibitors. However FDA did not approve Memantine for mild AD. Results of clinical trials have shown small but statistically significant improvements in mental functions and ability to perform daily activities in AD patients [34,35].

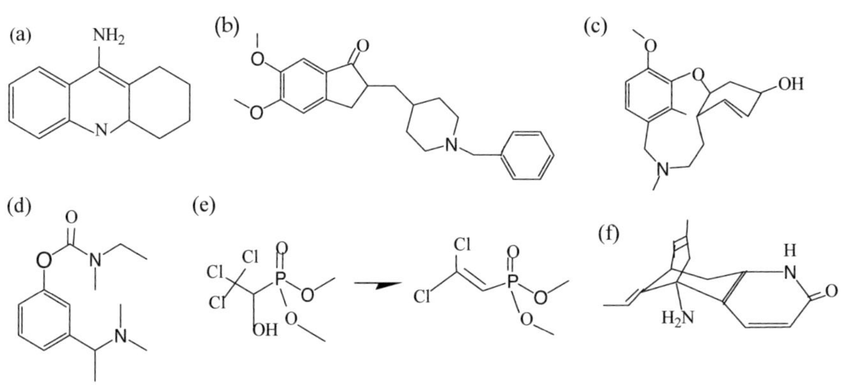

Figure 14. AChE inhibitors (a) Tacrine (b) Donepezil (c) Galantamine (d) Rivastigmine (e) Metrifonate (f) Huperzine

Several metal species like iron, zinc, copper, aluminum are reported to induce beta amyloid aggregation and neurotoxicity in the brain of AD patients; results of structural evidences showing interrelations between aluminum and Abeta, presence of iron and zinc in abnormal high concentrations in AD patients have triggered the idea of using metal chelators as therapeutic targets in the treatment of AD. Desferrioxamine (DFO) and Clioquinol are clinically proven metal chelators used to treat AD patients. DFO chelates with metal ions or aluminium and reduces its neocortical concentrations thereby delaying the progression of

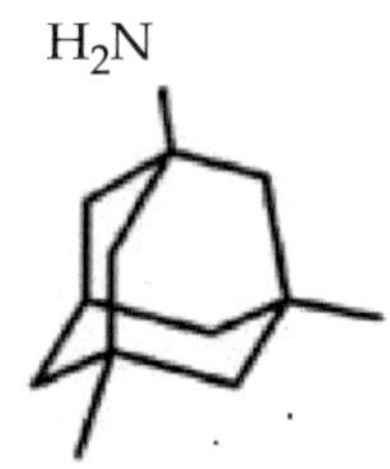

Figure 15. Memantine

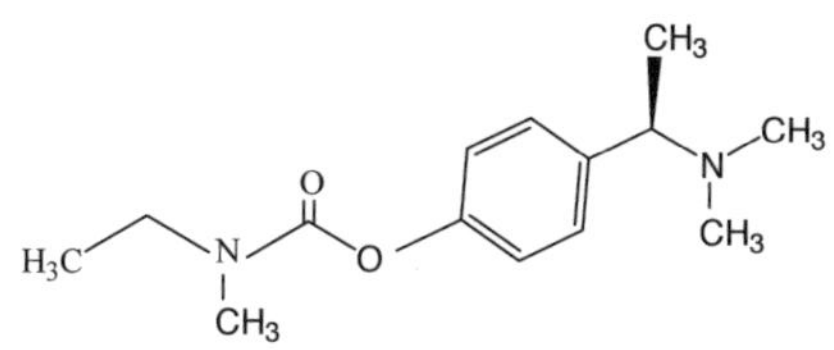

Figure 16. Rivastigmine

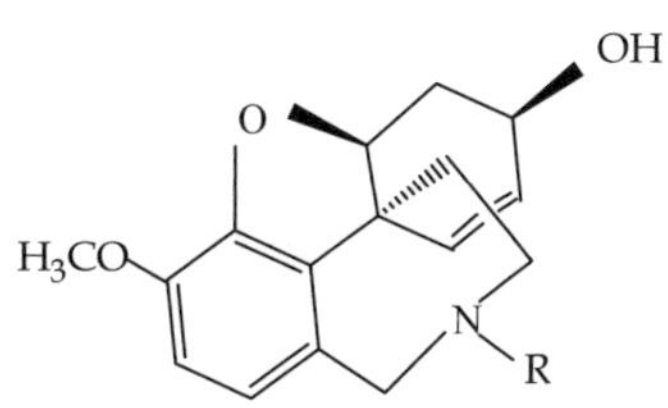

Figure 17. Galanthamine

dementia associated with AD and shows behavioral improvements. However the proper mechanism of action is not yet revealed. Transition metals like copper and zinc are found to be in high concentrations in the neo-cortical regions of the AD patients and these metals are mostly aggregated in the neurotic plaques potentiating beta amyloid aggregation and neuro-toxicity. Clioquinol chelates with these metals and reduces the beta amyloid aggregation in the brain, thus finding use as a therapeutic target in treating Alzheimer [35].

From the pathology of Alzheimer it is clear that several neurotransmitter systems, especially those regulating dopamine, serotonin, acetylcholine has a role in it. With the dysfunction of the dopaminergic system, there is increase in activity of type B monoamine oxidase, the enzyme responsible for degradation of dopamine. The increase in monoamine oxidase level is prominent in the brain platelets contributing to the severity of dementia. The drug Selegiline reversibly inhibits MAO-B; moreover it has a potent anti oxidative effect over the neurons of the brain and also protect against glutamate-receptor-mediated toxicity. Apart from MAO inhibition selegiline has a potent action in the recovery of damaged neurons involving a number of mechanisms like stimulation of neurite outgrowth, stimulation of gene expression in pre apoptotic neurons or stimulation of cytokine biosynthesis. Rasagiline, structurally similar to selegiline also shows neuro protective activities and is found to be ten times more

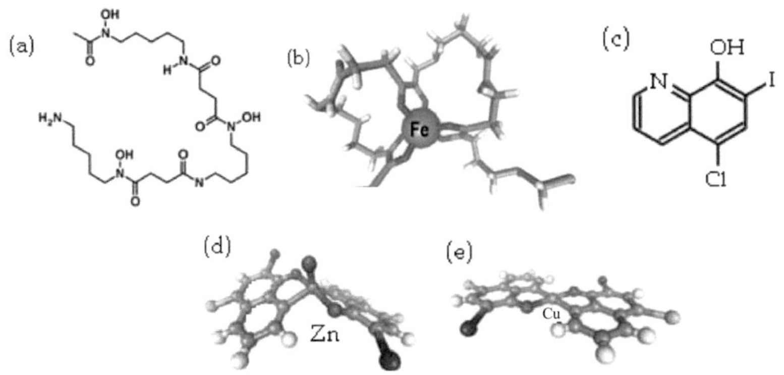

Figure 18. (a) Desferrioxamine (b) Ferrioxamine B (c) Clioquinol (d) Clioquinol Zn complex (e) Clioquinol Cu complex

active in inhibition of MAO-B. The propargylamine moiety in rasagiline is responsible for neuro protective activities. The drug Ladostigil, is the result of combination of active compounds from rasagiline (MAO-B inhibitor, neuroprotector) and rivastigmine (AChE inhibitor) thus finding application as a effective therapeutic agent in treating AD [33-35].

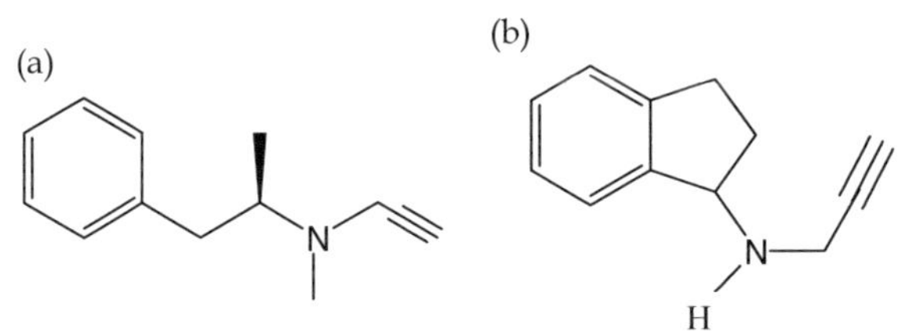

Figure 19. Monoamine oxidase inhibitors (a) Selegiline (b) Rasagiline

Oxidative damage to neurons has a significant role in the pathogenesis of AD; hence antioxidant therapy to prevent oxidative injury can be effective in preventing or retarding the progress of AD. Extracts from *Ginko biloba* named as Egb761 have been found to show cognitive improvement in AD patients and in those with multi-infarct dementia. Similarly Melatonin is found to have antiamyloidogenic activities and is found to reduce neuronal damage caused by reactive oxygen species in AD patients. Antioxidant therapy with vitamin E though reported in some cases but it does not improve cognitive impairment and its therapeutic use has not been established. Clinical trials with Idebenone, a co-enzyme Q10 analog have been found to attenuate Abeta-induced neurotoxicity and cognitive impairments. Dehydroevodiamine hydrochloride (DHED), a compound extracted from *Evodia rutaecarpa* showed AChE inhibitory activities, DHED protects neurons against hydrogen peroxide and glutamate. Moreover DHED decreases reactive oxygen species production and cell death induced by Abeta and carboxyterminal peptides of amyloid precursor proteins, thus improving cognitive impairments in AD. Metalloporphyrin antioxidants have been found to delay neuronal death resulting from increased mitochondrial oxidative stress; Mn-salen complexes have been found to be efficacious against oxidative stress [35].

http://dx.doi.org/10.5772/54915

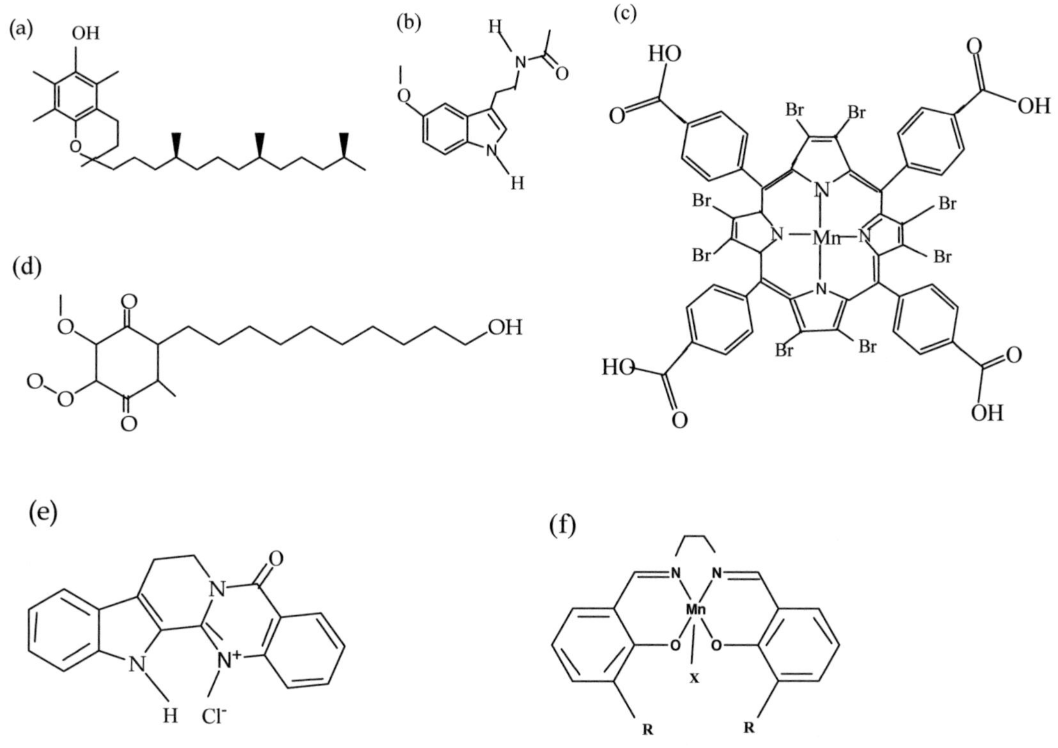

Figure 20. Antioxidants: (a)alpha tocopherol (b) Melatonin (c) Manganese (ш) beta-octabromo-meso tetrakis (4-carboxy phenyl) porphyrin (d) Idebenone (e) Dehydroevodiamine (f) Mn-salen

In AD, neuronal destruction is due to inflammation around Abeta plaques. Drugs under the NSAID groups have anti-inflammatory actions, and found to inhibit cyclooxygenase-1 and cyclooxygenase-2 which are responsible for the oxidation of arachidonic acids to prostaglandins; however due to adverse effects of some NSAIDs on cardiovascular systems, these group of drugs have not found routine use in AD treatment.

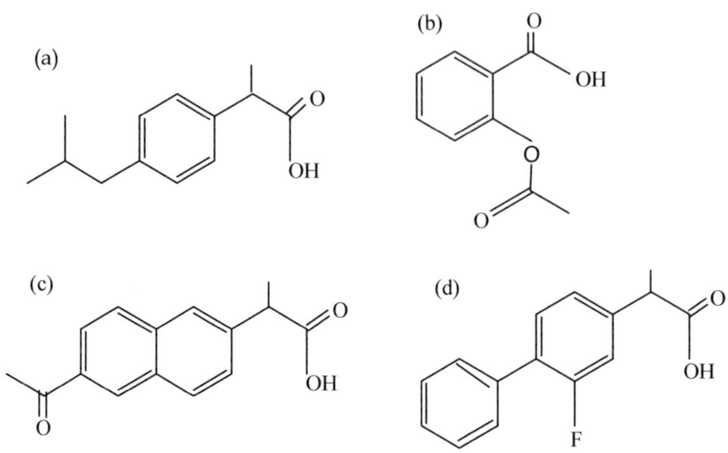

Figure 21. NSAIDs (a) Ibuprofen (b) Aspirin (c) Naproxen (d) Flubiprofen

6. Omega fatty acids in treating Alzheimer

Polyunsaturated fatty acids or PUFA have significant biological roles in cellular structure and function. PUFA are the key components of phospholipids, comprising cellular and intracellular membranes. They govern the growth and vitality through oxidation (metabolism of food to produce energy required for cellular processes), chemical activities and transportation. In addition to being the structural materials for bio-membranes, PUFA are required for generating and propagating electrical impulses; synthesis of eicosanoids, important signaling hormones with numerous complex functions. Amongst its wide range of actions include anti-inflammatory, anti-thrombotic and vasodilatory properties, balancing and counteracting pro-inflammatory, vasoconstrictor actions of eicosanoids; the cardiovascular benefits of n-3 PUFA are largely attributed to these eicosanoid properties, and at the same time having significant roles in brain function. Polyunsaturated fatty acids like alpha linoleic acids (ALA), linolenic acids (LA), eicosapentaenoic acids (EPA) or docosahexaenoic acids (DHA) are not synthesized in the body and hence must be supplied in the diet [36].

Lipids constitute approximately sixty percent of the dry weight of the brain. DHA and Arachidonic acids (AA) are the most highly concentrated PUFAs present in neural phospholipids, including sub cellular membranes. DHA is particularly concentrated at neural synapses, retina, brain and nervous system. Though there is a predominance of omega-6 fatty acids in circulation, in contrast to omega-3 fatty acids, however DHA predominates in these vital structures. The amount of DHA levels in the neural phospholipids depend on the amount of dietary intake rich in omega-3 fatty acids. Clinical studies have shown that insufficient omega-3 PUFA during early neural development shows decreased DHA content in the brain.

The n-3 PUFAs have significant biological mechanisms in brain function. Neurotransmitters such as dopamine and serotonin have a role in mental illness, research data have focused on associations between PUFA and central nervous system activity. Levels of n-3 PUFA have been associated with monoaminergic neurotransmitter levels. There are indications that PUFA are involved in the synthesis and activities of brain peptides, which are involved in modulating the activities of neurotransmitters. Evidence points to the role of eicosanoids in healthy brain functioning, and phospholipid membranes in neural cell signaling. Results of animal studies have shown that, n-3 deficiency is found to reduce phosphatidylserine (PS) levels in the brain, which is thought to play an important function in neural signaling activities. In alcoholics, DHA deficiency has predicted reduced 5-hydroxyindoleacetic acid (5-HIAA) concentrations in cerebrospinal fluid, an indicator of low serotonin turnover rate in the frontal cortex. Studies have further indicated that n-3 PUFA may affect receptor properties or activation of signal transduction by receptors. Electrical impulse conduction is dependent on the exchange of ions through the cell membrane, which relies on the fluidity and physiological structure of cell membranes. Furthermore, n-3 PUFA are also thought to influence gene expression of a range of enzymes required for important neural functions including synaptic transduction, ion channel formation, energy metabolism and formulation of proteins vital for brain development and function. Regular delivery of oxygen and nutrients via the blood is also vital for optimal brain function, and psychopathology is associated with both reduced cerebral blood flow and transportation of glucose, the brain's primary energy source, to brain regions as required. In this regard, n-3 PUFA are associated with production of nitric oxide, as well as anti-inflammatory and vasodilatory eicosanoids (notably PGI_2), and are known to assist in endothelial-dependent vasodilatation. They have also been associated with substantially increased transport of glucose across the blood-brain barrier. Therefore, it is also possible that their primary influence on brain function includes improved cerebral blood flow and blood-brain barrier integrity. This idea is supported by the fact that there's a high co-morbidity between cardiovascular disease and psychopathology, having a common underlying vascular pathology which can be mediated by lifestyle factors such as suboptimal levels of n-3 PUFA [36].

The mechanisms by which ω-3 fatty acids could interfere in AD patho physiologic features are not clear, but since anti-inflammatory effects are an important property of these fish oils rich in PUFA, they are applicable for AD also. Epidemiologic evidences have shown that administration of ω-3 fatty acid in patients with mild to moderate AD did not delay the rate of cognitive decline according to the MMSE or the cognitive portion of the Alzheimer Disease Assessment Scale but, positive effects were observed in a small group of patients with very mild AD. Increased intake of the ω-3 polyunsaturated fatty acids (primarily eicosapentaenoic acid (EPA), 20:5ω-3, and docosahexaenoic acid (DHA), 22:6ω-3) may be beneficial in reducing risk for AD. Increased fish consumption and diets supplemented with omega-3 fatty acids are found to exhibit a protective effect, cognitive improvement and enhancement of learning abilities. Animal studies on transgenic mouse model of AD with DHA-enriched diets significantly reduced total β-amyloid by 70% when compared with diets low in DHA or control chow diets [ext-link ext-link-type="bibr" rid="REF-NOC60062-9 REF-NOC60062-10"/].

However these findings cannot serve as a basis for general recommendations for treatment of AD with dietary DHA-rich fish oil preparations. Rather, larger cohort's studies in patients with mild cognitive impairment, including those at risk for AD are needed to further explore the potentiality of the ω-3 fatty acids in halting initial progression of the disease [36].

7. In silico drug design in Alzheimer

Though a number of FDA approved drugs are currently available for the treatment of Alzheimer but there are no such effective treatments to stop the insidious nerve cell death process once the disease begins. Available drugs can manage and ease some of the symptoms of the disease but the progression of the disease can in no way be slowed down by these treatments. In AD patients there is very less production of neurotransmitter acetylcholine due to the progressive damage of the cells producing acetylcholine. Most of the FDA approved drugs aim to prevent the breakdown of acetylcholine by inhibiting the enzyme acetyl cholinesterase. But in AD due to rapid destruction of nerve cells, the acetylcholine produced even though protected from further breakdown but the amount produced is significantly insufficient to transmit messages between the brain cells. This fact necessitates further new drug development.

In contrast to traditional drug discovery, "Rational Drug Design" has been found to be a more deterministic approach where the first necessary step is the identification of the molecular target critical to the disease process and then determine the molecular structure of the target molecule. In-silico drug design approach makes use of Computer Assisted Drug Design (CADD) tools to find a ligand (putative drug) that will interact with a receptor which represents the 'target site'. A ligand can bind to the receptor either by hydrophobic, electrostatic or hydrogen bonding interactions and solvation energies of the ligand and receptor sites are the important facts to be considered in this case.

The basics behind the pathology of AD is the presence of neuritic plaques containing amyloid-β-peptide (Aβ) and intra neuronal accumulation of tubule associated 'tau' protein. In order to target therapeutic strategies basing on molecular mechanisms for AD, new drug entities can be developed that will act directly on the Aβ or the amyloid precursor protein (APP) processing which may include vaccination with Aβ peptide, Aβ passive immunization. However clinical trials with a vaccine made of synthetic Aβ 1-42 showed the lateral development of encephalitis and hence the trial was put on hold though the concept exists. Passive immunization can be obtained by monoclonal antibodies against Aβ. New anti-amyloid agents to prevent fibrillizations can be designed by detailed characterizations of the proto fibrils and fibril formations. Another lucrative approach is to target the APP processing where the three major enzymes are to be targeted: alpha secretase, beta secretase and gamma secretase, the basic aim is to increase the alpha cleavage or to decrease the beta and gamma secretase activities. Nerve growth factors and neurotrophines can also act as important therapeutic targets. Growth factor gene therapy (though under clinical trial) where patient's fibroblasts transfected with NFG and transplanted to brain are expected to be effective in case of severe AD [37].

In in -silico drug design approach, computational docking techniques can be used to develop an effective drug to prevent the progression of Alzheimer disease. Here the 'TARGET' is the amyloid precursor protein (APP) and the 'LEAD COMPOUND' is the protease enzyme. By the aid of database search tools like FASTA, BLAST in Swissport, proteins having protease activity for b-APP can be identified. Next step is to identify the protease enzyme that cleaves the b-APP so as to prevent the formation of beta-amyloid peptide. Structural informations on b-APP is available from PDB (Protein Data Bank) with ID 1RW6. Soft wares like PASS, CASTp provides information about the active site for b-APP. Enzyme modeling can be done using packages like Swiss Model, Modeller etc. Specific interactions of these lead compounds with the active site of b-APP can be studied by docking programs like DOCK, AUTODOCK etc. The most effective protease enzyme with minimum energy conformation can be identified by the above procedure which will act as the potential drug in treating Alzheimer. Use of computational docking techniques help to explore a large number of compounds, study the binding characteristics of 'hits' and is found to be effective in reducing the time and monetary expenditure as associated with traditional drug development techniques [38].

8. Non-pharmacological approach

Virtually at this point of time there is no cure for Alzheimer. But apart from therapeutic interventions, attempts can be done to manage the disease and treat the symptoms by the care givers in a non-pharmacologic manner. Along with medications, physical exercise, social involvement as well as proper nutrition are essential in treating the symptoms of AD. The goal of non-pharmacologic treatment in AD though sounds simple but clinically remains a challenge where the care giver has a vital role to play; first thing is to provide a calm structured environment where the comfort, dignity of the afflicted person is maintained and the patient remains functioning as long as possible [39-41]. For AD patients the environment should be so arranged that maximize use of cognitive capacities of AD patients that are intact and compensate for those cognitive capacities that decline. Treatment in a non-pharmacologic manner aims to improve the quality of life to treat the disease symptoms. It is not a simple task for a care giver to increase functional independence, reduce the need for psychoactive medications, prolong life, reduce the need for restraints, reduce acute hospital admissions, reduce depression and improve morale. Alzheimer begins in the medial temporal lobe and spreads to other parts of the brain slowly destroying parietal, temporal and frontal lobes, cingulated cortex, hippocampus, amygdale, damaging the tempero-parieto-occipital association cortex leading to memory dysfunction, emotional disturbances, personality changes, visual, language and movement disorders. Due to damages in the frontal lobes AD patients will have difficulty in performing daily tasks; with the gradual progression of the disease hallucinations, delusions, paranoia, agitation, panic and denial are seen among the afflicted. Among the non-pharmacologic treatment domains include: properly mapped physical environment that removes fear and promotes safety, induce a sense of positive attitude or emotion among the afflicted persons by the care giver while helping in daily activities by helping them to perform the task but not to do the total task for them and make them even more dependent; change negative emotions and promote feelings of purpose and accomplishment. While treating AD patients in non-pharmacologic manner one of the major corner stone is how we understand the afflicted person and help him to understand himself [42-44]. The care giver must change his/her behavior & environment in order to change the behavior of the patient. A person in middle stage of AD should never be attempted to bring back to the realistic world but reduce his fear in all possible stages and help him to move into his sense of the world. Due to sensory impairment and lack of receptive and expressive language abilities non-verbal perceptual inputs which replace words like familiar music, known food smell, and known touch may be used and afflicted can be communicated with a look, tone or a hug to induce a feeling of care and safety. In case of negative behavior and aggression the triggering agent should be identified and eliminated. The ultimate outcome of such a treatment approach is to slow the rate of disease progression, delay institutionalization, improve the quality of life and reduce the need for medication [39]. Below in fig.22 a specially designed room is shown for sensory integration therapy.

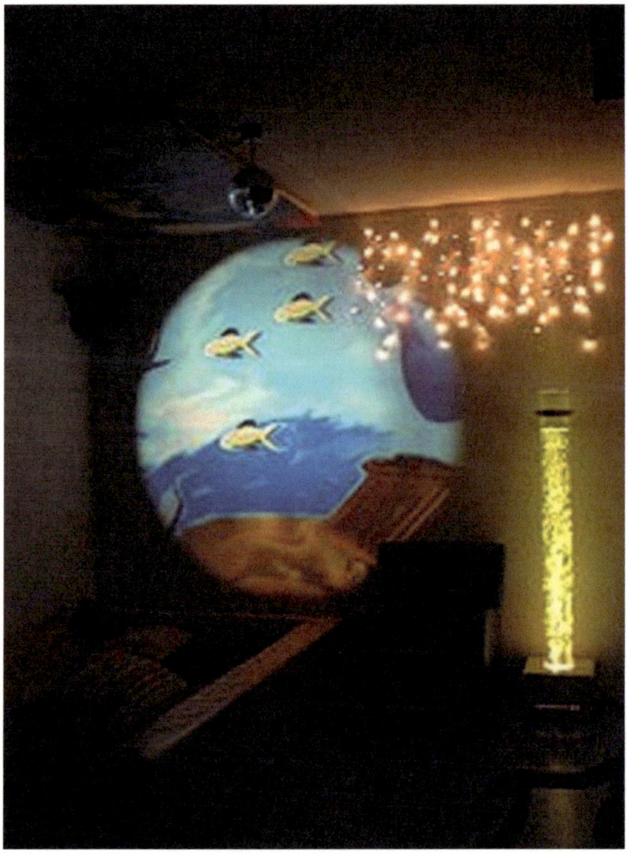

Figure 22. Specially designed room for sensory integration therapy (Snoezelen); an emotion oriented psychosocial intervention for people with dementia

9. Conclusions

There is an increasing emergency in finding a prevention or treatment for AD and dementia because of the aging of the populations and realizing the severity and complications associated with this deadly disease. Fortunately, AD and dementia research is now at a progressing stage. Availability of improved medical imaging technologies like CT scan, MRI, PET, use of biomarkers helps in early diagnosis of the disease, its progression and severity. Furthermore, pharmacological and non-pharmacological therapies could be directly tested both to prevent and delay the progression of amyloid in the brain and effects on brain morphology and cognitive decline. Pharmacological therapies that could delay the onset of dementia for several years could result in a substantial reduction in the prevalence of AD because the patients will die of another cause before they develop AD. A second and far more important approach will be the application of these new technologies to understand the etiology of AD. The identification of specific etiological factors is much more likely in the long term to have a major impact on the incidence, prevalence, and disability because of AD and dementia. Proper understanding the etiology of the disease is essential to develop hypothetical treatment approaches which can be further clinically established. Basing on in-silico drug design approaches it is essential to understand the molecular mechanisms of APP processing, role of folate and homocysteine in neuronal homeostasis. Main target should be to develop novel therapeutic agents via cost effective, eco-friendly methodologies. Along with specific drug therapy, lifestyle interventions and environmental variables are also to be targeted to reduce the incidence of AD. However in case of new drug research in Alzheimer, ability to utilize the technologies, clinical skills and financial resources to support research studies are of vital importance.

Author details

Analava Mitra* and Baishakhi Dey

*Address all correspondence to: analavamitra@gmail.com

School of Medical Science and Technology, IIT Kharagpur, India

References

[1] Basics of Alzheimer diseaseAlzheimer association (2011).

[2] Alzheimer Disease facts and FiguresAlzheimer's & Dementia. Alzheimer association (2011)., 7(2), 1-68.

[3] Yamasaki, T, Muranaka, H, Kaseda, Y, Mimori, Y, & Tobimatsu, S. Understanding the pathophysiology of Alzheimer disease and mild cognitive impairment: A mini review on fMRI and ERP studies. Neurology Research International (2011)., 20(12), 1-10.

[4] Gary, S. W. Barry RPV, Buckholtz PP, Dekosky NS, Ferris ST et al. Diagnosis and treatment of Alzheimer disease and related disorders: consensus statement of the American Association for Geriatric Psychiatry, the Alzheimer Association and the

American Geriatrics Society. Journal of the American Medical Association (1997). , 278(16), 1-9.

[5] Verghese, P. B, Castellano, J. M, & Holtzmann, D. M. Roles of Apolipoprotein E in Alzheimer's disease and Other Neurological Disorders. Lancet Neurology (2011). , 10(3), 241-252.

[6] Kuller, L. H, & Lopez, O. L. Dementia and Alzheimer's disease: A new direction. The 2010 Jay L. Foster Memorial Lecture. Alzheimer's Dement (2011). Doi:j.jalz. 2011.05.901, 7(5), 540-550.

[7] Guidelines for Alzheimer Disease ManagementCalifornia Workgroup on Guidelines for Alzheimer's disease Management (2008).

[8] Winslow, B. T, Onysko, M. K, Stob, C. M, & Hazlewood, K. A. Treatment of Alzheimer Disease. American Family Physician website www.aafp.org/afp.

[9] Alzheimer's disease and Dementia-A Growing ChallengeNational Academy on an Aging Society (2000).

[10] Bell, R. D, & Zloklovic, B. V. Neurovascular mechanisms and blood brain barrier disorder in Alzheimer's disease. Acta Neuropathologica (2009). Doi:s00401-009-0522-3, 118(1), 103-113.

[11] Alonzo, N. C, Hyman, B. T, Rebeck, G. W, & Greenberg, S. M. Progression of cerebral amyloid angiopathy: accumulation of amyloid-beta40 in affected vessels. Journal of Neuropathology and Experimental Neurology (1998). Doi:, 57, 353-359.

[12] Asahina, M, Yoshiyama, Y, & Hattori, T. Expression of matrix metalloproteinase-9 and urinary-type plasminogen activator in Alzheimer's disease brain. Clinical Neuropathology (2001). , 20, 60-63.

[13] Attems, J, Jellinger, K. A, & Lintner, F. Alzheimer's disease pathology influences severity and topographical distribution of cerebral amyloid angiopathy. Acta Neuropathologica (2005). Doi:s00401-005-1064-y., 110, 222-231.

[14] Attems, J, Quass, M, Jellinger, K. A, & Lintner, F. Topographical distribution of cerebral amyloid angiopathy and its effect on cognitive decline are influenced by Alzheimer disease pathology. Journal of Neurological Sciences (2007). Doi:10.1016/j.jns. 2007.01.013., 257, 49-55.

[15] Bailey, T. L, Rivara, C. B, Rocher, A. B, & Hof, P. R. The nature and effects of cortical microvascular pathology in aging and Alzheimer's disease. Neurological Research (2004). Doi:, 26, 573-578.

[16] Begley, D. J, & Brightman, M. W. Structural and functional aspects of the blood-brain barrier. Progress in Drug Research (2003). , 61, 39-78.

[17] Bell, R. D, Sagare, A. P, Friedman, A. E, et al. Transport pathways for clearance of human Alzheimer's amyloid beta-peptide and apolipoproteins E and J in the mouse

central nervous system. Journal of Cerebral Blood Flow and Metabolism (2007). , 27, 909-918.

[18] Corder, E. H, Saunders, A. M, Strittmatter, W. J, et al. Gene dose of apolipoprotein E type 4 allele and the risk of Alzheimer's disease in late onset families. Science. (1993). Doi:10.1126/science.8346443., 261, 921-923.

[19] Deane, R, Bell, R. D, Sagare, A, & Zlokovic, B. Z. Clearance of amyloid-beta peptide across the blood-brain barrier: implications for therapies in Alzheimer's disease. CNS and Neurological Disorders- Drug Targets (2009). Doi:

[20] Deane, R. Du Yan S, Submamaryan RK, et al. RAGE mediates amyloid-beta peptide transport across the blood-brain barrier and accumulation in brain. Nature Medicine (2003). Doi:nm890., 9, 907-913.

[21] Deane, R, Wu, Z, Sagare, A, et al. LRP/amyloid beta-peptide interaction mediates differential brain efflux of Abeta isoforms. Neuron. (2004). Doi:10.1016/j.neuron. 2004.07.017., 43, 333-344.

[22] Drzezga, A, Lautenschlager, N, Siebner, H, et al. Cerebral metabolic changes accompanying conversion of mild cognitive impairment into Alzheimer's disease: a PET follow-up study. European Journal of Nuclear Medicine and Molecular Imaging (2003). Doi:s00259-003-1194-1., 30, 1104-1113.

[23] Ervin, J. F, Pannell, C, Szymanski, M, Welsh-bohmer, K, Schmechel, D. E, & Hulette, C. M. Vascular smooth muscle actin is reduced in Alzheimer disease brain: a quantitative analysis. Journal of Neuropathology and Experimental Neurology (2004). , 63, 735-741.

[24] Grabowski, T. J, Cho, H. S, Vonsattel, J. P, Rebeck, G. W, & Greenberg, S. M. Novel amyloid precursor protein mutation in an Iowa family with dementia and severe cerebral amyloid angiopathy. Annals of Neurology (2001). Doi:10.1002/ana.1009., 49, 697-705.

[25] Jung, S. S, Zhang, W, & Van Nostrand, W. E. Pathogenic A beta induces the expression and activation of matrix metalloproteinase-2 in human cerebrovascular smooth muscle cells. Journal of Neurochemistry (2003). Doi:10.1046/j.1471-4159.2003.01745.x., 85, 1208-1215.

[26] Parks, J. K, Smith, T. S, Trimmer, P. A, & Bennett, J. P. Jr, Parker WD., Jr Neurotoxic Abeta peptides increase oxidative stress in vivo through NMDA-receptor and nitric-oxide-synthase mechanisms, and inhibit complex IV activity and induce a mitochondrial permeability transition in vitro. Journal of Neurochemistry (2001). Doi:10.1046/j. 1471-4159.2001.00112.x., 76, 1050-1056.

[27] Preston, S. D, Steart, P. V, Wilkinson, A, Nicoll, J. A, & Weller, R. O. Capillary and arterial cerebral amyloid angiopathy in Alzheimer's disease: defining the perivascu-

lar route for the elimination of amyloid beta from the human brain. Neuropathology and Applied Neurobiology (2003). Doi:10.1046/j.1365-2990.2003.00424.x., 29, 106-117.

[28] Rosenberg, G. A. Matrix metalloproteinases and their multiple roles in neurodegenerative diseases. Lancet Neurology (2009). Doi:S1474-4422(09)70016-X., 8, 205-216.

[29] Sagare, A, Deane, R, Bell, R. D, et al. Clearance of amyloid-beta by circulating lipoprotein receptors. Nature Medicine (2007). Doi:nm1635., 13, 1029-1031.

[30] Ushijima, Y, Okuyama, C, Mori, S, Kubota, T, Nakai, T, & Nishimura, T. Regional cerebral blood flow in Alzheimer's disease: Comparison between short term and long term donepezil therapy. Annals of Nuclear Medicine (2006). , 20(6), 425-429.

[31] Sugimoto, H, Yamanishi, Y, Limura, Y, & Kawakami, Y. Donepezil hydrochloride (E2020) and other Acetylcholinesterase Inhibitors. Current Medicinal Chemistry (2000). , 7-303.

[32] Orhan, G, Orhan, I, Oztekin, N. S, Fikri, A. K, & Sener, B. Contemporary Anticholinesterase Pharmaceuticals of Natural Origin and their Synthetic Analogues for the Treatment of Alzheimer Disease. Recent Patents on CNS Drug Discovery (2009). , 4, 43-51.

[33] Woodruff Pak DS, Vogel RW, Wenk GL. Mecamylamine Interactions with Galantamine and Donepezil: Effects on Learning, Acetylcholinesterase and Nicotinic Acetylcholine Receptors. Neuroscience (2003). , 117-439.

[34] Sugimoto, H. Structure-activity relationships of acetylcholinesterase inhibitors: Donepezil hydrochloride for the treatment of Alzheimer's disease. Journal of Pure and Applied Chemistry (1999). , 71(11), 2031-2037.

[35] Suh, W. H, Suslick, K. S, & Suh, Y. H. Therapeutic agents for Alzheimer Disease. Current Medicinal Chemistry-Central Nervous System Agents (2005). , 5-259.

[36] Sinn, N, & Milte, C. Howe PRC. Oiling the Brain: A Review of Randomized Controlled Trials of Omega-3 Fatty Acids in Psychopathology across the Lifespan. Nutrients (2010). , 2(2), 128-170.

[37] Religa, D, & Winblad, B. Therapeutic strategies for Alzheimer Disease based on new molecular mechanisms. Acta Neurobiol Express (2003). , 63-393.

[38] Kandavelmani, A. Alzheimer Disease: In silico Drug Design-An Endeavour. Bioinformatics India (2005). , 3(2), 25-28.

[39] Zeisel, J, & Raia, P. Non-pharmacological Treatment for Alzheimer Disease: A mind-brain approach. American Journal of Alzheimer Disease and Other Dementias (2000). , 15(6), 331-340.

[40] Weiner, M. F, & Gray, K. F. Balancing Psychosocial and Psychopharmacologic measures in Alzheimer Disease. The American Journal of Alzheimer's Care and Related Disorders and Research (1994). , 9(4), 6-12.

[41] Martichuski, D. K, & Bell, P. A. Treating excess disabilities in special care units: A Review of interventions. The American Journal of Alzheimer's Care and related disorders and Research (1993). , 5-8.

[42] Reisberg, B, Kenowsky, S, & Franssen, E. Souren LEM, Shulman E, Steinberg G, Aronstein Z, Auer S. Slowing the progression of Alzheimer Disease: Towards a Science of Alzheimer Disease care. Caring (1996). , 2(2), 2-4.

[43] Morton, I, & Bleathman, C. The effectiveness of validation therapy in dementia: a pilot study. International Journal of Geriatric Psychiatry (1991). , 6-327.

[44] Sclan, S, Saillon, A, Franssen, E, et al. The Behavioral Pathology in Alzheimer's disease Rating Scales (BEHAVE-AD): Reliability and Analysis of symptom category scores. International journal of Geriatric Psychiatry (1996). , 11-819.

Section 3

Pathopysiological Aspects of Other Neurodegenerative Diseases

Chapter 13

Other Dementias

Abhishek Shastri, Domenico Marco Bonifati and
Uday Kishore

Additional information is available at the end of the chapter

http://dx.doi.org/10.5772/53460

1. Introduction

The non-Alzheimer dementias (NAD) are a group of disorders that account for approximately 30 to 40 per cent of dementias worldwide [1-3]. Some of the common types of NAD are listed in Table 1.

2. Vascular dementia

The term vascular dementia (VaD) deals with cognitive impairment affecting daily activities required for living of vascular origin (ischemia, haemorrhage). However, VaD as a concept and disease entity is undergoing regular transformation. The term 'vascular cognitive impairment' (VCI) introduced in 1995 [4] is used to include any cognitive impairment from cerebrovascular disease (CVD) except major stroke. It was then proposed that the term VCI should include all forms of cognitive impairment associated with CVD [5] (Table 2). This term would include not only VaD but also mild cognitive impairment (MCI) with no dementia and dementia of mixed origin (Alzheimer's and vascular dementia) (see [6]). It has been argued that this classification does not fit the purpose of clinical differentiation and that this term should be restricted to MCI without dementia due to vascular cause [7]. However, some scholars are of the opinion that VCI is a research terminology and that clinicians should identify the condition and deal with the associated risk factors thereby avoiding progression to VaD [8].

The diagnostic criteria that characterise cognitive syndromes associated with vascular disease are usually based on two factors: demonstration of presence of a cognitive disorder by neuropsychological testing and history of clinical stroke or presence of vascular disease by neuroimaging that suggests a link between the cognitive disorder and vascular disease. The term VCI is not used for patients who have an active diagnosis of drug or alcohol dependence or for patients with delirium [9].

2.1. Epidemiology

VaD is considered to be the second most prevalent type of dementia worldwide accounting for about 15 to 20 % of the dementia cases [10]. Prevalence of VaD in Japan has been reported to be as high as 47 % [11]. 16 % of all cases of late-onset dementia (65 years or after) [12] and 18 % of all cases of early-onset dementia (below 65 years) [13] was found to be VaD. However, it must be kept in mind that establishing the exact epidemiology of VaD is not an easy task mainly due to difficulty in diagnosing clinically [14] and overlap of AD neuropathology (see [15]).

Some of the risk factors for developing VaD are hypertension [16] and metabolic factors like diabetes and obesity. Males are considered to be at a significantly higher risk of developing VaD [17]. The incidence rate of VaD was found to be two times higher than Alzheimer's disease for males in Japan [18]. The risk factors have been classified [19] and are listed in Table 3. Some of the protective factors found in the Canadian Study of Health and Aging include eating shellfish and regular exercise for women [20]. Antioxidants, which include vitamin E and C and also intake of fatty fish have been found to be protective against VCI [21].

a. Vascular dementia
• Vascular dementia of acute onset (post-stroke)
• Multi-infarct dementia
• Subcortical vascular dementia (Binswanger's disease)
• Mixed cortical and subcortical vascular dementia
• Other vascular dementia (CADASIL, vasculitis, post-cardiac arrest)
b. Dementia with Lewy Bodies
c. Frontotemporal dementia
d. Dementia in other diseases
• Pick's disease
• Creutzfeldt-Jakob disease
• Huntington's disease
• Parkinson's disease
• Human immunodeficiency virus (HIV) disease
e. Treatable or reversible dementias
• Normal pressure hydrocephalus
• Alcohol-related
• Neoplasia (glioma, meningioma, secondaries)
• Vitamin deficiencies (B12, folate, thiamine, nicotinic acid)
• Metabolic and endocrine (liver disease, hypothyroidism)

Table 1. Types of non-Alzheimer dementia

http://dx.doi.org/10.5772/53460

• VCI-no dementia
• Vascular dementia
• Mixed Alzheimer's disease and vascular dementia

Table 2. Vascular cognitive impairment (VCI)

1. Demographic
Age
Male sex
Lower educational level
2. Atherosclerosis
Hypertension
Cigarette smoking
Myocardial infarction
Diabetes mellitus
Hyperlipidemia
3. Genetic
CADASIL
Apolipoprotein E
4. Stroke-related
Volume of cerebral tissue loss
Bilateral cerebral infarction
Strategic infarction (thalamic, angular gyrus)
White matter disease

Table 3. Risk factors for vascular dementia according to reference [18]

2.2. Clinical features and pathophysiology

Firstly, to diagnose dementia, there should be a decline in memory and a decline in at least two cognitive skills such as orientation, social behaviour, verbal skills, attention, motor control, praxis, emotional control and executive functions (goal-directed behaviour and problem-solving skills). In VaD, the onset may be sudden or gradual, with stepwise progression. Since vascular component is involved, there may be focal neurological deficits such as hemiparesis or swallowing disturbances and dysarthria (pseudobulbar lesion symptoms). A history of transient ischaemic attacks is common. Depending on the site of the lesion, features such as motor aphasia, dyspraxia (due to left anterior cerebral artery ischemia) or psychosis (right middle cerebral artery) or amnesia and visual disturbances (posterior cerebral artery) may be seen. Other important associated features include gait disturbance which may be associated with a history of unsteadiness as well as frequent falls. It is vital to distinguish dementia of vascular origin from degenerative form of dementia. This is because VaD, when diagnosed at an early stage provides for chances to prevent or delay progression. Thus, treatment strategies may vary. For this purpose, clinicians use a scoring system called Hachinski ischaemic score [22]. A score of above six signifies dementia due to vascular cause. Some of the clinical criteria developed to assist in diagnosing VaD include State of California Alzheimer Disease Diagnostic and Treatment Centers (ADDTC) criteria [23], International Classification of Diseases (ICD-10) criteria [24], National Institute of Neurological Disorders and Stroke (NINDS)-Association Internationale pour la Recherche et l'Enseignement en Neurosciences (AIREN) criteria [25] and Diagnostic and Statistical Manual for Mental Disorders (DSM-IV) criteria [26].

The most widely followed or accepted criteria for diagnosis of VaD is the NINDS-AIREN criteria. According to this, both clinical and radiological criteria must be fulfilled. Clinical criteria include presence of dementia and CVD as well as a relation between the two features i.e. dementia should develop after and within 3 months of the stroke. Radiological criteria are based on topography and severity of vascular lesions. There should be either a large vessel stroke or multiple lacunar infarcts in basal ganglia or white matter lesions in periventricular regions. Large vessel lesions should be present in dominant hemisphere or in both the hemispheres while white matter lesions must involve at least 25 % of the cerebral white matter. However it was found that the neuroimaging criteria listed above does not always differentiate between stroke patients with and without dementia [27]. Definite vascular dementia is diagnosed by fulfilling the above mentioned criteria with histopathological evidence from brain biopsy or autopsy. Absence of other causes of dementia must be ruled out.

2.2.1. Post-stroke dementia

Post-stroke dementia (PSD) is the type of VaD developing after a stroke. Among patients who have experienced a first stroke, the prevalence of poststroke dementia (PSD) varies in relation to the interval after stroke, definition of dementia, location and size of the infarct. This includes a large-vessel lesion or single strategic lesion (thalamus or midbrain) (Figure 1). The cause of stroke may be haemorrhagic, or ischemic. The rate of dementia in people with stroke was found to be two times respect people without stroke [28]. Increasing age is significantly associated with PSD [29,30]. The severity of cognitive decline after a stroke is associated with increased risk of PSD [31]. Long-term mortality is 2 to 6 times higher in patients with PSD after adjustment for demographic factors, associated cardiac diseases, stroke severity, and stroke recurrence (for review, see [32]). Silent cerebral infarcts, white matter changes, and global and medial temporal lobe atrophy are associated with increased risk of PSD [32]. Dementia is severe in lesions involving thalamus or midbrain. After stroke, recovery of patient involving both physical and cognitive functions is variable.

2.2.2. Multi-infarct dementia

As the name suggests, there are multiple strokes occurring in the same patient (Figure 2). Sometimes these may even go undetected and may be noticed only after a major stroke. This causes the characteristic step-wise progression of the disease where there may be deterioration in cognitive abilities but also there may be periods of stability or even improvement of the patient. The severity of dementia increases with each stroke. The type of vessel involved

http://dx.doi.org/10.5772/53460

may be either large or small vessels or both. It is thought that the reason for multiple infarcts is due to underlying predisposing factors associated with VaD.

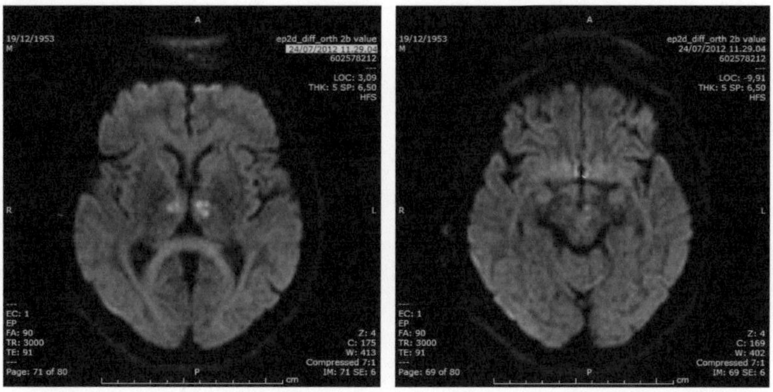

Figure 1. Brain MRI scan (DWI sequences) of a 59 years old man presenting with an acute onset of confusion, ideative and motor slowness and apathy with memory loss. A marked cognitive and motor slowness and apathy remained after 15 days from onset. MRI scan showed ischemic lesions in the medial part of both thalami and in the midbrain (top of the basilar syndrome).

2.2.3. *Binswanger's disease*

It is a type of subcortical ischaemic VaD. It is a progressive small vessel disease. Occlusion of small arteries (arterioles) leads to hypoperfusion and this in turn leads to white matter lacunes and necrosis [33]. Clinical features vary slightly where the patients develop a slowly progressing dementia. Brain imaging studies reveal increased white matter and periventricular lesions (Figure 3).

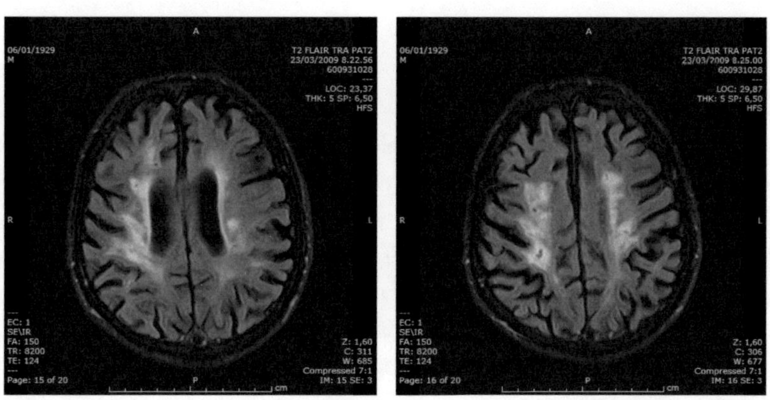

Figure 2. Brain MRI (FLAIR sequences) of a 80 years old man with a multi-infarct progressive dementia with bulbar symptoms. Multiple cortical and subcortical infarct are seen together with periventricular white matter changes and corticola atrophy.

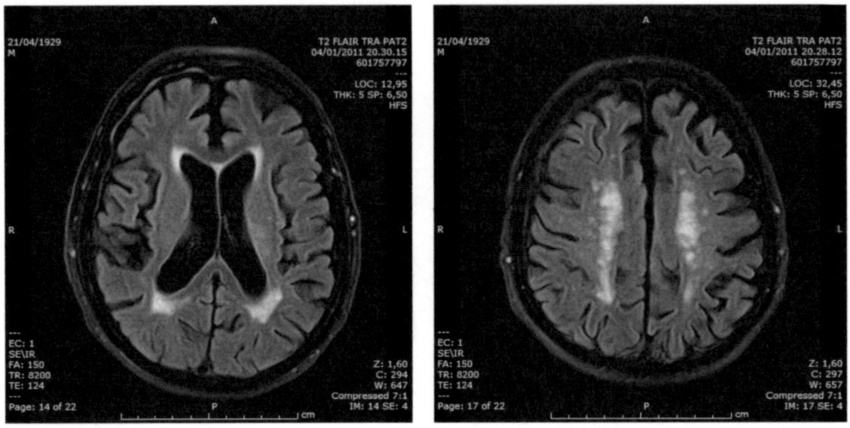

Figure 3. White matter changes and periventricular lesions observed in a 82 years old man with loss of memory and slowly progressive cognitive impairment. Brain atrophy is also present (mixed dementia)

2.2.4. Cerebral Autosomal Dominant Arteriopathy with Subcortical Infarcts and Leukoencephalopathy (CADASIL)

CADASIL is a familial form of vascular dementia. It is associated with migraine and is a subcortical ischaemic type of dementia. It is due to mutation in the *NOTCH3* gene on chromosome 19. It is the most common genetic form of VaD. The disease has an autosomal dominant type of inheritance. From the pathological point of view vascular lesions occur not only in vessels of the brain but also other organs. Hence, it can be diagnosed by skin biopsy and confirmed by immunohistochemistry with *NOTCH3* monoclonal antibody [34]. Brain imaging shows white matter lesions of necrosis and lacunae. A recessive form has also been described and mutations in the HTRA1 gene identified [35,36].

2.3. Neuropathology

The types of lesions seen in VaD are mainly infarctions. The infarctions may be present in the cortex and subcortical regions (complete infarctions) as well as the white matter and basal ganglia (lacunar infarctions). Cerebral amyloid angiopathy may be observed. Atrophy and sclerosis of hippocampus are also common [37]. A study was conducted on 135 post-mortem brains with dementia to conceptualize the natural history of cerebrovascular lesions (CVL) and operationalize it into a cerebrovascular staging system [38]. The authors rated the following CVL; in the frontal and temporal lobes: arteriosclerosis, amyloid angiopathy, perivascular hemosiderin leakage, perivascular spaces dilatation in deep and juxtacortical white matter, myelin loss and cortical infarcts; in the hippocampus: neuronal loss, perivascular spaces dilatation and presence of micro- and large infarcts; in the basal ganglia: arteriosclerosis, perivascular spaces dilatation, density of micro- and large infarcts, either lacunar or territorial.

http://dx.doi.org/10.5772/53460

2.4. Management

2.4.1. Investigations

Routine blood investigations and biochemistry including lipid and glucose levels as well as liver enzymes must be done in order to rule out treatable causes of dementia and identify risk factors such as hyperlipidemia and diabetes. The Mini-Mental State Examination is a brief but good way of screening for dementia. Executive function may be tested by Clock-Drawing Task. A proper history from the patient and/or informant must be obtained and should include history for unprovoked falls, TIA and urinary incontinence also. Computed tomography (CT) and Magnetic Resonance Imaging (MRI) are useful investigations to check for both large and small infarcts and white matter lesions. Other imaging techniques like Single Photon Emission Computed Tomography (SPECT) and Positron Emission Tomography (PET) may be done to assess blood flow. Population MRI studies have revealed high prevalence of overt small-vessel disease in the elderly population (23 % for silent lacunes and 95 % for incidental hyperintensities). These lesions are associated with an increased risk for stroke and dementia [39]. A thorough and complete neurological examination must be done to confirm signs of stroke. It is extremely important to conduct a good cardiovascular examination including measuring blood pressure and examining for presence of murmurs. Electrocardiogram to look for presence of fibrillation is essential.

2.4.2. Treatment

Since there are several risk factors associated with developing VaD, it is important to treat them or keep them in check. In people at risk for VCI, smoking cessation is mandatory. Lifestyle modification such as eating a low-fat diet, moderation in alcohol intake and regular exercise are reasonably effective. Hypertension, hyperglycemia and hypercholesterolaemia must be treated. Antiplatelet therapy is used and is effective in preventing further strokes. Primary prevention with antihypertensive drugs perindopril and indapamide has been shown to be effective in reducing risk of dementia and cognitive decline in patients with recurrent stroke [40]. Treatment of VaD is usually symptomatic. No specific drug has yet been recommended. Cholinesterase inhibitors (ChEI) such as donepezil have been found to be beneficial in improving cognition [41] but other ChEI such as galantamine[42] and rivastigmine [43] have been found to be ineffective. N-methyl-D-aspartate antagonist like memantine has been tried in trials but was also found to be ineffective [44].

2.5. Prognosis

The prognosis of VaD is generally poor. Most patients die within few years from onset. Death may be due to CVD or complications of dementia. Since there is no specific treatment recommended, it is very important to diagnose the disease at an early stage and stop it from progressing further. Preventive measures are also vital.

3. Dementia with lewy bodies

Dementia with Lewy Bodies (DLB) is a degenerative type of dementia (like AD). It is the second most common type of degenerative dementia (after AD). Lewy Bodies are inclusion bodies present in the cytoplasm containing a protein called ubiquitin. The first cases of DLB with cortical involvement were reported in 1961 [45]. The Lewy Body was seen in autopsy by neuropathological staining only as far as 1989 [46]. Over the years, DLB has been given several terminologies, namely diffuse Lewy body Disease [47], Lewy body dementia [48], Lewy body variant of AD [49], senile dementia of Lewy body type [50] and dementia associated with cortical Lewy bodies [51].

3.1. Epidemiology

The prevalence of DLB is about 0.1 to 5 % in the general population and about 10 to 20 % of all dementia cases [52-54]. The incidence is about 0.1 % a year in the general population and about 3 % a year of all new dementia diagnosed cases [55]. A French cohort study found that the incidence of DLB increases with age [56].

3.2. Clinical features and pathophysiology

The main feature is the presence of dementia which means impairment of cognition affecting normal day to day and social activities. Guidelines [57] suggest the core features as being fluctuation in level of cognition, detailed visual hallucinations that are recurrent and parkinsonism that is spontaneous. Any two of these core features indicate probable DLB while the presence of only one of the core features indicates possible DLB. Other psychiatric features may include depression, anxiety or apathy. There may also be a history of repeated falls given by the carers. Another interesting feature is the presence of Rapid Eye Movement sleep behaviour disorder (RBD) [58, 59]. RBD is a sleep disorder and is characterized by loss of muscle atonia during rapid eye movement as well as movement of limbs, with or without vocalization and dreaming. Carers often give a history that it is as though the patient is acting out his or her dreams. A recent study [60] found that inclusion of RBD as a core feature may help improve diagnosis of DLB.

On pathological examination, LB contain ubiquitin which is examined by immunohistochemistry. Increased presence of LB in the parahippocampus has been linked to increase in the severity of dementia [61]. DLB patholgy has been shown to be related to plaques in hippocampus and amygdala [62]. Another biomarker for diagnosis is α-synuclein (AS) immunohistochemistry [63]. Genetic mutation of AS has also been associated with DLB [64]. Diagnosis with AS staining was found to be more sensitive and more specific than ubiquitin staining [65]. Presence of LB in the temporal lobe has been shown to be related to visual hallucinations [66].

http://dx.doi.org/10.5772/53460

3.3. Management

3.3.1. Investigations

Clinically, dementia must be diagnosed. Other neuropsychiatric features such as depression, hallucinations and sleep disturbances must be identified. Proper history from carer or family member must be obtained. A complete psychiatric and neurological evaluation must be carried out. There are no specific diagnostic tests. MRI may show preservation of medial temporal lobe [67] or reduced amygdala volume [62]. SPECT may show hypoperfusion in occipital lobe [68]. Using SPECT with dopamine transporter imaging is turning out to be promising [69,70]. Imaging and findings of global amyloid deposition may also give a clue in diagnosis of LBD [71].

3.3.2. Treatment

Drugs used in treatment include levodopa viz. usually used to treat Parkinson's disease. A one year follow-up study has shown it to be acutely effective [72] but its use is debatable as it also lead to adverse effects most notably being hallucinations [73]. Another promising drug is memantine which was also found to be well tolerated [74]. A Cochrane review found cholinesterase inhibitors to be not useful in patients with DLB [75]. Other measures include education of carers and also reality orientation of patients.

3.4. Prognosis

The prognosis in DLB can be variable. Initial health and well-being may play a role in deciding the prognosis. When compared to AD, the prognosis has been found to be similar [76] as well as more severe [77]. No single factor have been identified that may dictate the outcome of disease progression [78].

4. Frontotemporal dementia

Frontotemporal dementia (FTD) is considered to be the second most common type of early-onset (before the age of 65) dementia. There is pathological involvement of frontal and temporal lobes of the brain. FTD consists of a behavioural variant (bvFTD) and a language variant. The language variant can be further divided into semantic dementia (SD) and progressive non-fluent aphasia (PNFA). Overlap of FTD with motor neuron disease (MND) is also seen clinically, pathologically and genetically [79]. The whole clinico-pathological spectrum is often referred to as frontotemporal lobar degeneration.

4.1. Epidemiology

The prevalence of FTD was found to be about 15 in 100,000 in UK involving age groups 45-64 years [80] while in the Netherlands it was found to be 9.4 per 100,000 in the age group 60-69 years [81]. The prevalence of early-onset AD and FTD was (be consistent between past and present verbs) found to be similar [80,82]. The incidence was found to be about 3.5 cases per 100000 person-years [83]. Average age of onset is around 50-60 years [80,81].

4.2. Clinical Features and pathophysiology

The core features are an insidious onset, decline in personal and social conduct as well as early emotional blunting and loss of insight [84]. The most common presenting symptoms are then changes in behaviour. Decrease in cognitive functions involving executive functions and speech is also observed. bvFTD is the most common of the subtypes [85] and is considered to be the most typical of FTD. It is associated with degeneration of frontal and temporal lobes [86] Other important features include behavioural disinhibition, apathy and loss of empathy [87]. SD is characterised by loss of ability to name and recognise words, objects and faces. It is associated with atrophy of left temporal lobe [88]. However, at least initially, speech in SD may be unhampered, fluent and grammatically correct [89]. In PNFA, speech is hampered and is grammatically incorrect but usually comprehension is preserved. This is associated with problems in language expression [89] and also with left temporal lobe atrophy and Broca's area degeneration [84,90]. FTD associated with MND has similar clinical presentations involving areas of language, memory and behavioural changes[91]. Genetic studies involving families where some members have FTD and others have MND have shown a repeat of hexanucleotide sequence GGGGCC in chromosome 9 open reading frame 72 region (*C9ORF72*) [92,93].

FTLD shows atrophy or degeneration of frontal and/or temporal lobes along with microvacuolation and neuronal loss in the cerebral cortex [94]. By the use of immunohistochemistry, FTLD is associated with the accumulation of microtubule-associated protein tau and trans-active response DNA-binding protein 43 (TDP-43). It can also be divided into two types (1) FTLD with tau-positive inclusions (FLTD-tau) and (2) FTLD with ubiquitin-positive and TDP-43-positive but tau-negative inclusions (FLTD-TDP) [95]. FLTD-tau mainly present as PNFA and overlap with Pick's disease while FLTD-TDP present mainly as SD and is associated with MND. Patients with bvFTD can show either of the two types of pathology [96,97]. Apart from TDP-43 involvement in MND, another protein called fused in sarcoma (FUS) is also associated with familial cases of dementia and MND [98].

4.3. Management

4.3.1. Investigations

MRI is the most useful investigation. Features of lobar atrophy may be observed. In bvFTD, there is involvement of frontal, temporal, cortical and subcortical areas (Figure 4). Hypoperfusion of these areas is also seen with SPECT and hypometabolism with PET. In the language variant, left temporal grey matter involvement is observed. Orbitofrontal cortex involvement is associated with behavioural changes in these patients. Also, cortical and subcortical hyoperfusion is found to be more marked on the left side [99]. A complete neuropsychological battery is necessary to fully characterise clinically these patients.

http://dx.doi.org/10.5772/53460

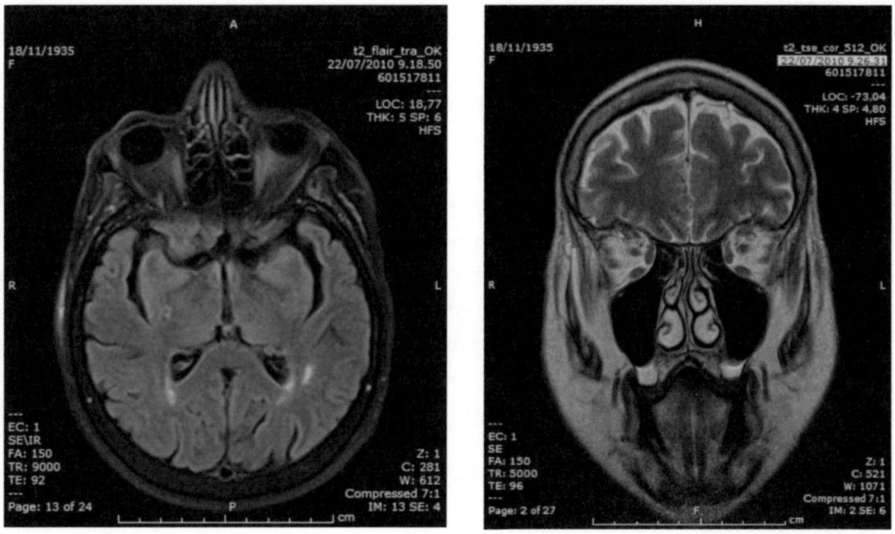

Figure 4. MRI brain scan (FLAIR and T2 sequences) of a 75 old woman with progressive FTD with mainly behavioural disturbances showing frontal and temporal lobe atrophy along with minor periventricular hyperintensities. She had deficit in executive and attention functions, aggressive behaviour and obsessive-compulsive disorder.

4.3.2. Treatment

No known or effective treatment exists for FTD. Treatment is mainly supportive or palliative. Multi-disciplinary management involving psychiatrist, physician, clinical psychologist and specialist nurse may be an effective way to treat patients with FTD.

4.4. Prognosis

The prognosis varies and to some extent depends on the type of FTD. The severity of the disease is more and clinical progression is faster in bvFTD [100]. In the language variant, the disease progression is slow with mainly impairment of language component for several years [89].

5. Dementia in other diseases

5.1. Dementia in Pick's disease

Pick's disease (PD) is a neurodegenerative disease. From the clinical point of view it overlaps with FTD but it is characterised by the presence of Pick bodies. These Pick bodies are argyrophilic, intraneuronal, cytoplasmic inclusions made up of three-repeat tau. Other features include circumscribed atrophy of frontal and temporal lobes, gliosis and loss of neurons [101] as it has seen in FTD. Clinically, patients present with symptoms similar to FTD such as those of bvFTD, PNFA and SD as mentioned previously. Therefore, it is difficult to distinguish FTD from PD clinically. Post-mortem clinical correlation studies have shown that PD is associated more closely with behavioural and language associated symptoms and not with motor disturbances [102]. The age of onset is around 45 to 65 years [103, 104]. There are no known risk factors associated with PD. 'Knife-edge' atrophy is observed pathologically in the cortex which implies sharp, circumscribed degeneration (also referred to as 'dried walnut' appearance) [105]. There may also be the presence of swollen, ballooned neurons in the cortex called as Pick cells although they are not always present. No specific treatment is available at present for PD.

5.2. Dementia in Creutzfeldt-Jakob disease

Creutzfeldt-Jakob disease (CJD) is a subacute fatal neurodegenerative disease. It is the most common of the prion diseases to affect humans. Prion proteins are infectious-like agents that cause diseases termed as transmissible spongiform encephalopathies. Prion proteins are found normally in the cells of central nervous system and immune system [106]. However, a misfolded form of this protein is considered to be pathologic. CJD occurs as sporadic, genetic, iatrogenic or juvenile variant forms. Clinical features associated with CJD are a rapidly progressive encephalopathy with dementia, cerebellar ataxia and myoclonus [107]. It progresses to stupor and coma in few months. The sporadic form of CJD (sCJD) accounts for about 85 % of all CJD cases [108, 109]. The average age of onset is around 60 years. Median time to death is about 5 months and 85-90 % of patients die within 1 year of onset [110-112]. In the familial form, mutations in the gene *PNRP* that encodes the prion protein are seen. Autosomal dominant inheritance is observed. Disease progression is slower than sCJD. Iatrogenic form of CJD occurs accidently during surgical or medical procedures. In the juvenile variant form of CJD (vCJD), the age of onset is around 30 years. Other features include early psychiatric features (depression, anxiety, apathy), delay in dementia and duration of illness of more than 6 months [113,114]. Pathologically all cases of CJD have features of neuronal loss, spongiform changes (vacuolation in grey matter) and astrogliosis [107]. Pathological prion proteins can be observed via immunohistochemistry [113].

5.3. Dementia in Huntington's disease

Huntington's disease (HD) is a genetic cause of dementia. It is inherited as an autosomal-dominant trait. The mutation in the *huntingtin* gene (chromosome 4) producing the disease was identified in 1993 [115]. Mutant protein called huntingtin has an abnormal CAG repeats (at least 36) on the coding sequence of this gene. HD is characterised by chorea (involuntary, jerky movement of limbs spreading to all muscles of body), behavioural and psychiatric changes (mainly psychoses and depression) along with dementia. The onset is around middle age (about 40 years). Cognitive changes mainly slowing of intellectual capabilities and decline of executive functions occur and may sometimes be detected even before onset of motor symptoms [116, 117]. Dementia is progressive and increases as the course of the dis-

http://dx.doi.org/10.5772/53460

ease advances. Pathological features include neostriatal (caudate and putamen) atrophy in early stages of disease [118] and presence of intranuclear inclusions of mutant huntingtin in neurons of the striatum region of the brain [119]. Management includes genetic counselling, regular neurological and neuropsychiatric evaluation. Treatment is mainly symptomatic.

5.4. Dementia in Parkinson's disease

Parkinson's disease (PD) is a neurodegenerative disease mainly associated with motor symptoms. However, dementia develops in about 40 % of the sufferers [120,121]. Dementia developing after diagnosis of PD is termed as Parkinson's disease dementia (PDD). The prevalence of PDD in PD after 8-10 years has been found to be nearly 75 % [122,123]. Risk factors for developing early dementia are old age and severity of motor symptoms [123]. Clinical diagnostic features associated with PDD are impairment in attention, executive functions and memory. Other behavioural features are apathy, hallucinations and delusions [124]. Sleep disorders like RBD may be present and has been found to be associated with increased risk of developing PDD [125]. There are no investigations to diagnose PDD but there is association with hippocampal and medial temporal lobe atrophy [126]. SPECT studies have found abnormalities in dopamine transporter and occipital region hypoperfusion [127]. Cholinergic deficits are also observed and treatment with cholinesterase inhibitors has been found to be useful in PDD [128]. Treatment is otherwise symptomatic. Prognosis varies but PDD sufferers have been found to have increased risk of mortality [129].

5.5. Dementia in HIV disease

The HIV-1 virus is known to cause AIDS and also other neurological disorders. These neurological disorders are known as HIV-associated neurocognitive disorders (HAND). The most severe form of HAND is HIV-associated dementia (HAD) [130]. The annual incidence of HAD in 1990's was 7 % [131]. However, with the advent of highly active antiretroviral therapy (HAART), the incidence has decreased by more than half to about 2 to 4% [132-134]. The clinical features as part of the diagnostic criteriae include dementia, no evidence for presence of delirium nor any other cause for dementia [130]. Neuroinflammation in brain is observed. Viral proteins that are released from infected glial cells activate uninfected microglial cells and astrocytes to secrete cytokines and neurotoxins. This causes neuronal cell death i.e. neurodegeneration [135,136]. To help in detecting HAD, a rating scale has been developed which tests timed fingertapping, alternating hand sequence test and recall of four items at 2 minutes [137]. HAART is used as treatment of HAD. The aim is to suppress the virus and its replication in plasma and CNS [138]. Some of the drugs used in HAART regimen are a combination of efavirenz, lamivudine and zidovudine. Other medications like memantine, valproic acid and selegiline listed under adjunctive therapies have not been found to be useful in HAD [139]. HAD is associated with increased mortality with median survival time after dementia found to be 6 months [131].

6. Conclusions

The NAD or other dementias form a vital part of the fight against dementia and its consequences. Even though AD forms the bulk of dementia cases, knowledge and understanding of NAD might play an important role in the much needed quest for cure or prevention of dementia. More cutting-edge research into these diseases and their pathogenesis will help combat the spread and probably even onset of dementia.

Author details

Abhishek Shastri[1*], Domenico Marco Bonifati[2] and Uday Kishore[1]

*Address all correspondence to: abhishek.shastri@brunel.ac.uk

*Address all correspondence to: domenicomarco.bonifati@apss.tn.it

1 Centre for Infection, Immunity and Disease Mechanisms, Brunel University, London, United Kingdom

2 Unit of Neurology, Department of Neurosciences, Santa Chiara Hospital, Trento, Italy

References

[1] Plassman BL, Langa KM, Fisher GG, Heeringa SG, Weir DR, Ofstedal MB, et al. Prevalence of dementia in the United States: the aging, demographics, and memory study. Neuroepidemiology 2007;29(1-2):125-132.

[2] Kalaria RN, Maestre GE, Arizaga R, Friedland RP, Galasko D, Hall K, et al. Alzheimer's disease and vascular dementia in developing countries: prevalence, management, and risk factors. Lancet Neurol 2008 Sep;7(9):812-826.

[3] Brookmeyer R, Evans DA, Hebert L, Langa KM, Heeringa SG, Plassman BL, et al. National estimates of the prevalence of Alzheimer's disease in the United States. Alzheimers Dement 2011 Jan;7(1):61-73.

[4] Bowler JV, Hachinski V. Vascular cognitive impairment: a new approach to vascular dementia. Baillieres Clin Neurol 1995 Aug;4(2):357-376.

[5] O'Brien JT, Erkinjuntti T, Reisberg B, Roman G, Sawada T, Pantoni L, et al. Vascular cognitive impairment. Lancet Neurol 2003 Feb;2(2):89-98.

[6] Moorhouse P, Rockwood K. Vascular cognitive impairment: current concepts and clinical developments. Lancet Neurol 2008 Mar;7(3):246-255.

[7] Roman GC, Sachdev P, Royall DR, Bullock RA, Orgogozo JM, Lopez-Pousa S, et al. Vascular cognitive disorder: a new diagnostic category updating vascular cognitive impairment and vascular dementia. J Neurol Sci 2004 Nov 15;226(1-2):81-87.

[8] Bowler JV. Vascular cognitive impairment. J Neurol Neurosurg Psychiatry 2005 Dec; 76 Suppl 5:v35-44.

[9] Chui HC, Mack W, Jackson JE, Mungas D, Reed BR, Tinklenberg J, et al. Clinical criteria for the diagnosis of vascular dementia: a multicenter study of comparability and interrater reliability. Arch Neurol 2000 Feb;57(2):191-196.

[10] van der Flier WM, Scheltens P. Epidemiology and risk factors of dementia. J Neurol Neurosurg Psychiatry 2005 Dec;76 Suppl 5:v2-7.

[11] Ikeda M, Hokoishi K, Maki N, Nebu A, Tachibana N, Komori K, et al. Increased prevalence of vascular dementia in Japan: a community-based epidemiological study. Neurology 2001 Sep 11;57(5):839-844.

[12] Lobo A, Launer LJ, Fratiglioni L, Andersen K, Di Carlo A, Breteler MM, et al. Prevalence of dementia and major subtypes in Europe: A collaborative study of population-based cohorts. Neurologic Diseases in the Elderly Research Group. Neurology 2000;54(11 Suppl 5):S4-9.

[13] Harvey RJ, Skelton-Robinson M, Rossor MN. The prevalence and causes of dementia in people under the age of 65 years. J Neurol Neurosurg Psychiatry 2003 Sep;74(9): 1206-1209.

[14] Mathias JL, Burke J. Cognitive functioning in Alzheimer's and vascular dementia: a meta-analysis. Neuropsychology 2009 Jul;23(4):411-423.

[15] Kalaria RN, Ballard C. Overlap between pathology of Alzheimer disease and vascular dementia. Alzheimer Dis Assoc Disord 1999 Oct-Dec;13 Suppl 3:S115-23.

[16] Sharp SI, Aarsland D, Day S, Sonnesyn H, Alzheimer's Society Vascular Dementia Systematic Review Group, Ballard C. Hypertension is a potential risk factor for vascular dementia: systematic review. Int J Geriatr Psychiatry 2011 Jul;26(7):661-669.

[17] Di Carlo A, Baldereschi M, Amaducci L, Lepore V, Bracco L, Maggi S, et al. Incidence of dementia, Alzheimer's disease, and vascular dementia in Italy. The ILSA Study. J Am Geriatr Soc 2002 Jan;50(1):41-48.

[18] Yoshitake T, Kiyohara Y, Kato I, Ohmura T, Iwamoto H, Nakayama K, et al. Incidence and risk factors of vascular dementia and Alzheimer's disease in a defined elderly Japanese population: the Hisayama Study. Neurology 1995 Jun;45(6):1161-1168.

[19] Gorelick PB. Risk factors for vascular dementia and Alzheimer disease. Stroke 2004 Nov;35(11 Suppl 1):2620-2622.

[20] Hebert R, Lindsay J, Verreault R, Rockwood K, Hill G, Dubois MF. Vascular dementia : incidence and risk factors in the Canadian study of health and aging. Stroke 2000 Jul;31(7):1487-1493.

[21] Perez L, Heim L, Sherzai A, Jaceldo-Siegl K, Sherzai A. Nutrition and vascular dementia. J Nutr Health Aging 2012 Apr;16(4):319-324.

[22] Hachinski VC, Iliff LD, Zilhka E, Du Boulay GH, McAllister VL, Marshall J, et al. Cerebral blood flow in dementia. Arch Neurol 1975 Sep;32(9):632-637.

[23] Chui HC, Victoroff JI, Margolin D, Jagust W, Shankle R, Katzman R. Criteria for the diagnosis of ischemic vascular dementia proposed by the State of California Alzheimer's Disease Diagnostic and Treatment Centers. Neurology 1992 Mar;42(3 Pt 1): 473-480.

[24] Hanisch UK, Kettenmann H. Microglia: active sensor and versatile effector cells in the normal and pathologic brain. Nat Neurosci 2007 Nov;10(11):1387-1394.

[25] Roman GC, Tatemichi TK, Erkinjuntti T, Cummings JL, Masdeu JC, Garcia JH, et al. Vascular dementia: diagnostic criteria for research studies. Report of the NINDS-AIREN International Workshop. Neurology 1993 Feb;43(2):250-260.

[26] Mathias JL, Burke J. Cognitive functioning in Alzheimer's and vascular dementia: a meta-analysis. Neuropsychology 2009 Jul;23(4):411-423.

[27] Ballard CG, Burton EJ, Barber R, Stephens S, Kenny RA, Kalaria RN, et al. NINDS AIREN neuroimaging criteria do not distinguish stroke patients with and without dementia. Neurology 2004 Sep 28;63(6):983-988.

[28] Ivan CS, Seshadri S, Beiser A, Au R, Kase CS, Kelly-Hayes M, et al. Dementia after stroke: the Framingham Study. Stroke 2004 Jun;35(6):1264-1268.

[29] Tatemichi TK, Desmond DW, Paik M, Figueroa M, Gropen TI, Stern Y, et al. Clinical determinants of dementia related to stroke. Ann Neurol 1993 Jun;33(6):568-575.

[30] Pohjasvaara T, Erkinjuntti T, Ylikoski R, Hietanen M, Vataja R, Kaste M. Clinical determinants of poststroke dementia. Stroke 1998 Jan;29(1):75-81.

[31] Henon H, Durieu I, Guerouaou D, Lebert F, Pasquier F, Leys D. Poststroke dementia: incidence and relationship to prestroke cognitive decline. Neurology 2001 Oct 9;57(7):1216-1222.

[32] Leys D, Henon H, Mackowiak-Cordoliani MA, Pasquier F. Poststroke dementia. Lancet Neurol 2005 Nov;4(11):752-759.

[33] Roman GC, Erkinjuntti T, Wallin A, Pantoni L, Chui HC. Subcortical ischaemic vascular dementia. Lancet Neurol 2002 Nov;1(7):426-436.

[34] Joutel A, Favrole P, Labauge P, Chabriat H, Lescoat C, Andreux F, et al. Skin biopsy immunostaining with a Notch3 monoclonal antibody for CADASIL diagnosis. Lancet 2001 Dec 15;358(9298):2049-2051.

[35] Hara K, Shiga A, Fukutake T, Nozaki H, Miyashita A, Yokoseki A, et al. Association of HTRA1 mutations and familial ischemic cerebral small-vessel disease. N Engl J Med 2009 Apr 23;360(17):1729-1739.

[36] Fukutake T. Cerebral autosomal recessive arteriopathy with subcortical infarcts and leukoencephalopathy (CARASIL): from discovery to gene identification. J Stroke Cerebrovasc Dis 2011 Mar-Apr;20(2):85-93.

[37] Kalaria RN, Kenny RA, Ballard CG, Perry R, Ince P, Polvikoski T. Towards defining the neuropathological substrates of vascular dementia. J Neurol Sci 2004 Nov 15;226(1-2):75-80.

[38] Deramecourt V, Slade JY, Oakley AE, Perry RH, Ince PG, Maurage CA, et al. Staging and natural history of cerebrovascular pathology in dementia. Neurology 2012 Apr 3;78(14):1043-1050.

[39] Pantoni L. Cerebral small vessel disease: from pathogenesis and clinical characteristics to therapeutic challenges. Lancet Neurol 2010 Jul;9(7):689-701.

[40] PROGRESS Collaborative Group. Effects of a perindopril-based blood pressure lowering regimen on cardiac outcomes among patients with cerebrovascular disease. Eur Heart J 2003 Mar;24(5):475-484.

[41] Roman GC, Salloway S, Black SE, Royall DR, Decarli C, Weiner MW, et al. Randomized, placebo-controlled, clinical trial of donepezil in vascular dementia: differential effects by hippocampal size. Stroke 2010 Jun;41(6):1213-1221.

[42] Craig D, Birks J. Galantamine for vascular cognitive impairment. Cochrane Database Syst Rev 2006 Jan 25;(1)(1):CD004746.

[43] Craig D, Birks J. Rivastigmine for vascular cognitive impairment. Cochrane Database Syst Rev 2005 Apr 18;(2)(2):CD004744.

[44] Kavirajan H, Schneider LS. Efficacy and adverse effects of cholinesterase inhibitors and memantine in vascular dementia: a meta-analysis of randomised controlled trials. Lancet Neurol 2007 Sep;6(9):782-792.

[45] Okazaki H, Lipkin LE, Aronson SM. Diffuse intracytoplasmic ganglionic inclusions (Lewy type) associated with progressive dementia and quadriparesis in flexion. J Neuropathol Exp Neurol 1961 Apr;20:237-244.

[46] Lennox G, Lowe J, Landon M, Byrne EJ, Mayer RJ, Godwin-Austen RB. Diffuse Lewy body disease: correlative neuropathology using anti-ubiquitin immunocytochemistry. J Neurol Neurosurg Psychiatry 1989 Nov;52(11):1236-1247.

[47] Kosaka K, Yoshimura M, Ikeda K, Budka H. Diffuse type of Lewy body disease: progressive dementia with abundant cortical Lewy bodies and senile changes of varying degree--a new disease? Clin Neuropathol 1984 Sep-Oct;3(5):185-192.

[48] Gibb WR, Esiri MM, Lees AJ. Clinical and pathological features of diffuse cortical Lewy body disease (Lewy body dementia). Brain 1987 Oct;110 (Pt 5)(Pt 5):1131-1153.

[49] Hansen L, Salmon D, Galasko D, Masliah E, Katzman R, DeTeresa R, et al. The Lewy body variant of Alzheimer's disease: a clinical and pathologic entity. Neurology 1990 Jan;40(1):1-8.

[50] Perry RH, Irving D, Blessed G, Fairbairn A, Perry EK. Senile dementia of Lewy body type. A clinically and neuropathologically distinct form of Lewy body dementia in the elderly. J Neurol Sci 1990 Feb;95(2):119-139.

[51] Stoll G, Jander S. Microglia. eLS: John Wiley & Sons, Ltd; 2001.

[52] Yamada T, Hattori H, Miura A, Tanabe M, Yamori Y. Prevalence of Alzheimer's disease, vascular dementia and dementia with Lewy bodies in a Japanese population. Psychiatry Clin Neurosci 2001 Feb;55(1):21-25.

[53] Stevens T, Livingston G, Kitchen G, Manela M, Walker Z, Katona C. Islington study of dementia subtypes in the community. Br J Psychiatry 2002 Mar;180:270-276.

[54] Rahkonen T, Eloniemi-Sulkava U, Rissanen S, Vatanen A, Viramo P, Sulkava R. Dementia with Lewy bodies according to the consensus criteria in a general population aged 75 years or older. J Neurol Neurosurg Psychiatry 2003 Jun;74(6):720-724.

[55] Zaccai J, McCracken C, Brayne C. A systematic review of prevalence and incidence studies of dementia with Lewy bodies. Age Ageing 2005 Nov;34(6):561-566.

[56] Perez F, Helmer C, Dartigues JF, Auriacombe S, Tison F. A 15-year population-based cohort study of the incidence of Parkinson's disease and dementia with Lewy bodies in an elderly French cohort. J Neurol Neurosurg Psychiatry 2010 Jul;81(7):742-746.

[57] McKeith IG, Dickson DW, Lowe J, Emre M, O'Brien JT, Feldman H, et al. Diagnosis and management of dementia with Lewy bodies: third report of the DLB Consortium. Neurology 2005 Dec 27;65(12):1863-1872.

[58] Ferman TJ, Boeve BF, Smith GE, Silber MH, Lucas JA, Graff-Radford NR, et al. Dementia with Lewy bodies may present as dementia and REM sleep behavior disorder without parkinsonism or hallucinations. J Int Neuropsychol Soc 2002 Nov;8(7): 907-914.

[59] Boeve BF, Silber MH, Ferman TJ. REM sleep behavior disorder in Parkinson's disease and dementia with Lewy bodies. J Geriatr Psychiatry Neurol 2004 Sep;17(3):146-157.

[60] Ferman TJ, Boeve BF, Smith GE, Lin SC, Silber MH, Pedraza O, et al. Inclusion of RBD improves the diagnostic classification of dementia with Lewy bodies. Neurology 2011 Aug 30;77(9):875-882.

[61] Harding AJ, Halliday GM. Cortical Lewy body pathology in the diagnosis of dementia. Acta Neuropathol 2001 Oct;102(4):355-363.

[62] Burton EJ, Mukaetova-Ladinska EB, Perry RH, Jaros E, Barber R, O'Brien JT. Neuropathological correlates of volumetric MRI in autopsy-confirmed Lewy body dementia. Neurobiol Aging 2012 Jul;33(7):1228-1236.

[63] Spillantini MG, Schmidt ML, Lee VM, Trojanowski JQ, Jakes R, Goedert M. Alpha-synuclein in Lewy bodies. Nature 1997 Aug 28;388(6645):839-840.

http://dx.doi.org/10.5772/53460

[64] Zarranz JJ, Alegre J, Gomez-Esteban JC, Lezcano E, Ros R, Ampuero I, et al. The new mutation, E46K, of alpha-synuclein causes Parkinson and Lewy body dementia. Ann Neurol 2004 Feb;55(2):164-173.

[65] Gomez-Tortosa E, Newell K, Irizarry MC, Sanders JL, Hyman BT. alpha-Synuclein immunoreactivity in dementia with Lewy bodies: morphological staging and comparison with ubiquitin immunostaining. Acta Neuropathol 2000 Apr;99(4):352-357.

[66] Harding AJ, Broe GA, Halliday GM. Visual hallucinations in Lewy body disease relate to Lewy bodies in the temporal lobe. Brain 2002 Feb;125(Pt 2):391-403.

[67] Watson R, Blamire AM, O'Brien JT. Magnetic resonance imaging in lewy body dementias. Dement Geriatr Cogn Disord 2009;28(6):493-506.

[68] Lobotesis K, Fenwick JD, Phipps A, Ryman A, Swann A, Ballard C, et al. Occipital hypoperfusion on SPECT in dementia with Lewy bodies but not AD. Neurology 2001 Mar 13;56(5):643-649.

[69] McKeith I, O'Brien J, Walker Z, Tatsch K, Booij J, Darcourt J, et al. Sensitivity and specificity of dopamine transporter imaging with 123I-FP-CIT SPECT in dementia with Lewy bodies: a phase III, multicentre study. Lancet Neurol 2007 Apr;6(4):305-313.

[70] O'Brien JT, McKeith IG, Walker Z, Tatsch K, Booij J, Darcourt J, et al. Diagnostic accuracy of 123I-FP-CIT SPECT in possible dementia with Lewy bodies. Br J Psychiatry 2009 Jan;194(1):34-39.

[71] Gomperts SN, Rentz DM, Moran E, Becker JA, Locascio JJ, Klunk WE, et al. Imaging amyloid deposition in Lewy body diseases. Neurology 2008 Sep 16;71(12):903-910.

[72] Lucetti C, Logi C, Del Dotto P, Berti C, Ceravolo R, Baldacci F, et al. Levodopa response in dementia with lewy bodies: a 1-year follow-up study. Parkinsonism Relat Disord 2010 Sep;16(8):522-526.

[73] Ballard C, Kahn Z, Corbett A. Treatment of dementia with Lewy bodies and Parkinson's disease dementia. Drugs Aging 2011 Oct 1;28(10):769-777.

[74] Aarsland D, Ballard C, Walker Z, Bostrom F, Alves G, Kossakowski K, et al. Memantine in patients with Parkinson's disease dementia or dementia with Lewy bodies: a double-blind, placebo-controlled, multicentre trial. Lancet Neurol 2009 Jul;8(7): 613-618.

[75] Rolinski M, Fox C, Maidment I, McShane R. Cholinesterase inhibitors for dementia with Lewy bodies, Parkinson's disease dementia and cognitive impairment in Parkinson's disease. Cochrane Database Syst Rev 2012 Mar 14;3:CD006504.

[76] Ballard C, O'Brien J, Morris CM, Barber R, Swann A, Neill D, et al. The progression of cognitive impairment in dementia with Lewy bodies, vascular dementia and Alzheimer's disease. Int J Geriatr Psychiatry 2001 May;16(5):499-503.

[77] Walker Z, Allen RL, Shergill S, Mullan E, Katona CL. Three years survival in patients with a clinical diagnosis of dementia with Lewy bodies. Int J Geriatr Psychiatry 2000 Mar;15(3):267-273.

[78] McKeith I, Mintzer J, Aarsland D, Burn D, Chiu H, Cohen-Mansfield J, et al. Dementia with Lewy bodies. Lancet Neurol 2004 Jan;3(1):19-28.

[79] Burrell JR, Kiernan MC, Vucic S, Hodges JR. Motor neuron dysfunction in frontotemporal dementia. Brain 2011 Sep;134(Pt 9):2582-2594.

[80] Ratnavalli E, Brayne C, Dawson K, Hodges JR. The prevalence of frontotemporal dementia. Neurology 2002 Jun 11;58(11):1615-1621.

[81] Rosso SM, Donker Kaat L, Baks T, Joosse M, de Koning I, Pijnenburg Y, et al. Frontotemporal dementia in The Netherlands: patient characteristics and prevalence estimates from a population-based study. Brain 2003 Sep;126(Pt 9):2016-2022.

[82] Borroni B, Alberici A, Grassi M, Rozzini L, Turla M, Zanetti O, et al. Prevalence and demographic features of early-onset neurodegenerative dementia in Brescia County, Italy. Alzheimer Dis Assoc Disord 2011 Oct;25(4):341-344.

[83] Mercy L, Hodges JR, Dawson K, Barker RA, Brayne C. Incidence of early-onset dementias in Cambridgeshire, United Kingdom. Neurology 2008 Nov 4;71(19): 1496-1499.

[84] Neary D, Snowden JS, Gustafson L, Passant U, Stuss D, Black S, et al. Frontotemporal lobar degeneration: a consensus on clinical diagnostic criteria. Neurology 1998 Dec; 51(6):1546-1554.

[85] Johnson JK, Diehl J, Mendez MF, Neuhaus J, Shapira JS, Forman M, et al. Frontotemporal lobar degeneration: demographic characteristics of 353 patients. Arch Neurol 2005 Jun;62(6):925-930.

[86] Neary D, Snowden J, Mann D. Frontotemporal dementia. Lancet Neurol 2005 Nov; 4(11):771-780.

[87] Rascovsky K, Hodges JR, Kipps CM, Johnson JK, Seeley WW, Mendez MF, et al. Diagnostic criteria for the behavioral variant of frontotemporal dementia (bvFTD): current limitations and future directions. Alzheimer Dis Assoc Disord 2007 Oct-Dec; 21(4):S14-8.

[88] Hodges JR, Patterson K, Oxbury S, Funnell E. Semantic dementia. Progressive fluent aphasia with temporal lobe atrophy. Brain 1992 Dec;115 (Pt 6)(Pt 6):1783-1806.

[89] Tambuyzer BR, Ponsaerts P, Nouwen EJ. Microglia: gatekeepers of central nervous system immunology. J Leukoc Biol 2009 Mar;85(3):352-370.

[90] Nestor PJ, Graham NL, Fryer TD, Williams GB, Patterson K, Hodges JR. Progressive non-fluent aphasia is associated with hypometabolism centred on the left anterior insula. Brain 2003 Nov;126(Pt 11):2406-2418.

http://dx.doi.org/10.5772/53460

[91] Lillo P, Hodges JR. Frontotemporal dementia and motor neurone disease: overlapping clinic-pathological disorders. J Clin Neurosci 2009 Sep;16(9):1131-1135.

[92] Renton AE, Majounie E, Waite A, Simon-Sanchez J, Rollinson S, Gibbs JR, et al. A hexanucleotide repeat expansion in C9ORF72 is the cause of chromosome 9p21-linked ALS-FTD. Neuron 2011 Oct 20;72(2):257-268.

[93] DeJesus-Hernandez M, Mackenzie IR, Boeve BF, Boxer AL, Baker M, Rutherford NJ, et al. Expanded GGGGCC hexanucleotide repeat in noncoding region of C9ORF72 causes chromosome 9p-linked FTD and ALS. Neuron 2011 Oct 20;72(2):245-256.

[94] Cairns NJ, Bigio EH, Mackenzie IR, Neumann M, Lee VM, Hatanpaa KJ, et al. Neuropathologic diagnostic and nosologic criteria for frontotemporal lobar degeneration: consensus of the Consortium for Frontotemporal Lobar Degeneration. Acta Neuropathol 2007 Jul;114(1):5-22.

[95] Mackenzie IR, Neumann M, Bigio EH, Cairns NJ, Alafuzoff I, Kril J, et al. Nomenclature and nosology for neuropathologic subtypes of frontotemporal lobar degeneration: an update. Acta Neuropathol 2010 Jan;119(1):1-4.

[96] Piguet O, Hornberger M, Mioshi E, Hodges JR. Behavioural-variant frontotemporal dementia: diagnosis, clinical staging, and management. Lancet Neurol 2011 Feb; 10(2):162-172.

[97] Rohrer JD, Lashley T, Schott JM, Warren JE, Mead S, Isaacs AM, et al. Clinical and neuroanatomical signatures of tissue pathology in frontotemporal lobar degeneration. Brain 2011 Sep;134(Pt 9):2565-2581.

[98] Mackenzie IR, Rademakers R, Neumann M. TDP-43 and FUS in amyotrophic lateral sclerosis and frontotemporal dementia. Lancet Neurol 2010 Oct;9(10):995-1007.

[99] Agosta F, Canu E, Sarro L, Comi G, Filippi M. Neuroimaging findings in frontotemporal lobar degeneration spectrum of disorders. Cortex 2012 Apr;48(4):389-413.

[100] Mioshi E, Hsieh S, Savage S, Hornberger M, Hodges JR. Clinical staging and disease progression in frontotemporal dementia. Neurology 2010 May 18;74(20):1591-1597.

[101] McKhann GM, Albert MS, Grossman S, Miller B, Dickson D, Trojanowski JQ. Clinical and Pathological Diagnosis of Frontotemporal Dementia. Report of the Work Group on Frontotemporal Dementia and Pick's Disease. Arch Neurol 2001;58:1803-1809.

[102] Yokota O, Tsuchiya K, Arai T, Yagishita S, Matsubara O, Mochizuki A, et al. Clinicopathological characterization of Pick's disease versus frontotemporal lobar degeneration with ubiquitin/TDP-43-positive inclusions. Acta Neuropathol 2009 Apr;117(4): 429-444.

[103] Binetti G, Locascio JJ, Corkin S, Vonsattel JP, Growdon JH. Differences between Pick disease and Alzheimer disease in clinical appearance and rate of cognitive decline. Arch Neurol 2000 Feb;57(2):225-232.

[104] Cohen BJ. Theory and Practice of Psychiatry. New York: Oxford University Press; 2003.

[105] Munoz DJ, Morris HR, Rossor M. Pick's Disease. In: Dickson DW, Weller RO (eds.) Neurodegeneration: The Molecular Pathology of Dementia and Movement Disorders, Second Edition. Blackwell Publishing Ltd.; 2011. p156-164.

[106] Aguzzi A, Heikenwalder M. Pathogenesis of prion diseases: current status and future outlook. Nat Rev Microbiol 2006 Oct;4(10):765-775.

[107] Sikorska B, Knight R, Ironside JW, Liberski PP. Creutzfeldt-Jakob Disease. In: Ahmad SI (ed.) Neurodegenerative Diseases. Landes Bioscience and Springer Science+Business Media; 2012. p76-90.

[108] Rosenbloom MH, Atri A. The evaluation of rapidly progressive dementia. Neurologist 2011 Mar;17(2):67-74.

[109] Aguzzi A, Calella AM. Prions: protein aggregation and infectious diseases. Physiol Rev 2009 Oct;89(4):1105-1152.

[110] Geschwind MD, Shu H, Haman A, Sejvar JJ, Miller BL. Rapidly progressive dementia. Ann Neurol 2008 Jul;64(1):97-108.

[111] Brown P, Gibbs CJ,Jr, Rodgers-Johnson P, Asher DM, Sulima MP, Bacote A, et al. Human spongiform encephalopathy: the National Institutes of Health series of 300 cases of experimentally transmitted disease. Ann Neurol 1994 May;35(5):513-529.

[112] Johnson RT, Gibbs CJ,Jr. Creutzfeldt-Jakob disease and related transmissible spongiform encephalopathies. N Engl J Med 1998 Dec 31;339(27):1994-2004.

[113] Johnson RT. Prion diseases. Lancet Neurol 2005 Oct;4(10):635-642.

[114] Heath CA, Cooper SA, Murray K, Lowman A, Henry C, MacLeod MA, et al. Validation of diagnostic criteria for variant Creutzfeldt-Jakob disease. Ann Neurol 2010 Jun; 67(6):761-770.

[115] A novel gene containing a trinucleotide repeat that is expanded and unstable on Huntington's disease chromosomes. The Huntington's Disease Collaborative Research Group. Cell 1993 Mar 26;72(6):971-983.

[116] Gil JM, Rego AC. Mechanisms of neurodegeneration in Huntington's disease. Eur J Neurosci 2008 Jun;27(11):2803-2820.

[117] Lovestone S. Alzheimer's Disease and Other Dementias (Including Pseudodementias). In: David AS, Fleminger S, Kopelman MD, Lovestone S, Mellers JDC (eds.) Lishman's Organic Psychiatry, Fourth Edition. Blackwell Publishing; 2009. p543-616.

[118] Sturrock A, Leavitt BR. The clinical and genetic features of Huntington disease. J Geriatr Psychiatry Neurol 2010 Dec;23(4):243-259.

[119] Ross CA, Poirier MA. Protein aggregation and neurodegenerative disease. Nat Med 2004 Jul;10 Suppl:S10-7.

[120] Emre M. Dementia associated with Parkinson's disease. Lancet Neurol 2003 Apr;2(4): 229-237.

[121] Perez F, Helmer C, Foubert-Samier A, Auriacombe S, Dartigues JF, Tison F. Risk of dementia in an elderly population of Parkinson's disease patients: A 15-year population-based study. Alzheimers Dement 2012 May 30.

[122] Aarsland D, Andersen K, Larsen JP, Lolk A, Kragh-Sorensen P. Prevalence and characteristics of dementia in Parkinson disease: an 8-year prospective study. Arch Neurol 2003 Mar;60(3):387-392.

[123] Aarsland D, Kurz MW. The epidemiology of dementia associated with Parkinson's disease. Brain Pathol 2010 May;20(3):633-639.

[124] Emre M, Aarsland D, Brown R, Burn DJ, Duyckaerts C, Mizuno Y, et al. Clinical diagnostic criteria for dementia associated with Parkinson's disease. Mov Disord 2007 Sep 15;22(12):1689-707; quiz 1837.

[125] Postuma RB, Bertrand JA, Montplaisir J, Desjardins C, Vendette M, Rios Romenets S, et al. Rapid eye movement sleep behavior disorder and risk of dementia in Parkinson's disease: A prospective study. Mov Disord 2012 May;27(6):720-726.

[126] Weintraub D, Doshi J, Koka D, Davatzikos C, Siderowf AD, Duda JE, et al. Neurodegeneration across stages of cognitive decline in Parkinson disease. Arch Neurol 2011 Dec;68(12):1562-1568.

[127] Rossi C, Volterrani D, Nicoletti V, Manca G, Frosini D, Kiferle L, Unti E, De Feo P, Bonuccelli U, Ceravolo R. "Parkinson-dementia" diseases: A comparison by double tracer SPECT studies. Parkinsonism and Related Disorders 2009 (15)762-766.

[128] Rolinski M, Fox C, Maidment I, McShane R. Cholinesterase inhibitors for dementia with Lewy bodies, Parkinson's disease dementia and cognitive impairment in Parkinson's disease. Cochrane Database Syst Rev 2012 Mar 14;3:CD006504.

[129] Levy G, Tang MX, Louis ED, Cote LJ, Alfaro B, Mejia H, et al. The association of incident dementia with mortality in PD. Neurology 2002 Dec 10;59(11):1708-1713.

[130] Antinori A, Arendt G, Becker JT, Brew BJ, Byrd DA, Cherner M, et al. Updated research nosology for HIV-associated neurocognitive disorders. Neurology 2007 Oct 30;69(18):1789-1799.

[131] McArthur JC, Hoover DR, Bacellar H, Miller EN, Cohen BA, Becker JT, et al. Dementia in AIDS patients: incidence and risk factors. Multicenter AIDS Cohort Study. Neurology 1993 Nov;43(11):2245-2252.

[132] Sacktor N. The epidemiology of human immunodeficiency virus-associated neurological disease in the era of highly active antiretroviral therapy. J Neurovirol 2002 Dec;8 Suppl 2:115-121.

[133] Mocroft A, Katlama C, Johnson AM, Pradier C, Antunes F, Mulcahy F, et al. AIDS across Europe, 1994-98: the EuroSIDA study. Lancet 2000 Jul 22;356(9226):291-296.

[134] Heaton RK, Clifford DB, Franklin DR,Jr, Woods SP, Ake C, Vaida F, et al. HIV-associated neurocognitive disorders persist in the era of potent antiretroviral therapy: CHARTER Study. Neurology 2010 Dec 7;75(23):2087-2096.

[135] Nath A. Human immunodeficiency virus (HIV) proteins in neuropathogenesis of HIV dementia. J Infect Dis 2002 Dec 1;186 Suppl 2:S193-8.

[136] del Palacio M, Alvarez S, Munoz-Fernandez MA. HIV-1 infection and neurocognitive impairment in the current era. Rev Med Virol 2012 Jan;22(1):33-45.

[137] Sacktor NC, Wong M, Nakasujja N, Skolasky RL, Selnes OA, Musisi S, et al. The International HIV Dementia Scale: a new rapid screening test for HIV dementia. AIDS 2005 Sep 2;19(13):1367-1374.

[138] McArthur JC, Brew BJ, Nath A. Neurological complications of HIV infection. Lancet Neurol 2005 Sep;4(9):543-555.

[139] Uthman OA, Abdulmalik JO. Adjunctive therapies for AIDS dementia complex. Cochrane Database Syst Rev 2008 Jul 16;(3)(3):CD006496.

Chapter 14

The Role of Epigenetics in Neurodegenerative Diseases

Luca Lovrečić, Aleš Maver, Maja Zadel and
Borut Peterlin

Additional information is available at the end of the chapter

http://dx.doi.org/10.5772/54744

1. Introduction

Neurodegenerative disorders are among the greatest challenges and among the most serious health problems that will have to be faced by the modern societies across the world, especially in light of increasing population age. They are incurable, progressive conditions resulting from continuous degeneration and death of nerve cells. Most of these disorders become more common with advancing age, including Alzheimer's disease and Parkinson's disease. The burden of these neurodegenerative diseases is growing inexorably as the population ages, with incalculable economic and human costs. According to a collaborative study of the World Health Organization, the World Bank and the Harvard School of Public Health (the Global Burden of Disease Study) dementia and other neurodegenerative diseases will be the eighth cause of disease burden for developed regions in 2020 [1, 2]. Moreover, they will become the world's second leading cause of death by 2050, overtaking cancer [2]. These future projections are of course only estimates, but they in combination with current state certainly support the fact that neurodegenerative diseases are of an increasing public concern

Although a minor subset of these disorders is caused by clearly defined genetic factors, for example Huntington's disease, the largest proportion arise due to a complex interplay of genetic and environmental factors. For this reason, delineation of specific risk factors, useful biomarkers, potential new therapeutic targets and agents and even definite diagnosis still remains difficult. Pathological characteristics in brain during the process of neurodegeneration show considerable overlap among different types of neurodegenerative cognitive and motor impairment [3]. Moreover, pathological findings do not neccessarily correlate with clinical findings, meaning that extensive neuropathology does not definitely imply a severly impared neurological function and, on the other hand, minor pathology may entail significantly impaired neurological function [4, 5]. Namely, neuropathological processes are not necessarily the cause of the underlying disease at the early disease stages, but may merely be the reflection of fundamental disease processes, yet unknown in majority of neurodegenerative disorders. Later, as disease progresses, neuropathological changes probably contribute to disease progression in a positive feedback loop.

Currently, there is no diagnostic test that can clearly indicate the presence, absence, or category of a neurodegenerative disease. Individual diagnosis is based on clinical evaluation of the symptoms and specific neuroimaging characteristics, and it often takes years to make one. The exceptions are monogenic diseases, such as Huntington's disease (HD), where specific genetic test confirms the diagnosis.

Another unexplained field is underlying mechanism in a majority of neurodegenerative diseases. Most are characterized by the aggregation of intracellular proteins, but it is not clear whether this is a primary mechanism or a consequence of another disturbed cell function. The potential mechanisms of neurodegeneration are innumerable, including primary effects of protein homeostasis, disturbed protein degradation, gene expression, transcriptional regulation, mitochondrial dysfunction, etc. There is the urgent need to better understand disease pathophysiology in order to improve early diagnosis and development of disease-modifying treatments.

In the recent decade, however, a role of epigenetic alterations in development of neurodegenerative diseases has been increasingly discussed. Epigenetic constitution presents a landscape where environmental factors may interact with genetic make-up of an individual. Additionally, the development of high-throughput technologies for genomic, trancriptomic and epigenomic profiling now offers insight into epigenetic alterations in neurodegeneration, as well as opportunity for an integrative view of its interactions with various 'omic' levels. Interpretation of epigenomic profiling results in the context of neurodegeneration and the methodology for integration of heterogeneous 'omic' data opens an array of novel biological and bioinformatic challenges and requires the development of novel approaches towards analysis of these data.

2. Neurodegenerative disorders

2.1. Common neurodegenerative disorders – Alzheimer and Parkinson disease

Parkinson's disease (PD) and Alzheimer disease (AD) are two most common neurodegenerative diseases. Both are very heterogeneous in regard to the causes (combination of genetic and environmental factors), wide range in the age at onset, vast variety in leading symptoms and presenting clinical manifestations, disease progression and responses to different therapies. Definitive clinical diagnosis is hard, although a number of clinical and neuropsychological tests are often employed when making it. AD is detected with approximately 85–90% accuracy and PD with approximately 75% accuracy. Despite endless number of research groups worldwide trying to uncover and explain the pathogenesis of both AD and PD, they still remain unexplained.

Ballard et all estimated in 2011[6] that 24 million people have dementia worldwide, majority attributable to AD. Namely, it is foreseen that more than 80 million people will have AD by 2040 [7], because of the population ageing and age-dependent incidence rate of AD. In order to improve development of disease-modifying treatment we need to understand the underlying pathophysiology of the disease. It is a progressive neurodegenerative disease which predominantly affects cortical and hippocampal neurons and leads to their irreversible loss [8]. Major clinical signs and symptoms include progressive impairment in memory, judgment, decision making, orientation to physical surroundings, and language. There are several neuropathological features in AD, but only 2 are considered essential for the diagnosis - β amyloid containing extracellular senile plaques and neurofibrillary tangles, composed of a hyperphosphorylated form of the microtubular protein tau. Others include synapse loss, neuron loss, atrophy, gliosis, degenerative changes in white matter, granulovacuolar degeneration, other protein aggregates [9].

PD was first described by James Parkinson in earyl 1800s as "shaking palsy". It is the second most prevalent neurodegenerative disease after AD. There are over 6 million people with PD worldwide (European Parkinson's Disease Association, EPDA). As elderly population increases, this estimate is predicted to double by the year 2040. The typical clinical signs are resting tremor, bradykinesia, muscle rigidity, and postural instability. The key neuropathological characteristics are the loss of neurons in the substantia nigra and the presence of neuronal protein aggregates termed Lewy bodies [10]. It is believed that approximately 5-20% of patients have monogenic PD with more than 10 genes being identified as causative. These gene defects in familial PD highlight the importance of genetic influences in this disease, however the majority of PD cases are considered sporadic and idiopathic nad thus believed to be largely influenced also by other factors. The current consensus suggests that PD develops from multiple risk factors including aging, genetic predisposition, and environmental exposure [11].

Important future challenge in the management AD and PD remains the establishment of early diagnosis or even identification of individuals prior to the onset of dementia in AD or resting tremor in PD. This implicates advancement in understanding disease pathogenesis and development of diagnostic approaches, including disease/process specific biomarkers.

2.2. Huntington disease – A model of genetic neurodegenerative disorder

Huntington disease is a late onset, autosomal dominant genetic disease - its cause is invariably trinucleotide expansion mutation, known for almost 2 decades [12]. Typical clinical signs are progressive motor impairment, cognitive decline and various psychiatric symptoms with the age of onset between 30 and 50 years. The disease is fatal after 15-20 years of progressive neurodegeneration [13]. So far, no effective treatment has been available to cure the disease or to even efficiently slow its progression. Although hyperkinesias and psychiatric symptoms respond well to pharmacotherapy, neuropsychological deficits and dementia remain untreatable [14]. There is no way of predicting the age at onset. Also, due to the insensitive clinical rating scales, it is not feasible to follow the disease progression over short time periods. Moreover, there are no specific measures to follow response to symptomatic treatment over short time periods. In addition, in the presymptomatic period when preventive treatment and slowing of neurodegeneration might be most effective, there are no measures/markers to monitor those responses and benefits.

The function of normal huntingtin in the cells and mutation mechanism that leads to neurodegeneration and typical signs are still not clear, despite the fact, that the responsible gene and mutation were already identified and characterized in 1993. Basic research created many different hypotheses about pathogenic mechanisms – they include disturbances in variety of biochemical pathways, such as accumulation of misfolded mutated proteins, apoptosis, protein degradation, intracellular signaling as well as oxidative stress, disturbed transcription regulation [15, 16] and epigenetic processes [17].

3. Epigenetic mechanisms

Increasing interest in epigenetics which is currently one of the most rapidly expanding fields in biomedical research has been accompanied by several breakthroughs like finding new histone variants and modifications, the discovery of the CpG island shores and most of all possibility of genome-wide analysis of epigenetic marks – epigenomic analysis – at single nucleotide resolution. The recognition of the role of epigenetics and how important it could be in human disease was first discussed in oncology and further extended to neurodevelopment and neurodegenerative diseases.

Changes in gene expression which are heritable are not always due to alterations in DNA sequence but are also attributable to epigenetic mechanisms. This could explain many cases where different phenotypes arise from the same genotype, such as monozygotic twins which are identical at DNA sequence level but have different DNA methylation and histone modification profiles [18] that possibly affect the penetrance for several complex diseases (cancer, autoimmune, neurodegenerative and cardiovascular diseases).

Studying epigenetic mechanisms made it possible to map epigenetic marks which are critical for regulating gene expression. The importance of epigenetics in maintaining normal development and in being one of the key factors in cellular differentiation can be explained by the observing how aberrant placement of epigenetic marks and mutations in the epigenetic machinery is involved in disease [19].

There are three distinct, yet highly interrelated, major mechanisms of epigenetic regulation (Figure 1) [20] :

1. **DNA methylation** refers to the addition of a methyl group to the 5-position of cytosine in the context of CpG dinucleotides to define the "fifth base of DNA."
2. **Histone modification** - The fundamental repeating unit of chromatin is the nucleosome comprised of an octamer of core histone proteins. Posttranslational modifications of the amino-terminal tails of histone proteins and the density of these proteins per unit length of DNA, can importantly affect chromatin structure and constitute a putative "histone code."

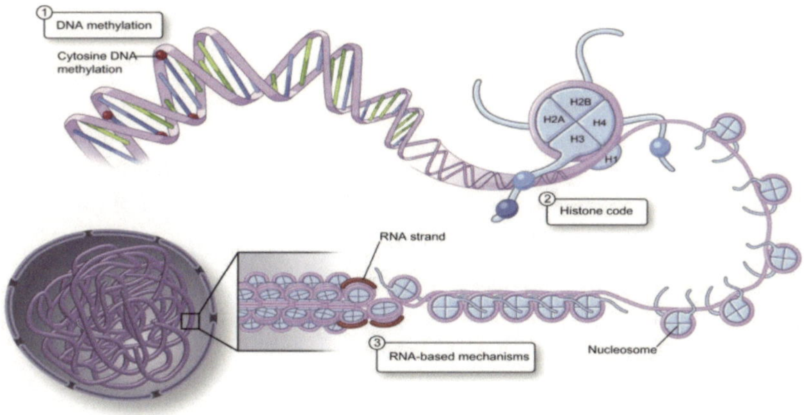

(Reproduced with permission, Yan, M. S. et al. J Appl Physiol 2010;109:916-926).

Figure 1. Schematic representation of 3 fundamental mechanisms of epigenetic gene regulation.

3. **RNA-based mechanisms** have also recently been shown to impact the higher-order structure of chromatin, such as small noncoding RNAs.

3.1. DNA methylation

This is the most widely studied epigenetic mechanism which consists of covalent addition of methyl group at the 5-position of cytosines followed by guanines (CpG dinucleotides) and is usually associated with gene silencing. CpG dinucleotides are generally clustered in regions called CpG islands defined as regions with G-C content of at least 50%. Human gene promoters are associated with CpG island in about 60%. In normal cells they are usually unmethylated and about 6% of them become methylated in a tissue-specific manner in differentiated tissue or during early development [21].

DNA methylation is not present only at CpG islands. Recently, a new term has been coined, CpG island shores which are regions of lower CpG density that are located close (≈ 2kb) to the CpG islands. Additionally, it seems that methylation of CpG island shores is closely related to the inactivation of transcription and is also found that most of tissue-specific methylation of DNA occurs not at CpG islands but CpG island shores [22].

DNA methylation can inhibit gene expression in direct or indirect ways. Indirect transcription inhibition is mediated through promoting activation of methyl-CpG-binding domain (MBD) proteins by methylated DNA, which inhibit transcription [23]. Direct transcriptional inhibition is possible by interruption of activity of DNA binding proteins from their target sites.

A significant portion of methylated CpG islands is also found in repetitive elements. This methylation is functional and needed because of protection from reactivation of endoparasitic sequences which can cause chromosomal instability, gene disruption and translocations [24]. Eventhough DNA methylation occurs mostly in CpG islands in mammals, non-CG methylation has recently been described in humans at CHG and CHH sites (H=A,C or T). The level of of non-CpG methylation decrease during differentiation and mechanisms of non-CpG methylation actually remains unclear at the moment [25].

Other epigenetic regulators linked to DNA methylation are DNA methylation enzyme DNA methyltransferases (DNMT) [26]. DNMT enzyme family mediates DNA methylation by catalyzing the transfer of a methyl group from an S-adenosyl-L-methionine to cytosine. In mammals there are five membrs of the DNMT family, but only three of them have methylatransferase activity – DNMT1, DNMT3a and DNMT3b.

The question that still remains unclear is how DNA methylation machinery is directed to specific sequences. Several proposed mechanisms imply there should be some interaction of DNMTs with other epigenetic factors.

3.2. Histone modifications

Another important epigenetic mark is histone modification. There are 4 groups of core histones H2A, H2B, H3 and H4 which form H2A and H2B dimers and one H3-H4 tetramer. Together they form nucleosome – fundamental unit of cromatin structure. These proteins provide a solid structure for DNA helix and also an interactive surface as N-terminal regions of histones protrude from the nucleosome and are susceptible to interactions with other proteins.

The residues at histone tails are subject to many post-translational modifications like acetylation, methylation, phosphorylation, SUMOylation and ADP-ribosylation [27]. Post-translational modifications are dynamic and reversible processes mediated by two antagonistic sets of enzyme-complexes that can attach or remove corresponding chemical groups. Acetylation at lysine residues is one of most thoroughly studied histone modifications and is associated with transcriptional activation [28]. Modifications are made by histone acetyl transferases (HATs) and can be reverted by histone deacetylase (HDACs).

As previously mentioned, there are interactions between all epigenetic marks. An interesting example of such interplay between histone modification and DNA methylation is relationship between DNA methyltransferase3 (DNMT3L) and H3K4 where DNMT3L specifically interacts with histone H3 tails inducing *de novo* DNA methylation [19].

3.3. RNA-based mechanisms - Noncoding RNA-mediated modulation of gene expression

RNA mediated post-transcriptional gene silencing (TGS) was first observed already in 1989 in tobacco plants [29] and later became known as an important epigenetic mechanism also in humans. It has also been shown in the last years that small RNAs are directed to the targeted promoter regions and this leads to modulation of silent state chromatin modifications [30]. In addition to gene silencing, there is evidence to suggest involvement of small RNAs in additional aspects of transcriptional regulation. These molecules may also activate certain genes, when targeted to promoter regions low in GC content [31]. One subtype of small RNAs are microRNAs, which excert their role on post-transcriptional level, probably by influencing the stability, compartmentalization and translation of mRNAs. In this way, expression of numerous genes is regulated related to different key biological processes cellular processes such as proliferation, morphogenesis, apoptosis and differentiation [32].

http://dx.doi.org/10.5772/54744

In addition to above described epigenetic mechanism, there is another mechanisms, tightly linked to both histone modifications and DNA methylation – **nucleosome positioning.**

Gene expression is also regulated by DNA packed into nucleosomes as these represent a barrier to transcription that blocks access of activators and transcription factors. For instance nucleosome displacement of about 30 bp at transcription start site (TSS) has been reported which leads to changes in RNA polymerase II activity [19]. Gene activation is highly correlated with loss of nucleosome directly upstream of the TSS, whereas the occlusion of TSS by a nucleosome is correlated with gene repression [33]. Nucleosomes can be destabilized or ejected in ATP-hydrolysis dependent manner by groups of large macromolecular complexes, known as chromatin remodeling complexes. There are four families – SWI/SNF, ISWI, CHD and INO80 [34].

In general very little is known about specific mechanisms of nucleosome positioning and further investigation will give us more insights into these processes.

4. Epigenetics and its role in neurodegeneration

Proper differentiation and function of the central nervous system cells are subject to significant influence of a variety of epigenetic modifications. It has been shown that substantial reorganization of the epigenome on the level of cytosine methylation and histone modifications occurs throughout early brain development and continuing through the process of aging [35].

Most notably, the association between epigenetic signature and neurologic disease has been established through observation of monogenic neurodevelopmental disorders resulting from mutations in genes coding for proteins directly involved in core processes of methylation and histone modification. While mutatations in the MECP2 gene, coding for Methyl-CpG-binding protein and related to Rett syndrome, are probably most widely known for association of dysfunctional epigenetic regulation and neurologic disease, mutations in several similar genes have recently been related to neurologic disesease occuring in a variety of age groups.

The role of epigenetic alterations in common neurodegenerative disorders, such as Huntington's, Parkinson's and Alzheimer's disease, on the other hand, has not been considered until recently. Specific disturbed epigenetic mechanisms and changes in all three neurodegeneration NDG disorders are shown in Figure 2.

Surprisingly, it has been shown in the recent decade, that inhibition of histone deacetylase enzymes (HDACs) confers neuroprotective effects in invertebrate and mouse models of Huntington's disease [36]. It is thought that observed beneficial effects of HDAC inhibitors results from re-stabilization of gene transcription, owing to a shift of histone acetylation equilibrium towards increased acetylation of histones, relaxation of DNA-chromatin complexes and subsequent increase of gene transcription. In addition to putative alleviation of symptoms observed in Huntington's disease, the potential benefit of HDAC inhibitors has been considered in a range of neurologic diseases, from monogenic neurologic diseases to common neurodegenerative disorders, such as Parkinson's and Alzheimer's disease[35].

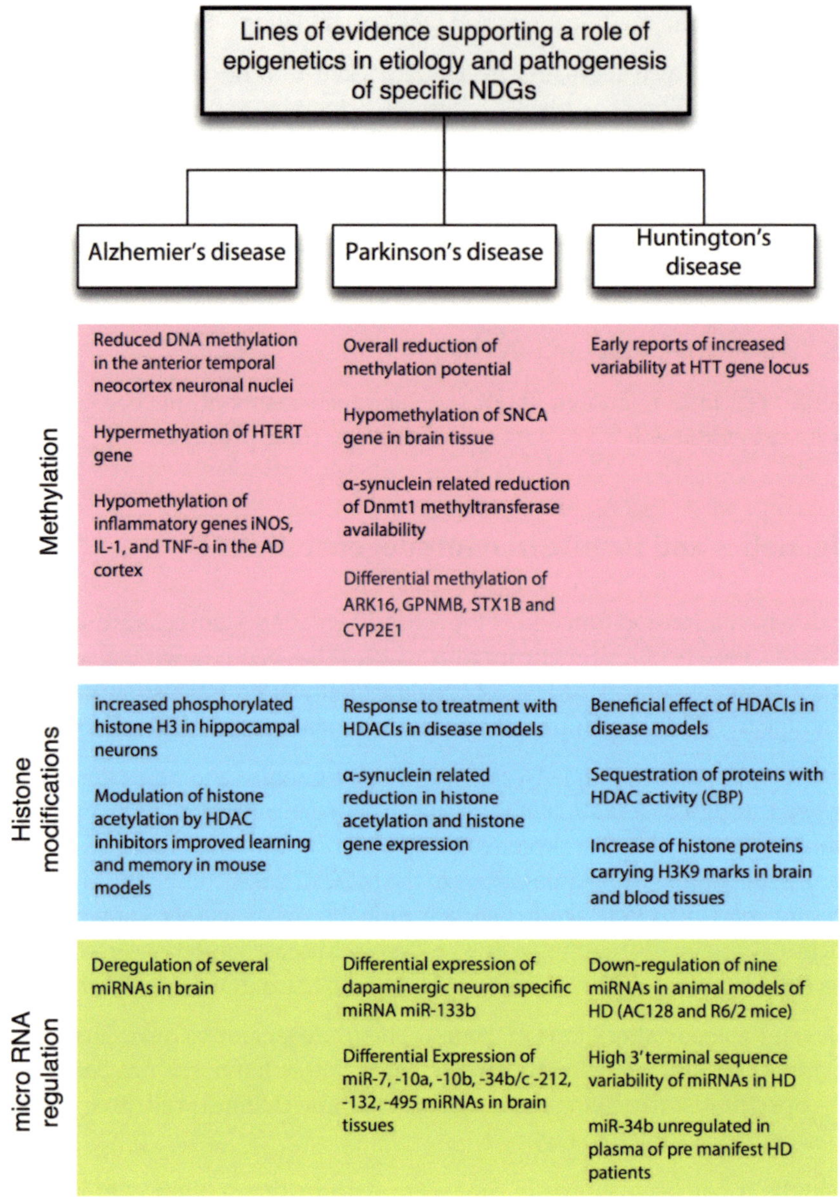

Figure 2. Key epigenetic changes in PD, AD and HD

Other line of evidence stems from the fact that a multitude of monogenic disorders, resulting from mutations in genes essential for proper epigenetic regulation, are characterized by symptoms that arise late in the course of life, such as cerebellar ataxia and hereditary neuropathy. This observation rose a possibility that common neurodegenerative disorders may

http://dx.doi.org/10.5772/54744

share pathogenetic mechanisms and be related to dysfunctions of methylation and histone modifications. It has been demonstrated that nuclei of brain cells from patients with Parkinson's disease contain reduced amounts of methyltransferase enzymes (most notably Dnmt1), leading to dysfunctional methylation of several genes playing a key role in PD pathogenesis, including synuclein-α gene, whose accumulation is observed in plaques of patients with PD [37]. It is also hypothesized that mitochondrial function, commonly perturbed in brain cells of patients with neurodegenerative disorders, is affected by methylation patterns of mitochondrial DNA [35].

Moreover, it was shown that protein aggregates constituting plaques found in brain cells of patients with Alzheimer's disease and Huntington's disease, contain sequestred proteins with histone acetyltranferase activity (notably CBP protein), potentially leading to reduced histone acetylation [38]. Increase of histone proteins carrying H3K9 marks has also been detected in blood and brain tissues of patients with Huntington's disease [39].

This novel evidence substantiates that epigenetic modifications may play a significant role in the etiology of neurodegenerative diseases and pathogenetic mechanisms involved in their propagation and may also present a great opportunity for therapeutic interventions.

4.1. Epigenetics in Parkinson's disease

Parkinson's disease (PD) is the second among most common neurodegenerative disorders and is characterized by progressive depletion of dopaminergic neurons within the substantia nigra, clinically manifesting as progressive symptoms of tremor, rigidity, bradykinesia and postural instability [40, 41]. PD belongs to a group of complex diseases and is hypothesized to arise consequentially to interaction of a multitude of genetic and environmental factors. Details of specific sites of genetic predisposition and environmental insults, however, remain largely unclear [42]. Nevertheless, discovery of monogenic forms of PD provided a great insight into specific physiologic pathways that, once perturbed, lead to destruction of dopaminergic neurons. A significant proportion of cases with familial forms of PD, following clear Mendelian inheritance has been identified. Here, causative mutations have been discovered, offering valuable insight into intricacies and key points of disease pathogenesis. To date, mutations in genes *SNCA* (encoding α-synuclein protein), *PARK2* (parkin), *PINK1* (PTEN-induced kinase protein 1), *UCHL1* (ubiquitin carboxyl-terminal hydrolase isozyme L1), *DJ1* (DJ-1 protein), and *LRRK2* (leucine-rich repeat serine/threonine-protein kinase 2) were identified as a cause of familial PD [41].

Perhaps the most studied gene in light of potential epigenetic alterations in PD is SNCA gene. Depositions of misfolded α-synuclein constitute a pathologic hallmark of Parkinson's disease (Lewy bodies) and co-locate with sites of neuronal loss. As α-synuclein toxic effects are primarily exerted in neuronal nuclei, it has been hypothesized that it perturbs the distribution and organization of DNA and histone epigenetic modifications [43]. Indeed, recent studies have demonstrated α-synuclein associates with histones and inhibits their acetylation, doing so through its association with Sirtuin-2 (Sirt2) histone deacetylase. Interestingly, in a *Drosophila* model of PD, targeted down-regulation of Sirt2 resulted in reduced α-synuclein toxicity [44]. Additionally, other histonic modifications have been related to increased or decreased death of neurons in PD. Treatment with MPTP (1-methyl-4-phenyl-1,2,3,6-tetrahydropyridine), commonly used in animal models to provoke PD symptoms, has been assocated with increased presence of H3 histonic marks, which has been reverted after treatment with levo-dopa [45]. In a *C. elegans* model of PD, where overexpression of SNCA was stimulated, reduced expression of nine genes coding for histone proteins was observed [46]. In addition, a recent study has linked a mutation (A53T) in SNCA gene to monoallelic silencing of transcription form mutated allele, which was shown to result from histonic modifications at that site [47].

On the other hand, the role of DNA methylation in PD is currently unclear. It has been shown that metabolism of one-carbon compounds required for normal methylation is perturbed in PD [48]. Several studies have already pointed to the possibility of altered SNCA promoter gene methylation in relation to neuropsychiatric disorders [49]. Methylation of SNCA intron 1 has been associated with decrease in SNCA transcription and reduction of methylation at this site was observed at several brain regions affected in PD (including *substantia nigra*) [50]. This observation was further substantiated in analyses of other parts of the gene, where hypomethylation was also detected [51]. These results raise the possibility that increase in α-synuclein production may result from increased SNCA expression, potentially as a consequence of reduced methylation status of this gene. Additionally, α-synuclein has been shown to sequester DNA methyltransferase 1 (DNMT1), resulting in decreased overall methylation of genes in brain tissues of PD patients [37]. A study investigating larger set of genes, has revealed that other genes besides SNCA are characterized by differential methylation in PD (ARK16, GPNMB, and STX1B) [52]. Recently, these investigations have been expanded to global epigenomic scale of methylation in postmortem brain samples and a novel gene characterized by hypomethylation in PD was identified (CYP2E1, the cytochrome P450, family 2, subfamily E, polypeptide 1). In accordance, increased expression of the same gene has also been detected. Interestingly, CYP2E1 knock-out mice models have also been shown to be protected from MPTP toxic effects [53].

The role of miRNA regulatory system has also been implicated and surveyed in the context of PD. Initial study, performed by Kim et al, reported a detection of miRNA molecule (miR-133b) with expression specific to midbrain dopaminergic neurons and reduction of expression level in PD patients' midbrain tissue samples [54]. Differences in expression of several other microRNAs have been detected in early symptomatic mouse models of PD (miR-10a, -10b, -212, -132, -495) [55]. In addition, miR-7 has been found to repress expression of SNCA gene in two independent studies where it was demonstrated that its expression levels were reduced in MPTP cell culture and animal models [56, 57]. A global miRNA profiling approach in PD brain samples revealed downregulation of miR-34b/c, which has an important role in regulation of mitochondrial function. This deregulation was particularly notable in patients early in disease course, who have not yet been subjected to PD treatment modalities [58]. In another study, alterations of miRNAs could even be detected in blood samples from PD patients in regard to affection and pre- and post-treatment status. Their expression levels could be used to distinguish patients from controls based on blood expression profiles [59].

These lines of evidence provide support for the possibility that a proportion of pathways leading to PD could be better understood by incorporating epigenetic regulome into the our current disease models. In addition, epigenetic alterations provide novel treatment targets, allowing re-stabilization of perturbed cellular mechanisms. Most notably, histone deacetylase inhibitors (HDACIs), currently already approved for treatment of haematologic malignancies, have been shown to rescue α-synuclein- induced toxicity in models in vitro and in vivo. Several new forms of HDACIs and DNA-demethylating drugs are currently in preclinical testing stage and provide an array of new opportunities to benefit patients with PD [60].

4.2. Epigenetics in Alzheimer disease

Alzheimer disease, as discussed above, is the leading couse of dementia world wide. It is characterized by dementia that typically begins with subtle and poorly recognized failure of memory and slowly becomes more severe and, eventually, incapacitating. Other findings include confusion, poor judgment, language disturbance, agitation, withdrawal, and hallucinations. As is true for PD, AD is believed to be a complex disease, combining the effects of genetic and environmental factors. On the other hand, approximately 25% of all AD is familial, 95% of which is late-onset (age >60-65 years) and 5% is early-onset (age <60 years). In familial AD definite causative genes and mutations are known, offering important models for studying disease pathogenesis. To date, mutations in three genes are undoubtfully linked to AD – Presenilin-1 (*PSEN1*), Presenilin-2 (*PSEN2*) and Amyloid beta A4 protein (*APP*). Others remain to be discovered. This is also true for the cause of sporadic AD, which can in part be attributable to epigenetic mechanisms.

Epigenetics is an emerging field in the light of potential impact on development of neurodegenerative diseases. It is a mechanism independant of DNA sequence with effects on gene transcription, yet in specific way it is heritable. It is well known that epigenetic modifications alter transcriptional activity of thousands of genes and simultaneously of many different cellular pathways in individually specific manner, dependant also on environmental factors and yet unknown co-factors. In this way epigenetics might constitute a crossroad for diverse pathophysiological mechanisms and risk factors contributing to development of Alzheimer disease. In addition, epigenetics may explain a part of mechanism by which AD in a first degree relative means an increased risk of "sporadic" disease, since epigenetic impressions are passed from generation to generation. Different mechanism have been implicated – DNA methylation, histone acetylation, miRNAs.

4.2.1. DNA methylation in AD

An important suggestive evidence of the role of epigenetic modifications in AD was a study on monozygotic twins discordant for AD, where status of DNA methylation in temporal neocortex neuronal nuclei was significantly altered in the AD twin [61].

It has been shown this year in genome-wide DNA methylation study that more than 900 CpG sites representing 918 unique genes might be associated with late onset AD. The best candidate gene turned out to be a Transmembrane Protein 59 (TMEM59), whose promoter was hypomethylated in AD [62]. Interestingly, TMEM59 was previously linked to amyloid precursor protein shedding, which is a central regulatory point in the production of amyloid β peptid in AD [63]. Regulation of amyloid precursor protein shedding is still not clear and mostly unknown at the molecular level.

Another gene candidate shown to be differentially methylated is mRNA componentof telomerase HTERT (human telomerase reverse transcriptase), potentially involved in higher telomerase activity and immune dysfunctions in AD pathogenesis [64]. Disturbances in inflammatory regulation and response has been widely accepted and studied in AD for more than a decade. Numerous studies have proven this connection, for example, inflammatory mediators and signs of oxidative stress were described mostly in regions of beta-amyloid peptide deposits and neurofibrillary tangles [65]. Also, *in vitro* and *in vivo* studies on connection between pro-inflammatory cytokines and processing and production of the beta-amyloid peptid shown important influence [66]. In addition, whole genome expression studies showed widespread transcriptional alterations - decreased neurotrophic support and activated apoptotic and neuroinflammatory signaling in AD brain [67]. Specific studies on DNA methylation have added to this hypothesis by detecting hypomethylation of iNOS, IL-1, and TNF-α in the AD brain [65].

4.2.2. Hystone modification in AD

Another pathway of epigenetic regulation of transcription and other functions in cells is chromatin acetylation and deacetylation of histone proteins. Many studies associated histone hypoacetylation and transcriptional dysfunction with many different neurodegenerative conditions, including AD [68], Parkinson's disease [69] and Huntington's disease [70]. Direct evidence of disturbed histone modifications in AD was proposed in a study where elevated levels of phosphorylated histone H3 in AD hippocampal neurons were found and dislocalised to neuronal cytoplasm, as opposed to the nucleus as in actively dividing cells [71]. On the other hand, a recent study using novel proteomic approaches showed that histone acetylation is significantly lower in AD temporal lobe as compared to aged controls [72].

Using HDAC inhibitors to manipulate histone acetylation in several animal models of AD showed important potential of these molecules as treatment options. For example, valproic acid, which has HDAC1 inhibitor activity, decreased the production of amyloid-beta precursor protein and reduced plaque burden in the brains of Alzheimer's disease transgenic mouse model [73]. Another study reported beneficial role of phenylbuthyrate in cognitive impairment and neuropathology in AD. Using sodium 4-phenylbutyrate to treat Tg2576 mice it was shown that it reversed spatial memory loss and normalized levels of phosphorylated tau in the hippocampus. At the same time, it failed to change amyloid-beta precursor level [74]. This is in concordance with earlier studies which have shown that changes in amyloid-beta precursor levels are not necessarily associated with improvement in learning and memory performance [75, 76].

Another important finding was that increased histone acetylation induced sprouting of dendrites, increased number of synapses and reinstated learning behaviour and access to long-term memories, after already present brain atrophy and neuronal loss in a mouse model [77]. The author suggested that histone deacetylase inhibitors might be potential therapeutic agents for AD nad other neurodegenerative diseases where learning and memory impairment is present.

As it seems, histone modifications happen and have an important role in AD and AD animal models. Still, the underlying mechanisms and regulation and post-modification pathways are complex and not fully understood yet.

4.2.3. miRNA in AD

Micro RNAs (miRNAs) are post-transcriptional regulators that bind to complementary sequences on target mRNAs. This usually results in translational repression or target degradation and gene silencing. It is assumed that human genome might encode approximatelly 1000 miRNAs. miRNAs have been linked to posttranscriptional control of amyloid precursor protein expression [78], namely negative regulatory control by miR-101 and miR-16 [79]. The study clearly demonstrated that amyloid precursor protein is a target of miR-16 and that abnormally low expression of miR-16 might directly lead to protein accumulation in AD mice. Also, miRNAs are equally involved in the regulation of neuronal mRNA alternative splicing [80]. Smith et al have shown that miR-124 is down-regulated in AD brain and at the same time, its underexpression in neurons is associated with inclusion of exons 7 and 8 to amyloid precursor protein. To contribute to this finding, they have also shown that ectopic expression of miR-124 reversed these effects in cultured neurons.

At present, miRNAs are hot topic and the full complement of miRNA that participate in the regulation of precursor protein expression, splicing and potential other steps in its accumulation are yet to be discovered.

4.3. Epigenetics in Huntington's disease

Huntington's disease (HD) is caused by dominant mutation with expanded number of glutamine codons within an existing poly-glutamine (polyQ) repeat sequence of a gene encoding for protein huntingtin (htt). Normal htt has 36 polyQ repeats and aberrant has more than 39 polyQ repeats. In case of 36-39 polyQ repeats we have an "intermediate allele" with incomplete penetrance and greater probability of becoming pathogenic if there is family history of Huntington's disease.

It has been shown in brain of mouse models [16] and in blood and brain of patients with HD that changes in gene expression occur very early in the disease course [81]. Gene transcription is regulated by complex interplay of different protein complexes, including transcription factors and histones, which in turn are regulated by covalent modifications such as acetylation, methylation and phosphorylation. Histone acetylation, which promotes transcription, is reduced in models of HD [82] and, on the other hand, histone methylation, which inhibits transcription, is increased [83]. Moreover, histone methylation was shown to be increased in HD patients, suggesting important role in disease pathogenesis [39].

Further evidence was provided by the use of histone acetylase inhibitors (HDACi), sodium butyrate and phenylbutyrate which increased survival of R6/2 mice. Also, improved motor performance and to some extend reversed alteration in gene expression and hypoacetylation at selected promoters in cerebellum of R6/2 mice was reported [82]. The exact mode of histone acetylation and methylation in HD is still unknown, but HDACs might be a potentially promising treatment. One of HDAC inhibitors, sodium phenylbutyrate, is already approved in the treatment of urea cycle disorders and is under investigation for treatment of various refractory cancers, amyotrophic lateral sclerosis and spinobulbar muscular atrophy. A dose-finding study of this compound in human HD has already been conducted to determine the tolerability of the compound in patients with HD [84].

Another epigenetic mechanism, implicated in HD, is also disturbed miRNAs levels. Several miRNAs are significantly misregulated in HD brains compared with healthy controls. Five miRNAs, miR-9, miR-9*, miR-29b, miR-124a and miR-132 are significantly disregulated in HD cortex [85]. Interestingly, miR-9/miR9* are important in regulation of transcriptional repressor REST, which is mislocalized in brains neurons of patients with HD [86]. Together with other transcriptional factors it acts to regulate neuronal gene expression. How this is related to HD progression and potential for treatment remains yet to be elucidated.

In addition to human HD, an important role of miRNAs has also been shown in cell models of HD and linked directly to mutated protein huntingtin. Huntingtin has been shown to be the target of several miRNAs, miR-214, miR-150, miR-146a and miR-125b. Their expression reduced the expression of mutated protein. This regulation of huntingtin by miRNAs might provide a new approach to modulate HD [87].

5. Conclusion

Neurodegenerative diseases are becoming one of the most important public health issue in the developed world due to the population ageing. It is of paramount importance to improve our knowledge on pathophysiology of the group of these diseases with the aim to improve diagnostics, development of disease-modifying treatment and preventive measures. The most important field is early diagnosis with accurate risk estimates and potential preventive treatment. Numerous research groups and initiatives are working with this same goal in order to improve above mentioned issues.

Global epigenetic changes, with downstream effect on numerous genes and different biological pathways, appear to be involved in synchronous cellular response and alterations that direct development, aging, and, in some cases, even disease. Epigenetic modifications in the patho-psysiology of neurodegenerative diseases are lately becoming more and more important and widely discussed. This field is expected to provide important molecular mechanisms that will contribute to understanding of the pathogenesis, treatment response and even development of new therapeutic targets in the field of neurodegenerative disorders.

DNA methylation, histone modifications and small noncoding RNA regulation are different epigenetic mechanisms directly or indirectly linked to transcriptional activity and post-translational modifications, such as alternative splicing. It has already been proposed and well accepted that these epigenetic alterations with consequent transcriptional dysregulation might be an important marker of disease status and its progression in many neurodegenerative diseases. The disruption of normal transcriptional pathways through altered epigenetic status triggers signaling cascades linked with a number of pathological mechanisms.

In this chapter we have shortly reviewed epigenetic role in Parkinson's disease, Alzheimer disease and Huntington's diseases. Epigenetic characteristics show an important role and certain specifics in all three. Moreover, the epigenetic modifications that have been reported in PD and AD, are in some points similar to trends in normal aging. Therefore, in addition to giving us insight to pathogenesis of neurodegeneration, they might also explain why aging by itself is a risk factor for developing neurodegenerative disorder.

Instead of studying preselected genes or regions and their epigenetic characteristics, whole-genome epigenetic status, so-called epigenome should be studied. With the knowledge on direct impact of epigenetic to transcriptional dysregulation, it would be of great importance to conduct epigenomic studies in tandem with transcriptomic (genome-wide gene expression profiling) studies. Only with this approach is one able to directly validate functional effects of epigenetic changes on gene expression. True, research on the epigenetic components and mechanisms associated with neurodegeneration is still in its beginning and future will provide additional essential information.

Last but not least - epigenetic modification is a reversible characteristic while genetic mutation is not. Influencing and tightly regulating epigenetic modification is therefore theoretically very promising candidate method from a therapeutic perspective of neurodegenerative diseases. It is well known that certain therapeutic compounds can influence and change the DNA methylation status and transcriptional activity accordingly. Though, one has to bear in mind, that in general, epigenetic mechanisms exert effects on many genes simultaneously and the same is also true for currently known effective epigenetic therapeutics.

Author details

Luca Lovrečić*, Aleš Maver, Maja Zadel and Borut Peterlin

*Address all correspondence to: lucalovrecic@gmail.com

Clinical Institute of Medical Genetics, University Medical Center Ljubljana, Slovenia

References

[1] C.J.L. Murray, A.D.L., *The Global Burden of Disease*, 1996, World Health Organisation: Geneva.

[2] Menken, M., T.L. Munsat, and J.F. Toole, *The global burden of disease study: implications for neurology.* Arch Neurol, 2000. 57(3): p. 418-20.

[3] Schneider, J.A., et al., *Mixed brain pathologies account for most dementia cases in community-dwelling older persons.* Neurology, 2007. 69(24): p. 2197-204.

[4] *Pathological correlates of late-onset dementia in a multicentre, community-based population in England and Wales. Neuropathology Group of the Medical Research Council Cognitive Function and Ageing Study (MRC CFAS).* Lancet, 2001. 357(9251): p. 169-75.

[5] Prohovnik, I., et al., *Dissociation of neuropathology from severity of dementia in late-onset Alzheimer disease.* Neurology, 2006. 66(1): p. 49-55.

[6] Ballard, C., et al., *Alzheimer's disease.* Lancet. 377(9770): p. 1019-31.

[7] Forlenza, O.V., B.S. Diniz, and W.F. Gattaz, *Diagnosis and biomarkers of predementia in Alzheimer's disease.* BMC Med. 8: p. 89.

[8] McKhann, G., et al., *Clinical diagnosis of Alzheimer's disease: report of the NINCDS-ADRDA Work Group under the auspices of Department of Health and Human Services Task Force on Alzheimer's Disease.* Neurology, 1984. 34(7): p. 939-44.

[9] Hyman, B.T., et al., *National Institute on Aging-Alzheimer's Association guidelines for the neuropathologic assessment of Alzheimer's disease.* Alzheimers Dement, 2012. 8(1): p. 1-13.

[10] Spillantini, M.G., et al., *Alpha-synuclein in Lewy bodies.* Nature, 1997. 388(6645): p. 839-40.

[11] Gao, H.M. and J.S. Hong, *Gene-environment interactions: key to unraveling the mystery of Parkinson's disease.* Prog Neurobiol, 2011. 94(1): p. 1-19.

[12] *A novel gene containing a trinucleotide repeat that is expanded and unstable on Huntington's disease chromosomes. The Huntington's Disease Collaborative Research Group.* Cell, 1993. 72(6): p. 971-83.

[13] Harper, P.S., *Huntington's disease*. Major Problems in Neurology1996, London: W.B. Saunders Company Ltd.

[14] Bonelli, R.M. and P. Hofmann, *A systematic review of the treatment studies in Huntington's disease since 1990.* Expert Opin Pharmacother, 2007. 8(2): p. 141-53.

[15] Harjes, P. and E.E. Wanker, *The hunt for huntingtin function: interaction partners tell many different stories.* Trends Biochem Sci, 2003. 28(8): p. 425-33.

[16] Sugars, K.L. and D.C. Rubinsztein, *Transcriptional abnormalities in Huntington disease.* Trends Genet, 2003. 19(5): p. 233-8.

[17] He, F. and P.K. Todd, *Epigenetics in nucleotide repeat expansion disorders.* Semin Neurol, 2011. 31(5): p. 470-83.

[18] Kaminsky, Z.A., et al., *DNA methylation profiles in monozygotic and dizygotic twins.* Nat Genet, 2009. 41(2): p. 240-5.

[19] Portela, A. and M. Esteller, *Epigenetic modifications and human disease.* Nat Biotechnol, 2010. 28(10): p. 1057-68.

[20] Yan, M.S., C.C. Matouk, and P.A. Marsden, *Epigenetics of the vascular endothelium.* J Appl Physiol, 2010. 109(3): p. 916-26.

[21] Straussman, R., et al., *Developmental programming of CpG island methylation profiles in the human genome.* Nat Struct Mol Biol, 2009. 16(5): p. 564-71.

[22] Irizarry, R.A., et al., *The human colon cancer methylome shows similar hypo- and hypermethylation at conserved tissue-specific CpG island shores.* Nat Genet, 2009. 41(2): p. 178-86.

[23] Esteller, M., *Epigenetic gene silencing in cancer: the DNA hypermethylome.* Hum Mol Genet, 2007. 16 Spec No 1: p. R50-9.

[24] Esteller, M., *Cancer epigenomics: DNA methylomes and histone-modification maps.* Nat Rev Genet, 2007. 8(4): p. 286-98.

[25] Laurent, L., et al., *Dynamic changes in the human methylome during differentiation.* Genome Res, 2010. 20(3): p. 320-31.

[26] Espada, J., et al., *Epigenetic disruption of ribosomal RNA genes and nucleolar architecture in DNA methyltransferase 1 (Dnmt1) deficient cells.* Nucleic Acids Res, 2007. 35(7): p. 2191-8.

[27] Kouzarides, T., *Chromatin modifications and their function.* Cell, 2007. 128(4): p. 693-705.

[28] Santos-Rosa, H., et al., *Histone H3 tail clipping regulates gene expression.* Nat Struct Mol Biol, 2009. 16(1): p. 17-22.

[29] Matzke, M.A., et al., *Reversible methylation and inactivation of marker genes in sequentially transformed tobacco plants.* EMBO J, 1989. 8(3): p. 643-9.

[30] Kim, D.H., et al., *Argonaute-1 directs siRNA-mediated transcriptional gene silencing in human cells.* Nat Struct Mol Biol, 2006. 13(9): p. 793-7.

[31] Janowski, B.A., et al., *Activating gene expression in mammalian cells with promoter-targeted duplex RNAs.* Nat Chem Biol, 2007. 3(3): p. 166-73.

[32] Carthew, R.W., *Gene regulation by microRNAs.* Curr Opin Genet Dev, 2006. 16(2): p. 203-8.

[33] Schones, D.E., et al., *Dynamic regulation of nucleosome positioning in the human genome.* Cell, 2008. 132(5): p. 887-98.

[34] Ho, L. and G.R. Crabtree, *Chromatin remodelling during development.* Nature, 2010. 463(7280): p. 474-84.

[35] Jakovcevski, M. and S. Akbarian, *Epigenetic mechanisms in neurological disease.* Nat Med, 2012. 18(8): p. 1194-204.

[36] Steffan, J.S., et al., *Histone deacetylase inhibitors arrest polyglutamine-dependent neurodegeneration in Drosophila.* Nature, 2001. 413(6857): p. 739-43.

[37] Desplats, P., et al., *Alpha-synuclein sequesters Dnmt1 from the nucleus: a novel mechanism for epigenetic alterations in Lewy body diseases.* J Biol Chem, 2011. 286(11): p. 9031-7.

[38] Nucifora, F.C., Jr., et al., *Interference by huntingtin and atrophin-1 with cbp-mediated transcription leading to cellular toxicity.* Science, 2001. 291(5512): p. 2423-8.

[39] Ryu, H., et al., *ESET/SETDB1 gene expression and histone H3 (K9) trimethylation in Huntington's disease.* Proc Natl Acad Sci U S A, 2006. 103(50): p. 19176-81.

[40] Lees, A.J., J. Hardy, and T. Revesz, *Parkinson's disease.* Lancet, 2009. 373(9680): p. 2055-66.

[41] Mayeux, R., *Epidemiology of neurodegeneration.* Annu Rev Neurosci, 2003. 26: p. 81-104.

[42] Klein, C. and A. Westenberger, *Genetics of Parkinson's disease.* Cold Spring Harb Perspect Med, 2012. 2(1): p. a008888.

[43] Kontopoulos, E., J.D. Parvin, and M.B. Feany, *Alpha-synuclein acts in the nucleus to inhibit histone acetylation and promote neurotoxicity.* Hum Mol Genet, 2006. 15(20): p. 3012-23.

[44] Outeiro, T.F., et al., *Sirtuin 2 inhibitors rescue alpha-synuclein-mediated toxicity in models of Parkinson's disease.* Science, 2007. 317(5837): p. 516-9.

[45] Nicholas, A.P., et al., *Striatal histone modifications in models of levodopa-induced dyskinesia.* J Neurochem, 2008. 106(1): p. 486-94.

[46] Vartiainen, S., et al., *Identification of gene expression changes in transgenic C. elegans overexpressing human alpha-synuclein.* Neurobiol Dis, 2006. 22(3): p. 477-86.

[47] Voutsinas, G.E., et al., *Allelic imbalance of expression and epigenetic regulation within the alpha-synuclein wild-type and p.Ala53Thr alleles in Parkinson disease.* Hum Mutat, 2010. 31(6): p. 685-91.

[48] Obeid, R., et al., *Methylation status and neurodegenerative markers in Parkinson disease.* Clin Chem, 2009. 55(10): p. 1852-60.

[49] Qureshi, I.A. and M.F. Mehler, *Advances in epigenetics and epigenomics for neurodegenerative diseases.* Curr Neurol Neurosci Rep, 2011. 11(5): p. 464-73.

[50] Jowaed, A., et al., *Methylation regulates alpha-synuclein expression and is decreased in Parkinson's disease patients' brains.* J Neurosci, 2010. 30(18): p. 6355-9.

[51] Matsumoto, L., et al., *CpG demethylation enhances alpha-synuclein expression and affects the pathogenesis of Parkinson's disease.* PLoS One, 2010. 5(11): p. e15522.

[52] *A two-stage meta-analysis identifies several new loci for Parkinson's disease.* PLoS Genet, 2011. 7(6): p. e1002142.

[53] Kaut, O., I. Schmitt, and U. Wullner, *Genome-scale methylation analysis of Parkinson's disease patients' brains reveals DNA hypomethylation and increased mRNA expression of cytochrome P450 2E1.* Neurogenetics, 2012. 13(1): p. 87-91.

[54] Kim, J., et al., *A MicroRNA feedback circuit in midbrain dopamine neurons.* Science, 2007. 317(5842): p. 1220-4.

[55] Gillardon, F., et al., *MicroRNA and proteome expression profiling in early-symptomatic alpha-synuclein(A30P)-transgenic mice.* Proteomics Clin Appl, 2008. 2(5): p. 697-705.

[56] Junn, E., et al., *Repression of alpha-synuclein expression and toxicity by microRNA-7.* Proc Natl Acad Sci U S A, 2009. 106(31): p. 13052-7.

[57] Doxakis, E., *Post-transcriptional regulation of alpha-synuclein expression by mir-7 and mir-153.* J Biol Chem, 2010. 285(17): p. 12726-34.

[58] Minones-Moyano, E., et al., *MicroRNA profiling of Parkinson's disease brains identifies early downregulation of miR-34b/c which modulate mitochondrial function.* Hum Mol Genet, 2011. 20(15): p. 3067-78.

[59] Margis, R. and C.R. Rieder, *Identification of blood microRNAs associated to Parkinsonis disease.* J Biotechnol, 2011. 152(3): p. 96-101.

[60] Kazantsev, A.G. and L.M. Thompson, *Therapeutic application of histone deacetylase inhibitors for central nervous system disorders.* Nat Rev Drug Discov, 2008. 7(10): p. 854-68.

[61] Mastroeni, D., et al., *Epigenetic differences in cortical neurons from a pair of monozygotic twins discordant for Alzheimer's disease.* PLoS One, 2009. 4(8): p. e6617.

[62] Bakulski, K.M., et al., *Genome-wide DNA methylation differences between late-onset Alzheimer's disease and cognitively normal controls in human frontal cortex.* J Alzheimers Dis, 2012. 29(3): p. 571-88.

[63] Selkoe, D.J. and D. Schenk, *Alzheimer's disease: molecular understanding predicts amyloid-based therapeutics.* Annu Rev Pharmacol Toxicol, 2003. 43: p. 545-84.

[64] Silva, P.N., et al., *Promoter methylation analysis of SIRT3, SMARCA5, HTERT and CDH1 genes in aging and Alzheimer's disease.* J Alzheimers Dis, 2008. 13(2): p. 173-6.

[65] Akiyama, H., et al., *Inflammation and Alzheimer's disease.* Neurobiol Aging, 2000. 21(3): p. 383-421.

[66] Blasko, I., et al., *TNFalpha plus IFNgamma induce the production of Alzheimer beta-amyloid peptides and decrease the secretion of APPs.* FASEB J, 1999. 13(1): p. 63-8.

[67] Colangelo, V., et al., *Gene expression profiling of 12633 genes in Alzheimer hippocampal CA1: transcription and neurotrophic factor down-regulation and up-regulation of apoptotic and pro-inflammatory signaling.* J Neurosci Res, 2002. 70(3): p. 462-73.

[68] Stilling, R.M. and A. Fischer, *The role of histone acetylation in age-associated memory impairment and Alzheimer's disease.* Neurobiol Learn Mem, 2011. 96(1): p. 19-26.

[69] Chuang, D.M., et al., *Multiple roles of HDAC inhibition in neurodegenerative conditions.* Trends Neurosci, 2009. 32(11): p. 591-601.

[70] Sadri-Vakili, G. and J.H. Cha, *Mechanisms of disease: Histone modifications in Huntington's disease.* Nat Clin Pract Neurol, 2006. 2(6): p. 330-8.

[71] Ogawa, O., et al., *Ectopic localization of phosphorylated histone H3 in Alzheimer's disease: a mitotic catastrophe?* Acta Neuropathol, 2003. 105(5): p. 524-8.

[72] Zhang, K., et al., *Targeted proteomics for quantification of histone acetylation in Alzheimer's disease.* Proteomics, 2012. 12(8): p. 1261-8.

[73] Su, Y., et al., *Lithium, a common drug for bipolar disorder treatment, regulates amyloid-beta precursor protein processing.* Biochemistry, 2004. 43(22): p. 6899-908.

[74] Ricobaraza, A., et al., *Phenylbutyrate ameliorates cognitive deficit and reduces tau pathology in an Alzheimer's disease mouse model.* Neuropsychopharmacology, 2009. 34(7): p. 1721-32.

[75] Malm, T.M., et al., *Pyrrolidine dithiocarbamate activates Akt and improves spatial learning in APP/PS1 mice without affecting beta-amyloid burden.* J Neurosci, 2007. 27(14): p. 3712-21.

[76] Dodart, J.C., et al., *Immunization reverses memory deficits without reducing brain Abeta burden in Alzheimer's disease model.* Nat Neurosci, 2002. 5(5): p. 452-7.

[77] Fischer, A., et al., *Recovery of learning and memory is associated with chromatin remodelling.* Nature, 2007. 447(7141): p. 178-82.

[78] Long, J.M. and D.K. Lahiri, *Current drug targets for modulating Alzheimer's amyloid precursor protein: role of specific micro-RNA species.* Curr Med Chem, 2011. 18(22): p. 3314-21.

[79] Liu, W., et al., *MicroRNA-16 targets amyloid precursor protein to potentially modulate Alzheimer's-associated pathogenesis in SAMP8 mice.* Neurobiol Aging, 2012. 33(3): p. 522-34.

[80] Smith, P., et al., *In vivo regulation of amyloid precursor protein neuronal splicing by microRNAs.* J Neurochem, 2011. 116(2): p. 240-7.

[81] Borovecki, F., et al., *Genome-wide expression profiling of human blood reveals biomarkers for Huntington's disease.* Proc Natl Acad Sci U S A, 2005. 102(31): p. 11023-8.

[82] Ferrante, R.J., et al., *Histone deacetylase inhibition by sodium butyrate chemotherapy ameliorates the neurodegenerative phenotype in Huntington's disease mice.* J Neurosci, 2003. 23(28): p. 9418-27.

[83] Gardian, G., et al., *Neuroprotective effects of phenylbutyrate in the N171-82Q transgenic mouse model of Huntington's disease.* J Biol Chem, 2005. 280(1): p. 556-63.

[84] Hogarth, P., L. Lovrecic, and D. Krainc, *Sodium phenylbutyrate in Huntington's disease: a dose-finding study.* Mov Disord, 2007. 22(13): p. 1962-4.

[85] Packer, A.N., et al., *The bifunctional microRNA miR-9/miR-9* regulates REST and CoREST and is downregulated in Huntington's disease.* J Neurosci, 2008. 28(53): p. 14341-6.

[86] Zuccato, C., et al., *Widespread disruption of repressor element-1 silencing transcription factor/neuron-restrictive silencer factor occupancy at its target genes in Huntington's disease.* J Neurosci, 2007. 27(26): p. 6972-83.

[87] Sinha, M., J. Ghose, and N.P. Bhattarcharyya, *Micro RNA -214,-150,-146a and-125b target Huntingtin gene.* RNA Biol, 2011. 8(6): p. 1005-21.

Chapter 15

Plasma Membrane Channels Formed by Connexins or Pannexins in Microglia: Possible Role in the Inflamed Brain

Juan A. Orellana

Additional information is available at the end of the chapter

http://dx.doi.org/10.5772/54306

1. Introduction

In a healthy brain, microglia exhibit a resting surveillance state associated with active exploration of their environment for exogenous or endogenous signals representing a threat to the homeostasis [1-5]. When physiological balance is impaired in the central nervous system (CNS), resting phenotype of microglia shift to a reactive phenotype with different degrees of activation according to the nature of the stimuli and the context. During intense CNS inflammation, rather than show a repair-orientated activity profile, reactive microglia constitute a source of toxic factors and participate in the recruitment of non-resident brain cells involved in the innate immune response, which worsen brain damage. The brain performs exceptionally complex and dynamic tasks that depend on the coordinated interaction of glial cells, therefore it is conceivable that impairment of intercellular signaling and coordination among microglia could play an important role on several CNS disorders. In vertebrate cells, this synchronization is in part mediated by gap junctions [6-10]. They are aggregates of intercellular channels termed gap junction channels that allow direct, but selective, cytoplasmic continuity between contacting cells, promoting the exchange of ions (allowing eletrical coupling), metabolites (e.g., ADP, glucose, glutamate and glutathione) and second messengers (e.g., cAMP and IP_3)[11-16]. Whereas a gap junction channel is formed by the serial docking of two hemichannels each one contributed by one of two adjacent cells, each hemichannel is composed by six protein subunits termed connexins (Fig. 1). The latter belong to a highly conserved protein family encoded by 21 genes in human and 20 in mouse with orthologs in other vertebrate species [17-19]. Connexins are abundantly expressed in cells of the CNS, and they are named after their predicted molecular mass expressed in kDa, so that connexin43 (Cx43) has a molecular mass of ~43 kDa.

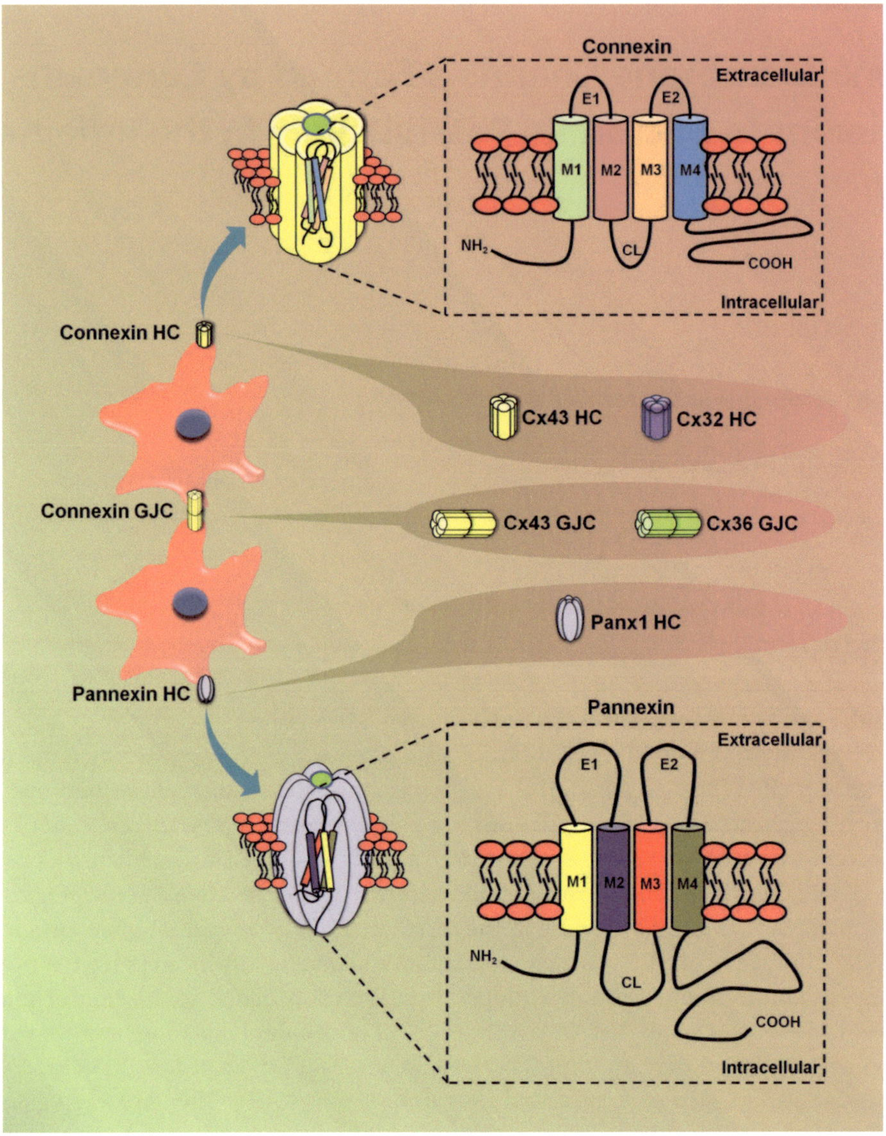

Figure 1. Diagram illustrating basic structures of gap junction channels and hemichannels formed by connexins or pannexins in microglia. Connexins and pannexins share similar membrane topology, with four α-helical transmembrane domains (M1-M4) connected by two extracellular loops (E1 and E2), one cytoplasmic loop (CL) where both amino (NH2)- and caboxy (COOH)-termini are intracellular. Top and bottom center show hemichannels formed by six connexin or pannexin subunits each, respectively. The middle center shows a connexin gap junction channel, at a close contact between two microglia. A hemichannel is formed by six connexins or pannexins that oligomerize laterally leaving a central pore in the activated state (open). Under resting conditions hemichannels remain preferentially closed, but they can be activated by diverse physiological and pathological conditions, offering a diffusional transmembrane route between the intra and extracellular milieu. In addition, it is depicted the types of hemichannels and gap junction channels expressed by microglia. This figure includes only the available information obtained under in vivo and/or in vitro studies using more than one experimental approach.

http://dx.doi.org/10.5772/54306

For a long time the main function attributed to connexin hemichannels was the formation of gap junction channels. Nevertheless, in the last decade, the presence of functional connexin hemichannels in nonjunctional membranes has been demonstrated by several experimental approaches [20-24]. These channels serve like aqueous pores permeable to ions and small molecules that permit diffusional exchange between the intra and extracellular compartments, allowing cellular release of relevant quantities of autocrine/paracrine signaling molecules (e.g., ATP, glutamate, NAD^+ and PGE_2) to the extracellular milieu [25-30], as well as uptake of small molecules (e.g., glucose) [31]. One decade ago, a new gene family of gap junction proteins composed by three members was discovered in chordates [32, 33]. These proteins are the chordate homologs of innexins (the gap junction proteins of non chordates), and were denominated pannexins (panx1, 2 and 3) because apparently they are present in all eumetazoans except echinoderms [34] (Fig. 1). It has been suggested that gap junctional intercellular communication occur via Panx3 in osteoblasts [35], whereas other studies have shown that overexpression of exogenous Panx1 could form gap junctions *in vitro* [33, 36, 37]. Nevertheless, the absence of ultrastructural evidences for gap junction formation and demonstration of functional communication mediated by other endogenously expressed pannexins indicate that they apparently act mainly as hemichannels [38].

Current knowledge regarding brain hemichannels state that, under physiological conditions, they have a low activity, but enough to ensure the release of paracrine substances necessary for diverse functions of the CNS, including ischemic tolerance [39, 40], establishment of adhesive interactions [41]; fear memory consolidation [42], glucosensing [30], chemoreception [43], blood-brain barrier permeability [44], neuronal migration [45, 46] and metabolic autocrine regulation [47]. Nevertheless, under acute or chronic neurodegeneration dysregulation of hemichannel properties could be critical on the beginning and maintenance of homeostatic imbalances observed in diverse brain diseases [48-50]. Pioneering findings from Paul and colleagues showed that Xenopus oocytes transfected with Cx46 mRNA exhibited non-selective cation currents associated to depolarization and cell lysis within 24 h [51]. From then on, several studies supported the idea that dysregulated opening of hemichannels is incompatible with normal cell life. In the CNS, the first convincing evidence of hemichannel opening was provided by Contreras and colleagues, whose work showed that opening of Cx43 hemichannels accelerate astroglial cell death induced by ischemia-like conditions [52]. Such increased hemichannel activity induced by ischemia-like conditions has been observed in neurons [40, 53-55], oligodendrocytes [56], and also in brain cells subjected to other pro-inflammatory conditions [48]. Up to now, it is believed that sustained hemichannel opening contributes to increased intracellular Ca^{2+} concentration ($[Ca^{2+}]_i$), which in turn may favor even more the hemichannel activity (De Vuyst et al., 2007, Schalper et al., 2008), inducing Ca^{2+} and Na^+ intracellular overload (Fig. 2).

Under these conditions, ionic (or electrolyte) imbalance leads to an osmotic imbalance that results in cell swelling and plasma membrane breakdown. Calcium overload induced in part by hemichannel opening may also activate phospholipase A_2, with the subsequent generation of arachidonic acid and activation of cyclooxygenase/lipoxygenase pathways leading to increased free radicals, lipid peroxidation and further plasma membrane damage. Possibly, exacerbated or uncontrolled hemichannel opening could lead to cellular damage by several ways: 1) High increase of $[Ca^{2+}]_i$ by Ca^{2+} entry through hemichannels, 2) cellular swelling by increased entry of Na^{2+} and Cl^- through hemichannels, 3) release of metabolic products essential to cell viability as glucose, NAD^+ or glutathione via hemichannels and 4) alternatively, spread of toxic molecules released by hemichannels (e.g., glutamate) could affect the viability of healthy neighboring cells.

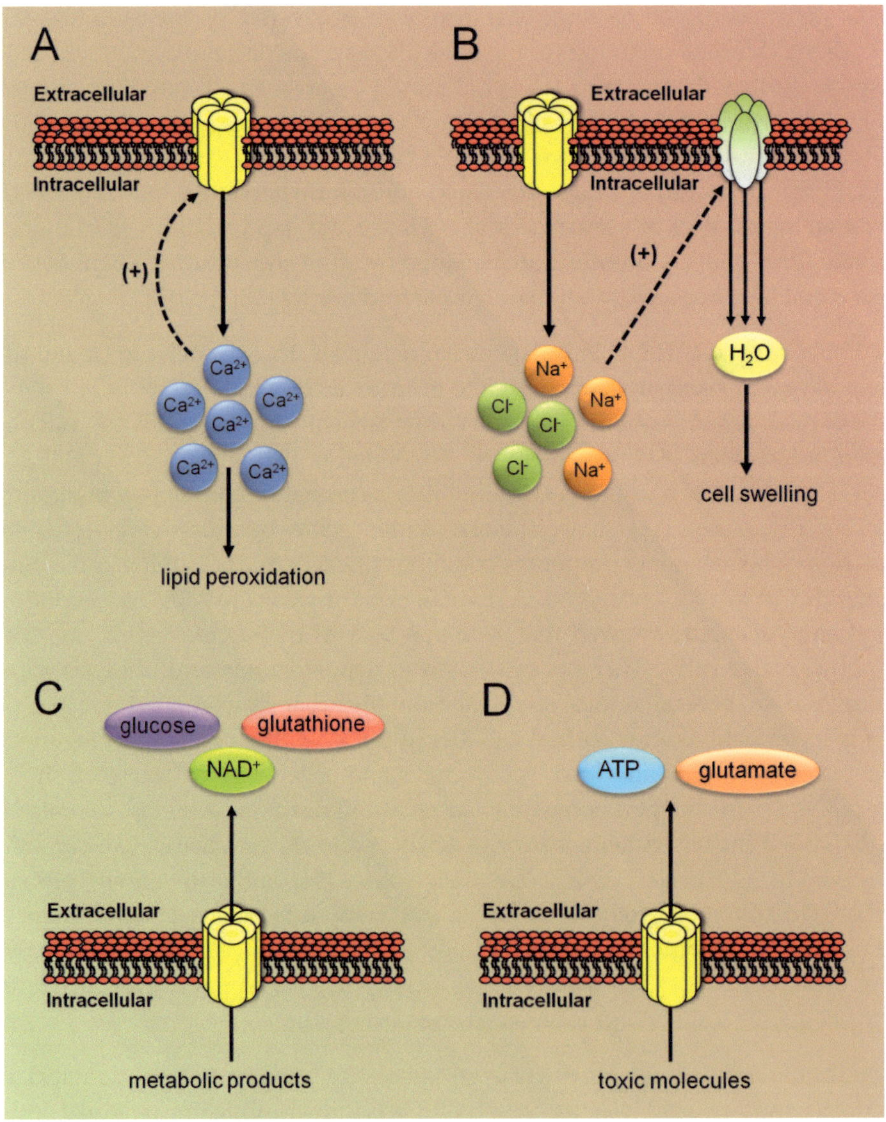

Figure 2. Dysregulated opening of hemichannels induces cell damage by different mechanisms. Under normal conditions, hemichannels (yellow channels) exhibit a low activity. However, upon exposure to inflammatory conditions, hemichannels undergo a dysregulation proccess leading to an uncontrolled opening which further results in cellular

damage by various mechanisms. (A) Ca^{2+} entry through hemichannels activate phospholipase A_2, with the subsequent generation of arachidonic acid and activation of cyclooxygenase/lipoxygenase pathways leading to increased free radicals, lipid peroxidation and further plasma membrane damage. Note that increased levels of $[Ca^{2+}]_i$ may activate even more hemichannel opening as demonstrated previously [57, 58]. (B) Na^{2+} and Cl^- entry through hemichannels could produce cellular swelling by increased influx of H_2O via aquoporins (green channels). (C) Release of essencial metabolic products via hemichannels (eg., glucose, NAD^+ or glutathione) could increase cell vulnerability. (D) Release via hemichannels of molecules that in high amounts are toxic (e.g., ATP and glutamate) could affect the viability of healthy neighboring cells and spread damage.

Taking into account that hemichannels participate in the paracrine signaling among brain cells, the current chapter attempts to review and discuss the role of gap junction channels and hemichannels in microglia on normal and inflamed brain.

2. Gap junction channels in microglia

In a resting surveillance state, microglia express almost undetectable levels of Cx43 and Cx36 [59-65]. Nevertheless, when microglia are subjected to pro-inflammatory conditions, they exhibit expression of Cx43 and are able to form gap junction channels among them, as evaluated by dye-coupling experiments. In fact, Cx43 expression and gap junctional communication is induced in microglia by LPS, TNF-α plus IFN-γ [61], calcium ionophore plus PMA [66], or Staphylococcus aureus-derived peptidoglycan [64]. Despite the above, cultured human or mouse microglia treated with LPS, granulocyte-macrophage colony-stimulating factor, INF-γ or TNF-α do not exhibit modifications in connexin expression [60, 63]. Recently has been showed that resting microglia exhibit detectable levels of surface and total Cx43, whereas upon treatment with amyloid-β peptide (Aβ) a high increase in Cx43 expression is observed (Orellana 2011a). The discrepancy in the above mentioned studies may be related to different types of animal used to obtain brain tissue, dissimilar methods to take out cells and different culture conditions.

The ability to establish gap junctional communication among microglia, requires a rise in $[Ca^{2+}]_i$ [66], while cAMP, cGMP or activation of PKC have been ruled out as possible inductors gap junction-mediated coupling [66]. In this regard, different degrees of microglial activation may trigger intracellular pathways that further result in a specific pattern of expression of gap juntion proteins. Communication via gap junctions may allow to activated microglia to recruit resting microglia at the site of injury, resulting in more damage or repair depending on the circumstances. Interestingly, microglia stimulated with cytokines or LPS exhibit reduced levels of Cx43 expression and gap junctional communication in astrocytes when both cell types are in co-culture or when conditioned media from activated microglia is used [31, 55, 59, 60, 67, 68]. Interestingly, gap junctions among dendritic cells ensure sharing of antigenic peptides [69-74], suggesting the possibility that these channels in microglia also could coordinate the CNS immune response. Importantly, recently it has been shown that the release of TNF-α and IL-1β by microglia depend on the activity of gap junction channels, because secretion of those cytokines was partially blocked by a gap junction blocker, α-glicirretinic acid [75]. Thus, it was proposed that gap junction channels play a key role into coordinate the microglial mediated inflammation.

3. Hemichannels in microglia

Up to now only few studies have documented the expression of functional hemichannels in microglia. Contrary to the expectations regarding as Cx43 the most possible protein to form hemichannels in microglia, TNF-α treatment was shown to induce release of glutamate through a pathway inhibited by a Cx32 (^{32}Gap27), but not Cx43 (^{43}Gap27) mimetic peptide [76]. Moreover, surface levels of Cx32 were increased in microglia treated with TNF-α. Noteworthy, the increased neuronal death associated with the release of glutamate was inhibited completely with the ^{32}Gap27 mimetic peptide [76]. Later, the same group of authors proposed that glutamate released via Cx32 hemichannels play a key role in neuronal damage originated by brain ischemia [77] and experimental autoimmune encephalomyelitis [78]. Accordingly, microglial cells from Mecp2 null mice, a model of a neurodevelopmental disorder known as Rett syndrome, promote neuronal death through glutamate release via a cell membrane pathway inhibited by ^{32}Gap27 and ^{32}Gap24, two Cx32 hemichannel mimetic peptides [79]. It is relevant to kept in mind that these and other mimetic peptides are homologous to extracellular domains of the respective connexin sequences, but their effects on hemichannel activity have not been documented, thereby some studies have questioned their specificity [80-82]. The use of cell cultures derived from connexin null mice and/or performing knockdown of the respective connexin, along the appropriate use of mimetic peptides could ensure the involvement of Cx32 hemichannels in these studies.

Almost two years ago, the opening of Cx43 and Panx1 hemichannels, evaluated by dye uptake and macroscopic cell membrane currents, were shown to be increased in microglia by $A\beta_{25-35}$ exposure (Orellana et al. 2012a). These observations were confirmed by using microglial cultures from Cx43 KO mice and Panx1 mimetic peptides. These currents were recorded at negative holding potential (-60 mV) in the presence of external divalent cations, suggesting that opening of microglial hemichannels may occur in Alzheimer's disease (AD). Importantly, ATP and glutamate released from microglia treated with $A\beta_{25-35}$ trigger hemichannel opening in neurons causing deleterious effects on them [83]. Supporting the idea of hemichannels as possible regulators in damage observed in AD, a novel putative hemichannel blocker (INI-0602) that crosses the blood brain barrier was recently shown to inhibit *in vivo* the LPS-induced glutamate release from microglia and to improve memory deficits in APP/PS1 mice [84]. Due the pharmacological pattern of this response," it was proposed the involvement of Cx32 hemichannels. However, the possible implication of other hemichannel forming proteins or even other channels was not ruled out and studies on the specificity of INI-0602 require further demonstration using, for example, *in vivo* experiments with $Cx32^{-/-}$ microglia or knockdown of Cx32. To demonstrate the participation of hemichannels in this disease it is necessary to analyze the functional state of microglial hemichannels in brain slices from AD model mice (APP/PS1) by using patch-clamp and membrane permeability assays.

http://dx.doi.org/10.5772/54306

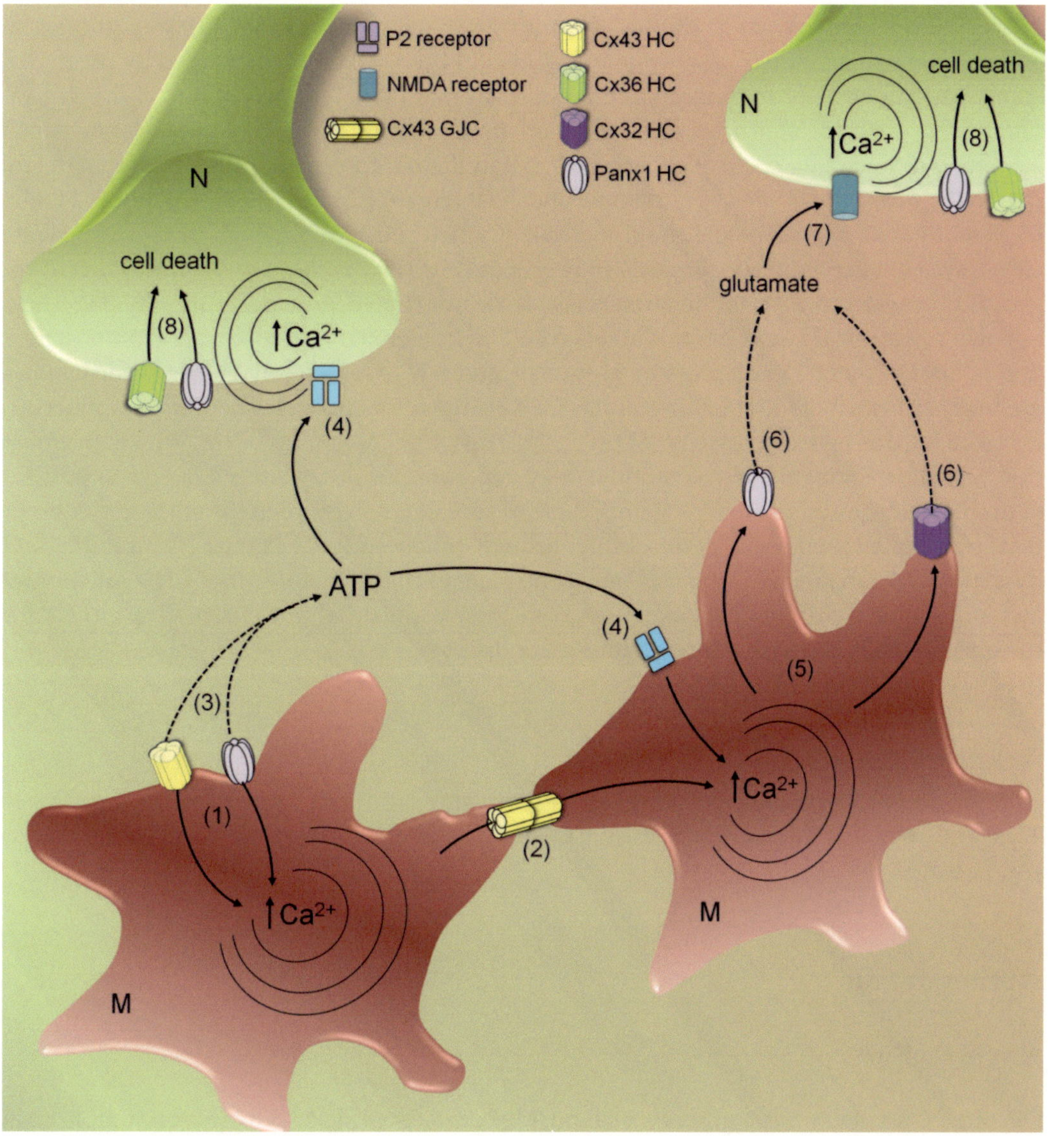

Figure 3. Role of microglial cell hemichannels and gap junction channels during neuroinflammation. Chronic or acute inflammation increases hemichannel (HC) activity in microglia allowing the influx of Ca^{2+} (1) and its spread to neighbor cells through gap junctions (GJCs) (2) raising the intracellular free Ca^{2+} concentration ($[Ca^{2+}]_i$). HC opening induced by inflammation in microglia leads to ATP release (3), which diffuses through the extracellular space and activates membrane purinergic (P2) receptors (4). High levels of $[Ca^{2+}]_i$ (5) allow the release of glutamate through microglial cell HCs (6) and further activation of neuronal NMDA receptors (7). P2 and NMDA receptor activation in neurons increase the activity of neuronal Panx1 and Cx36 HCs, affecting electrochemical and Ca^{2+} imbalance in neurons, which leads to cell death (8).

4. Conclusions

Microglial cells are known to play a relevant role in neuronal survival [3]. In pathological situations, dysregulation of connexin- and pannexin-based channels expressed by microglia, contribute importantly to determine the neuronal fate [48, 50]. Microgliosis and brain inflammation are associated with most, if not all, brain injuries and pathologies. Hemichannel activation in microglia could play a crucial role in the reinforcement of the neuronal death, due to their capacity to release glutamate and ATP (Fig. 3) [55, 76, 83, 85]. Opening of Cx43, Cx32 and Panx1 hemichannels could increase $[Ca^{2+}]_i$ in microglia, which further propagate Ca^{2+} waves via gap junction channels to neighbor cells (Fig. 3). Moreover, in distant microglia, Ca^{2+} waves can activate hemichannels, as demonstrated previously [57, 58, 86]. Then, opening of neuronal Panx1 hemichannels could be triggered by the rise in $[Ca^{2+}]_i$ via activation of NMDA and P2X receptors by glutamate and ATP, respectively. Panx1 hemichannels are likely to contribute to the intracellular Ca^{2+} overload that activates neurotoxic intracellular cascades during excitotoxicity [87] (Fig. 3). Thus, the prevention of hemichannel activation under pro-inflammatory conditions may represent an unexplored strategy to prevent neuronal damage and death. Altogether these observations strengthen the emerging concept that unregulated membrane permeability through enhanced hemichannel permeability and dysfunctional gap junction channels may contribute to the development of CNS pathologies and connexins as well as pannexins might represent potential and alternative targets for therapeutic intervention in neuroinflammatory diseases.

Acknowledgements

This work was partially supported by CONICYT 79090028 and FONDECYT 11121133 (to JAO) grants.

Author details

Juan A. Orellana

Departamento de Neurología; Escuela de Medicina, Pontificia Universidad Católica de Chile, Santiago, Chile

References

[1] Kettenmann, H, et al. *Physiology of microglia.* Physiol Rev, (2011). , 461-553.

[2] Block, M. L, & Hong, J. S. *Microglia and inflammation-mediated neurodegeneration: multiple triggers with a common mechanism.* Prog Neurobiol, (2005). , 77-98.

[3] Block, M. L, Zecca, L, & Hong, J. S. *Microglia-mediated neurotoxicity: uncovering the molecular mechanisms.* Nat Rev Neurosci, (2007). , 57-69.

[4] Hanisch, U. K. *Microglia as a source and target of cytokines.* Glia, (2002). , 140-155.

[5] Streit, W. J. *Microglia as neuroprotective, immunocompetent cells of the CNS.* Glia, (2002). , 133-139.

[6] Saez, J. C, et al. *Plasma membrane channels formed by connexins: their regulation and functions.* Physiol Rev, (2003). , 1359-1400.

[7] Sohl, G, & Willecke, K. *Gap junctions and the connexin protein family.* Cardiovasc Res, (2004). , 228-232.

[8] Laird, D. W. *The gap junction proteome and its relationship to disease.* Trends Cell Biol, (2010). , 92-101.

[9] Goodenough, D. A, & Paul, D. L. *Gap junctions.* Cold Spring Harb Perspect Biol, (2009). , a002576.

[10] Evans, W. H, De Vuyst, E, & Leybaert, L. *The gap junction cellular internet: connexin hemichannels enter the signalling limelight.* Biochem J, (2006). , 1-14.

[11] Saez, J. C, et al. *cAMP delays disappearance of gap junctions between pairs of rat hepatocytes in primary culture.* Am J Physiol, (1989). Pt 1): , C1-11.

[12] Connors, B. W, & Long, M. A. *Electrical synapses in the mammalian brain.* Annu Rev Neurosci, (2004). , 393-418.

[13] Goldberg, G. S, Lampe, P. D, & Nicholson, B. J. *Selective transfer of endogenous metabolites through gap junctions composed of different connexins.* Nat Cell Biol, (1999). , 457-459.

[14] Kam, Y, et al. *Transfer of second messengers through gap junction connexin 43 channels reconstituted in liposomes.* Biochim Biophys Acta, (1998). , 384-388.

[15] Lawrence, T. S, Beers, W. H, & Gilula, N. B. *Transmission of hormonal stimulation by cell-to-cell communication.* Nature, (1978). , 501-506.

[16] Niessen, H, et al. *Selective permeability of different connexin channels to the second messenger inositol 1,4,5-trisphosphate.* J Cell Sci, (2000). Pt 8): , 1365-1372.

[17] Cruciani, V, & Mikalsen, S. O. *The connexin gene family in mammals.* Biol Chem, (2005). , 325-332.

[18] Abascal, F, & Zardoya, R. *Evolutionary analyses of gap junction protein families.* Biochim Biophys Acta, (2012).

[19] Willecke, K, et al. *Structural and functional diversity of connexin genes in the mouse and human genome.* Biol Chem, (2002). , 725-737.

[20] Goodenough, D. A, & Paul, D. L. *Beyond the gap: functions of unpaired connexon channels.* Nat Rev Mol Cell Biol, (2003). , 285-294.

[21] Stout, C, Goodenough, D. A, & Paul, D. L. *Connexins: functions without junctions.* Curr Opin Cell Biol, (2004)., 507-512.

[22] Saez, J. C, et al. *Connexin-based gap junction hemichannels: gating mechanisms.* Biochim Biophys Acta, (2005)., 215-224.

[23] Schalper, K. A, et al. *Currently used methods for identification and characterization of hemichannels.* Cell Commun Adhes, (2008)., 207-218.

[24] Saez, J. C, et al. *Cell membrane permeabilization via connexin hemichannels in living and dying cells.* Exp Cell Res, (2010)., 2377-2389.

[25] Bruzzone, S, et al. *Connexin 43 hemi channels mediate Ca2+-regulated transmembrane NAD+ fluxes in intact cells.* FASEB J, (2001)., 10-12.

[26] Ye, Z. C, et al. *Functional hemichannels in astrocytes: a novel mechanism of glutamate release.* J Neurosci, (2003)., 3588-3596.

[27] Cherian, P. P, et al. *Mechanical strain opens connexin 43 hemichannels in osteocytes: a novel mechanism for the release of prostaglandin.* Mol Biol Cell, (2005)., 3100-3106.

[28] Stout, C. E, et al. *Intercellular calcium signaling in astrocytes via ATP release through connexin hemichannels.* J Biol Chem, (2002)., 10482-10488.

[29] Braet, K, et al. *Pharmacological sensitivity of ATP release triggered by photoliberation of inositol-1,4,5-trisphosphate and zero extracellular calcium in brain endothelial cells.* J Cell Physiol, (2003)., 205-213.

[30] Orellana, J. A, et al. *Glucose increases intracellular free Ca(2+) in tanycytes via ATP released through connexin 43 hemichannels.* Glia, (2012)., 53-68.

[31] Retamal, M. A, et al. *Cx43 hemichannels and gap junction channels in astrocytes are regulated oppositely by proinflammatory cytokines released from activated microglia.* J Neurosci, (2007)., 13781-13792.

[32] Panchin, Y, et al. *A ubiquitous family of putative gap junction molecules.* Curr Biol, (2000)., R473-R474.

[33] Bruzzone, R, et al. *Pannexins, a family of gap junction proteins expressed in brain.* Proc Natl Acad Sci U S A, (2003)., 13644-13649.

[34] Shestopalov, V. I, & Panchin, Y. *Pannexins and gap junction protein diversity.* Cell Mol Life Sci, (2008)., 376-394.

[35] Ishikawa, M, et al. *Pannexin 3 functions as an ER Ca(2+) channel, hemichannel, and gap junction to promote osteoblast differentiation.* J Cell Biol, (2011)., 1257-1274.

[36] Lai, C. P, et al. *Tumor-suppressive effects of pannexin 1 in C6 glioma cells.* Cancer Res, (2007)., 1545-1554.

[37] Vanden AbeeleF., et al., *Functional implications of calcium permeability of the channel formed by pannexin 1.* J Cell Biol, (2006)., 535-546.

[38] MacVicarB.A. and R.J. Thompson, *Non-junction functions of pannexin-1 channels.* Trends Neurosci, (2010). , 93-102.

[39] Lin, J. H, et al. *A central role of connexin 43 in hypoxic preconditioning.* J Neurosci, (2008). , 681-695.

[40] Schock, S. C, et al. *ATP release by way of connexin 36 hemichannels mediates ischemic tolerance in vitro.* Biochem Biophys Res Commun, (2008). , 138-144.

[41] Cotrina, M. L, Lin, J. H, & Nedergaard, M. *Adhesive properties of connexin hemichannels.* Glia, (2008). , 1791-1798.

[42] Stehberg, J, et al. *Release of gliotransmitters through astroglial connexin 43 hemichannels is necessary for fear memory consolidation in the basolateral amygdala.* FASEB J, (2012).

[43] Wenker, I. C, et al. *Regulation of ventral surface CO2/H+-sensitive neurons by purinergic signalling.* J Physiol, (2012). Pt 9): , 2137-2150.

[44] De Bock, M, et al. *Connexin channels provide a target to manipulate brain endothelial calcium dynamics and blood-brain barrier permeability.* J Cereb Blood Flow Metab, (2011). , 1942-1957.

[45] Liu, X, et al. *Gap junctions/hemichannels modulate interkinetic nuclear migration in the forebrain precursors.* J Neurosci, (2010). , 4197-4209.

[46] Liu, X, et al. *Connexin 43 controls the multipolar phase of neuronal migration to the cerebral cortex.* Proc Natl Acad Sci U S A, (2012). , 8280-8285.

[47] Kawamura, M, Jr, D. N, & Ruskin, S. A. Masino, *Metabolic autocrine regulation of neurons involves cooperation among pannexin hemichannels, adenosine receptors, and KATP channels.* J Neurosci, (2010). , 3886-3895.

[48] Orellana, J. A, et al. *Modulation of brain hemichannels and gap junction channels by pro-inflammatory agents and their possible role in neurodegeneration.* Antioxid Redox Signal, (2009). , 369-399.

[49] Orellana, J. A, et al. *Hemichannels in the neurovascular unit and white matter under normal and inflamed conditions.* CNS Neurol Disord Drug Targets, (2011). , 404-414.

[50] Orellana, J. A, et al. *Glial hemichannels and their involvement in aging and neurodegenerative diseases.* Rev Neurosci, (2012). , 163-177.

[51] Paul, D. L, et al. *Connexin46, a novel lens gap junction protein, induces voltage-gated currents in nonjunctional plasma membrane of Xenopus oocytes.* J Cell Biol, (1991). , 1077-1089.

[52] Contreras, J. E, et al. *Metabolic inhibition induces opening of unapposed connexin 43 gap junction hemichannels and reduces gap junctional communication in cortical astrocytes in culture.* Proc Natl Acad Sci U S A, (2002). , 495-500.

[53] Thompson, R. J, & Zhou, N. and B.A. MacVicar, *Ischemia opens neuronal gap junction hemichannels.* Science, (2006). , 924-927.

[54] Thompson, R. J, et al. *Activation of pannexin-1 hemichannels augments aberrant bursting in the hippocampus.* Science, (2008)., 1555-1559.

[55] Orellana, J. A, et al. *ATP and glutamate released via astroglial connexin 43 hemichannels mediate neuronal death through activation of pannexin 1 hemichannels.* J Neurochem, (2011)., 826-840.

[56] Domercq, M, et al. receptors *mediate ischemic damage to oligodendrocytes*. Glia, (2010). p. 730-40., 2X7.

[57] Schalper, K. A, et al. *Connexin 43 hemichannels mediate the Ca2+ influx induced by extracellular alkalinization.* Am J Physiol Cell Physiol, (2010)., C1504-C1515.

[58] De Vuyst, E, et al. *Connexin hemichannels and gap junction channels are differentially influenced by lipopolysaccharide and basic fibroblast growth factor.* Mol Biol Cell, (2007)., 34-46.

[59] Rouach, N, et al. *Brain macrophages inhibit gap junctional communication and downregulate connexin 43 expression in cultured astrocytes.* Eur J Neurosci, (2002)., 403-407.

[60] Meme, W, et al. *Proinflammatory cytokines released from microglia inhibit gap junctions in astrocytes: potentiation by beta-amyloid.* FASEB J, (2006)., 494-496.

[61] Eugenin, E. A, et al. *Microglia at brain stab wounds express connexin 43 and in vitro form functional gap junctions after treatment with interferon-gamma and tumor necrosis factor-alpha.* Proc Natl Acad Sci U S A, (2001)., 4190-4195.

[62] Parenti, R, et al. *Immunocytochemical and RT-PCR analysis of connexin36 in cultures of mammalian glial cells.* Arch Ital Biol, (2002)., 101-108.

[63] Dobrenis, K, et al. *Human and mouse microglia express connexin36, and functional gap junctions are formed between rodent microglia and neurons.* J Neurosci Res, (2005)., 306-315.

[64] Garg, S, & Md, M. Syed, and T. Kielian, *Staphylococcus aureus-derived peptidoglycan induces Cx43 expression and functional gap junction intercellular communication in microglia.* J Neurochem, (2005)., 475-483.

[65] Lee, I. H, et al. *Glial and neuronal connexin expression patterns in the rat spinal cord during development and following injury.* J Comp Neurol, (2005)., 1-10.

[66] Martinez, A. D, et al. *Identification of second messengers that induce expression of functional gap junctions in microglia cultured from newborn rats.* Brain Res, (2002)., 191-201.

[67] Faustmann, P. M, et al. *Microglia activation influences dye coupling and Cx43 expression of the astrocytic network.* Glia, (2003)., 101-108.

[68] Hinkerohe, D, et al. *Effects of cytokines on microglial phenotypes and astroglial coupling in an inflammatory coculture model.* Glia, (2005)., 85-97.

[69] Neijssen, J, et al. *Cross-presentation by intercellular peptide transfer through gap junctions.* Nature, (2005)., 83-88.

[70] Matsue, H, et al. *Gap junction-mediated intercellular communication between dendritic cells (DCs) is required for effective activation of DCs.* J Immunol, (2006)., 181-190.

[71] Corvalan, L. A, et al. *Injury of skeletal muscle and specific cytokines induce the expression of gap junction channels in mouse dendritic cells.* J Cell Physiol, (2007)., 649-660.

[72] Handel, A, et al. *Gap junction-mediated antigen transport in immune responses.* Trends Immunol, (2007)., 463-466.

[73] Mendoza-naranjo, A, et al. *Functional gap junctions facilitate melanoma antigen ransfer and cross-presentation between human dendritic cells.* J Immunol, (2007)., 6949-6957.

[74] Pang, B, et al. *Direct antigen presentation and gap junction mediated cross-presentation during apoptosis.* J Immunol, (2009)., 1083-1090.

[75] Eugenin, E. A, et al. *The Role of Gap Junction Channels During Physiologic and Pathologic Conditions of the Human Central Nervous System.* J Neuroimmune Pharmacol, (2012).

[76] Takeuchi, H, et al. *Tumor necrosis factor-alpha induces neurotoxicity via glutamate release from hemichannels of activated microglia in an autocrine manner.* J Biol Chem, (2006)., 21362-21368.

[77] Takeuchi, H, et al. *Blockade of microglial glutamate release protects against ischemic brain injury.* Exp Neurol, (2008)., 144-146.

[78] Shijie, J, et al. *Blockade of glutamate release from microglia attenuates experimental autoimmune encephalomyelitis in mice.* Tohoku J Exp Med, (2009)., 87-92.

[79] Maezawa, I, et al. *Rett syndrome astrocytes are abnormal and spread MeCP2 deficiency through gap junctions.* J Neurosci, (2009)., 5051-5061.

[80] Wang, J, et al. *Modulation of membrane channel currents by gap junction protein mimetic peptides: size matters.* Am J Physiol Cell Physiol, (2007)., C1112-C1119.

[81] Dahl, G. *Gap junction-mimetic peptides do work, but in unexpected ways.* Cell Commun Adhes, (2007)., 259-264.

[82] Evans, W. H, & Leybaert, L. *Mimetic peptides as blockers of connexin channel-facilitated intercellular communication.* Cell Commun Adhes, (2007)., 265-273.

[83] Orellana, J. A, et al. *Amyloid beta-induced death in neurons involves glial and neuronal hemichannels.* J Neurosci, (2011)., 4962-4977.

[84] Takeuchi, H, et al. *Blockade of gap junction hemichannel suppresses disease progression in mouse models of amyotrophic lateral sclerosis and Alzheimer's disease.* PLoS One, (2011)., e21108.

[85] Kang, J, et al. *Connexin 43 hemichannels are permeable to ATP.* J Neurosci, (2008)., 4702-4711.

[86] Sanchez, H. A, et al. *Metabolic inhibition increases activity of connexin-32 hemichannels permeable to Ca2+ in transfected HeLa cells.* Am J Physiol Cell Physiol, (2009). , C665-C678.

[87] Szydlowska, K, & Tymianski, M. *Calcium, ischemia and excitotoxicity.* Cell Calcium, (2010). , 122-129.

Chapter 16

Influence of Obesity on Neurodegenerative Diseases

Rana Awada , Avinash Parimisetty and
Christian Lefebvre d'Hellencourt

Additional information is available at the end of the chapter

http://dx.doi.org/10.5772/53671

1. Introduction

Obesity is one of the greatest public health challenges of the 21st century. Obesity prevalence has been increasing globally at an alarming rate, particularly among children. The progressively increased prevalence of obesity over the past decades among children, as well as adults, is not limited to the US and other industrialized nations but is also evident in developing countries [1].The World Health Organization (WHO) estimated the prevalence of obesity at more than 1 billion overweight adults, with at least 500 million reaching the level of obese. As this continues to increase, by 2015, WHO estimates the number of overweighed adults will balloon to 2.3 billion with more than 700 million obese. Worldwide, obesity is currently responsible for 2–8% of health care costs and approximately 10–13% of deaths [2].

Fundamental causes of the current obesity epidemic are associated with sedentary lifestyles, increased consumption of energy-dense foods high in saturated fats and sugars and reduced physical activity. All of which correlate with the profound changes occurring in behavioral patterns of communities across societies as a consequence of increased urbanization and industrialization and often the disappearance of traditional lifestyles [3]. However, it is now appreciated that the progression to obesity represents a complex interaction of genetics, metabolism, as well as diet and physical activity level.

Clinically, obesity is defined by measurements of body mass index [4] or waist circumference and waist to hip ratio [5]. Body mass index (BMI) is a simple index weight-to-height defined as a person's weight in kilograms divided by the square of his/her height in meters (kg/m^2). According to WHO guidelines, a BMI 25 kg/m^2 identifies overweight and a BMI of 30 kg/m^2 or higher identifies an individual as obese. Physiologically, obesity is an excessive accumulation of fat in adipose tissue in the form of triglycerides, which can negatively affect health. Obesity is associated with number of metabolic disorders, increased expression of pro-inflammatory markers and elevated risk for various disease including type 2 diabetes, cardiovascular disease, gastrointestinal disorders, respiratory difficulties, and various types of cancer [6]. In a more general nature, it has been suggested that obesity may accelerate the normal process of aging [7] (figure 1).

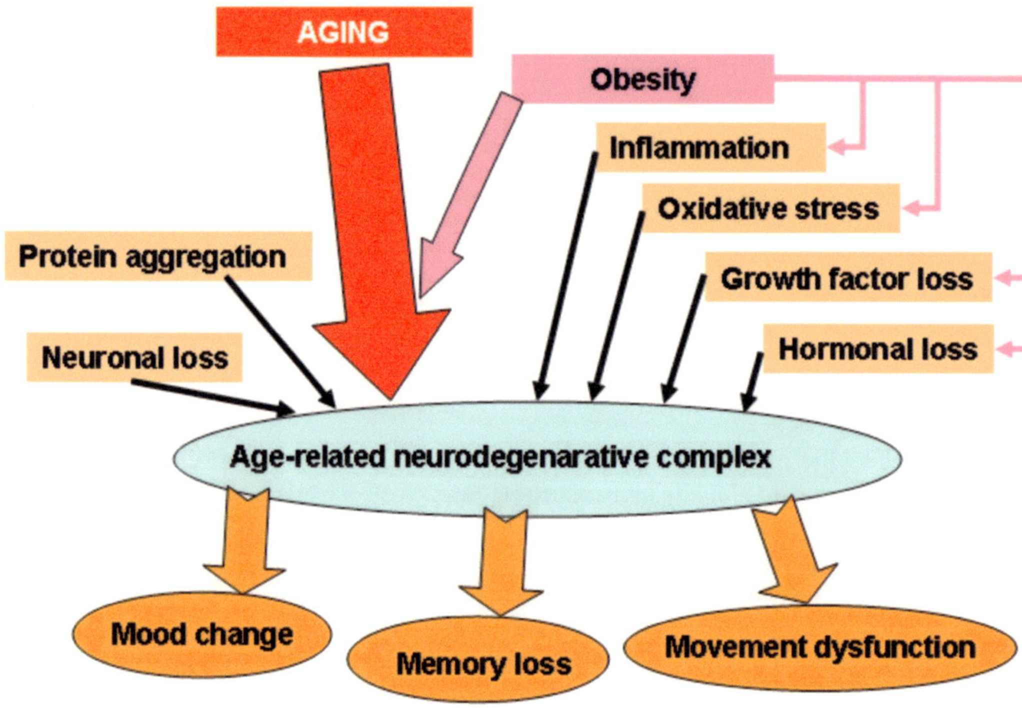

Figure 1. Obesity accelerates age and age related pathologies. Adapted from [8]

2. Obesity and inflammatory mediators

Adipose tissue has long been regarded as tissue storage of fat in the form of triglycerides; however, it is now recognized as an endocrine tissue producing a number of different factors, including inflammatory-related factors, acting at a physiological level [9].

Two forms of adipose tissues exist in mammals: the brown fat and the white fat (figure 2).

Brown adipose tissue is involved in the regulation of the body temperature. In humans, until recently, it was thought that brown fat was only present in the newborn and infant [12]. The extensive use of positron emission tomography (PET) in cancer medical imaging has changed this dogma. An evaluation of fluorodeoxyglucose PET (FDG PET) data from adult cancer patients indicated a high level of glucose consumption in specific body regions corresponding to brown fat [10], presumably in order to maintain normal body temperature

http://dx.doi.org/10.5772/53671

within an air conditioned room as this was not observed when patients were in a warm environment. White adipose tissue (WAT) is a source of energy involved in heat insulation and mechanical cushion. WAT represents around 15-20% of body weight and in obese individuals it increases up to 50%. WAT is composed of several different cell types, including preadipocytes, mature adipocytes, macrophages, endothelial cells which are involved in WAT homeostasis (Figure 3) [13, 14]. It is worth noting the presence of stem cells in the WAT, which are extensively studied for their potential in therapeutic reparation and even for the treatment of obesity and metabolic disorders [15-17].

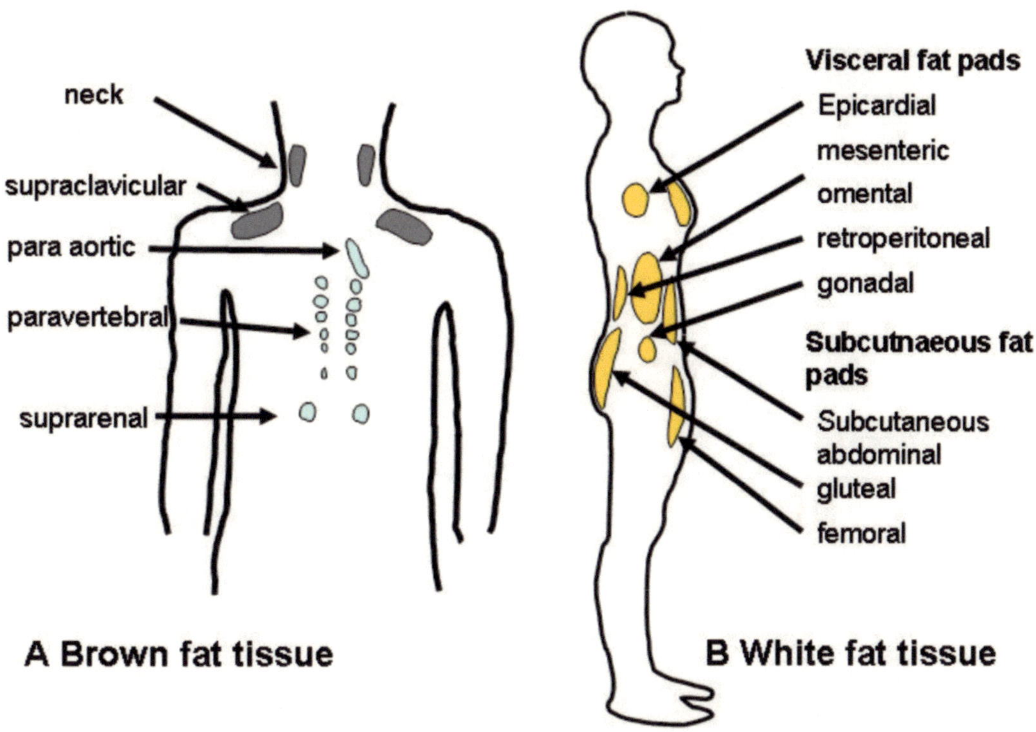

Figure 2. Brown fat (A) and white fat (B) tissue distribution in adult from [10, 11]

Different functional properties have been identified for WAT depending upon location in the subcutaneous or visceral areas. For example, a correlation exists between visceral obesity and increased risk of insulin resistance and cardiovascular diseases, while an increase of subcutaneous fat is associated with favorable plasma lipid profiles [11]. Adipose tissue was not usually thought of as an immune or inflammatory organ based upon studies demonstrating that loss of adipose tissue is associated with a decrease in markers of inflammation. It is now well accepted however, that adipose tissue is a key player in the development of inflammation [19]. Excess fat tissue in the obese environment contributes to a low-grade chronic inflammation [20] with elevated production of pro-inflammatory cytokines, such as tumor necrosis factor alpha (TNFα), interleukin -6 (IL-6) and IL-1 [21, 22]. The visceral adipocytes significantly contribute in this role as they are metabolically active and produce a higher level of pro-inflammatory cytokines [11, 23-25].

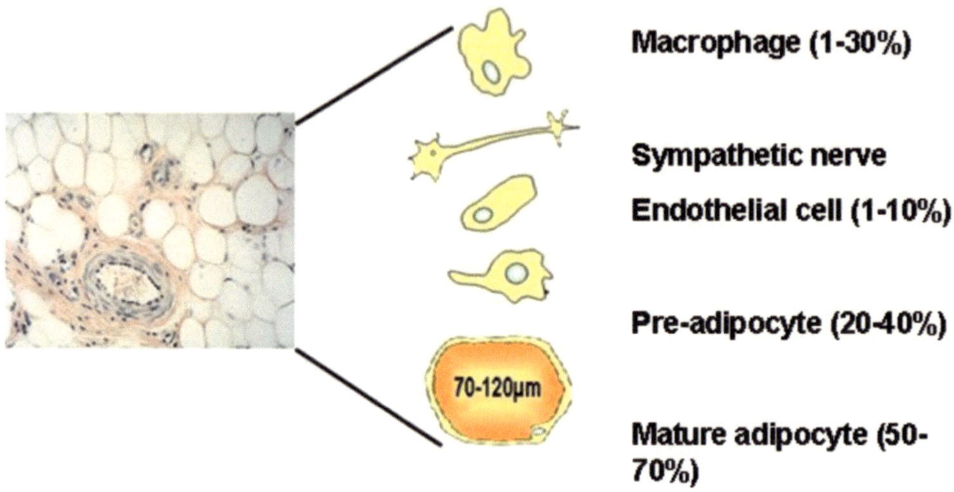

Figure 3. Cells present in the fat tissue adapted from [13, 18]

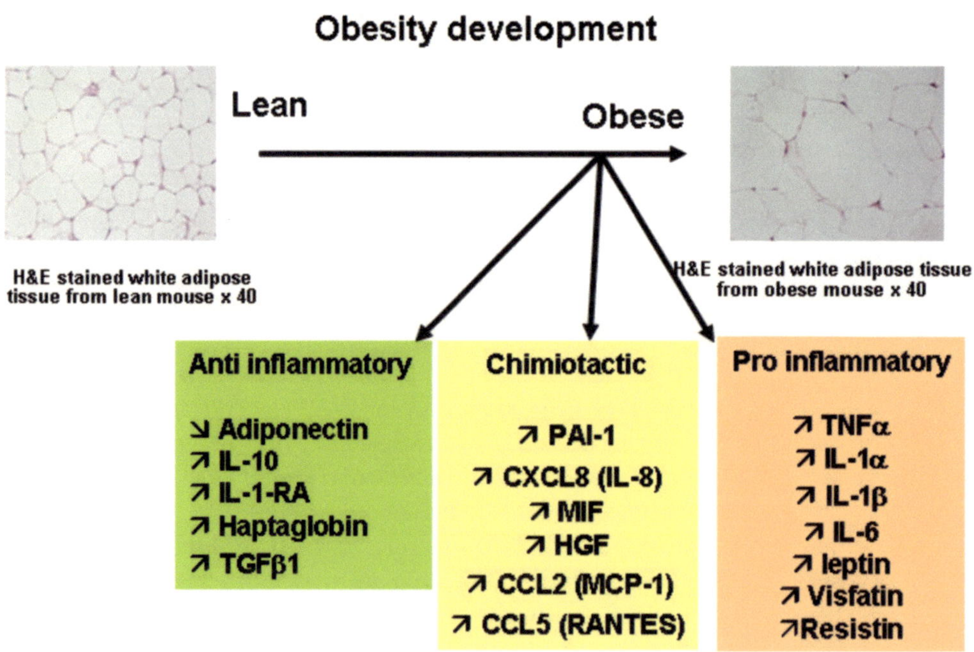

Figure 4. Inflammatory factors produced by WAT in obese situations. [26-35]

WAT is considered as an important organ in the regulation of many pathological processes by producing several inflammatory factors including, chemokines, cytokines and adipokines (also named adipocytokines). During the development of obesity expression of these factors is modified (figure 4).

Adipocytes secrete various chemo-attractants that recruit monocytes into the WAT. Obese adipose tissue exhibits an increased expression of Monocyte Chemoattractant Protein 1 (MCP-1) and of its receptor CCR2. The signaling of MCP1 / CCR2 has a direct impact on the development of obesity (for review see [36]). CCL-2, another chemokine with capability to recruit macrophages, has also a high level of expression in obese adipose tissue; however, it does not appear to be critical for adipose tissue macrophage recruitment [37]. Several other chemokines are also likely to play a role in the recruitment of monocytes/macrophages into the adipose tissue, such as MCP2, MCP4, migration inhibitory factor (MIF), macrophage inflammatory protein-1α (MIP-1α), MIP-1β, or MIP2-α [26, 38]. The adipocytes are not alone in the elevated inflammatory condition of obesity in that the number of macrophages is also higher in the obese environment thus, providing an additional cellular source of inflammatory factors [19].

Experimental animal studies have served a critical role in advancing our knowledge with regards to the biological relationship between adipose tissue, obesity, and inflammation. The first study to show a link between obesity and inflammation was the work of Hotamisligil and colleagues in 1993 in which they demonstrated that TNFα expression was up-regulated in adipose tissue of genetically obese mice [39]. Additional work reported that the number of bone-marrow derived macrophages present in white adipose tissue directly correlated with obesity [19]. In addition to macrophages, it has been demonstrated that pre-adipocytes and mature adipocytes also produce inflammatory factors. The mechanisms that initiate and trigger the inflammation are not yet totally elucidated, but different hypothesis have been proposed. A number of factors could trigger an inflammatory response and among them the saturated fatty acids may play a contributing role. For example, palmitate, an abundant nutritional fatty acid, could bind to the inflammation-related toll like receptors (TLR) leading to activation of a signalling cascade and the activation of the transcription factor NF-kB (nuclear factor kappa-light-chain-enhancer of activated B cells) [40]. NF-kB is involved in many cellular processes including immune and inflammatory responses. Upon activation and nuclear translocation, NF-kB can further induce the production of inflammatory cytokines, including TNF and IL-1. An alternative, but as relevant a process, is the recognition of a diverse range of stress and damage signals by inflammasomes. These are a group of protein complexes including the Nod-Like Receptor (NLR) proteins that can directly activate caspase-1 leading to the secretion of pro-inflammatory cytokines and pyroptotic cell death (for review see [41]).

Recently inflammasomes and their activation of down-stream events have been shown to play a major role in the development of obesity, insulin resistance, and diabetes [42, 43]. Another hypothesis linking inflammation and obesity is supported by Burcelin's group and involves the intestinal flora equilibrium. In this model, a high fat diet is proposed to increase the gram-negative bacteria proportion in the intestine; this increases intestine permeability and the absorption of lipopolysacharide (LPS; the wall component of the gram-negative bacteria). Upon this increased absorption, TLR activation leads to an up-regulation of the inflammatory response [44, 45]. These two hypotheses are not mutually exclusive but rather it is likely that the two mechanisms coexist. While the classic localization of TLRs is on macrophages our laboratory and others have shown the presence of functional Toll-like receptors (TLRs) on human adipocytes including the expression of TLR type 2 (TLR2) and TLR type 4 (TLR4) [46, 47] providing evidence for the potential of an adipocyte receptor-mediated response.

Adipokines are defined as soluble mediators that are mainly, but not exclusively, produced by adipocytes and exert their biological function in an autocrine, paracrine or systemic manner. Over 50 adipokines have been identified, and they generally function as hormones to influence energy homeostasis and feeding [22, 48]. The following sections will focus on a review of two specific adipokines (leptin and adiponectin) and an additional factor (autotaxin) produced by WAT. Information is presented supporting that these factors and their activation may provide an important link between obesity and related inflammatory disorders.

Leptin was identified in 1994 as the 16 kDa protein product of the obese (ob) gene [49]. It displays immune-regulatory effects by increasing the production of pro-inflammatory cytokines by macrophages [50]. It is best known as an important regulator of energy balance through its actions in the brain to suppress appetite and increase energy expenditure [51]. Leptin in the blood enters the brain via a transport mechanism that can be saturated [52]. Upon entry it is believed to act primarily on the hypothalamic centers thus possibly providing a target for its effects upon appetite. In addition to the hypothalamus, leptin receptors (OBR) are widely expressed in numerous extra-hypothalamic regions of the brain, including the hippocampus, cerebellum, amygdala, and brain stem [53]. There are many splice variants of the receptor; those with short cytoplasmic domains are expressed in multiple tissues while the one with long cytoplasmic domains (OB-Rb) are expressed in specific brain regions. OB-Rb stimulates the JAK/STAT3 pathway and PI3K which are necessary for the leptin effects on food intake and hepatic glucose metabolism [54, 55].

Adiponectin, a prototypic adipocytokine is an anti-inflammatory adipokine secreted by adipocytes [56-58]. It plays a major role in regulation of insulin sensitivity and in obesity the levels of adiponectin are diminished due to a decreased release from WAT [59]. A deficiency in adiponectin is associated with exaggerated inflammatory response in patients with critical illness, including sepsis [32, 60] and with the development of a proinflammatory phenotype in in animal models of polymicrobial sepsis [61, 62]. Further studies demonstrated that adiponectin deficiency is associated with increased leukocyte and platelet adhesion as well as blood brain barrier dysfunction with cecal ligation and puncture induced sepsis in mice [63].

Autotaxin (ATX), also known as ectonucleotide pyrophosphatase phosphodiesterase-2 (ENPP2), is a secreted enzyme with lysophospholipase D (lysoPLD) activity involved in hydrolysis of lysophosphatidylcholine (LPC) into lysophosphatidic acid (LPA) [64]. LPA is bioactive phospholipid involved in numerous biological activities, including cell proliferation, differentiation, and migration acting via specific G-protein coupled receptors [65]. The LPA strongly influences proliferation and differentiation of pre-adipocytes *via* the activation of LPA1 receptor [66, 67]. Anti-inflammatory properties for LPA have been suggested based upon the ability to inhibit, in mice, the LPS-induced inflammatory response of macrophages [68]. The expression of ATX is up-regulated during adipogenesis [69, 70] as well as in adipocytes from obese-diabetic db/db mice and in adipose tissue obtained from glucose-intolerant obese women subjects [69, 71]. The role of ATX in inflammation is less clear, but LPA seems to demonstrate some anti-inflammatory properties as it inhibits LPS-induced inflammation in cultured macrophages and in mice. Based upon these findings, it has been suggested that in addition to its role in cancer and LPA production, ATX may be involved in adipose tissue development and/or obesity-associated pathologies such as diabetes.

3. Influence of obesity on CNS

It is only relatively recently that the concept that obesity could have an effect on the brain has been emerging. Associations between obesity and various neurological disorders have been reported including sleep apnea, anxiety, manic depressive disorders, increased risk of developing cerebrovascular accident (CVA), and other neurological disorders [18, 72]. Additional consideration has been raised that obesity may be linked to various progressive and aging-related neurodegenerative diseases such as Parkinson's disease, Alzheimer's disease (AD), and autoimmune nervous system diseases like multiple sclerosis.

Over the last decade, a number of magnetic resonance imaging (MRI) and computed tomography (CT) studies have reported alterations in brain morphology of overweight/obese individuals. Initial studies demonstrated a higher BMI and/or waist-to-hip ratio in middle-aged individuals associated with a reduction in whole brain volume [73-75]. A similar association was observed with temporal lobe atrophy in elderly women [76] with additional evidence of hippocampal atrophy [77]. Debette et al. [78] reported a link between abdominal fat and reduced brain volume in otherwise healthy middle-aged adults. This study reported an inverse association between various obesity indicators (BMI, waist circumference, waist-to-hip ratio, and abdominal fat) and brain volume as determined by structural MRI of 733 participants. Independent of other obesity indicators, waist-to-hip ratio was found to be associated with increased temporal horn volume. Pannacciulli et al., 2006 reported gray matter reductions in the left postcentral gyrus, bilateral putamen, and right cerebellar regions in obese individuals as detected using voxel-based morphometry [79]. Gender differences have been suggested with a male-specific association between increasing BMI and smaller cerebellum, midbrain, frontal, termporal, and parietal cortex [74]. In a cohort of 95 obese women between the ages of 52 and 92, gray matter reductions were reported in the left orbitofrontal, right inferior frontal, right precentral gyri, and right cerebellar regions [80]. In contrast, increased volumes in white matter in the frontal, temporal, and parietal lobes were also reported [80]. In a cross-sectional study of normal elderly individuals showing no sign of cognitive deficit, tensor-based morphometry unveiled atrophy in the white and gray matter of the frontal lobes, anterior cingulate gyrus, hippocampus, and thalamus in both male and female subjects with a high BMI (BMI > 30) as compared to individuals with a normal BMI (18.5–25) [81]. Upon further investigation, the brain volume reduction in gray and white matter was found to be associated with a common variant of the fat mass and obesity associated (*FTO*) gene [82]. Three-dimensional MRI brain maps of 206 healthy elderly participants showed an association between brain volume and the risk allele of the *FTO* gene known to be strongly associated with higher body-mass index. Participants who carried at least one copy of the allele had marked reductions in the volume of various brain structures compared to average volumes in non-carriers and in the general population. Carriers of the allele had, on average, an 8% deficit in the frontal lobe, 12% deficit in the occipital lobe (percentage units are expressed in terms of the average volumes seen in the general population of carriers and non-carriers). A reduction in temporal lobe volume was observed in participants with a higher BMI, but not in carriers of the risk allele. A pronounced effect of BMI was seen in carriers of the FTO allele showing volume deficits in all the other lobes of the brain, as well as in the brain stem and cerebellum. The authors proposed as a strong hypothesis that "BMI affects brain structure and that FTO exerts some additive detectable effect over and above whatever the BMI of the person happens to be" [82].

The possible relationship between neurodegeneration and obesity in animal models and in humans has been studied now for over a decade with a primary focus on the possibility that obesity and related metabolic disorders exacerbate neurodegeneration and thereby, promote cognitive decline and increase vulnerability to brain injury [73]. Based upon the identification of hereditary neurodegenerative disorders associated with obesity such as Alstrom, Bardet-Biedl or Prader-Willi syndromes, some studies have addressed the possibility that neurodegeneration in the brain may be a causal factor for obesity [83]. A more recent association between obesity and neurological function is based upon correlations with biological processes of oxidative stress and inflammation. While the causal nature of these processes to neurodegeneration has not been definitively established, it is widely accepted that neuroinflammation and oxidative stress responses occur with clinical manifestation of the disease. Given the recent reports of adipokines within the body fat and the elevation of these inflammatory factors with stimulation, a more direct linkage between obesity and various human diseases, including neurodegenerative disease, has been hypothesized. In the past decade, a linkage has been demonstrated between being overweight in middle age and increased risk for AD and other forms of dementia [84, 85]. However, as to date, the exact nature of the elevated risk has not been identified and characterized. There however, have been a number of hypotheses put forth, many including a role for inflammation. As previously stated, WAT can produce an array of inflammatory-related factors, for which expression levels may be modified in obesity. It has been proposed that an obesity-related chronic low-grade inflammation can serve to change the environment leading to a priming the brain for subsequent insults leading to a heightened inflammatory response and possibly exacerbation of the damage (figure 5).

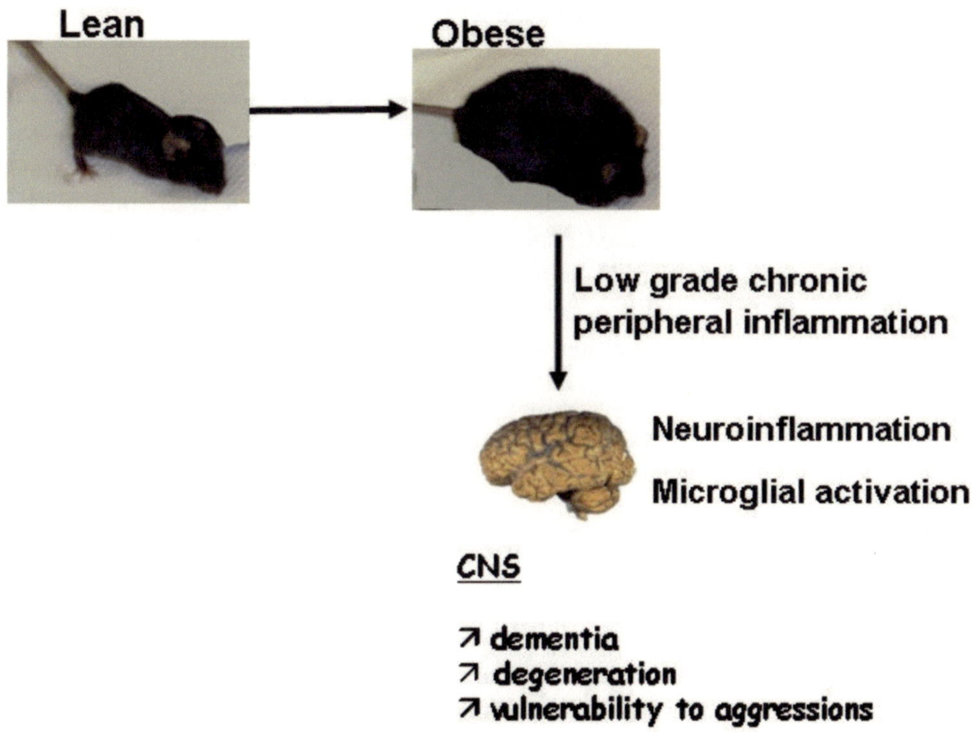

Figure 5. low grade chronic inflammation affect the response of the brain to later injury.

Obesity has a major negative impact on cognitive function due to vascular defects, impaired insulin metabolism and signaling pathway or a defect in glucose transport mechanisms in brain [86]. As shown in figure 4, leptin level is increased in obesity but there is also evidence that leptin signaling may become less effective in obesity, provoking a leptin-resistance status [87-89]. Thus, obesity, as it relates to leptin, may be due to a lack of leptin or of its receptor(s) but may also be a consequence of a signaling defect. Interestingly, leptin has protective effects in the brain both *in vitro* and *in vivo* and thus, has been suggested to be a good candidate as a link between obesity and neurodegeneration [90]. Similar to leptin, ATX is increased in obesity. LPA receptors are present in the CNS but the potential effect of ATX on oxidative stress or neuroinflammation was not known. In a recent study, Awada et al. [91] demonstrated that ATX synthesis and secretion by the brain immune cell, the microglia, have a protective effect by mitigating intracellular oxidation. These data suggests a novel anti-oxidant role for ATX in the brain. In contrast, adiponectin level is lowered with obesity [92]. In the CNS, adiponectin has been shown to improve cerebrovascular injury in mice [93, 94]. A deficiency in adiponectin in the mouse increases the severity of seizure activity [95] while presence of adiponectin provides a level of protection to hippocampal neurons against kainic acid-induced excitotoxicity [96]. It is likely that other factors produced by the WAT could have some effects on the CNS and further investigations are needed to decipher this complex network.

4. Susceptibility of the CNS to obesity in animal studies

Animal models of obesity have been very useful and important for understanding the regulation of food intake and imbalance in energy expenditure. The initial models examined spontaneous single gene mutations leading to the loss of the gene function [97]. The first of these models described is the agouti mouse [98, 99]. In addition to rats, other species have been used to study obesity related issues. These include, pigs, chicken, and even bats [97, 100, 101]. As several genes have been found to be involved in energy balance regulation, the advancement of methods for the overexpression or silencing of genes has allowed for a dramatic increase in the number of mouse models of obesity.

There is a growing body of evidence that nutrition could affect the inflammatory status of the brain [102, 103]. High dietary fat is a significant risk for cerebral oxidative stress development, neuronal inflammation, vascular dementia, AD, and Parkinson disease [104-108]. High fat diet induces a rapid (24 hours) temporary inflammation in the CNS, which can potentially progress to a chronic condition in obese mice as well as in human and leads to gliosis and mediobasal hypothalamus neuronal injury [109].

In genetic murine model of obesity, an increased susceptibility of CNS to trauma has been observed; obesity is an aggravating factor in chemical-induced neurodegeneration. In mice deficient for the leptin gene (ob/ob), the effects of two neurotoxicants are exacerbated, methamphetamine (METH), which affects dopaminergic neurons and kainic acid (KA), affecting the hippocampus [110]. The ob/ob mice are also more susceptible to seizure induced by the gamma-aminobutyric acid A receptor (GABAAR) antagonist, pentylenetetrazol (PTZ) [111].

It is now known that in distinct neurogenic sites of the brain the presence of stem/progenitor cells allows for the generation of new neurons over the full lifespan [112]. This process is influenced by a number of factors including cytokines, hormones, growth factors, and exercise [112-116]. The regulatory effects of growth factors demonstrate a level of specificity for brain regions with brain-derived neurotrophic factor (BDNF) showing prominent effects in the hippocampus while ciliary neurotrophic factor (CNTF) induces neurogenesis in the hypothalamus. In this case the neurogenesis occurs in the satiety centers inducing a persistent weight loss [117]. More importantly, with regards to inflammatory factors, injury to the brain such as ischemia [118], epilepsy [119], or chemically induced neurodegeneration [120] induce an increase in neurogenesis. This induction has been termed "injury-induced neurogenesis". A relationship between adult neurogenesis and obesity has been demonstrated in the decrease in the turnover of new neurons in the hypothalamic arcuate nucleus (region playing a key role in body weight regulation) in obese mice (high fat diet or ob/ob) [121]. While the research effort targeted toward this area of the effects of nutrition or obesity on adult neurogenesis is in its infancy, it is likely that a link similar to what has been found with neurodegeneration, may be found for molecules such as Omega 3 fatty acids, flavonoids, and polyphenols [122-124].

5. Conclusion

It is now well accepted that obesity is associated with several pathologies including neuropathies and the ability of the nervous system to repair following injury. While further research is needed in characterizing the nature of the effect of obesity on the nervous system there are current studies suggesting that such effects can be modified. For example, resveratrol or ursolic acid have been shown to attenuate obesity-associated nervous system inflammation resulting in an improvement of memory deficits in mice fed a high-fat diet. [125, 126]. Given the accelerated increase in obesity and neurodegenerative diseases as well as the influence of childhood health status and adult disease, there is a critical need to better understand the relationship between obesity and the nervous system. Identification of the critical factors underlying the various changes seen in the brain and its response to injury as a function of age, nutritional status, and body mass, i.e., obesity will lay the foundation for developing therapeutic interventions that will be applicable to the human population.

Acknowledgements

We would like to thanks Dr. G. Jean Harry (NTP/NIEHS/NIH) for her comments and edition. We would like to thank the 'Region La Reunion', Europe (CPER/FEDER) for its funding supports. AP is funded by fellowships from 'Conseil Régional de La Réunion'.

Author details

Rana Awada , Avinash Parimisetty and Christian Lefebvre d'Hellencourt*

*Address all correspondence to: Christian.Lefebvre-d-Hellencourt@univ-reunion.fr

Groupe d'Etude sur l'Inflammation Chronique et l'Obesité (GEICO), EA 4516, Plateforme CYROI, UFR Santé, Université de La Réunion, Ile de La Réunion, France

References

[1] Prentice AM. The emerging epidemic of obesity in developing countries. Int J Epidemiol 2006; 35(1) 93-9

[2] World Health Organisation (WHO). Obesity in Europe. http://www.euro.who.int/obesity. 2008

[3] Obesity: preventing and managing the global epidemic. Report of a WHO consultation. World Health Organ Tech Rep Ser 2000; 894(i-xii, 1-253

[4] Mei Z, Grummer-Strawn LM, Pietrobelli A, Goulding A, Goran MI and Dietz WH. Validity of body mass index compared with other body-composition screening indexes for the assessment of body fatness in children and adolescents. Am J Clin Nutr 2002; 75(6) 978-85

[5] Eckel RH, Grundy SM and Zimmet PZ. The metabolic syndrome. Lancet 2005; 365(9468) 1415-28

[6] Haslam DW and James WP. Obesity. Lancet 2005; 366(9492) 1197-209

[7] Tzanetakou IP, Katsilambros NL, Benetos A, Mikhailidis DP and Perrea DN. "Is obesity linked to aging?": adipose tissue and the role of telomeres. Ageing Res Rev 2012; 11(2) 220-9

[8] Granholm AC, Boger H and Emborg ME. Mood, memory and movement: an age-related neurodegenerative complex? Curr Aging Sci 2008; 1(2) 133-9

[9] Harwood HJ, Jr. The adipocyte as an endocrine organ in the regulation of metabolic homeostasis. Neuropharmacology 2012; 63(1) 57-75

[10] Nedergaard J, Bengtsson T and Cannon B. Unexpected evidence for active brown adipose tissue in adult humans. Am J Physiol Endocrinol Metab 2007; 293(2) E444-52

[11] Wronska A and Kmiec Z. Structural and biochemical characteristics of various white adipose tissue depots. Acta Physiol (Oxf) 2012; 205(2) 194-208

[12] Cannon B and Nedergaard J. Brown adipose tissue: function and physiological significance. Physiol Rev 2004; 84(1) 277-359

[13] Hauner H. Secretory factors from human adipose tissue and their functional role. Proc Nutr Soc 2005; 64(2) 163-9

[14] Hauner H. The new concept of adipose tissue function. Physiology & Behavior 2004; 83(4) 653-8

[15] Cawthorn WP, Scheller EL and MacDougald OA. Adipose tissue stem cells meet preadipocyte commitment: going back to the future. J Lipid Res 2011; 53(2) 227-46

[16] Tran TT and Kahn CR. Transplantation of adipose tissue and stem cells: role in metabolism and disease. Nat Rev Endocrinol 2010; 6(4) 195-213

[17] Roche R, Hoareau L, Mounet F and Festy F. Adult stem cells for cardiovascular diseases: the adipose tissue potential. Expert Opin Biol Ther 2007; 7(6) 791-8

[18] Palaniyandi R, Awada R, Harry GJ and Lefebvre d'Hellencourt C. White fat tissue, obesity and possible role in neurodegeneration in Harry GJ and Tilson HA (ed) White fat tissue, obesity and possible role in neurodegeneration. Book 2010

[19] Weisberg SP, McCann D, Desai M, Rosenbaum M, Leibel RL and Ferrante AW, Jr. Obesity is associated with macrophage accumulation in adipose tissue. J Clin Invest 2003; 112(12) 1796-808

[20] Greenberg AS and Obin MS. Obesity and the role of adipose tissue in inflammation and metabolism. Am J Clin Nutr 2006; 83(2) 461S-5S

[21] Moschen AR, Kaser A, Enrich B, Mosheimer B, Theurl M, Niederegger H and Tilg H. Visfatin, an adipocytokine with proinflammatory and immunomodulating properties. J Immunol 2007; 178(3) 1748-58

[22] Tilg H and Moschen AR. Adipocytokines: mediators linking adipose tissue, inflammation and immunity. Nat Rev Immunol 2006; 6(10) 772-83

[23] Van Harmelen V, Reynisdottir S, Eriksson P, Thorne A, Hoffstedt J, Lonnqvist F and Arner P. Leptin secretion from subcutaneous and visceral adipose tissue in women. Diabetes 1998; 47(6) 913-7

[24] Fain JN, Madan AK, Hiler ML, Cheema P and Bahouth SW. Comparison of the release of adipokines by adipose tissue, adipose tissue matrix, and adipocytes from visceral and subcutaneous abdominal adipose tissues of obese humans. Endocrinology 2004; 145(5) 2273-82

[25] Lafontan M and Langin D. Lipolysis and lipid mobilization in human adipose tissue. Prog Lipid Res 2009; 48(5) 275-97

[26] Tilg H and Moschen AR. Role of adiponectin and PBEF/visfatin as regulators of inflammation: involvement in obesity-associated diseases. Clin Sci (Lond) 2008; 114(4) 275-88

[27] Berndt J, Kloting N, Kralisch S, Kovacs P, Fasshauer M, Schon MR, Stumvoll M and Bluher M. Plasma visfatin concentrations and fat depot-specific mRNA expression in humans. Diabetes 2005; 54(10) 2911-6

[28] Azuma K, Katsukawa F, Oguchi S, Murata M, Yamazaki H, Shimada A and Saruta T. Correlation between serum resistin level and adiposity in obese individuals. Obes Res 2003; 11(8) 997-1001

[29] Sartipy P and Loskutoff DJ. Monocyte chemoattractant protein 1 in obesity and insulin resistance. Proc Natl Acad Sci U S A 2003; 100(12) 7265-70

[30] Madani R, Karastergiou K, Ogston NC, Miheisi N, Bhome R, Haloob N, Tan GD, Karpe F, Malone-Lee J, Hashemi M, Jahangiri M and Mohamed-Ali V. RANTES release by human adipose tissue in vivo and evidence for depot-specific differences. Am J Physiol Endocrinol Metab 2009; 296(6) E1262-8

[31] Chiellini C, Santini F, Marsili A, Berti P, Bertacca A, Pelosini C, Scartabelli G, Pardini E, Lopez-Soriano J, Centoni R, Ciccarone AM, Benzi L, Vitti P, Del Prato S, Pinchera A and Maffei M. Serum haptoglobin: a novel marker of adiposity in humans. J Clin Endocrinol Metab 2004; 89(6) 2678-83

[32] Hillenbrand A, Knippschild U, Weiss M, Schrezenmeier H, Henne-Bruns D, Huber-Lang M and Wolf AM. Sepsis induced changes of adipokines and cytokines - septic patients compared to morbidly obese patients. BMC Surg 2010; 10(26

[33] Bell LN, Ward JL, Degawa-Yamauchi M, Bovenkerk JE, Jones R, Cacucci BM, Gupta CE, Sheridan C, Sheridan K, Shankar SS, Steinberg HO, March KL and Considine RV. Adipose tissue production of hepatocyte growth factor contributes to elevated serum HGF in obesity. Am J Physiol Endocrinol Metab 2006; 291(4) E843-8

[34] Fain JN. Release of inflammatory mediators by human adipose tissue is enhanced in obesity and primarily by the nonfat cells: a review. Mediators Inflamm 2010; 2010(513948

[35] Meier CA, Bobbioni E, Gabay C, Assimacopoulos-Jeannet F, Golay A and Dayer JM. IL-1 receptor antagonist serum levels are increased in human obesity: a possible link to the resistance to leptin? J Clin Endocrinol Metab 2002; 87(3) 1184-8

[36] Panee J. Monocyte Chemoattractant Protein 1 (MCP-1) in obesity and diabetes. Cytokine 2012;

[37] Clement S, Juge-Aubry C, Sgroi A, Conzelmann S, Pazienza V, Pittet-Cuenod B, Meier CA and Negro F. Monocyte chemoattractant protein-1 secreted by adipose tissue induces direct lipid accumulation in hepatocytes. Hepatology 2008; 48(3) 799-807

[38] Gonzalez-Castejon M and Rodriguez-Casado A. Dietary phytochemicals and their potential effects on obesity: a review. Pharmacol Res 2011; 64(5) 438-55

[39] Hotamisligil GS, Shargill NS and Spiegelman BM. Adipose expression of tumor necrosis factor-alpha: direct role in obesity-linked insulin resistance. Science 1993; 259(5091) 87-91

[40] Shi H, Kokoeva MV, Inouye K, Tzameli I, Yin H and Flier JS. TLR4 links innate immunity and fatty acid-induced insulin resistance. J Clin Invest 2006; 116(11) 3015-25

[41] Strowig T, Henao-Mejia J, Elinav E and Flavell R. Inflammasomes in health and disease. Nature 481(7381) 278-86

[42] Stienstra R, Tack CJ, Kanneganti TD, Joosten LA and Netea MG. The inflammasome puts obesity in the danger zone. Cell Metab 2012; 15(1) 10-8

[43] Stienstra R, van Diepen JA, Tack CJ, Zaki MH, van de Veerdonk FL, Perera D, Neale GA, Hooiveld GJ, Hijmans A, Vroegrijk I, van den Berg S, Romijn J, Rensen PC, Joosten LA, Netea MG and Kanneganti TD. Inflammasome is a central player in the induction of obesity and insulin resistance. Proc Natl Acad Sci U S A 2011; 108(37) 15324-9

[44] Cani PD, Bibiloni R, Knauf C, Waget A, Neyrinck AM, Delzenne NM and Burcelin R. Changes in gut microbiota control metabolic endotoxemia-induced inflammation in high-fat diet-induced obesity and diabetes in mice. Diabetes 2008; 57(6) 1470-81

[45] Nicholson JK, Holmes E, Kinross J, Burcelin R, Gibson G, Jia W and Pettersson S. Host-gut microbiota metabolic interactions. Science 2012; 336(6086) 1262-7

[46] Bes-Houtmann S, Roche R, Hoareau L, Gonthier MP, Festy F, Caillens H, Gasque P, Lefebvre d'Hellencourt C and Cesari M. Presence of functional TLR2 and TLR4 on human adipocytes. Histochem Cell Biol 2007; 127(2) 131-7

[47] Meijer K, de Vries M, Al-Lahham S, Bruinenberg M, Weening D, Dijkstra M, Kloosterhuis N, van der Leij RJ, van der Want H, Kroesen BJ, Vonk R and Rezaee F. Human primary adipocytes exhibit immune cell function: adipocytes prime inflammation independent of macrophages. PLoS ONE 2011; 6(3) e17154

[48] Ahima RS and Osei SY. Adipokines in obesity. Front Horm Res 2008; 36(182-97

[49] Zhang Y, Proenca R, Maffei M, Barone M, Leopold L and Friedman JM. Positional cloning of the mouse obese gene and its human homologue. Nature 1994; 372(6505) 425-32

[50] Loffreda S, Yang SQ, Lin HZ, Karp CL, Brengman ML, Wang DJ, Klein AS, Bulkley GB, Bao C, Noble PW, Lane MD and Diehl AM. Leptin regulates proinflammatory immune responses. Faseb J 1998; 12(1) 57-65

[51] Friedman JM and Halaas JL. Leptin and the regulation of body weight in mammals. Nature 1998; 395(6704) 763-70

[52] Banks WA, Kastin AJ, Huang W, Jaspan JB and Maness LM. Leptin enters the brain by a saturable system independent of insulin. Peptides 1996; 17(2) 305-11

[53] Elmquist JK, Bjorbaek C, Ahima RS, Flier JS and Saper CB. Distributions of leptin receptor mRNA isoforms in the rat brain. J Comp Neurol 1998; 395(4) 535-47

[54] Buettner C, Pocai A, Muse ED, Etgen AM, Myers MG, Jr. and Rossetti L. Critical role of STAT3 in leptin's metabolic actions. Cell Metab 2006; 4(1) 49-60

[55] Gautron L and Elmquist JK. Sixteen years and counting: an update on leptin in energy balance. J Clin Invest 2011; 121(6) 2087-93

[56] Ohashi K, Ouchi N and Matsuzawa Y. Anti-inflammatory and anti-atherogenic properties of adiponectin. Biochimie 2012;

[57] Ouchi N and Walsh K. Adiponectin as an anti-inflammatory factor. Clin Chim Acta 2007; 380(1-2) 24-30

[58] Robinson K, Prins J and Venkatesh B. Clinical review: adiponectin biology and its role in inflammation and critical illness. Crit Care 2011; 15(2) 221

[59] Arita Y, Kihara S, Ouchi N, Takahashi M, Maeda K, Miyagawa J, Hotta K, Shimomura I, Nakamura T, Miyaoka K, Kuriyama H, Nishida M, Yamashita S, Okubo K, Matsubara K, Muraguchi M, Ohmoto Y, Funahashi T and Matsuzawa Y. Paradoxical

decrease of an adipose-specific protein, adiponectin, in obesity. Biochem Biophys Res Commun 1999; 257(1) 79-83

[60] Venkatesh B, Hickman I, Nisbet J, Cohen J and Prins J. Changes in serum adiponectin concentrations in critical illness: a preliminary investigation. Crit Care 2009; 13(4) R105

[61] Uji Y, Yamamoto H, Tsuchihashi H, Maeda K, Funahashi T, Shimomura I, Shimizu T, Endo Y and Tani T. Adiponectin deficiency is associated with severe polymicrobial sepsis, high inflammatory cytokine levels, and high mortality. Surgery 2009; 145(5) 550-7

[62] Teoh H, Quan A, Bang KW, Wang G, Lovren F, Vu V, Haitsma JJ, Szmitko PE, Al-Omran M, Wang CH, Gupta M, Peterson MD, Zhang H, Chan L, Freedman J, Sweeney G and Verma S. Adiponectin deficiency promotes endothelial activation and profoundly exacerbates sepsis-related mortality. Am J Physiol Endocrinol Metab 2008; 295(3) E658-64

[63] Vachharajani V, Cunningham C, Yoza B, Carson J, Jr., Vachharajani TJ and McCall C. Adiponectin-deficiency exaggerates sepsis-induced microvascular dysfunction in the mouse brain. Obesity (Silver Spring) 2012; 20(3) 498-504

[64] Umezu-Goto M, Kishi Y, Taira A, Hama K, Dohmae N, Takio K, Yamori T, Mills GB, Inoue K, Aoki J and Arai H. Autotaxin has lysophospholipase D activity leading to tumor cell growth and motility by lysophosphatidic acid production. J Cell Biol 2002; 158(2) 227-33

[65] Ishii I, Fukushima N, Ye X and Chun J. Lysophospholipid receptors: signaling and biology. Annu Rev Biochem 2004; 73(321-54

[66] Simon MF, Daviaud D, Pradere JP, Gres S, Guigne C, Wabitsch M, Chun J, Valet P and Saulnier-Blache JS. Lysophosphatidic acid inhibits adipocyte differentiation via lysophosphatidic acid 1 receptor-dependent down-regulation of peroxisome proliferator-activated receptor gamma2. J Biol Chem 2005; 280(15) 14656-62

[67] Valet P, Pages C, Jeanneton O, Daviaud D, Barbe P, Record M, Saulnier-Blache JS and Lafontan M. Alpha2-adrenergic receptor-mediated release of lysophosphatidic acid by adipocytes. A paracrine signal for preadipocyte growth. J Clin Invest 1998; 101(7) 1431-8

[68] Fan H, Zingarelli B, Harris V, Tempel GE, Halushka PV and Cook JA. Lysophosphatidic acid inhibits bacterial endotoxin-induced pro-inflammatory response: potential anti-inflammatory signaling pathways. Mol Med 2008; 14(7-8) 422-8

[69] Ferry G, Tellier E, Try A, Gres S, Naime I, Simon MF, Rodriguez M, Boucher J, Tack I, Gesta S, Chomarat P, Dieu M, Raes M, Galizzi JP, Valet P, Boutin JA and Saulnier-Blache JS. Autotaxin is released from adipocytes, catalyzes lysophosphatidic acid

synthesis, and activates preadipocyte proliferation. Up-regulated expression with adipocyte differentiation and obesity. J Biol Chem 2003; 278(20) 18162-9

[70] Gesta S, Simon MF, Rey A, Sibrac D, Girard A, Lafontan M, Valet P and Saulnier-Blache JS. Secretion of a lysophospholipase D activity by adipocytes: involvement in lysophosphatidic acid synthesis. J Lipid Res 2002; 43(6) 904-10

[71] Boucher J, Quilliot D, Praderes JP, Simon MF, Gres S, Guigne C, Prevot D, Ferry G, Boutin JA, Carpene C, Valet P and Saulnier-Blache JS. Potential involvement of adipocyte insulin resistance in obesity-associated up-regulation of adipocyte lysophospholipase D/autotaxin expression. Diabetologia 2005; 48(3) 569-77

[72] Whitmer RA. The epidemiology of adiposity and dementia. Curr Alzheimer Res 2007; 4(2) 117-22

[73] Bruce-Keller AJ, Keller JN and Morrison CD. Obesity and vulnerability of the CNS. Biochim Biophys Acta 2009; 1792(5) 395-400

[74] Taki Y, Kinomura S, Sato K, Inoue K, Goto R, Okada K, Uchida S, Kawashima R and Fukuda H. Relationship between body mass index and gray matter volume in 1,428 healthy individuals. Obesity (Silver Spring) 2008; 16(1) 119-24

[75] Ward MA, Carlsson CM, Trivedi MA, Sager MA and Johnson SC. The effect of body mass index on global brain volume in middle-aged adults: a cross sectional study. BMC Neurol 2005; 5(23

[76] Gustafson D, Lissner L, Bengtsson C, Bjorkelund C and Skoog I. A 24-year follow-up of body mass index and cerebral atrophy. Neurology 2004; 63(10) 1876-81

[77] Jagust W, Harvey D, Mungas D and Haan M. Central obesity and the aging brain. Arch Neurol 2005; 62(10) 1545-8

[78] Debette S, Beiser A, Hoffmann U, Decarli C, O'Donnell CJ, Massaro JM, Au R, Himali JJ, Wolf PA, Fox CS and Seshadri S. Visceral fat is associated with lower brain volume in healthy middle-aged adults. Ann Neurol 2010; 68(2) 136-44

[79] Pannacciulli N, Del Parigi A, Chen K, Le DS, Reiman EM and Tataranni PA. Brain abnormalities in human obesity: a voxel-based morphometric study. Neuroimage 2006; 31(4) 1419-25

[80] Walther K, Birdsill AC, Glisky EL and Ryan L. Structural brain differences and cognitive functioning related to body mass index in older females. Hum Brain Mapp 2010; 31(7) 1052-64

[81] Raji CA, Ho AJ, Parikshak NN, Becker JT, Lopez OL, Kuller LH, Hua X, Leow AD, Toga AW and Thompson PM. Brain structure and obesity. Hum Brain Mapp 2010; 31(3) 353-64

[82] Ho AJ, Stein JL, Hua X, Lee S, Hibar DP, Leow AD, Dinov ID, Toga AW, Saykin AJ, Shen L, Foroud T, Pankratz N, Huentelman MJ, Craig DW, Gerber JD, Allen AN,

Corneveaux JJ, Stephan DA, DeCarli CS, DeChairo BM, Potkin SG, Jack CR, Jr., Weiner MW, Raji CA, Lopez OL, Becker JT, Carmichael OT and Thompson PM. A commonly carried allele of the obesity-related FTO gene is associated with reduced brain volume in the healthy elderly. Proc Natl Acad Sci U S A 2010; 107(18) 8404-9

[83] Ristow M. Neurodegenerative disorders associated with diabetes mellitus. J Mol Med 2004; 82(8) 510-29

[84] Gustafson D. Adiposity indices and dementia. Lancet Neurol 2006; 5(8) 713-20

[85] Gustafson D, Rothenberg E, Blennow K, Steen B and Skoog I. An 18-year follow-up of overweight and risk of Alzheimer disease. Arch Intern Med 2003; 163(13) 1524-8

[86] Naderali EK, Ratcliffe SH and Dale MC. Obesity and Alzheimer's disease: a link between body weight and cognitive function in old age. Am J Alzheimers Dis Other Demen 2009; 24(6) 445-9

[87] Myers MG, Jr., Heymsfield SB, Haft C, Kahn BB, Laughlin M, Leibel RL, Tschop MH and Yanovski JA. Challenges and opportunities of defining clinical leptin resistance. Cell Metab 2012; 15(2) 150-6

[88] St-Pierre J and Tremblay ML. Modulation of leptin resistance by protein tyrosine phosphatases. Cell Metab 2012; 15(3) 292-7

[89] Shimizu H, Oh IS, Okada S and Mori M. Leptin resistance and obesity. Endocr J 2007; 54(1) 17-26

[90] Doherty GH. Obesity and the ageing brain: could leptin play a role in neurodegeneration? Curr Gerontol Geriatr Res 2011; 2011(708154

[91] Awada R, Rondeau P, Gres S, Saulnier-Blache JS, Lefebvre d'Hellencourt C and Bourdon E. Autotaxin protects microglial cells against oxidative stress. Free Radic Biol Med 2012; 52(2) 516-26

[92] Hu E, Liang P and Spiegelman BM. AdipoQ is a novel adipose-specific gene dysregulated in obesity. J Biol Chem 1996; 271(18) 10697-703

[93] Chen B, Liao WQ, Xu N, Xu H, Wen JY, Yu CA, Liu XY, Li CL, Zhao SM and Campbell W. Adiponectin protects against cerebral ischemia-reperfusion injury through anti-inflammatory action. Brain Res 2009; 1273(129-37

[94] Nishimura M, Izumiya Y, Higuchi A, Shibata R, Qiu J, Kudo C, Shin HK, Moskowitz MA and Ouchi N. Adiponectin prevents cerebral ischemic injury through endothelial nitric oxide synthase dependent mechanisms. Circulation 2008; 117(2) 216-23

[95] Lee EB, Warmann G, Dhir R and Ahima RS. Metabolic dysfunction associated with adiponectin deficiency enhances kainic acid-induced seizure severity. J Neurosci 2012; 31(40) 14361-6

[96] Jeon BT, Shin HJ, Kim JB, Kim YK, Lee DH, Kim KH, Kim HJ, Kang SS, Cho GJ, Choi WS and Roh GS. Adiponectin protects hippocampal neurons against kainic acid-induced excitotoxicity. Brain Res Rev 2009; 61(2) 81-8

[97] Speakman J, Hambly C, Mitchell S and Krol E. Animal models of obesity. Obes Rev 2007; 8 Suppl 1(55-61

[98] Dickies MM. A new viable yellow mutation in the house mouse. J Hered 1962; 53(84-6

[99] Yen TT, Gill AM, Frigeri LG, Barsh GS and Wolff GL. Obesity, diabetes, and neoplasia in yellow A(vy)/- mice: ectopic expression of the agouti gene. Faseb J 1994; 8(8) 479-88

[100] Dietrich HM. Housing, breeding and selecting chickens of the Obese strain (OS) with spontaneous autoimmune thyroiditis. Lab Anim 1989; 23(4) 345-52

[101] Hen G, Yosefi S, Simchaev V, Shinder D, Hruby VJ and Friedman-Einat M. The melanocortin circuit in obese and lean strains of chicks. J Endocrinol 2006; 190(2) 527-35

[102] Keller JN. Special issue: Reciprocal interactions between diet, metabolism, and the nervous system. Foreword. Biochim Biophys Acta 2009; 1792(5) 393-4

[103] Zhang L, Bruce-Keller AJ, Dasuri K, Nguyen AT, Liu Y and Keller JN. Diet-induced metabolic disturbances as modulators of brain homeostasis. Biochim Biophys Acta 2009; 1792(5) 417-22

[104] Kalmijn S. Fatty acid intake and the risk of dementia and cognitive decline: a review of clinical and epidemiological studies. J Nutr Health Aging 2000; 4(4) 202-7

[105] Hida K, Wada J, Eguchi J, Zhang H, Baba M, Seida A, Hashimoto I, Okada T, Yasuhara A, Nakatsuka A, Shikata K, Hourai S, Futami J, Watanabe E, Matsuki Y, Hiramatsu R, Akagi S, Makino H and Kanwar YS. Visceral adipose tissue-derived serine protease inhibitor: a unique insulin-sensitizing adipocytokine in obesity. Proc Natl Acad Sci U S A 2005; 102(30) 10610-5

[106] Bousquet M, St-Amour I, Vandal M, Julien P, Cicchetti F and Calon F. High-fat diet exacerbates MPTP-induced dopaminergic degeneration in mice. Neurobiol Dis 2012; 45(1) 529-38

[107] Choi JY, Jang EH, Park CS and Kang JH. Enhanced susceptibility to 1-methyl-4-phenyl-1,2,3,6-tetrahydropyridine neurotoxicity in high-fat diet-induced obesity. Free Radic Biol Med 2005; 38(6) 806-16

[108] Morris JK, Bomhoff GL, Stanford JA and Geiger PC. Neurodegeneration in an animal model of Parkinson's disease is exacerbated by a high-fat diet. Am J Physiol Regul Integr Comp Physiol 299(4) R1082-90

[109] Thaler JP, Yi CX, Schur EA, Guyenet SJ, Hwang BH, Dietrich MO, Zhao X, Sarruf DA, Izgur V, Maravilla KR, Nguyen HT, Fischer JD, Matsen ME, Wisse BE, Morton

GJ, Horvath TL, Baskin DG, Tschop MH and Schwartz MW. Obesity is associated with hypothalamic injury in rodents and humans. J Clin Invest 2012; 122(1) 153-62

[110] Sriram K, Benkovic SA, Miller DB and O'Callaghan JP. Obesity exacerbates chemically induced neurodegeneration. Neuroscience 2002; 115(4) 1335-46

[111] Erbayat-Altay E, Yamada KA, Wong M and Thio LL. Increased severity of pentylenetetrazol induced seizures in leptin deficient ob/ob mice. Neurosci Lett 2008; 433(2) 82-6

[112] Ming GL and Song H. Adult neurogenesis in the mammalian brain: significant answers and significant questions. Neuron 2011; 70(4) 687-702

[113] Anderson MF, Aberg MA, Nilsson M and Eriksson PS. Insulin-like growth factor-I and neurogenesis in the adult mammalian brain. Brain Res Dev Brain Res 2002; 134(1-2) 115-22

[114] Ciaroni S, Cuppini R, Cecchini T, Ferri P, Ambrogini P, Cuppini C and Del Grande P. Neurogenesis in the adult rat dentate gyrus is enhanced by vitamin E deficiency. J Comp Neurol 1999; 411(3) 495-502

[115] Valente T, Hidalgo J, Bolea I, Ramirez B, Angles N, Reguant J, Morello JR, Gutierrez C, Boada M and Unzeta M. A diet enriched in polyphenols and polyunsaturated fatty acids, LMN diet, induces neurogenesis in the subventricular zone and hippocampus of adult mouse brain. J Alzheimers Dis 2009; 18(4) 849-65

[116] van Praag H, Christie BR, Sejnowski TJ and Gage FH. Running enhances neurogenesis, learning, and long-term potentiation in mice. Proc Natl Acad Sci U S A 1999; 96(23) 13427-31

[117] Kokoeva MV, Yin H and Flier JS. Neurogenesis in the hypothalamus of adult mice: potential role in energy balance. Science 2005; 310(5748) 679-83

[118] Bachner D, Ahrens M, Betat N, Schroder D and Gross G. Developmental expression analysis of murine autotaxin (ATX). Mech Dev 1999; 84(1-2) 121-5

[119] Bengzon J, Kokaia Z, Elmer E, Nanobashvili A, Kokaia M and Lindvall O. Apoptosis and proliferation of dentate gyrus neurons after single and intermittent limbic seizures. Proc Natl Acad Sci U S A 1997; 94(19) 10432-7

[120] Harry GJ, McPherson CA, Wine RN, Atkinson K and Lefebvre d'Hellencourt C. Trimethyltin-induced neurogenesis in the murine hippocampus. Neurotox Res 2004; 5(8) 623-7

[121] McNay DE, Briancon N, Kokoeva MV, Maratos-Flier E and Flier JS. Remodeling of the arcuate nucleus energy-balance circuit is inhibited in obese mice. J Clin Invest 2012; 122(1) 142-52

[122] Dias GP, Cavegn N, Nix A, do Nascimento Bevilaqua MC, Stangl D, Zainuddin MS, Nardi AE, Gardino PF and Thuret S. The role of dietary polyphenols on adult hippo-

campal neurogenesis: molecular mechanisms and behavioural effects on depression and anxiety. Oxid Med Cell Longev 2012; 2012(541971

[123] Stangl D and Thuret S. Impact of diet on adult hippocampal neurogenesis. Genes Nutr 2009; 4(4) 271-82

[124] Zainuddin MS and Thuret S. Nutrition, adult hippocampal neurogenesis and mental health. Br Med Bull 2012;

[125] Jeon BT, Jeong EA, Shin HJ, Lee Y, Lee DH, Kim HJ, Kang SS, Cho GJ, Choi WS and Roh GS. Resveratrol attenuates obesity-associated peripheral and central inflammation and improves memory deficit in mice fed a high-fat diet. Diabetes 2012; 61(6) 1444-54

[126] Lu J, Wu DM, Zheng YL, Hu B, Cheng W, Zhang ZF and Shan Q. Ursolic acid improves high fat diet-induced cognitive impairments by blocking endoplasmic reticulum stress and IkappaB kinase beta/nuclear factor-kappaB-mediated inflammatory pathways in mice. Brain Behav Immun 2011; 25(8) 1658-67

Chapter 17

Electro-Physiological Approaches to Monitoring Neuro-Degenerative Diseases

Manuel J. Rojas, Camilo Orozco and Francisco Olea

Additional information is available at the end of the chapter

http://dx.doi.org/10.5772/55228

1. Introduction

Electrical brain activity is recorded by means of a variety of techniques, including different approaches, for instance surface field electrodes among others. Additionally, specific local neuronal responses are suitable for recording. As an example, those known as evoked response potentials allow to determine whether neural pathways and neuronal groups are performing properly.

Neuro-degenerative diseases involve lost of integrity of a number of neuronal nuclei; in turn, this represents significant changes in electrical brain activity that might be compared with unaltered individuals. Several experiments have shown the potential usefulness of evoked response potentials ERP brain correlates as bio-markers, diagnostic and prognostic tools of some neurodegenerative diseases. Also, neuropsychological tests have demonstrated correlations with electrophysiological findings, and are helpful to detect early cognitive decline or disease progression in neurodegenerative diseases.

Electrodiagnostic examination should make available useful information for researchers and physicians. Furthermore, it could help to the correct diagnosis of the illness, its differential diagnosis to the identification of the pathophysiological abnormalities probably responsible for the pathology

2. Electro-physiological techniques

- Surface electrode cortical EEG:

The electroencephalogram EEG is usually described in terms of its rhythmic activity, which is helpful in relating the EEG to the brain function [1]. Neuronal activity during information processing is represented by oscillations within local or widespread neuronal networks. These oscillations can be recorded by means of surface electrodes over the skull. The rhythmic activity in EEG is commonly divided in specific frequency bands: 0.5–4Hz (delta), 4–8Hz (theta), 8–10Hz (alpha 1), 10–12Hz (alpha 2), 12–30Hz (beta), and 30–100Hz (gamma) [2]. The FFT decomposes the EEG time series into a voltage by frequency spectral graph commonly called the "power spectrum", with power being the square of the EEG magnitude, and magnitude being the integral average of the amplitude of the EEG signal, measured from(+) peak-to-(-)peak), across the time sampled, or epoch [3]. As a result of this procedure the quantitative electroencephalogram QEEG is obtained [4], [5].

- Recording deep brain electrodes

Local field potential and action potentials can be captured by means of very fine conductive electrodes for research and surgical monitoring purposes [6], [7]. In addition, deep brain electrodes implanted into the brain are used to apply electrical stimulation in order to treat disorders that have electrical generators [6].

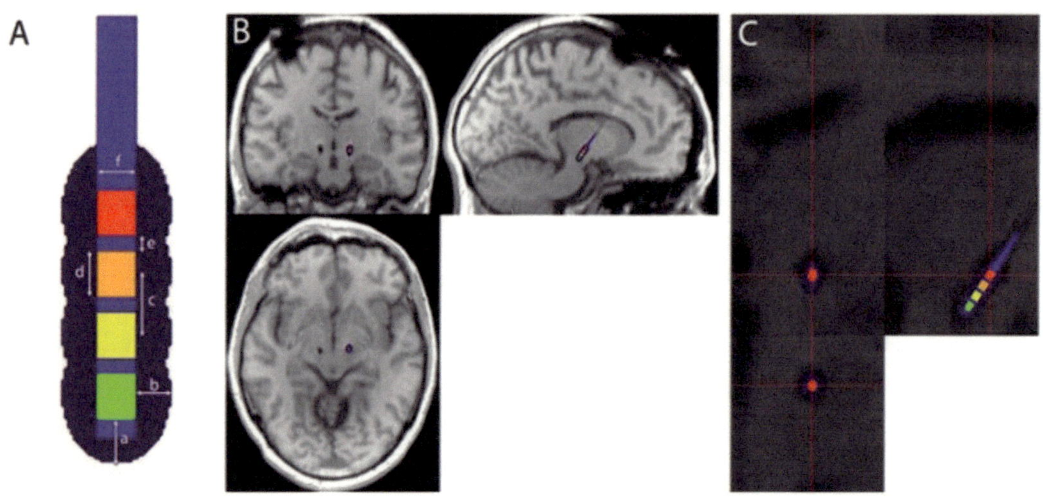

*Figure authorized for publication by the corresponding author from: Rodriguez-Oroz MC et al. Brain. 2011 Jan;134(Pt 1):36-49.

Figure 1. Deep brain electrodes to treat Parkinson's disease: (A) Electrode with four active contacts (0, 1, 2 and 3 from ventral to dorsal and each 1.5 mm high at 0.5 mm intervals; total length 7.5 mm) was placed at the selected coordinates in the subthalamic nucleus with the most ventral contact (contact 0) placed in the ventral part of the nucleus *

3. Alzheimer electroencephalographic patterns

The electroencephalogram EEG measures neuronal activity, and is an objective way to assess the degree of cognitive disturbance. Researchers have investigated how well cognitive function in dementia assessed by psychometric tests correlates with electrical brain activity (EEG). Results from such an experimental approach shows a slowing of the EEG, and an increase of dipole strength in the slow frequency bands, a more anterior equivalent dipole of alpha- and beta-activity, correlated with increasing cognitive deterioration in AD patients [8].

Relative power in different EEG frequency bands from EEG signals have been used in order to improve the diagnosis of AD. Frequency bands between 4 and 30 Hz have been systematically tested; the relative power of a certain frequency band is obtained by dividing the power of this frequency band by the power of the total frequency band. The frequency band 4-7 Hz is the optimal frequency range for detecting AD [9]. Progressive atrophy of hippocampus correlates with decreased cortical alpha power in AD patients. Moreover, the small hippocampal volume is measured in magnetic resonance imaging of the AD subjects [10], [11]. Additionally, the power of occipital, parietal, and temporal alpha sources is low in AD patients [10].

A promising study by Kann demonstrated the implication of the fast neuronal network oscillations in the gamma range (~30-90 Hz) in complex brain functions. Sensory processing, memory formation and, consciousness are brain functions highly vulnerable to neurodegenerative pathologies [12].

Cortical pathology in AD is related to decreasing fast frequency power; whereas increased slow frequency EEG power is observed in mixed dementia compared to AD. The quantitative EEG contributes to a better understanding of the electrical brain pattern in AD [13]. Slowing on qEEG is a marker for subsequent rate of cognitive and functional decline in mildly demented AD patients. Frequency bands analysis of EEG recordings from AD subjects shows lower parieto-occipital beta values, and higher frontocentral and parieto-occipital theta values. Additionally, lower parieto-occipital beta values are related to more decline in activities of daily living [14], [15]. Also, connectivity between frontal and parietal sites in AD patients is reduced, thus, resulting in significant decreased of coherence in the left fronto-parietal EEG [16].

In some cases there is no correlation between the increase of delta waves in the electroencephalogram, and the severity of mental deterioration of the AD patients, but this facts correlate by taking in account the intensity of delta waves rather than just their presence. The delta waves generated with participation of the cortex, thalamus, and brainstem seems to be more variable in different stages of AD. Measures of the theta activity discriminated between mild, marked, and severe cases of AD to some extent. The cognitive and EEG changes are probably related to atrophy of the cholinergic neurons in the hippocampal structures [17].

EEG recordings at rest and during visual stimulation processed by means of Fast Fourier Transform (FFT) are helpful to determine intra- and inter-hemispheric coherence in AD patients. Those studies have shown statistically significant phase dispersion especially at occipital and parietal regions in AD [18]. Coherence analysis of the EEG during photic stimulation also is low in AD patients, irrespective of the stimulus frequency, due to a failure of normal stimulation-related brain activation. What is more, when coherence analysis is done from recordings of the brain´s left hemisphere and the right one, impairment of interhemispheric functional connectivity is found [15].

4. Alzheimer diagnosis

A combination of computed techniques to analyze EEG recordings, such as the Higuchi fractal dimension (HFD), spectral entropy (SE), spectral centroid (SC), spectral roll-off (SR), and zero-crossing rate (ZCR), results in a AD diagnostic accuracy of 78%. HFD is a quantitative measure of time series complexity derived from fractal theory. Among spectral measures, SE measures the level of disorder in the spectrum, SC is a measure of spectral shape, and SR is frequency sample below which a specified percent of the spectral magnitude distribution is contained. Lastly, ZCR is simply the rate at which the signal changes signs. Even though, the individual accuracies ranged from 60-66%, that itself is not enough to be clinically useful alone. Combining these features and training a support vector machine (SVM) represent a novel alternative computed technique to reach high diagnostic accuracy for AD [19].

An electrophysiological marker in the early detection of neurodegeneration is found in the EEG pattern during stimulation for visual evoked potentials (VEP) in mild AD patients. In mild AD the altered activity concentrates on deep structures of the left hemisphere, say hippocampus and midbrain [20]. Visual evoked potentials in diagnosed Alzheimer patients (ApoE epsilon4 carriers) have significantly longer peak latencies and a trend to higher interpeak latencies of late potential components. However, potential amplitudes are similar in carriers and no carriers. It appears that the ApoE epsilon4 allele mainly promotes neuronal dysfunction [21]. In an ERPs lexical-decision task AD patients do not display repetition priming for words repeated at long lags [22].

Neuropathological findings in AD correlate with sensory-affective dissociation. Pain anticipation and autonomic reactivity depend on both the cognitive status and the frequency bands of the electroencephalogram, especially delta and theta frequencies. The painful stimulation perception is well preserved in AD, however, the affective and cognitive functions, which are related to both anticipation and autonomic reactivity are very affected [23].

A helpful tool to confirm an AD diagnosis is the electrophysiological correlate of minipolymyoclonus and a bi-frontal negativity in the EEG that precedes the myoclonic jerk. This electrophysiological fact may reflect activity of a subcortical generator. [24].

Quantitative relative power analysis of magnetoencephalography recordings can find widespread abnormalities in oscillatory brain dynamics in AD patients. In the delta band the AD patients have a consistently higher relative power, especially in the right occipital area. Delta activity is increased in AD patients, whereas alpha, and beta activity was decreased. Particularly the beta band (13–30 Hz) shows a very significant decrease in relative power in

AD. In the theta band the significant decrease in relative power of the left temporal region. In the beta band, all separate cortical regions demonstrated a significant decrease of relative power in AD [25]. Furthermore, the auto mutual information (AMI) provides a measure of future points predictability from past points in the magnetoencephalogram (MEG). Studies analyzing the (MEG) background activity in patients with AD, using the AMI reveals that the absolute values of the averaged decline rate of AMI is lower in AD patients than in control subjects. Thus, based on this kind of analysis is suggested that neuronal dysfunction in AD is associated with differences in the dynamical processes underlying the MEG recording [26].

REM sleep is a behavioral state characterized by atonia, and high frequency-low amplitude EEG among other features. Polysomnographic studies have found AD patients with REM sleep with-out atonia. The lack of atonia during REM sleep might involve alteration of the extrapyramidal motor control [27]. During quiet sleep in healthy human EEG there are components that consist of a brief negative high-voltage peak, usually greater than 100 μV, followed by a slower positive complex around 350 and 550 ms and at 900 ms a final negative peak, known as K-complex [28]; they are generated in response to external stimuli such as sounds, touches on the skin [29], and internal ones such as inspiratory interruptions [30]. They also occur in widespread cortical locations [28] though they tend to predominate over the frontal parts of the brain [31]. K-complexes synchronize the thalamocortical network during sleep, producing sleep oscillations such as spindles and delta waves [32]. Additionally, it has been suggested that K-complexes play an important role in memory consolidation [33]. In patients with Alzheimer disease, the electroencephalogram during wakefulness shows pathologic signs of abundant, delta activity. AD patients produced significantly fewer evoked K-complexes and had substantially smaller N550 amplitudes than controls. Even though observed increases in pathologic delta-frequency electroencephalographic activity, patients with Alzheimer disease have an impaired capacity to generate normal physiologic delta responses such as K-complexes during quiet sleep [34].

5. Alzheimer early detection

The progressive deterioration of AD patient progresses is caused by the loss of functional connectivity within neocortical association areas. Much more sensitive methods to identify early alterations of neuronal networks makes possible to predict the onset of AD. Diffuse slowing is correlated with the cognitive decline. This is a method to extract meaningful EEG parameters for the early diagnosis and staging of Alzheimer's disease [35]. Also, a clear difference between AD patients carrying the ApoE epsilon4 allele and no carriers is detected in the EEG; neurophysiological endophenotype of non-demented individuals at genetic risk for AD have increased excitability and dysfunction of deep brain and alpha rhythm-generating structures even decades before the first clinical symptoms of presumable dementia. Under hyperventilation the presence of the epsilon4 allele in AD relatives is associated with the manifestation of synchronous high-voltage delta-, theta-activity and sharp-waves, pronounced decrease in alpha and increase in delta and theta relative powers [36]. Mildly demented AD patients have an increase of relative delta power in the left side, and a decrease for relative alpha power in the right side; this preserves a linear correlation, and allows to predicting activity daily living ADL loss timing, and general behavioral and cognitive deterioration in mild Alzheimer's disease [5]. The delta relative power in the left side predicts both the loss of ADL and death, whereas right theta predicted the onset of incontinence [37]. In addition, the qEEG measures is correlated with neuropsychological test scores related to abilities that are impaired in the early stages of disease, such as delayed recall and verbal fluency [11].

Prognosis of early AD onset can be done by means of calculating the REO/REC power ratio; this tool takes the spectral analysis of the EEG recorded under awake resting eyes closed (REC) and open (REO) conditions. Demented AD patients show an increased REO/REC power ratio in the 6.5-12 Hz band. Patients lacking a dominant peak in the 6.5-12 Hz band, but with high power in 1-6.5 Hz band have an earlier age of disease onset [38].

Increased risk of mortality in AD is associated with higher theta, lower alpha, and lower beta activity in the parieto-occipital EEG. Also, higher theta activity in the fronto-central EEG has a prognosis value. Decreases of beta and alpha activity on quantitative spectral EEG are independent predictors of mortality in patients with early Alzheimer disease [39].

IFAST (implicit function as squashing time) is an artificial neural networks (ANNs) assembly; it is capable of compressing the temporal sequence of EEG data into spatial invariants. This model represents spatial features of the EEG patterns at scalp surface by means of filtering EEG tracks according to four different frequency ranges (0.12 Hz, 12.2 - 29.8 Hz; 30.2 - 40 Hz, and Notch Filter 48 - 50 Hz). The spatial content of the EEG voltage is extracted by IFAST step-wise procedure using ANNs. The data input for the classification operated by ANNs are the connections weights of a nonlinear auto-associative ANN trained to reproduce the recorded EEG tracks. This method allows distinguish between mild cognitive impairment (MCI) stable and MCI subjects who will convert to Alzheimer's disease (MCI/AD), with a high degree of accuracy. Eyes-closed resting EEG data in individual MCI/AD subjects show significant differences in the 10-12 Hz band when compared to MCI subjects [40].

Event-modulated EEG dynamic analysis makes it possible to investigate the functional activation of neocortical circuits [41]. Evoked Response Potentials (ERP) brain correlates are useful preclinical markers to identify individuals at risk for AD. Additionally, the ERP measures can predict its presence. Asymptomatic PSEN1 mutation carriers have greater occipital positivity, but less positivity in frontal regions than control subjects. Those differences are more evident during the 200-300 msec period of the ERP. It seems like carriers rely more upon perceptual details of the items to distinguish between them, while control subjects may use frontally mediated processes to distinguish between studied and unstudied visual items [42].

An electrophysiological marker in the early detection of neurodegeneration is found in the EEG pattern during stimulation for visual evoked potentials VEP in mild AD patients compared to Elderly controls, and MCI. Elderly controls have a neural pattern with a right–left dominance; in MCI this pattern seems to be displaced from right hemisphere to the left one, while in mild AD the activity concentrates on deep structures of this hemisphere (hippocampus and midbrain). Mild AD and MCI were more active for beta and gamma band, but at the same time beta and alpha band are more active than theta band. Elderly controls showed dominance of gamma and beta band in all significant areas. Mild AD and MCI have different neural patterns but show virtually similar frequency band activations, while elderly people differ from them in space and frequency bands [20].

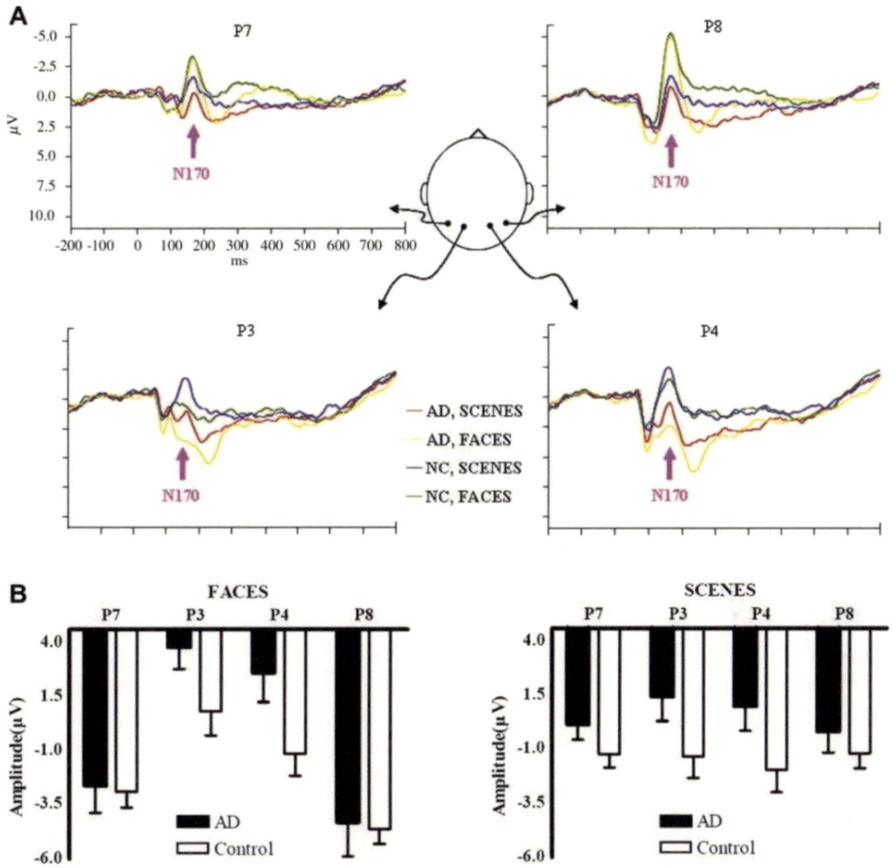

* Figure authorized for publication by the corresponding author from: Cheng PJ, Pai MC. Clin Neurophysiol. 2010 Sep; 121(9):1519-25

Figure 2. Event-related potential study: Comparison between alzheimer diseases patients and normal control patients: (A) N170 at the four electrode sites; (B) the amplitudes of N170 between groups and types, AD: Alzheimer's disease. *

Visual ERP features have shown that different neural regions are responsible for the early visual processing in the structural encoding of scenes and faces. P100 is a part of the evoked response suitable to examine basic visual processing, N170 brings information about structural encoding, and N250 is related to familiarity. The pattern of P100 and that of N170 suggest that mild Alzheimer disease patients maintain basic visual processing and structural encoding abilities, and scene recognition is impaired earlier than face recognition in the course of

Alzheimer disease [43]. There is a diminished N400 component during a semantic categorization task in elderly subjects which suggest that due to the difficulty in accessing information there are deficient associative connections within the semantic network [44]. Auditory sensory and cognitive cortical potentials in persons with familial Alzheimer disease (FAD) mutations are abnormal approximately 10 years before dementia will be manifest. FAD mutation carriers had significantly longer latencies of the N100, P200, N200, and P300 components, and smaller slow wave amplitudes. Longer event-related potential latencies suggest slowing of cortical information processing in FAD mutation carriers [45]. The P300 latency is very useful in diagnosis, since it is found to be altered in cases with AD at an early stage, with very little cognitive degeneration [46].

6. Parkinson electroencephalographic patterns

Recordings in humans as a result of functional neurosurgery have revealed a tendency for basal ganglia neurons to oscillate and synchronize their activity, giving rise to a rhythmic population activity, manifest as oscillatory local field potentials. The most important activity is synchronized oscillation in the beta band (13-30 Hz), which has been picked up at various sites within the basal ganglia-cortical loop in PD. Dopaminergic medication and movement suppress this activity, with the timing and degree of suppression closely correlating with behavioral performance. for that reason synchronization in the beta band has been hypothesized to be essentially antikinetic in nature and pathophysiologically relevant to bradykinesia [47].

Post-movement beta synchronization is an increase in EEG beta power after movement termination. Parkinson patients have longer movement duration than controls, and also execute longer movement with their left hand, unrelated to the side of tremor. In Parkinson patients post-movement beta synchronization is significantly smaller contralateral to the tremulous hand movement. The post-movement beta synchronization has anterior shifting in Parkinson-patients; whilst in tremor dominant Parkinson's disease the asymmetric decrease of post-move beta synchronization is related to the laterality of tremor rather than bradykinesia [48].

Local Field Potentials LFP recording beta oscillatory activity is generated largely within the dorsal portion of the sub thalamic nucleus STN and can produce synchronous oscillatory activity of the local neuronal population. Recent studies suggest that beta (15-30 Hz) oscillatory activity in the subthalamic nucleus (STN) is severely increased in PD, and may interfere with movement execution [49].

Parkinson's disease is known to result from basal ganglia dysfunction. Electrophysiological recordings show abnormal synchronous oscillatory activity in the cortico-basal ganglia network in parkinsonian patients and animals. Also, it has been recorded an altered response pattern during movement execution in the pallidum of parkinsonian animals. In Parkinson animal models, spontaneous correlated activity increased later, after animals became severely bradykinetic, whereas synchronous oscillatory activity appeared only after major motor symptoms developed. Thus, causality between the emergence of synchronous oscillations in the pallidum and main parkinsonian motor symptoms seems unlikely. Consequently, the pathological disruption of movement-related activity in the basal ganglia appears to be a better correlate at least to bradykinesia and is probably the best responsible candidate for this motor symptom [50].

The observation of a voluntary movement executed by another person is associated with an alpha and beta EEG desynchronization over the motor cortex, thought to reflect activity from the human "mirror neuron" system. Movement observation is accompanied by bilateral beta reduction in subthalamic power and cortico-STN coherence in PD, which is smaller than the decrease observed during movement execution, but significant when compared with control conditions. Movement observation is accompanied by changes in the beta oscillatory activity of the STN, similar to those observed in the EEG. These changes suggest that the basal ganglia might be engaged by the activity of the human mirror system [51].

The difficulty that patients have in initiating voluntary movement in the absence of any external cues might be due to the fact that the amplitude of movement-related cortical potential is equal to those prior to random-choice movements. The implication is that processes involved in self-selection of movement are abnormal in Parkinson's disease [52].

Parkinson disease patients show deficits in simple visuo-perceptual functions. Moreover, PD patients had impairment in tasks requiring set shifting from one reaction to another that may suggest frontal lobe dysfunction. The memory deficit in PD may derive from lowered motivation or initiating behavior [53].

Looking for electrophysiological correlates of perceptual categorization in Parkinson's disease, visual event-related potentials (ERPs) in a natural scene categorization task become a suitable tool. In healthy control subjects, there is a significant early difference (150-250 ms poststimulus) between ERPs elicited by pictures containing animals and scenes without animals. In spite of relatively preserved basic-level visual functions, this is not the case in untreated PD patients. These results move up the possibility for striatal contributions to visual categorization and may present a novel protocol for further clinical studies [54].

It has been reported an oscillatory theta-alpha activity in the ventral subthalamic nucleus associated with impulse control disorders ICD in patients with Parkinson's disease. This activity is distinct from that associated with L-dopa-induced dyskinesias LID and is also coherent with EEG activity recorded in frontal areas. The activity recorded in PD patients with impulse control disorders come out from the associative-limbic area (ventral subthalamic area), which is coherent with premotor frontal cortical activity. Patients with impulse control disorders display theta-alpha (4-10 Hz) activity (mean peak: 6.71 Hz) that is generated 2-8 mm below the intercommissural line. In PD the oscillatory activity of the subthalamic nucleus recorded through the electrodes implanted for deep brain stimulation displays dopamine-dependent changes whereby the OFF to ON motor state is signalled by a marked reduction in beta band activity [55]. Thus, dopaminergic side effects in Parkinson's disease are associated with oscillatory activity in the theta-alpha band, but at different frequencies and with different topography for the motor (dyskinesias) and behavioural (abnormal impulsivity) manifestations [6]. Diffuse lesions correlate with slowing of the EEG in patients with severe cognitive impairment [56], [57], [58]. All patients with dementia have an increase in slow waves in all the EEEG electrodes recording. In addition, all PD patients present diffuse slowing in the EEG with increased delta power [57].

Movement disorders in PD are due to the imbalance of inhibitory and excitatory processes involving motor cortical and subcortical neuronal circuits together with a nigrostriatal dopamine deficit [59]. A paired-pulse paradigm is usually used to study postexcitatory inhibition effect related to sensory gating mechanisms and synaptic processes in neurotransmitters release. There are two mechanisms that might explain paired-pulse inhibition phenomena. The first mechanism is the decrease in release probability of excitatory neurotransmitters from terminals of afferent axons. Another possible mechanism of the decrement of the second response on paired stimulation is connected with synaptically released GABA from terminals of inhibitory interneurons [60]. As the paired-pulse facilitation, paired-pulse inhibition is considered to be a form of a short-term synaptic plasticity. The investigation of cortical evoked potentials to paired-pulse sensory stimulation may provide additional information about mechanisms of neurological disturbances in PD [60].

7. Parkinson diagnosis

When individuals performed a reaching motor task (catching a ball in free fall), beta band asymmetry is observed. This result show a pattern of asymmetry in the somatosensory cortex, associated with a preparatory mechanism. With respect to task moment, after the ball's fall, the asymmetry is reduced. Moreover, the difference in asymmetry between the regions is related to a supposed specialization of areas (i.e., temporal and central). The temporal region is associated with cognitive processes involved in the motor action (i.e., explicit knowledge). On the other hand, the central sites are related to the motor control mechanisms per se (i.e., implicit knowledge). The premotor cortex shows a decrease on neural activity in the contralateral hemisphere (i.e., to the right hand). This finding is in agreement with others suggesting a participation of the frontal cortex in the planning of the apprehension task. This sensorimotor paradigm may be added to the inventory of tasks used to study clinical conditions such as depression, alzheimer and Parkinson diseases [61].

The corpus callosum (CC) is the morphological correlate of inter-hemispheric connectivity. Its integrity is of great importance for motor function and inter-hemispheric coordination of bimanual movements. Callosal fiber tracts are highly vulnerable as they are involved in number of neurodegenerative disease like parkinsonian syndromes and amyotrophic lateral sclerosis, even at early stages of the diseases. Transcraneal magnetic stimulation of the transcallosal inhibition may be performed by measurement of the ipsilateral silent period (iSP). The most common finding is a loss or a prolongation of the iSP latency [62].

As PD progresses, components of the autonomic, limbic, and somatomotor systems become damaged [63]. The substantia nigra and other regions of nuclear gray matter in the midbrain and forebrain become the focus of initially slight and then severe pathologic changes. At certain point, most individuals probably cross the threshold to the symptomatic phase of the illness, the pathologic process comes to involve the neocortex, and the disease is manifested in all its clinical magnitude. These diffuse lesions correlate with slowing of the EEG in patients with severe cognitive impairment [56], [57], [58].

The auditory evoked potentials of different latencies are useful in the evaluation of cognitive changes associated to PD. Middle latency auditory evoked potentials are abnormal in most PD patient. P300 is absent significantly more often in PD patients with cognitive impairment [64].

Parkinson Early Detection:

Spectral ratio is the sum of the power values in the alpha and beta waves divided by the sum of the values in the slow waves. Since, all patients with dementia have an increase in slow waves in all the EEEG electrodes recording, the spectral ratios decrease have significant predictive value in PD at all electrode locations except for the frontal pole. In addition, all PD patients present diffuse slowing in the EEG giving to delta power significance as predictive electrophysiological biomarker for dementia in PD [57]. ERP is also useful tool for the evaluation of neuropsychological impairments in PD. In the classic oddball task P300 is elicited by target. Even though, P300b findings in PD have shown inconsistent results, prolonged P300b latency in PD patients with dementia have been consistently observed [65].

The hazard of developing dementia is 13 times higher for those with low background rhythm frequency (lower than the grand median of 8.5 Hz) than for those with high background rhythm frequency. The QEEG measures of background rhythm frequency and relative power in the band are potential predictive biomarkers for dementia incidence in PD [57].

8. Huntington electroencephalographic patterns

Huntington's disease (HD) is an autosomal dominant inherited neurodegenerative disorder, with neurodegeneration mainly affecting the striatum. In Nogo as opposed to Go trials two fronto-central ERP components are elicited: the Nogo-N2 and Nogo-P3. These components are supposed to depend on (medial) prefrontal regions, especially the anterior cingulate cortex (ACC). In HD the Nogo-P3 demonstrates a strong attenuation, while the Nogo-N2 does not differ from controls. The decline in inhibition is likely mediated via a dysfunction in the ACC, which is known to be dysfunctional in HD. Moreover, the decline in response inhibition in HD is gene-associated. The differentially affected Nogo-components suggest that they rely on different neuronal circuits, even within the ACC. For HD this suggests that this structure is not entirely dysfunctional [66].

Cognition is affected early in Huntington disease, and in HD animal models there is evidence that this reflects abnormal synaptic plasticity. HD gene carriers and controls respond differently to theta burst stimulation, with controls having more inhibition than HD gene carriers. However, there is no difference between pre-manifest and early symptomatic HD gene carriers. Motor cortex plasticity is abnormal in HD gene carriers but is not closely linked to the development of motor signs of HD [67]. In vivo recording of field potentials in the dorsomedial striatum evoked by stimulation of the prelimbic cortex in rats shows an altered plasticity, with higher paired-pulse facilitation, enhanced short-term depression, as well as stronger long-term potentiation after theta burst stimulation. This is a behavioral and electrophysiological evidence of a presymptomatic alteration of prefrontostriatal processing in an animal model for Huntington disease and suggests that supra-second timing may be the earliest cognitive dysfunction in HD [68].

The onset of Huntington disease (HD) might be atypical. Rarely, there is severe cognitive impairment and diffuse cortical atrophy before the onset of motor manifestations or symptoms of an extrapyramidal movement disorder. Thus, especial consideration must there be for patients with early dementia of unknown etiology [69].

The visually evoked potential is abnormal in patients with Huntington disease. Both early and late wave components are affected, and the averaged amplitude for the patients is reduced in comparison with normal control subjects. Despite striking attenuation and disorganization of the complex, latency of initial wave components is normal. The abnormality is not present in patients with a variety of other nonfocal cerebral disorders nor in children of patients with Huntington disease [70]. There are marked impairments of patients with HD in early visual sensory processing (early components). The early visual components show a significant latency shift (delay of about 50 milliseconds) in HD. In the search paradigms the P3 components differentiating target and standard stimuli is virtually absent in HD as is the ERP effect indexing word recognition. This is accompanied by a marked delay in search times and lower hit rates in the search tasks and grossly reduced recognition accuracy in the memory task. Deficits in visual search might be due to an impairment to deploy attentional resources across the visual field and/or an inability to control eye movements [71].

9. Huntington diagnosis

Huntington disease usually causes cognitive decline previously to motor symptoms. Studies performed in a HD animal model to assess this issue suggest that normal plasticity in prefrontostriatal circuits may be necessary for reliable and precise timing behavior. Furthermore, the behavioral analysis revealed poorer temporal sensitivity as early as 4 months of age, well before detection of overt motor deficits. At a later symptomatic age, animals were impaired in their temporal discriminative behavior [68].

10. Huntington early detection

It is well known that HD affects cognition earlier than motor system. The motor-evoked potential to burst stimulation is a suitable tool to evaluate motor synaptic plasticity. This might bring out clues about motor control decline related to HD before having symptoms of abnormal motor behavior [67].

Author details

Manuel J. Rojas*, Camilo Orozco and Francisco Olea

*Address all correspondence to: marojasba@unal.edu.co

Animal Health Department, National University of Colombia, Bogota, Colombia

References

[1] Brismar T. The human EEG--physiological and clinical studies. Physiol Behav. 2007 Sep;92(1-2):141-7.

[2] Nunez PL, Srinivasan R. A theoretical basis for standing and traveling brain waves measured with human EEG with implications for an integrated consciousness. Clin Neurophysiol. 2006 Nov;117(11):2424-35.

[3] Murali S, Vladimir KV. Analysis of fractal and fast fourier transform spectra of human electroencephalograms induced by odors. Int J Neurosci. 2007 Oct;117(10):1383-401.

[4] Soininen H, Reinikainen K, Partanen J, Mervaala E, Paljärvi L, Helkala EL, et al. Slowing of the dominant occipital rhythm in electroencephalogram is associated with low concentration of noradrenaline in the thalamus in patients with Alzheimer's disease. Neurosci Lett. 1992 Mar;137(1):5-8.

[5] Nobili F, Copello F, Vitali P, Prastaro T, Carozzo S, Perego G, et al. Timing of disease progression by quantitative EEG in Alzheimer' s patients. J Clin Neurophysiol. 1999 Nov;16(6):566-73.

[6] Rodriguez-Oroz MC, López-Azcárate J, Garcia-Garcia D, Alegre M, Toledo J, Valencia M, et al. Involvement of the subthalamic nucleus in impulse control disorders associated with Parkinson's disease. Brain. 2011 Jan;134(Pt 1):36-49.

[7] Rojas MJ, Navas JA, Rector DM. Evoked response potential markers for anesthetic and behavioral states. Am J Physiol Regul Integr Comp Physiol. 2006 Jul;291(1):R189-96.

[8] Dierks T, Frölich L, Ihl R, Maurer K. Correlation between cognitive brain function and electrical brain activity in dementia of Alzheimer type. J Neural Transm Gen Sect. 1995;99(1-3):55-62.

[9] Elgendi M, Vialatte F, Cichocki A, Latchoumane C, Jeong J, Dauwels J. Optimization of EEG frequency bands for improved diagnosis of Alzheimer disease. Conf Proc IEEE Eng Med Biol Soc. 2011;2011:6087-91.

[10] Babiloni C, Frisoni GB, Pievani M, Vecchio F, Lizio R, Buttiglione M, et al. Hippocampal volume and cortical sources of EEG alpha rhythms in mild cognitive impairment and Alzheimer disease. Neuroimage. 2009 Jan;44(1):123-35.

[11] Duffy FH, McAnulty GB, Albert MS. Temporoparietal electrophysiological differences characterize patients with Alzheimer's disease: a split-half replication study. Cereb Cortex. 1995 1995 May-Jun;5(3):215-21.

[12] Kann O, Huchzermeyer C, Kovács R, Wirtz S, Schuelke M. Gamma oscillations in the hippocampus require high complex I gene expression and strong functional performance of mitochondria. Brain. 2011 Feb;134(Pt 2):345-58.

[13] Schreiter Gasser U, Rousson V, Hentschel F, Sattel H, Gasser T. Alzheimer disease versus mixed dementias: an EEG perspective. Clin Neurophysiol. 2008 Oct;119(10): 2255-9.

[14] Claus JJ, Kwa VI, Teunisse S, Walstra GJ, van Gool WA, Koelman JH, et al. Slowing on quantitative spectral EEG is a marker for rate of subsequent cognitive and functional decline in early Alzheimer disease. Alzheimer Dis Assoc Disord. 1998 Sep; 12(3):167-74.

[15] Wada Y, Nanbu Y, Koshino Y, Yamaguchi N, Hashimoto T. Reduced interhemispheric EEG coherence in Alzheimer disease: analysis during rest and photic stimulation. Alzheimer Dis Assoc Disord. 1998 Sep;12(3):175-81.

[16] Güntekin B, Saatçi E, Yener G. Decrease of evoked delta, theta and alpha coherences in Alzheimer patients during a visual oddball paradigm. Brain Res. 2008 Oct; 1235:109-16.

[17] Kowalski JW, Gawel M, Pfeffer A, Barcikowska M. The diagnostic value of EEG in Alzheimer disease: correlation with the severity of mental impairment. J Clin Neurophysiol. 2001 Nov;18(6):570-5.

[18] Celesia GG, Villa AE, Brigell M, Rubboli G, Bolcioni G, Fiori MG. An electrophysiological study of visual processing in Alzheimer's disease. Electroencephalogr Clin Neurophysiol. 1993 Sep;87(3):97-104.

[19] Staudinger T, Polikar R. Analysis of complexity based EEG features for the diagnosis of Alzheimer's disease. Conf Proc IEEE Eng Med Biol Soc. 2011;2011:2033-6.

[20] Haupt M, González-Hernández JA, Scherbaum WA. Regions with different evoked frequency band responses during early-stage visual processing distinguish mild Alzheimer dementia from mild cognitive impairment and normal aging. Neurosci Lett. 2008 Sep;442(3):273-8.

[21] Rosengarten B, Paulsen S, Burr O, Kaps M. Effect of ApoE epsilon4 allele on visual evoked potentials and resultant flow coupling in patients with Alzheimer. J Geriatr Psychiatry Neurol. 2010 Sep;23(3):165-70.

[22] Schnyer DM, Allen JJ, Kaszniak AW, Forster KI. An event-related potential examination of masked and unmasked repetition priming in Alzheimer's disease: implications for theories of implicit memory. Neuropsychology. 1999 Jul;13(3):323-37.

[23] Benedetti F, Arduino C, Vighetti S, Asteggiano G, Tarenzi L, Rainero I. Pain reactivity in Alzheimer patients with different degrees of cognitive impairment and brain electrical activity deterioration. Pain. 2004 Sep;111(1-2):22-9.

[24] Hallett M, Wilkins DE. Myoclonus in Alzheimer's disease and minipolymyoclonus. Adv Neurol. 1986;43:399-405.

[25] de Haan W, Stam CJ, Jones BF, Zuiderwijk IM, van Dijk BW, Scheltens P. Resting-state oscillatory brain dynamics in Alzheimer disease. J Clin Neurophysiol. 2008 Aug;25(4):187-93.

[26] Gómez C, Hornero R, Fernández A, Abasolo D, Escudero J, López M. Magnetoencephalogram background activity analysis in Alzheimer's disease patients using auto mutual information. Conf Proc IEEE Eng Med Biol Soc. 2006;1:6181-4.

[27] Gagnon JF, Petit D, Fantini ML, Rompré S, Gauthier S, Panisset M, et al. REM sleep behavior disorder and REM sleep without atonia in probable Alzheimer disease. Sleep. 2006 Oct;29(10):1321-5.

[28] Cash SS, Halgren E, Dehghani N, Rossetti AO, Thesen T, Wang C, et al. The human K-complex represents an isolated cortical down-state. Science. 2009 May;324(5930): 1084-7.

[29] ROTH M, SHAW J, GREEN J. The form voltage distribution and physiological significance of the K-complex. Electroencephalogr Clin Neurophysiol. 1956 Aug;8(3): 385-402.

[30] Webster KE, Colrain IM. Multichannel EEG analysis of respiratory evoked-potential components during wakefulness and NREM sleep. J Appl Physiol. 1998 Nov;85(5): 1727-35.

[31] McCormick L, Nielsen T, Nicolas A, Ptito M, Montplaisir J. Topographical distribution of spindles and K-complexes in normal subjects. Sleep. 1997 Nov;20(11):939-41.

[32] Amzica F, Steriade M. Cellular substrates and laminar profile of sleep K-complex. Neuroscience. 1998 Feb;82(3):671-86.

[33] Tononi G, Cirelli C. Sleep function and synaptic homeostasis. Sleep Med Rev. 2006 Feb;10(1):49-62.

[34] Crowley K, Sullivan EV, Adalsteinsson E, Pfefferbaum A, Colrain IM. Differentiating pathologic delta from healthy physiologic delta in patients with Alzheimer disease. Sleep. 2005 Jul;28(7):865-70.

[35] Strik WK, Chiaramonti R, Muscas GC, Paganini M, Mueller TJ, Fallgatter AJ, et al. Decreased EEG microstate duration and anteriorisation of the brain electrical fields

in mild and moderate dementia of the Alzheimer type. Psychiatry Res. 1997 Oct; 75(3):183-91.

[36] Ponomareva NV, Korovaitseva GI, Rogaev EI. EEG alterations in non-demented individuals related to apolipoprotein E genotype and to risk of Alzheimer disease. Neurobiol Aging. 2008 Jun;29(6):819-27.

[37] Rodriguez G, Nobili F, Arrigo A, Priano F, De Carli F, Francione S, et al. Prognostic significance of quantitative electroencephalography in Alzheimer patients: preliminary observations. Electroencephalogr Clin Neurophysiol. 1996 Aug;99(2):123-8.

[38] Signorino M, Pucci E, Belardinelli N, Nolfe G, Angeleri F. EEG spectral analysis in vascular and Alzheimer dementia. Electroencephalogr Clin Neurophysiol. 1995 May; 94(5):313-25.

[39] Claus JJ, Ongerboer de Visser BW, Walstra GJ, Hijdra A, Verbeeten B, van Gool WA. Quantitative spectral electroencephalography in predicting survival in patients with early Alzheimer disease. Arch Neurol. 1998 Aug;55(8):1105-11.

[40] Buscema M, Grossi E, Capriotti M, Babiloni C, Rossini P. The I.F.A.S.T. model allows the prediction of conversion to Alzheimer disease in patients with mild cognitive impairment with high degree of accuracy. Curr Alzheimer Res. 2010 Mar;7(2):173-87.

[41] Giannakopoulos P, Missonnier P, Kövari E, Gold G, Michon A. Electrophysiological markers of rapid cognitive decline in mild cognitive impairment. Front Neurol Neurosci. 2009;24:39-46.

[42] Quiroz YT, Ally BA, Celone K, McKeever J, Ruiz-Rizzo AL, Lopera F, et al. Event-related potential markers of brain changes in preclinical familial Alzheimer disease. Neurology. 2011 Aug;77(5):469-75.

[43] Cheng PJ, Pai MC. Dissociation between recognition of familiar scenes and of faces in patients with very mild Alzheimer disease: an event-related potential study. Clin Neurophysiol. 2010 Sep;121(9):1519-25.

[44] Castañeda M, Ostrosky-Solis F, Pérez M, Bobes MA, Rangel LE. ERP assessment of semantic memory in Alzheimer's disease. Int J Psychophysiol. 1997 Dec;27(3):201-14.

[45] Golob EJ, Ringman JM, Irimajiri R, Bright S, Schaffer B, Medina LD, et al. Cortical event-related potentials in preclinical familial Alzheimer disease. Neurology. 2009 Nov;73(20):1649-55.

[46] Fernández- Lastra A, Morales-Rodríguez M, Penzol-Díaz J. [Neurophysiological study and use of P300 evoked potentials for investigation in the diagnosis and of follow-up of patients with Alzheimer s disease]. Rev Neurol. 2001 2001 Mar 16-31;32(6): 525-8.

[47] Brown P. Bad oscillations in Parkinson's disease. J Neural Transm Suppl. 2006 (70): 27-30.

[48] Szirmai I, Tamás G, Takáts A, Pálvölgyi L, Kamondi A. [Electrophysiologic investigation of cerebral cortex in the subtypes of Parkinson disease]. Ideggyogy Sz. 2002 May;55(5-6):182-9.

[49] Weinberger M, Mahant N, Hutchison WD, Lozano AM, Moro E, Hodaie M, et al. Beta oscillatory activity in the subthalamic nucleus and its relation to dopaminergic response in Parkinson's disease. J Neurophysiol. 2006 Dec;96(6):3248-56.

[50] Leblois A, Meissner W, Bioulac B, Gross CE, Hansel D, Boraud T. Late emergence of synchronized oscillatory activity in the pallidum during progressive Parkinsonism. Eur J Neurosci. 2007 Sep;26(6):1701-13.

[51] Alegre M, Rodríguez-Oroz MC, Valencia M, Pérez-Alcázar M, Guridi J, Iriarte J, et al. Changes in subthalamic activity during movement observation in Parkinson's disease: is the mirror system mirrored in the basal ganglia? Clin Neurophysiol. 2010 Mar;121(3):414-25.

[52] Touge T, Werhahn KJ, Rothwell JC, Marsden CD. Movement-related cortical potentials preceding repetitive and random-choice hand movements in Parkinson's disease. Ann Neurol. 1995 Jun;37(6):791-9.

[53] Hartikainen P, Helkala EL, Soininen H, Riekkinen P. Cognitive and memory deficits in untreated Parkinson's disease and amyotrophic lateral sclerosis patients: a comparative study. J Neural Transm Park Dis Dement Sect. 1993;6(2):127-37.

[54] Antal A, Kéri S, Dibó G, Benedek G, Janka Z, Vécsei L, et al. Electrophysiological correlates of visual categorization: evidence for cognitive dysfunctions in early Parkinson's disease. Brain Res Cogn Brain Res. 2002 Apr;13(2):153-8.

[55] Brown P. Oscillatory nature of human basal ganglia activity: relationship to the pathophysiology of Parkinson's disease. Mov Disord. 2003 Apr;18(4):357-63.

[56] Morita A, Kamei S, Mizutani T. Relationship between slowing of the EEG and cognitive impairment in Parkinson disease. J Clin Neurophysiol. 2011 Aug;28(4):384-7.

[57] Klassen BT, Hentz JG, Shill HA, Driver-Dunckley E, Evidente VG, Sabbagh MN, et al. Quantitative EEG as a predictive biomarker for Parkinson disease dementia. Neurology. 2011 Jul;77(2):118-24.

[58] Serizawa K, Kamei S, Morita A, Hara M, Mizutani T, Yoshihashi H, et al. Comparison of quantitative EEGs between Parkinson disease and age-adjusted normal controls. J Clin Neurophysiol. 2008 Dec;25(6):361-6.

[59] Ridding MC, Inzelberg R, Rothwell JC. Changes in excitability of motor cortical circuitry in patients with Parkinson's disease. Ann Neurol. 1995 Feb;37(2):181-8.

[60] Chu Z, Hablitz JJ. GABA(B) receptor-mediated heterosynaptic depression of excitatory synaptic transmission in rat frontal neocortex. Brain Res. 2003 Jan;959(1):39-49.

[61] Velasques B, Machado S, Portella CE, Silva JG, Basile LF, Cagy M, et al. Electrophysiological analysis of a sensorimotor integration task. Neurosci Lett. 2007 Oct;426(3): 155-9.

[62] Wittstock M. [Neurophysiological analysis of interhemispheric motor tracts in neurodegenerative diseases]. Fortschr Neurol Psychiatr. 2009 Aug;77 Suppl 1:S42-4.

[63] Braak H, Ghebremedhin E, Rüb U, Bratzke H, Del Tredici K. Stages in the development of Parkinson's disease-related pathology. Cell Tissue Res. 2004 Oct;318(1): 121-34.

[64] Nojszewska M, Pilczuk B, Zakrzewska-Pniewska B, Rowińska-Marcińska K. The auditory system involvement in Parkinson disease: electrophysiological and neuropsychological correlations. J Clin Neurophysiol. 2009 Dec;26(6):430-7.

[65] Kamei S. [Electroencephalogram and event-related potential analyses in Parkinson disease]. Brain Nerve. 2012 Apr;64(4):433-43.

[66] Beste C, Saft C, Andrich J, Gold R, Falkenstein M. Response inhibition in Huntington's disease-a study using ERPs and sLORETA. Neuropsychologia. 2008 Apr;46(5): 1290-7.

[67] Orth M, Schippling S, Schneider SA, Bhatia KP, Talelli P, Tabrizi SJ, et al. Abnormal motor cortex plasticity in premanifest and very early manifest Huntington disease. J Neurol Neurosurg Psychiatry. 2010 Mar;81(3):267-70.

[68] Höhn S, Dallérac G, Faure A, Urbach YK, Nguyen HP, Riess O, et al. Behavioral and in vivo electrophysiological evidence for presymptomatic alteration of prefrontostriatal processing in the transgenic rat model for huntington disease. J Neurosci. 2011 Jun;31(24):8986-97.

[69] Cooper DB, Ales G, Lange C, Clement P. Atypical onset of symptoms in Huntington disease: severe cognitive decline preceding chorea or other motor manifestations. Cogn Behav Neurol. 2006 Dec;19(4):222-4.

[70] Ellenberger C, Petro DJ, Ziegler SB. The visually evoked potential in Huntington disease. Neurology. 1978 Jan;28(1):95-7.

[71] Münte TF, Ridao-Alonso ME, Preinfalk J, Jung A, Wieringa BM, Matzke M, et al. An electrophysiological analysis of altered cognitive functions in Huntington disease. Arch Neurol. 1997 Sep;54(9):1089-98.

Chapter 18

Oxidative Changes and Possible Effects of Polymorphism of Antioxidant Enzymes in Neurodegenerative Disease

Eva Babusikova, Andrea Evinova, Jozef Hatok,
Dusan Dobrota and Jana Jurecekova

Additional information is available at the end of the chapter

http://dx.doi.org/10.5772/54619

1. Introduction

Frequency of neurodegenerative diseases increase significantly with the age. In the present, average age is increasing and the number of people over 60 years increases as well. Ageing is a physiological process; however it seems to be linked with an increasing risk of origin and development of several diseases including neurodegenerative disorders such as Alzheimer's disease, Parkinson's disease, and Huntington's disease. Exact mechanisms of ageing are still unclear but experimental evidences support a hypothesis that ageing changes are consequences of increasing oxidative damage of organs, tissues, cells and all biomolecules. Oxidative damage is elevated when production of reactive oxygen species is increased compared to the physiological condition or a defence ability of organism against attacks of reactive oxygen species is decreased. Oxidation of specific proteins could play a key role in age associated damage. A relationship between protein aggregation, oxidative stress and neurodegeneration remains unclear although neurodegenerative diseases are connected with an origin of protein deposits. It assumes that protein oxidation and generation of protein aggregates generate a base for a loss of cell function and a reduced ability aged organisms to resist to physiological stress. Accumulation of modified proteins, disturbance of ion homeostasis, lipid and DNA modifications, and impairment of energy production are some of the crucial mechanisms linking ageing to neurodegeneration. In addition mitochondrial dysfunction plays a key role in neurology. Damage of mitochondrial electron transport may be an important factor in the pathogenesis of neurodegenerative diseases, such as Alzheimer's, Parkinson's, and Huntington's diseases.

Oxygen is vital for all aerobic organisms and reactive oxygen species (ROS) are formed in cells as a consequence of aerobic metabolism. Moreover mitochondrial respiration is associated with inevitable electron leak, resulting in a non-stop production of reactive oxygen species, such as superoxide anion radical, hydrogen peroxide and hydrogen radical. Universal nature of reactive oxygen species is underlined by the presence of superoxide dismutase in all aerobic organisms. Genes involved in detoxification of reactive oxygen species are highly conserved among eukaryotes and their deficiency could be limit of several diseases and life span. Oxidative stress is a unique pathophysiological condition resulting from the disrupted balance between oxidants and antioxidants. Increased level of reactive oxygen species may cause oxidative damage of all four biomolecules: nucleic acids, proteins, lipids, saccharides. A progressive grow of oxidative damage is the result of increasing production of reactive oxygen species and this damage may contribute to the origin and development of several diseases including neurodegenerative diseases, but on the other hand oxidative damage can be the consequence of them as well (fig. 1). Cells possess defence systems: enzymatic and non-enzymatic against ROS. The most important enzymatic antioxidants are: superoxide dismutase, catalase and glutathione peroxidase but many others enzymes have antioxidant potential.

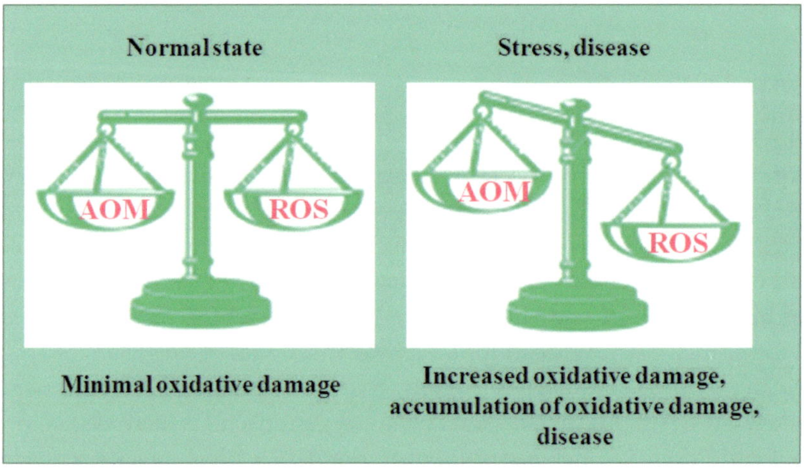

Figure 1. Reactive oxygen species in the development of disease. As a consequence of imbalance between reactive oxygen species (ROS) and antioxidant mechanisms (AOM) on the side of reactive oxygen species, oxidative stress is increasing. Increased level of reactive oxygen species causes increased oxidative damage of biomolecules, an accumulation of damage, and the development of many diseases.

2. Oxidative damage

Reactive oxygen species (ROS) are necessary for human life. The main characteristics of ROS are their high effectiveness in a small concentration and their extremely highly reactivity. ROS are oxidants which can be produced endogenously and exogenously. Potential harmful ROS generate in cells under normal physiological conditions in different metabolic pathways and cell compartments (fig. 2).

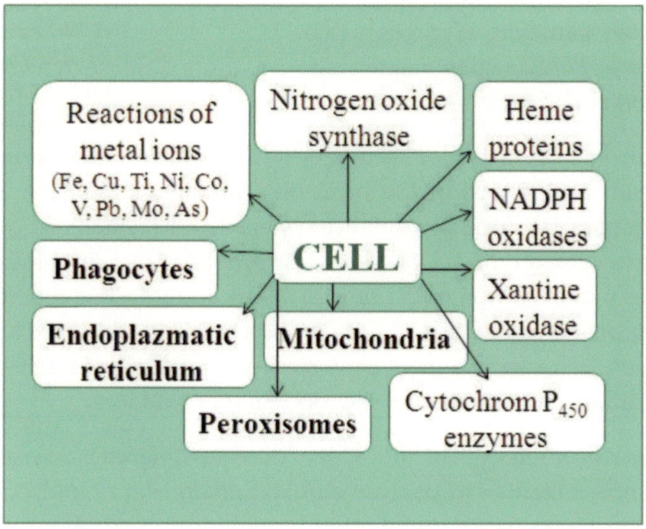

Figure 2. The main endogenous sources of reactive oxygen species (ROS) in cell. Organelles such as mitochondria, peroxisomes, phagocytes and endoplasmic reticulum and enzymes produce ROS during a pursuance their physiologic roles in cell and during metabolism of several components.

Four from the endogenous sources (mitochondria, phagocytes, peroxisomes, and cytochrome P_{450} enzymes) are responsible for origin of the majority of oxidants produced by cells [5]. The main endogenous sources of reactive oxygen species are mitochondria which produce reactive oxygen species continuously. Mitochondria serve mainly as producers of energy. In normal aerobic respiration mitochondria utilize oxygen that is reduced by serial steps whereby is produced water. Mitochondria are the major producer of reactive oxygen species via incomplete reduction of oxygen by electrons leaked out of the respiratory chain in the animal and human cells. Mitochondrial oxidative damage can lead to the release of greater amount of reactive oxygen species and cause increased oxidative damage of mitochondrial, cytoplasmic and nuclear components what subsequently may lead to dysfunctional mitochondria. Damage of mitochondrial electron transport may be an important factor in the pathogenesis of many diseases.

Phagocyting cells are another important endogenous source of oxidants. The main function of phagocytosis is the defence of host organisms against pathogens. Neutrophils and another phagocytes attack pathogens by mixture of reactive oxygen species: singlet oxygen ($O_2^{\bullet -}$), nitric oxide ($^{\bullet}NO$), hydrogen peroxide (H_2O_2), hypochlorous acid (HClO) [129]. Chronic virus, bacterial or parasite infection results in chronic increased phagocyting activity and finally chronic inflammation, which is a main risk factor for development of several diseases [5], and raising oxidative damage.

Peroxisomes are organelles from the microbody family and are present in almost all eukaryotic cells. They participate in the β-oxidation of fatty acids and in the metabolism of many others metabolites. Certain enzymes within peroxisome, by using molecular oxygen, remove hydrogen atoms from specific organic substrates, in an oxidative reaction, producing hydrogen peroxide. Hydrogen peroxide is degraded by catalase, another enzyme in peroxisome. Peroxisomes contain also xanthine oxidase which produces singlet oxygen and hydrogen peroxide.

Microsomal cytochrome P_{450} enzymes are a very large and diverse superfamily of hemoproteins identified from all lineages of life including humans, mammals, birds, fish, plants, bacteria. They form one of the primary defence system against xenobiotic compounds usually plant origin. Human cytochrome P_{450} enzymes are primarily membrane-associated proteins, located in the inner mitochondrial membrane or in the endoplasmic reticulum of cells. They modify thousands of endogenous and exogenous compounds by univalent oxidation or reduction. Induction of these enzymes protects before acute oxidative effects of foreign compounds or chemicals but also results in production of oxidants.

Although cells possess complex net of antioxidant defence, defence is not completely effective. Small fractions of pro-oxidants escape from elimination and cause molecular damage. Some of these damages are irreversible therefore they are accumulated in time and they make base of functional decline associated with age. Disruption of a balance between the level of reactive species generated during normal cellular metabolism and the level of endogenous antioxidant, either due to increased generation of ROS or decreased level of antioxidants, leads to oxidative damage and to several pathological conditions, including accelerated ageing and neurodegenerative disorders.

Exact mechanisms of reasons for origin of some neurodegenerative diseases are still unclear but experimental evidences support a hypothesis that ageing is a major risk and ageing changes are consequences of increasing oxidative damage. One of the basic problems is the analysis of mechanisms that are base of damage. ROS are effective in a very small concentrations and their half-life is very short. We still do not have sensitive instruments for measurement ROS (concentration and localisation) in living systems. Usually effects of ROS are determined indirect, by several markers of oxidative damage (fig. 3). Both localisation and kind of damage are necessary for understanding of neurodegeneration. Oxidative damage may by the most important contribution to ageing and age-related diseases. Literature is full of controversy results. Oxidative modification of proteins, saccharides, nucleic acid (nuclear and mitochondrial) and lipid peroxidation were observed in different tissues, cells, compartments, including mitochondria with advancing of age. There is no detail information how the higher availability of reactive oxygen species could be translated to an accumulation of oxidized biomolecules so far.

An accumulation of oxidized proteins, disturbance of ion homeostasis, modifications of lipids, saccharides, proteins and nucleic acids, and impairment of energy production are some of the crucial mechanisms linking ageing to neurodegeneration. Brain is particularly sensitive to reactive oxygen species attack and to oxidative damage consequence of several factors:

- Brain has a high content of unsaturated fatty acid (especially 20:4 and 22:6 fatty acids).
- Brain has high oxygen consumption (20% of using oxygen is consumed by brain).
- In the brain is high concentration of iron and ascorbate (key elements responsible for membrane lipid peroxidation).
- Brain is to poor of antioxidants and defence mechanisms.

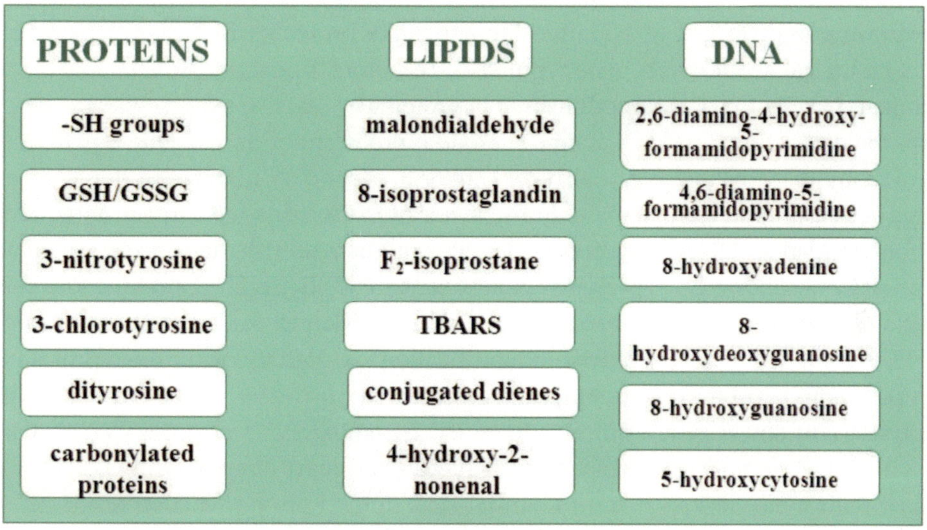

Figure 3. Markers of oxidative damage. Proteins, lipids and DNA are main targets of reactive oxygen species (ROS). These molecules generate a spectrum of molecules in the condition of oxidative stress which may be estimated for example in plasma, serum, bronchoalveolar lavage fluid, tissues and in exhalated breath condensate and reflect a danger of ROS for a subject in consequence of origin and development of several diseases.

Exclusive using of glucose as a source of energy by brain is responsible for high oxygen concentrations which are necessary for normal brain function. A predominant quantity of reactive oxygen species (90-95%) is generated during aerobic metabolism as a by-product in an electron transport chain of mitochondria. Mitochondrial dysfunction plays a key role in neurology [8]. A decline in respiratory chain Complex I and Complex IV activity is associated with ageing [38]. Damage of mitochondrial electron transport may be an important factor in the pathogenesis of neurodegenerative. Increased oxidative stress in consequence of unproportional ROS production is considered a main feature in the pathogenesis of neurodegenerative diseases [16, 141]. Apoptosis is an important mechanism of neuronal loss in age-related neurodegenerative diseases [38, 141]. Neuronal apoptosis in age-associated neurodegenerative disorders can be triggered by oxidative damage of proteins, lipids and DNA, metabolic compromise resulting from impaired glucose metabolism and mitochondrial dysfunction, and over activation of glutamate receptors resulting in disruption of neuronal calcium homeostasis. Several different kind of oxidative protein and lipid damages were observed in brain during ageing as well as increased generation of reactive oxygen species [59, 138, 144, 153, 154]. Increasing protein oxidation and lipid peroxidation can participate on the age-related brain cell dysfunction. There are many studies demonstrated elevated concentration of different ROS and decreased antioxidant status during ageing and in neurodegenerative disorders but majority of them are determined on animal models or cell lines. We are still limited in human studies especially in the case of neurodegenerative disorders; and ethnicity, environment and life style may be responsible for controversial results.

2.1. Protein oxidation

One of the important targets of oxidative damage can be proteins which play elementary roles such as biological accelerators, gene regulators, receptors, transport proteins and structural components of cells. Oxidative modification of proteins by reactive oxygen species or by other reactive molecules (e.g. products of lipid peroxidation) is implicated in aetiology or development of many diseases and it can also contribute to secondary damage of other molecules. Damage of DNA repair enzymes could raise levels of DNA oxidative damage and increase of mutation frequency. DNA polymerase damage might result in decreasing of fidelity in replicating DNA. Endogenous proteins are very sensitive to free radical modification as by by-products of normal metabolic processes or after exposition to oxidative stress *in vivo* or *in vitro* [48, 64, 86]. ROS-associated protein modification can lead to loss of biological functions and to the change of protein forms. Modified proteins have increased sensitivity to intracellular proteolysis [176] and they are quickly degraded by endogenous proteases, particularly by multi-catalytic system [45]. Reactive oxygen species can react directly with proteins or they can react with molecules such as saccharides and lipids forming reactive products, which consecutively attack proteins. Reactions are often influenced by redox cycle of metal cations, particularly by iron and copper. Proteins can go through many covalent changes after exposing to oxidants [98]. Some of this alternations result from direct attacks of ROS on protein molecule; meanwhile another changes are produced indirectly [110]. Protein oxidation can lead to the amino acid side chain residues oxidation. All protein amino acid residues are sensitive to oxidative damage by hydroxyl radical that is generated by radiation but no all products generated during oxidation of some amino acid residues were absolutely characterised. However, tyrosine, phenylalanine, tryptophan, histidine, methionine and cysteine are preferred target of $^{\bullet}OH$ attack [38]. In consequence of $^{\bullet}OH$ attack of side chains in presence of oxygen can form hydroperoxides, alcohols and carbonyl compounds [39]. Proteins can contain after ROS attack new functional groups (hydroxyl and carbonyl groups) [22]. Protein oxidation can lead to the breaking of peptide bounds (formation of products with lower molecular weight) and to the formation of protein-protein cross-links (formation of products with higher molecular weight) and to the protein netting. These changes can result in different secondary effects including protein fragmentation, aggregation and unfolding. These processes are ordinarily connected with loss or change of protein activity and function [11, 102]. Increased oxidative damage of proteins result in:

- an increased production of reactive oxygen species [77],
- a decreased capacity to scavenge reactive oxygen species,

- an increased sensitivity of damaged proteins to become oxidized as a consequence of transcriptional and translational errors [1],
- a decreased levels or activities of the proteasome or proteases which degrade oxidized proteins [24].

2.2. Lipid peroxidation

Lipid peroxidation is an example of oxidative damage of cell membranes, lipoproteins and other lipid containing structures. This oxidative damage is degenerative process, which affects cellular membranes under conditions of oxidative stress [136]. Membranes are particularly sensitive to oxidative damage because they are rich on two or more carbon-carbon double bonds -C=C- [148]. During lipid peroxidation, polyunsaturated higher fatty acids are damaged in auto-catalytic, uncontrolled process which result is production of hydroperoxides of membrane lipids and wide spectrum of secondary metabolites including different aldehydes. Aldehyde products of lipoperoxidation may interact with mitochondrial membrane lipids and can change physiochemical state of membrane [150]. The major components of biological membranes are lipids and proteins. The amount of proteins is increasing with the number of functions that are on membranes performed. Lipid peroxidation can therefore cause damage of membrane proteins as well as lipids. Lipoproteins are also target of oxidative damage. Lipid hydroperoxides are primary products of lipid peroxidation. Dissociation of hydroperoxides is important from toxicological point of view for two reasons:

- new radicals are generated and ramify radical reactions,
- non-radical products are produced which can be also biologically active.

It was found, that lipid peroxidation produces: unsaturated aldehydes, malondialdehyde, 4-hydroxy-2-nonenal (HNE) and other products that are cytotoxic and mutagenic and can damaged other biomolecules [91]. Malondialdehyde arises largely from peroxidation of polyunsaturated fatty acids with more than two double bonds and it can also arise enzymatically during eicosanoid metabolism. 4-hydroxy-2-nonenal has toxic property like cell growth inhibition, genotoxicity, chemotaxic activity and able ability to modify lipoproteins and promote atherosclerosis [51]. It is able react with nucleofil components largely with metabolites and proteins contained thiol groups [50]. Effect of HNE is depending on its concentration. Lipid peroxidation can be overly destructive process in living system. It damages biological membrane thereby are changed their biophysiological properties. Aldehyde products of lipoperoxidation reacted with mitochondria membrane lipids and can change physiochemical state of membrane [28]. Peroxidation of membrane phospholipids is accompanied by change structural and functional characteristics of membranes. Lipid peroxidation impacts also function of proteins that are component of biological membranes. Consequence of near physiological junction lipids and proteins can lead oxidative damage of mitochondrial proteins to form proteins cross linkage, protein degradation or to lose of their function [166]. Oxidative damage can be established into proteins with reaction with aldehydes arisen during lipid peroxidation. For example HNE or malondialdehyde can react with ε-amino group of lysine, with thiol group of cysteine and with imidazol group of histidine [16].

2.3. Oxidative damage of DNA

Nucleic acids are particularly sensitive to oxidative damage. There is increasing evidence that ROS are involved in the development of cancer, not only by direct effects on DNA but also by affecting signal transduction, cell proliferation, cell death and intracellular communication. ROS can damage DNA by direct chemical attack of purine and pyrimidine bases and deoxyribose sugars and also by indirect mechanisms. There is a known more than 20 product of oxidative damage of the nucleic acids.

Superoxide, nitric oxide or hydrogen peroxide at physiologically relevant levels do not react with any of DNA or RNA bases or with the ribose or deoxyribose sugars at significant rates. Particularly hydroxyl radical is known to cause chemical modifications of DNA through the formation of one strand and two strands breaks and cross linkages with other molecules. Different saccharides radicals of DNA can arise by abstraction of a hydrogen atom from 2`deoxyribose because all positions in saccharides are susceptible to oxidative damage. Hydroxyl radical reacts with aromatic rings therefore also nitrogen bases of nucleic acids are modified. C5-C6 double bonds of pyrimidines and carbon atoms C4, C5, and C8 of purines are the most sensitive position to oxidative effect of hydroxyl radical and hydroxyl radical abstract electron and no hydrogen atom [169]. In consequence of ROS attack to nuclear proteins are generated protein radicals and radicals of base react under formation of DNA-protein cross-linking.

Mitochondrial DNA (mtDNA) is excessively sensitive on an oxidative damage because mtDNA is situated near inner mitochondrial membrane, where are formed ROS. Mitochondrial DNA is small and is not protected by histones like nuclear DNA. Mitochondria are able repair an oxidative damage of mtDNA and that base excise repair pathway plays a dominant role in mtDNA repair [36]. Damage of mtDNA can be potentially more important like damage of nuclear DNA because all mitochondrial genome code genes which are expressed whereas nuclear DNA includes great number of untranscribed sequences [166]. Linnane and co-workers [101] assume that accumulation of somatic mutations mtDNA is the main origin of human ageing and degenerative diseases.

3. Antioxidant defence

In consequence, imbalance between pro-oxidant and antioxidant in favour of pro-oxidants and their harmful effects, oxidative stress is increased. Cells possess antioxidant defence systems: enzymatic and non-enzymatic [15]. Antioxidants can work at various levels:

- protection the organism from the formation of reactive oxygen species,
- elimination of reactive oxygen species by conversion to un-radical molecules or to less reactive ROS,
- reparation of damaged molecules and cell structures,
- removing of oxidised molecules.

The most important enzymatic antioxidants are: superoxide dismutase, catalase and glutathione peroxidase. Superoxide dismutase (SOD, EC 1.15.1.1) is universal enzymatic antioxidant. This enzyme is extremely efficient and catalyses the neutralization of superoxide anion to oxygen and hydrogen peroxide. There are three major families of superoxide dismutase, depending on the metal cofactor: Cu/Zn (which binds both copper and zinc), Fe and Mn types (which bind either iron or manganese), and the Ni type, which binds nickel. In humans three form of SOD are present: cytoplasmic Cu/Zn-SOD (SOD1), mitochondrial Mn-SOD (SOD2), and extracellular Cu/Zn-SOD (ECSOD, SOD3). Catalase (CAT, EC 1.11.1.6) is a common antioxidant enzyme responsible for controlling hydrogen peroxide concentrations in cells. Catalase as an intracellular antioxidant enzyme catalyzes the decomposition of two molecules of hydrogen peroxide into one molecule of oxygen and two of water and its activity is genetically determined. Glutathione peroxidases (GPXs, EC 1.11.1.9) are family of enzymes ubiquitously distributed which have peroxidase activity whose main biological role is to protect the organism from oxidative damage. Glutathione peroxidases reduce hydrogen peroxide to water and reduced glutathione and lipid hydroperoxides to their corresponding alcohols, water and reduced glutathione. Four types of GPXs have been identified: cellular GPX, gastrointestinal GPX, extracellular GPX, and phospholipid hydroperoxide GPX [161]. Other an essential part of defence mechanism is a super-family of enzymes called glutathione transferases (GSTs, EC 2.5.1.18). These enzymes are involved in the cellular detoxification of various electrophilic xenobiotic substances such as chemical carcinogens, environmental pollutants, drugs and antitumor agents. These enzymes also inactivate endogenous α,β-unsaturated aldehydes, quinone, epoxides, and hydroperoxides formed as secondary metabolites during oxidative damage. GSTs may reduce reactive oxygen species to less reactive metabolites and protect organism against consequences of lipid peroxidation. Heme oxygenase (heat shock protein 32, HO; EC 1.14.99.3) plays an important role in organism defence to oxidative stress [114] and inflammation [111]. There are known three isoforms of HO: HO-1, HO-2, and HO-3. HO-1 is activated by a lot of inflammatory mediators, reactive oxygen species and by other stimuli [109, 135]. Upregulation of HO-1 is accepted as a sensitive marker of oxidative stress. Oxidative modified DNA can be repaired by several enzymes such as glycosylases: 8-oxoguanine-DNA-glysocylase (OGG1, EC 4.2.99.18), Nei-like protein 1 and 2 (NEIL, EC 4.2.99.18); Apurinic/apyrimidinic endonuclease 1 (APE 1, EC 4.2.99.18), X ray repair cross-complementing group 1 (XRCC 1, EC 4.2.99.18) and poly(ADP-ribose) polymerase-1 (PARP 1, EC 2.4.2.30). OGG1 removes 8-oxoguanine paired with a cytosine. Human *OGG1* gene consists of eight exons which can be alternatively spliced to produce different isoforms. The most abundant mRNAs of OGG1 are type 1a and 2a. These two isoforms are ubiquitously expressed in human tissues.

4. Alzheimer`s disease

Ageing is the main risk factor of neurodegenerative disorders. Approximately 5% of people in age 65 years have Alzheimer`s disease (AD) and the prevalence of this disease increases with increasing age from 19% to 30% after 75 years of age. Overall, 90-95% of Alzheimer`s disease represents a sporadic form and 5-10% represents familiar form. Alzheimer`s disease is neurodegenerative disorder characterised by cognitive failures, impairment of memory and by dramatic changes in behaviour. AD symptoms may include:

- loss of memory,
- difficulty in finding the right words or understanding what people are saying,
- difficulty in performing previously routine tasks, and activities,
- problems with language,
- personality and mood changes.

Although the cause or causes of Alzheimer's disease are not yet known, most experts agree that AD, like other common chronic conditions, probably develops as a result of multiple factors rather than a single cause.

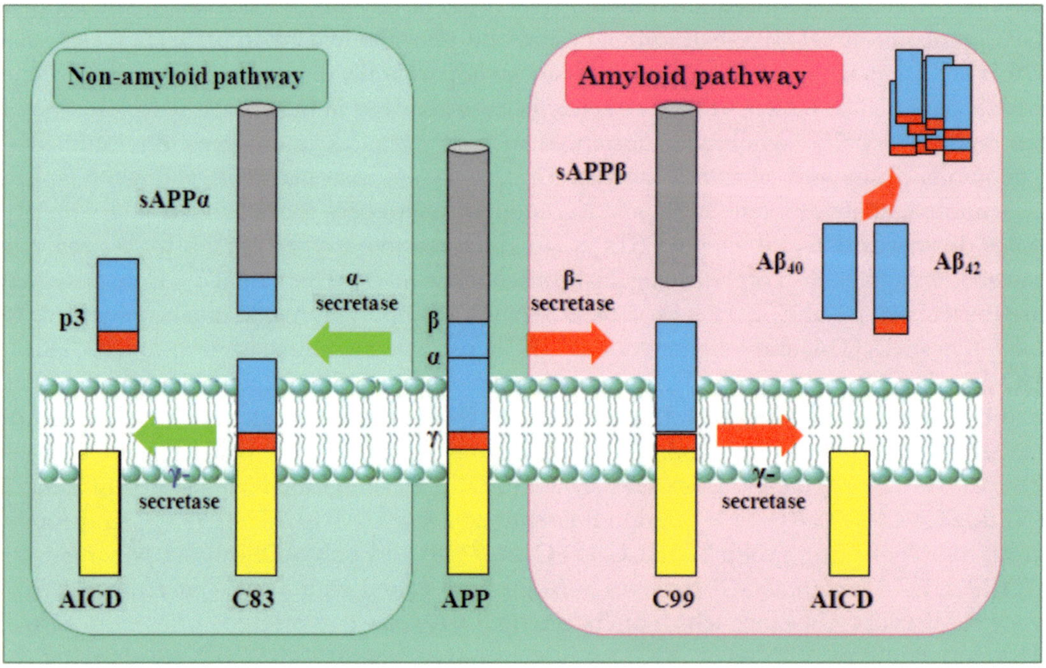

Figure 4. Processing of amyloid precursor protein (APP). Non-amyloid pathway of APP starts by α-secretase cleavage and continues by γ-secretase. Non toxic a soluble fragment of amyloid precursor protein (sAPPα), a small peptide (p3) and an amyloid intracellular domain (ACID) are produced. Amyloid pathway starts with β–secretase cleavage and after that it continues by γ–secretase. A soluble fragment of amyloid precursor protein (sAPPβ), a toxic amyloid β peptide (Aβ) and an amyloid intracellular domain are generated. Amyloid β peptide can be degradated or accumulated and therefore can be responsible for generation of amyloid plaques.

For Alzheimer`s disease many neurochemical and pathological changes are characteristic such as gliosis, tissue atrophy caused by loss of synapses which is the most striking in frontal and temporal parts of brain cortex and by formation of two main protein clusters in extracellular and intracellular region of brain. Extracellular deposits or senile amyloid plaques occur the most frequently in neocortex. Primary they are consisting of 4 kDa, 40-42 amino acid polypeptide chain called amyloid β peptide (Aβ) [66]. Intracellular deposits represent neurofibrillar tangles which are generated from filaments of microtubullar hyperphosphorylated tau protein [4, 70, 99]. Amyloid plaques are example of a specific damage that is characteristic for AD while neurofibrillar tangles are present in different neurodegenerative pathological situations [134]. Created aggregates are involved in a process which leads to progressive degeneration and to neuron death. In the past decade, a significant body of evidence has pointed the attention to the amyloid processing of amyloid precurcor protein - "amyloid cascade" (fig. 4). This event is the major causative factor in AD.

Pathogenesis of AD is complex and involves many molecular, cellular, biochemical and physiological pathologies [9]. Alzheimer`s disease is a characteristic process with identifiable clinical state which are in a continuity with normal ageing process. It is a multifactorial disease and genetic as well as environmental factors are included in its pathogenesis. Whereas majority of AD is sporadic 5% is caused by mutations (familiar AD). There was observed a large loss of synapses and a neuronal death in a part of brain which is crucial for cognitive function including cerebral cortex, entorhinal cartex and hippocampus. Senile plaques created by deposits of amyloid fibres were localized in the brain.

4.1. Oxidative damage and Alzheimer`s disease

Reactive oxygen species probably play an important role in the generation of amyloid plaques, the development of neurofibrillary tangles and the neurodegenerative process itself. Age-related accumulation of reactive oxygen species results in damage to nuclear and mitochondrial DNA, lipids (lipid peroxidation), proteins (protein oxidation), and sugars (advanced glycosylation end products). Oxidative damage caused by reactive oxygen species can account for the vastly heterogeneous nature of Alzheimer`s disease. Several different kind of oxidative protein and lipid damages were observed in brain during ageing as well as increased generation of reactive oxygen species [1, 24, 136, 147, 150]. We have found increased lipid peroxidation, accompanied by accumulation of conjugates of lipid peroxidation products with proteins, formation of dityrosines, loss of sulfhydryl groups and change in ANS (fluorescent probe 1-anilino-8-naphthalenesulfonate) in the ageing rat brain [7]. Keller et al. [91] observed that 4-hydroxy-2-nonenal damage a glutamate transport in synaptosome and mitochondrial function in brain. Increasing lipid peroxidation can participate on the age-related brain cell dysfunction. Recently, several reports have suggested that mitochondrial abnormalities and oxidative stress play a role in sporadic Alzheimer`s disease [26, 89, 132, 158, 181]. In brain tissue from Alzheimer`s disease patients, there are increased levels of markers of oxidative stress, including oxidized proteins, membrane lipids, and DNA [121, 127, 147, 148]. Oxidative modification of biomolecules is a marking process for the targeting of proteases. In the process of ageing there is a marked decrease in protease activity, damaged molecules can be cumulated with age and it may contribute to the age-related neurodegenerative diseases, including Alzheimer`s disease.

Brain and cerebral blood vessel deposits of amyloid β peptide are the main signs of Alzheimer`s disease. Experimental and clinical studies showed an causal relationship between an accumulation of amyloid β peptide and origin of Alzheimer`s disease [25, 63, 73]. An abnormal production of amyloid β peptide or disturbed amyloid β peptide degradation can cause a pathological accumulation of amyloid β peptide and subsequent production of amyloid plaques [182]. It is suggested hypothesis that amyloid β peptide cause neuronal damage and cognitive failure via the generation of reactive oxygen species, mitochondrial oxidative damage, synaptic failure, and by inflammation changing in the brains of Alzheimer`s disease patients [133, 140, 158, 160]. Several *in vitro* studies have shown that synthetic amyloid β peptide facilitates the production of reactive oxygen species [12, 78, 132]. It was observed increased levels of soluble amyloid precursor protein in plasma and cerebrospinal fluid with advancing age [88, 106]. Increased level of soluble amyloid precursor protein may be a sorce of amyloid β peptide in the brain and vessels. Pluta et al. [126] demonstrated a transit of amyloid β peptide through the blood brain barrier. Expression of amyloid precursor protein, α-secretase, β-secretase, enothelin-converting enzyme, neprilysin as well as insulin-degrading enzyme was demonstrated at the brain barrier system [35]. It is possible that 80% of amyloid plaques in transgenic models Alzheimer`s disease [44] and 90% of human amyloid plaques is in a contact with capillaries [87]. Transit of amyloid β peptide or fragments of amyloid precursor protein from blood to the endothelial cells and brain parenchyma can cause changes in the vascular elasticity [127, 162] or can have direct pathological implications in the brain tissue. Changes in the brain blood vessels after brain attack or during the ageing process can cooperate in the pathogenesis and development of Alzheimer`s disease. Beta-secretase (BACE1) expression and its mediated β-site amyloid precursor protein cleavage activity appear to be tightly coupled to mitochondrial function. Beta-secretase upregulation may be a common consequence in various potential Alzheimer`s disease-related etiological conditions that involve energy insufficiency and/or oxidative stress [174]. *Post mortem* analysis of Alzheimer`s disease patients showed increased level of β-secretase [100, 163] and it can be responsible for an accumulation of amyloid plaques [179] and amyloid cascade. Reactive oxygen species that are generated due to ageing can activate β-secretase and facilitate the cleavage of amyloid precursor protein. Amyloid β peptide can be toxic for organism not only for its accumulation and amyloid plaques generation but also for possibility to increase oxidative stress and oxidative damage, to inhibit complexes of respiratory chain in mitochondria, and to inhibit enzymes of Krebs cycle [117, 132, 133, 147, 148]. However clear and exact mechanisms interface between amyloid β peptide and increased oxidative damage are unknown. Oxidative damage of amyloid degrading enzymes can be result of pathological changes of Alzheimer`s disease as well as a contributing factor to amyloid β peptide accumulation and generation of amyloid plaques. During ageing we observed protein and lipid oxidative damage that was caused by increased production of reactive oxygen species and insufficient or inadequate antioxidant defence. Age-related increasing production of reactive oxygen species could be one of a key factor leading to the age-related diseases, including neurodegenerative disease. Elevated oxidative damage and accumulation of amyloid deposits can have repercussion on deepened oxidative damage, preference of amyloid processing of amyloid precursor protein and development of Alzheimer`s disease.

4.2. Alzheimer`s disease and polymorphism in antioxidant enzymes

Oxidative damage is one of the mechanisms which results in stimulation of the amyloid pathway of APP processing therefore genes of antioxidant enzymes could present another group of candidate genes. Superoxide dismutase represents the most important part of an active antioxidant defence. The genes encoding SOD1, SOD2, SOD3 are located in different chromosomes and in all of them polymorphisms have been described. *SOD1* is encoded on 21q22.1, *SOD2* on 6q25.3, and *SOD3* on 4p16.3-q21. Regulation of *SOD* genes plays a crucial role in balancing the reactive oxygen species concentration. In *SOD1* has been observed substitution of A to C at the non-coding position 35. This polymorphism influence SOD1 activity [56]. Substitution T to C at position 24, resulting in a valine to alanine substitution at amino acid 16 has been identified in *SOD2*. In *SOD3* gene has been identified three single nucleotide polymorphism: alanine to threonine substitution at amino acid 40, phenylalanine to cysteine at amino acid 131, and finally the most studied polymorphism which represents substitution of arginine to glycine at amino acid 213. It has been observed no linkage between AD polymorphism in *SOD1* [37, 105]. It was observed that three polymorphisms in *SOD2* can be associated with development of AD [173].

Catalase is a common antioxidant enzyme responsible for controlling hydrogen peroxide concentrations in cells. The catalase gene is located on chromosome 11p13. There are known different polymorphisms of this enzyme in coding regions [67, 93] and in non-coding regions as well [27, 58, 68, 93, 164, 180]. A common polymorphism in the promoter region of the catalase gene consists of a C to T substitution at position -262 in the 5' region [58], which is thought to result in reduced activity. Catalase gene polymorphism does not confirm a protective role in AD patients.

Glutathione transferases have historically also been called glutathione-S-transferases, and it is this latter name that gives rise to the widely used abbrevation, GST. Three major families of proteins the cytosolic, mitochondrial and microsomal (membrane-associated proteins in eicosanoids and glutathione metabolism, MAPEG) are known. In some organisms expression of *GSTs* are upregulated by exposure to prooxidants [6, 41, 167]. Seven classes of cytosolic glutathione transferases are recognising in mammals (Alpha, Mu, Pi, Sigma, Theta, Omega, and Zeta) [76]. At least 16 cytosolic GST subunits exist in human and display polymorphisms, and this is probably to contribute to interindividual differences in responses to diseases and xenobiotics. *GSTM1* is one of the genes encoding the Mu class of enzymes. Gene for GSTM1 has been mapped to glutathione transferase mu gene cluster on chromosome 1p13.3. Three polymorphisms of *GSTM1* have been identified: a substitution (*GSTM1A* and *GSTM1B*) and a deletion [131, 175]. The alleles of the substitution variant differ by C to G transition at base position 534, resulting in a lysine to asparagine substitution at amino acid 172 [34, 75]. There is no evidence to date that *GSTM1A* and *GSTM1B* alleles are functionally different from one another; thus these alleles are typically categorized together as a single functional phenotype. Other polymorphism is a deletion – *GSTM1* null variant that results in a lack of functional gene product and null genotype of GSTM1 was shown as a risk factor in Italian AD patients. The *GSTT1* gene is located at 22q11.2. Absence of both alleles for this gene represents null variant analogous to *GSTM1*. Deletion of whole gene results in the lack of enzymatic activity [152].

Gene for GSTP1 is one of the most intensive studying genes of glutathione transferase family and has been mapped on chromosome 11q13 and comprising nine exons. There are known two polymorphisms of *GSTP1*: substitution of isoleucine to valine at amino acid 105 and alanine to valine at amino acid 114, demonstrating different catalytic efficiencies due to changes in the active site [3]. Polymorphism in *GSTP1* may represent risk factor for AD and with advancing age [125, 151]. Presence of gene for GSTM1 and GSTT1 could be a protective factor [125, 157].

The *GPX1* gene is located in the 3p21 locus; the pro198leu polymorphism involves a change of thymine (T) for cytosine (C), which leads to the substitution of leucine (leu) for proline (pro), whose recessive allele leu has been linked to 70% reduction of enzyme activity. The leucine allele of *GPX1* may be a possible risk factor [118].

Subjects carrying the *HO-1* (-413) TT genotype might show a higher AD risk due to their genetic inability to induce a more effective HO-1 protective response [83]. Authors showed that an AD risk effect of *HO-1* (−413) TT genotype is only apparent in the presence of liver X receptor (LXR) LXR-β (intron 2) TT, LXR-β (intron 5) AA, or LXR-β (intron 7) TT genotypes. No genetic association between AD and polymorphisms of heme oxygenase 1 and 2 were observed in a Japanese population [143]. A (GT)n repeat in the human HO-1 gene promoter region is highly polymorphic, although no particular alleles are associated with AD or PD [92].

The DNA base excision repair (BER) pathway is the major pathway responsible for removing oxidative DNA damage caused by oxidative reagents and alkylation and thus protects cells against the toxic effects of endogenous and exogenous agents and this pathway is of particular importance in postmitotic tissues such as brain. The first step in the BER pathway is recognition and removal of the damaged base by a DNA glycosylase. A variety of glycosylases have evolved to recognize oxidized bases, which are commonly formed by reactive oxygen species generated during cellular metabolism. One of them is 8-oxoguanine-DNA-glysocylase (OGG1). The most common polymorphism of *OGG1* is in this gene substitution of serine (Ser) for cysteine (Cys) at codon 326 in exon 7. The variant homozygote is associated with reduced enzymatic activity [94]. Allele and genotype frequencies of *OGG1* were equally distributed between AD patients and healthy subjects [32, 115]. The Arg46Gln polymorphism of *OGG1* is also not associated with the pathogenesis of AD [47]. Mao et al. [104] identified in AD patients deletion in *OGG1* and their results suggest that defects in OGG1 may be important in the pathogenesis of AD in a significant fraction of AD.

Apurinic/apyrimidinic endonuclease 1 (APE1) is an enzyme involved in BER pathway. Its main role in the repair of damaged or mismatched nucleotides in DNA is to create a nick in the phosphodiester backbone of the AP site created when DNA glycosylase removes the damaged base. There are four types of AP endonucleases that have been classified according to their sites of incision. Genetic polymorphism has been identified in *APE1* gene and associated with cancer risk. One of the most studied polymorphism is Asp148Glu. No association was found in AD patients [115].

X-ray repair cross-complementing-1 (XRCC) is a protein, which plays a coordinating role for consecutive stages of the BER system and interacts with several proteins of BER including

http://dx.doi.org/10.5772/54619

hOGG1, APE1, DNA polymerase β (pol β) and DNA ligase IIIα [115]. XRCC1 is recruited to the site of repair till the last stage of ligation, regulating and coordinating the whole process. More than 60 single nucleotide polymorphisms (SNPs) XRCC1 polymorphisms are known but the most common polymorphisms in *XRCC1* gene are: Arg149Trp, Arg280His, and Arg399Gln, and are associated with decreased function of XRCC1. It is unlikely that the XRCC1 Arg194Trp polymorphism plays a major role in the pathogenesis of late-onset AD in elderly Han Chinese [130] but positive association was found in Turkish population [46]. Arg280His, and Arg399Gln were not associated with AD [115].

5. Parkinson´s disease

Parkinson´s disease (PD) was firstly described by James Parkinson in 1817. It is the second most common neurodegenerative disease which affects approximately 1% of the human population aged 65 and more [80]. PD is slowly progressed disorder characterized by selective degeneration and loss of dopaminergic neurons in the *substantia nigra* (SN) *pars compacta* region of the midbrain, as well as with the appearance of intracytoplasmic inclusions known as Lewy bodies [30]. Among clinical symptoms of the disease belong rigidity, resting tremor, bradykinesia and postural imbalance [139]. Beside motor dysfunctions, as the major clinical features, non-motor symptoms, such as sleep disturbances, dementia and depression may be present as well [177].

Familiar PD represents only 5-10% of the total cases of PD. Recently, several gene mutations have been linked with rare familiar forms of PD (e.g. α-synuclein, parkin, nuclear receptor-related 1). The most important in early-onset familiar PD is the parkin gene [40]. So far no genetic changes are definitely connected with sporadic or idiopathic form of the disease. However, the prevalent form of PD appears to be multifactorial and a combination of environmental and genetic factors, together with ageing, may contribute to the development of the disease. Biochemical abnormalities that have been detected in sporadic PD include: oxidative stress [108, 124, 168], mitochondrial and proteasomal dysfunction [116, 142] and glutathione depletion [10, 177].

5.1. Oxidative damage and Parkinson´s disease

Although the primary cause of PD is still unknown, oxidative stress together with mitochondrial dysfunction are thought to be significantly implicated in the neurodegenerative process. Excessive formation of reactive oxygen and nitrogen species in PD may damage cellular components such as lipids, proteins and DNA. Increased lipid peroxidation, measured by increased amounts of malondialdehyde [42] and 4-hydroxynonenal, as well as increase in the extent of protein oxidation and elevated concentration of 8-hydroxy-2´-deoxyguanosine, a product of DNA oxidation [84], in SN provides direct evidence of oxidative damage [43].

Since majority of all oxygen is used in mitochondria, electron transport chain is major source of free radicals. Recent research confirmed that about 1-2% of total molecular oxygen is converted into reactive oxygen species [23]. Post-mortem studies on patients with

PD have revealed a specific decrease in the activity of NADPH dehydrogenase (complex I). The alterations in complex I activity were not detected in other regions of the brain, as well as in other neurodegenerative diseases [142]. Complex I deficiency could contribute to neurodegeneration in PD not only due to decreased ATP synthesis but also increased ROS production [11, 137]. Van der Walt et al. [165] also published that the 10398G polymorphism within NADH dehydrogenase 3 may provide significant protection against developing PD in Caucasian populations.

Alternatively, ROS may arise during metabolism of dopamine. Autooxidation of dopamine and its polymerization into neuromelanin produces electrophilic semiquinones and quinones, which can contribute to ROS production, especially superoxide anion radicals [60]. It is also known that dopamine is able to coordinate iron and generate Fe^{2+}, providing an important source of hydroxyl and superoxide radical production [13]. In generally, elevated iron levels were observed in *substantia nigra* in PD [149]. A major source of increased iron levels during PD is microglial activation which induces iron release and free radical production [123]. Free iron may promote already mentioned autooxidation of dopamine [14]. Oxidative stress induced by elevated levels of free iron also appears to promote α-synuclein (a prominent component of Lewy bodies) aggregation, the major histopathological hallmark of PD [75].

Important role in protection of dopaminergic neurons against oxidative stress plays the antioxidant molecule glutathione (GSH). GSH removes H_2O_2, which is produced during cellular metabolism. Perry et al. [121] firstly reported decreased levels of total GSH in autopsied brains from PD patients. Total GSH is reported to be decreased by 40-50% specifically in nigral dopaminergic neurons [119]. GSH depletion also appears to correlate with the severity of the disease and is the earliest known marker of oxidative stress and indicator of degeneration of nigral neurons [85]. On the other hand, Mythri et al. [108] observed 3-5 fold increase in total GSH levels in all the non-SN regions of tested PD brains compared to control samples. On the contrary, they found no significant changes in the levels of protein carbonyls, as markers of protein oxidation, or nitrosative stress markers. According to these results, they expected that specific signals from the degenerating dopaminergic SN neurons might induce elevated levels of GSH and such prevent oxidative damage [108]. Beside GSH, other antioxidant activities are altered in the SN. The levels of antioxidant enzymes, such as superoxide dismutase, catalase, glutathione peroxidase and glutathione reductase, were found to be changed in SN [168].

5.2. Parkinson´s disease and polymorphism in antioxidant enzymes

Current research shows that ROS and oxidative damage are part of pathological processes during PD, but it remains to be determined whether this is a primary event or a consequence of other cellular dysfunctions. Analysis of polymorphisms of detoxifying enzymes may help to clarify whether PD may be caused by a genetic predisposition to oxidative stress.

Among antioxidant enzymes, superoxide dismutase (SOD) represents the first line of defence. From three different SOD isoenzymes, SOD2 appears to be the most relevant in PD because of its mitochondrial localization. Several research groups confirmed that *SOD2* (Ala9Val) polymorphism is not significantly associated with PD in Caucasian population [52, 69, 146]. On the other hand, some studies, especially on Asian population, found higher Ala allele frequency in the group of PD patients [57, 172]. Observed results might be explained by ethnic differences in genotypes frequencies.

Little is known about the association of catalase polymorphisms and PD. However, Parboosingh et al. [113] observed no connection between mutations of catalase gene and PD.

Glutathione transferases (GST) are the most studied phase II detoxification enzymes. Activity of GST was observed to be reduced in substantia nigra of PD [145]. Studies of *GST* polymorphisms and PD yielded mixed results. Several studies confirmed positive association between *GSTM1* and *GSTT1* null genotypes and higher risk of PD [120, 157]. On the other hand, other studies found no association [90, 171]. Similarly, *GSTP1* was detected to have only a minor role in PD [90,, 171]. However, Wahner et al. [90] noted a 32% risk reduction among Caucasian PD patients carrying at least one *GSTO1* and *GSTO2* variant allele.

Markedly elevated expression of heme oxygenase 1 was observed in PD and it has been shown that its overexpression may protect neurons against oxidative stress-induced toxicity [81]. However, Funke et al. [61] found no association of (GT)n fragment length polymorphism in the promoter region, as well as three other coding SNPs with PD.

Since increased 8-oxo-guanine levels have been observed in PD patients, still more attention is paid to analysis of genetic polymorphisms of oxoguanine DNA glycosylase (OGG1), which removes oxidized guanine from DNA. Coppede et al. [33] published that *hOGG1* Ser326Cys polymorphism is not associated with sporadic form of PD.

6. Huntington`s disease

Huntington`s disease (HD) is an autosomal dominant inherited neurodegenerative disorder of the central nervous system. Worldwide prevalence of HD is 5 to 8 per 100,000 people with no gender preponderance [74]. HD is characterized by cognitive and memory dysfunctions, weight loss, and choreiform movements. It is caused by an expansion of a polymorphic three nucleotide repeat sequence CAG in the exon 1 of the gene coding for the protein huntingtin (htt) on chromosome 4 (4p16.3) [82]. Wild type htt may exert a variety of intracellular functions such as: protein trafficking, vesicle transport and anchoring to the cytoskeleton, clathrine-mediated endocytosis, postsynaptic signaling, transcriptional regulation, and anti-apoptotic function [65]. For instance, htt is involved in fast axonal transport, enhancing vesicular transport of brain-derived neurotrophic factor along microtubules [62, 159]. The protein htt consists of a series of CAG repeats coding for glutamine residues (polyQ) followed by two short stretches of prolines. Normally, the number of the polyglutamine repeats is 10-29 (median, 18). By contrast, HD patients have expanded numbers of CAG repeats, from 39 to 121 (median, 44). Expanded repeats cause a conformational change in the htt promoting the formation of intracellular aggregates, mainly in medium spiny neurons where the expression of huntingtin is elevated. The number of CAG repeats is inversely correlated with the age of disease onset, and disease progression is rapid in patients with more CAG expansion [96]. In brain, the most remarkable changes are found within the striatum, there is a gradual atrophy of the caudate nucleus and putamen [170].

6.1. Oxidative damage and Huntington`s disease

The generation of reactive oxygen species and the consequent oxidative stress is thought to play a pivotal role in the neurodegeneration observed in HD [53, 71] (Ferrante, Grunewald). Several lines of evidence suggest that not only increased oxidative stress, but also protein metabolism impairment, mitochondrial dysfunction, and they interplay contribute to neuronal dysfunction in HD [18, 19, 112, 128].

DNA fragmentation is significantly increased in human HD patients and correlates with the length of CAG repeats [20]. The oxidation of DNA leads to the formation of the metabolite 8-hydroxy-2`-deoxyguanosine (OHdG) which is a direct result of free radical activity [128]. Significant increases of OHdG levels, coming from nuclear DNA, occur in the caudate nucleus and parietal cortex in postmortem tissue of HD patients [18, 128]. In addition, increased oxidative damage to DNA is present in serum from HD patients [29, 79. Moreover, the improvement of elevated OHdG by creatine treatment suggests OHdG as a promising peripheral biomarker [79]. These findings are in consensus with the elevated levels of OHdG that occur in other neurodegenerative diseases in which oxidative stress is implicated as a pivotal pathogenic mechanism [55]. Nevertheless, some research groups have not confirmed changes in OHdG levels in HD patients [2].

Elevated levels of malondialdehyde (MDA), a marker of lipid peroxidation, have been documented in HD brain [72]. Elevated levels of MDA have also been shown in the peripheral blood of HD patients, and preliminary results suggest that the levels of lipid peroxidation (MDA level) appear to be correlated to disease severity [29, 155]. Reduced activities of erythrocyte glutathione peroxidase and Cu/Zn-superoxid dismutase in HD patients implicate that the defense mechanism is impaired in peripheral blood cells of HD. Because of ubiquitous expression of huntingtin, the peripheral abnormalities may reflect the same consequences to mutant huntingtin in the brain [29]. An abnormal accumulation of lipofuscin, product of unsaturated fatty acid lipid peroxidation, has been proven in HD patients [17]. Supplemental markers of oxidative damage, as for example inducible form of heme oxygenase, 3-nitrotyrosine, and above mentioned malondialdehyde, are elevated in human HD striatum and cortex compared with age-matched control brain specimens [19, 54].

The primary source of reactive oxygen species in neurons is mitochondria. Mitochondrial dysfunction in HD is closely associated with oxidative stress. In was first reflected that here was an energetic impairment in HD, because HD patients exhibit profound weight loss despite continual caloric intake [20, 21]. Lowered glucose utilization in striatum of HD patients early stages prior to pronounced striatal atrophy [97]. Mitochondrial functional abnormalities were observed, such is a defect in succinate dehydrogenase in the caudate of postmortem HD brains. Subsequent studies confirmed that there was a significant decrease in complex II activity in the caudate nucleus, in complex III activity in the caudate and putamen, and of complex IV in the putamen of HD brains [18, 72, 103].

Plasma lipid peroxide and lactate concentrations as indicators of oxidative stress and mitochondrial dysfunction, were significantly elevated in HD patients. On contrary, aspartate and glutamate aminopeptidase activities were significantly reduced in HD patients. These changes may be related to the progression of the disease [49].

6.2. Polymorphisms and Huntington`s disease

Besides CAG repetition in huntingtin gene, there are 2 genetic polymorphisms in the full-length htt gene. One of them, named CCG polymorphism is located in the first proline-rich fragment, second one is delta 2642 glutamic acid polymorphism. Previous studies have shown that alleles with 7 or 10 repeats are predominant in CGG polymorphism, but the distribution from among ethnics is variable. In western population is strong association between the 7 repeat CCG allele and HD [156]. On contrary, in Japanese population has been shown association with the 10 repeat CCG allele and HD [107]. Latest study performed on Chinese population compared the clinical features between the 7 and 10 repeats CCG alleles, but did not find any statistical significant results [178].

It was proposed a model that somatic expansion of CAG repeats in HD cells might contribute to disease onset and progression of HD and is mediated by the DNA repair oxoguanine glycosylase 1 (OGG1) enzyme [95]. This enzyme removes 8-oxoguanine from the DNA. Study of the *hOGG1* Ser326Cys polymorphism performed on 91 patients showed that bearers of mutant Cys allele appear to have an increased number of the CAG repeats of the expanded HD allele. Since this is the first evidence of an association between the hOGG1 genotype and both CAG repeat length and age at onset of the HD, for confirmation, further studies are required [31].

7. Conclusions

Population ages therefore neurodegenerative diseases are in a centre of interest. Several studies showed that missing antioxidant genes may have negative effect on central nervous system and may represent a risk for development of neurodegenerative diseases. Unfortunately majority of results are from animals and cell tissue studies. Animal studies, in vitro and ex vivo studies are full of positive effects of single antioxidant gene overexpression such as superoxide dismutase, catalase and antioxidant therapy may represent promising treatment. Molecular and genetic analyses represent a new potential for neurodegenerative diseases studying. The role of gene polymorphisms and many others gene polymorphisms as risk factors for the occurrence of neurodegenerative diseases are still controversial. Moreover impact of gene polymorphisms can depend on several different factors, especially for neurodegenerative diseases, such as ethnicity, social environment, life style. We need new studies for clear determination of antioxidant gene polymorphisms. Moreover multiple genotype analyses are necessary as well because a single gene polymorphism can be without relationship to increased risk of neurodegenerative disorders but the combination of gene polymorphisms may have significant effect, positive or negative.

Acknowledgements

Project was supported by grants VEGA 1/0071/11 and Ministry of Health 2007/57- UK-17.

Author details

Eva Babusikova, Andrea Evinova, Jozef Hatok, Dusan Dobrota and Jana Jurecekova

Comenius University in Bratislava, Jessenius Faculty of Medicine in Martin, Department of Medical Biochemistry, Martin, Slovakia

References

[1] Agarwal S, Sohal RS. Relationship between susceptibility to protein oxidation, aging, and maximum life span potential of different species. Experimental Gerontology (1996); 31(3), 387-392.

[2] Alam ZI, Halliwell B, Jenner P. No evidence for increased oxidative damage to lipids, proteins, or DNA in Huntington's disease. Journal of Neurochemistry, 2000; 75(2), 840–846.

[3] Ali-Osman F, Akande O, Antoun G, Mao JX, Buolamwini J. Molecular cloning, characterization, and expression in Escherichia coli of full-length cDNAs of three human glutathione S-transferase Pi gene variants. Evidence for differential catalytic activity of the encoded proteins. The Journal of Biological Chemistry, 1997; 272(15), 10004-10012.

[4] Alonso AC, Li B, Grundke-Iqbal I, Iqbal K. Mechanis, of tau-induced neurodegeneration in Alzheimer disease and related tauopathies. Current Alzheimer Research, 2008; 5(4), 375-384.

[5] Ames BN, Shigenaga MK, Hagen TM. Oxidants, antioxidants, and the degenerative diseases of aging. Proceedings of the National Acadademy of the Sciences of the United States of America, 1993; 90(17), 7915-7922.

[6] An JH, Blackwell TK. SKN-1 links C. elegans mesendodermal specification to a conserved oxidative stress response. Genes and Development, 2003; 17(15), 1882-1893.

[7] Babusikova E, Hatok J, Dobrota D., Kaplan P. Age-related oxidative modifications of proteins and lipids in rat brain. Neurochemical Research, (2007); 32(8), 1351-1356.

[8] Babusikova E., Jesenak M. Mitochondria and Ageing: Do Mitochondria Play a Key Role? In: Svensson OL. (ed.) Mitochondria: Structure, Functions and Dysfunctions. New York: Nova Science; 2011. p377-410.

[9] Babusikova E., Evinova A., Jurecekova J., Jesenak M., Dobrota D. Alzheimer's disease: Definition, molecular and genetic factors. In: Chang R.Ch.-Ch. (ed.) Understanding of neurodegenerative diseases. Rijeka: InTech; 2011. p3-28.

[10] Barath S, Hsu M, Kaur D, Rajagopalan, Andersen JK. Glutathione, iron and Parkinson´s disease. Biochemical Pharmacology, 2002; 64(5-6), 1037-1048.

[11] Beal MF. Mitochondria take center stage in aging and neurodegeneration. Annals of Neurology, 2005; 58(4), 495-505.

[12] Behl C, Davis JB, Lesley R, Schubert B. Hydrogen peroxide mediates amyloid beta protein toxicity. Cell, 1994; 77(6), 817-827

[13] Ben-Shachar D, Youdim MBH. Iron, melanin and dopamine interaction:relevance to Parkinson´s disease. Progress in Neuro-Psychopharmacology and Biological Psychiatry, 1993; 17(1), 139-150.

[14] Berg D, Gerlach M, Youdim MB, Double KL, Zecca L, Riederer P, Becker G. Brain iron pathways and their prevalence to Parkinson´s disease. Journal of Neurochemistry, 2001; 79(2), 225-236.

[15] Bergendi L, Benes L, Durackova Z, Ferencik M. Chemistry, physiology and pathology of free radicals. Life Sciences 1999; 65(18-19), 1865-1874.

[16] Berlett BS, Stadtman ER. Protein oxidation in aging, disease, and oxidative stress. The Journal of Biological Chemistry, 1997; 272(33), 20313-20316.

[17] Braak H, Braak E. Allocortical involvement in Huntington's disease. Neuropathology and Applied Neurobiology, 1992; 18(6), 539–547.

[18] Browne SE, Bowling AC, Macgarvey U, Baik MJ, Berger SC, Muqit MM, Bird ED, Beal MF. Oxidative damage and metabolic dysfunction in Huntington's disease: Selective vulnerability of the basal ganglia. Annals of Neurology, 1997; 41(5), 646–653.

[19] Browne SE, Ferrante RJ, Beal MF. Oxidative stress in Huntington's disease. Brain Pathology, 1999; 9, 147–163.

[20] Browne SE, Beal MF. The energetics of Huntington's disease, Neurochemical Research, 2004; 29(3), 531–546.

[21] Browne SE. Mitochondria and Huntington's disease pathogenesis. Insight from Genetic and Chemical Models, Annals of the New York Acadademy of Sciences. 2008;1147, 358–382.

[22] Byrne E. Does mitochondrial respiratory chain dysfunction have a role in common neurodegenerative disorders? Journal of Clinnal Neuroscience, 2002; 9(5), 497-501.

[23] Cadenas E, Davies KJ. Mitochondrial free radical generation, oxidative stress, and aging. Free Radical Biology and Medicine, 2000; 29(3-4), 222-230.

[24] Cakatay U, Telci A, Kayali R, Tekeli R, Akcay T, Sivas A. Relation of oxidative protein damage and nitrotyrosine levels in the aging rat brain. Experimental Gerontology, 2001; 36(2), 221-229.

[25] Carr DB, Goate A, Phil D, Morris JC. Current concepts in the pathogenesis of Alzheimer s disease. The American Journal of Medicine, 1997; 103(3A), 3S-10S.

[26] Cash AD, Perry G, Ogawa O, Raina AK, Zhu X, Smith MA. Is Alzheimer's disease a mitochondrial disorder? The Neuroscientist: A Review Journal Bringing Neurobiology, Neurology and Psychiatry, 2002; 8(5), 489-896.

[27] Casp C., She JX, McCormack WT. Genetic association of the catalase gene (CAT) with vitiligo susceptibility. Pigment Cell Research, 2002; 15(1), 62-66.

[28] Chen JJ, Bertrand H, Yu BP. Inhibition of adenine nucleotide translocator by lipid peroxidation products. Free Radical Biology and Medicine, 1995; 19(5), 583-390.

[29] Chen CM, Wu YR, Cheng ML, Liu JL, Lee YM, Lee PW, Soong BW, Chiu DTY. Increased oxidative damage and mitochondrial abnormalities in the peripheral blood of Huntington's disease patients. Biochemical and Biophysical Research Communications, 2007; 359(2), 335–340.

[30] Chinta JS, Andersen JK. Redox imbalance in Parkinson´s disease. Biochimica et Biophysica Acta, 2008; 1780(11), 1362-1367.

[31] Coppede F, Geravolo R, Migheli F, Fanucchi f, Frosini D, Siciliano G, Bonuccelli U, Migliore L. The hOGG1 Ser326Cys polymorphism is not associated with sporadic Parkinson's disease. Neuroscience Letters, 2010; 473(3), 248-451.

[32] Coppedè F, Mancuso M, Lo Gerfo A, Manca ML, Petrozzi L, Migliore L, Siciliano G, Murri L. A Ser326Cys polymorphism in the DNA repair gene hOGG1 is not associated with sporadic Alzheimer's disease. Neuroscience Letters, 2007; 414(3), 282-285.

[33] Coppede F,Migheli F, Ceravolo R, Bregant E, Rocchi A, Petrozzi L, Unti E, Lonigro R, Siciliano G, Migliore L. The hOGG1 Ser326Cys polymorphism and Huntington's disease. Toxicology, 2010; 278(2), 199–203.

[34] Cotton SC, Sharp L, Little J, Brockton N. Glutathione S-transferase polymorphisms and colorectal cancer: a HuGE review. American Journal of Epidemiology, 2000; 151(1), 7-32.

[35] Crossgrove JS, Smith EL, Zheng W. Macromolecules involved production and metabolism of beta-amyloid at the brain barriers. Brain Research, 2007; 1138, 187-195.

[36] Croteau DL, Bohr VA. Repair of oxidative damage t nuclear and mitochondrial DNA in mammalian cells. The Journal of Biological Chemistry, 1997; 272(41), 25409-25412.

[37] David F, Intrator S, Foncin JF, Salmon D, Lucotte G. Absence of a close linkage between Alzheimer's disease and the polymorphic probe coding for superoxide dismutase 1. Comptes Rendus de l'Académie des Sciences - Series III, 1988; 306(1), 1-4.

[38] Davies KJA. Protein damage and degeneration by oxygen radicals. The Journal of Biological Chemistry, 262, 1987; 9895-9901.

[39] Davies MJ, Fu S, Wang H, Dean RT. Stable markers of oxidant damage to proteins and their application in the study of human disease. Free Radical Biology and Medicine, 1999; 27(11-12), 1151-1163.

[40] Dekker MC, Bonifati V, van Duijn CM. Parkinson's disease: piecing together a genetic jigsaw. Brain, 2003; 126(pt 8), 1722-1733.

[41] Desikan R, A-H-Mackerness S, Hancock JT, Neill SJ. Regulation of the Arabidopsis trancriptome by oxidative stress. Plant Physiology, 2001; 127(1), 159-172.

[42] Dexter DT, Cater AE, Wells FR, Javoy-Agid F, Agid Y, Lees A, Jenner P, Marsden CD. Basal lipid peroxidation in substantia nigra is increased in Parkinson's disease. Journal of Neurochemistry, 1989; 52(2), 381-389.

[43] Dexter DT, Holley AE, Flitter WD, Slatter TF, Wells FR, Daniel SE, Lees AJ, Jenner P, Marsden CD. Increased levels of lipid hydroperoxides in parkinsonian substamtia nigra:an HPLC and ESR study. Movement Disorders, 1994; 9(1), 92-97.

[44] Dickstein DL, Biron KE, Ujiie M, Pfeifer CG, Jeffries AR, Jefferies WA. Abeta peptide immunization restored blood-brain barrier integrity in Alzheimer disease. FASEB J. 2006; 20(3), 426-433.

[45] DiMauro S, Tanji K, Bonilla E, Pallotti F, Schon EA. Mitochondrial abnormalities in muscle and other aging cells: classification, causes, and effects. Muscle Nerve, 2002; 26(5), 597-607.

[46] Doğru-Abbasoğlu S, Aykaç-Toker G, Hanagasi HA, Gürvit H, Emre M, Uysal M. (2007). The Arg194Trp polymorphism in DNA repair gene XRCC1 and the risk for sporadic late-onset Alzheimer's disease. Neurologal Sciences, 2007; 28(1), 31-34.

[47] Dorszewska J, Kempisty B, Jaroszewska-Kolecka J, Rózycka A, Florczak J, Lianeri M, Jagodziński PP, Kozubski W. Expression and polymorphisms of gene 8-oxoguanine glycosylase 1 and the level of oxidative damage in peripheral lood lymphocytes of patients with Alzheimer's disease. DNA Cell Biology, 2009; 28(11), 579-588.

[48] Dukan S, Farewell A, Ballesteros M, Taddei F, Radman M, Nyström T. Protein oxidation in response to increased transcriptional or translational errors. Proceedings of the National Acadademy of the Sciences of the United States of America, 2000; 97(11), 5746-5749.

[49] Duran R, Barrero FJ, Morales B, Luna JD, Ramirez M, Vives F. Oxidative stress and plasma aminopeptidase activity in Huntington's disease. Journal of Neural Transmission, 2010; 117(3), 325–332.

[50] Eaton P, Li J-M, Hearse DJ, Shattock MJ. Formation of 4-hydroxy-2-nonenal-modified proteins in ischemic rat heart. The American Journal of Physiology, 1999; 276(3), H935-H943.

[51] Esterbauer H, Schaur RJ, Zollner H. Chemistry and biochemistry of 4-hydroxynonenal, malondialdehyde and related aldehydes. Free Radical Biology and Medicine, 1991; 11(1), 81-128.

[52] Farin FM, Hitosis Y, Hallagan SE, Kushleika J, Woods JS, Janssen PS, Smith-Weller T, Franklin GM, Swanson PD, Checkoway H. Genetic polymorphism of superoxid dismutase in Parkinson´s disease. Movement Disorders, 2001; 16(4), 705-707.

[53] Ferrante RJ, Beal MF, Kowall NW. Mechanisms of neuronal degeneration in Huntington's disease. In: The Basal Ganglia IV: New Ideas and Data on Structure and Function. G. Percheron, Js. Mckenzie & J. Feger, Eds. Plenum Press. New York, 1994. p149–161

[54] Ferrante RJ, Kowall NW, Hersch SM, et al. 1996. Immunohistochemical localization of markers of oxidative injury in Huntington's disease. 26th Annual Meeting of the Society for Neuroscience. Washington, DC.

[55] Ferrante RJ, Browne SE, Shinobu LA. Bowling AC, Baik MJ, MacGarvey U, Kowall NW, Brown RH Jr, Beal MF. Evidence of increased oxidative damage in both sporadic and familial amyotrophic lateral sclerosis. Journal of Neurochemistry, 1997; 69(5), 2064–2074.

[56] Flekac M, Skrha J, Hilgertova J, Lacinova Z, Jarolimkova M. Gene polymorphisms of superoxide dismutases and catalase in diabetes mellitus. BMC Medical Genetics, 2008; 9(30)

[57] Fong CS, Wu RM, Shieh JC, Chao YT, Fu YP, Kuao CL, Cheng CW. Pesticide exposure on southwestern Taiwanese with MnSOD and NQO1 polymorphisms is associated with increased risk of Parkinson's disease. Clinica Chimica Acta, 2007; 378(1-2), 136-141.

[58] Forsberg L, Lyrenäs L, de Faire U, Morgenstern R. A common functional C-T substitution polymorphism in the promoter region of the human catalase gene influences transcription factor binding, reporter gene transcription and its correlated to blood catalase levels. Free Radical Biology and Medicine, 2001; 30(5), 500-505.

[59] Fu S, Davies J, Dean RT. Molecular aspects of free radical damage to proteins. In: Aruoma OI, and Halliwell B. (eds.) Molecular biology of free radicals in human diseases, 1998. p29-56.

[60] Fukae J, Mizuno Y, Hattori N. Mitochondrial dysfunction in Parkinson´s disease. Mitochondrion, 2007; 7(1-2), 58-62.

[61] Funke C, Tomiuk J, Riess O, Berg D, Soehn AS. Genetic analysis of heme oxygenase-1 (HO-1) in German Parkinson's disease patients. Journal of Neural Transmission, 2009; 116(7), 853-859.

[62] Gauthier LR, Charrin BC, Borrell-Pages M, Dompierre JP, Rangone H, Cordelières FP, De Mey, J, MacDonald ME, Lessmann V, Humbert S, Saudou F. Huntingtin controls neurotrophic support and survival of neurons by enhancing BDNF vesicular transport along microtubules. Cell, 2004; 118 (1), 127–138.

[63] Ghiso J, Frangione B. Amyloidosis and Alzheimer`s disease. Advanced Drug Delivery Reviews, 2002; 54(12), 1539-1551.

[64] Giulivi C, Davies KJA. Dityrosine: a marker for oxidatively modified proteins and selective proteolysis. Methods Enzymology, 1994; 233, 363-371.

[65] Gil JM, Rego AC. Mechanisms of neurodegeneration in Huntington`s disease. European Journal of Neurosciene, 2008; 27(11), 2803-2820.

[66] Glenner GG, Wong CW. Alzheimer`s disease: initial report of the purification and characterization of a novel cerebrovascular amyloid protein. Biochemical and Biophysical Research Communications, 1984; 120(3), 885-889.

[67] Goth L. Genetic heterogeneity of the 5' uncoding region of the catalase gene in Hungarian acatalasemic and hypocatalasemic subjects. Clinica Chimica Acta, 1998; 271(1), 73-78.

[68] Goth L, Vitai M, Rass P, Sükei E, Pay A. Detection of a novel familial catalase mutation (Hungarian type D) and the possible risk of inherited catalase deficiency for diabetes mellitus. Electrophoresis, 2005; 26(9), 1646-1649.

[69] Grasbon-Frodl EM, Kosel S, Riess O, Muller U, Mehraein P, Graeber MB. Analysis of mitochondrial targeting sequence and coding region polymorphisms of manganese superoxide dismutase gene in German Parkinson disease patients. Biochemical and Biophysical Research Communications, 1999; 255(3), 749-752.

[70] Grundke-Iqbal I, Iqbal K, Tung YC, Quinlan M, Wisniewski HM, Binder LI. Abnormal phosphorylation of the microtubule-associated protein tau (tau) in Alzheimer cytoskeletal pathology. Proceedings of the National Acadademy of the Sciences of the United States of America, 1986; 83(13), 4913-4917.

[71] Grunewald T, Beal MF. Bioenergetics in Huntington's disease. Annals of the New York Acadademy of Sciences, 1999; 893, 203–213.

[72] Gu M, Gash MT, Mann VM, Javoy-Agid F, Cooper JM, Schapira AH. Mitochondrial defect in Huntington's disease caudate nucleus, Annals of Neurology, 1996; 39(3), 385–389.

[73] Hardy J, Selkoe DJ. The amyloid hypothesis of Alzheimer s disease: progress and problems on the road to therapeutics. Science, 2002; 297 (5580), 353-356.

[74] Harper PS. The epidemiology of Huntington's disease. Human Genetics, 1986; 89, 365–376.

[75] Hashimoto M, Hsu LJ, Xia Y, Takeda A, Sisk A, Sundsmo M, Masliah E. Oxidative stress induced amyloid-like aggregate formation of NACP/alpha-synuclein in vitro. NeuroReport, 1999; 10(4), 717-721.

[76] Hayes JD, Pulford DJ. The glutathione S-transferase supergene family: regulation of GST and the contribution of the isoenzymes to cancer chemoprotection and drug resistance. Critical Reviews in Biochemistry and Molecullar Biology, 1995; 30(6), 445-600.

[77] Hengartner MO. The biochemistry of apoptosis. Nature, 2000; 407(6805), 770-776.

[78] Hensley K, Carney JM, Mattson MP, Aksenova M, Harris M, Wu JF, Floyd RA, Butterfield DA. A model for beta-amyloid aggregation and neurotoxicity based on free radical generation by the peptide: relevance to Alzheimer disease. Proceedings of the National Acadademy of the Sciences of the United States of America, 1994; 91(8), 3270-3274.

[79] Hersch SM, Gevorkian S, Marder K, Moskowitz C, Feigin A, Cox M, Como P, Zimmerman C, Lin M, Zhang L, Ulug AM, Beal MF, Matson W, Bogdanov M, Ebbel E, Zaleta A, Kaneko Y, Jenkins B, Hevelone N, Zhang H, Yu H, Schoenfeld D, Ferrante R, Rosas HD. Creatine in Huntington disease is safe, tolerable, bioavailable in brain and reduces serum 8OH2'dG. Neurology, 2006; 66(2), 250–252.

[80] Huang Y, Cheung L, Rowe D, Halliday G. Genetic contribution to Parkinson´s disease. Brain Research Reviews, 2004; 46(1), 44-70.

[81] Hung SY, Liou HC, Kang KH, Wu RM, Wen CC, Fu WM. Overexpression of heme oxygenase-1 protects dopaminergic neurons against 1-methyl-4-phenylpyridinium-induced neurotoxicity. Molecular pharmacology, 2008; 74(6), 1564-1575.

[82] Huntington'sDiseaseCollaborativeResearchGroup. A novel gene containing a trinucleotide repeat that is expanded and unstable on Huntington's disease chromosomes. Cell, 1993; 72, 971–983.

[83] Infante J, Rodriguez- Rodriguez E, Mateo I, Llorca J, Vazquez-Higuera JL, Berciano J, Combarros O. Gene-gene interaction between heme oxygenase-1 and liver X receptor-β and Alzheimer`s disease risk. Neurology of Aging, 2010; 31(4), 710-714.

[84] Jenner P. Oxidative stress in Parkinson´s disease. Annals of Neurology, 2003; 53(3), S26-S38.

[85] Jenner P. Presymptomatic detection of Parkinson´s disease. Journal of Neural Transmission, 1993; 40, 23-36.

[86] Kanungo MS. A model for ageing. The Journal of Theoretical Biology, 1975; 53(2), 253-261.

[87] Kawai M, Kalaria RN, Harik SI, Perry G. The relationship of amyloid plaques to cerebral capillaries in Alzheimer`s disease. The American Journal of Pathology, 1990; 137(6), 1435-1446.

[88] Kawarabayashi T, Younkin LH, Saido TC, Shoji M, Ashe KH, Younkin SG. Age-dependent changes in brain, CSF, and plasma amyloid (beta) protein in the Tg2576 transgenic mouse model of Alzheimer`s disease. Journal of Neuroscience, 2001; 21(2), 372-381.

[89] Keil U, Bonert A, Marques CA, Scherping I, Weyermann J, Strosznajder JB, Müller-Spahn F, Haass C, Czech C, Pradier L, Müller W E, Eckert A. Amyloid beta-induced changes in nitric oxid production and mitochondrial activity lead to apoptosis. The Journal of Biological Chemistry, 2004; 279(48), 50310-50320.

[90] Kelada SN, Stapleton PL, Farin FM, Bammler TK, Eaton DL, Smith-Weller T, Franklin GM, Swanson PD, Longstreth Jr. WT, Checkoway H. Glutathione S-transferases M1, T1 and P1 polymorphisms and Parkinson's disease. Neurosciense Letters, 2003; 337(1), 5-8.

[91] Keller JN, Mark RJ, Bruce AJ, Blanc E, Rothstein JD, Uchida K, Waeg G, Mattson MP. 4-hydroxynonenal, an aldehydic product of membrane lipid peroxidation, impairs glutamate transport and mitochondrial function in synaptosomes. Neuroscience, 1997; 80(3), 685-696.

[92] Kimpara T, Takeda A, Watanabe K, Itoyama Y, Ikawa S, Watanabe M, Arai H, Sasaki H, Higuchi S, Okita N, Takase S, Saito H, Takahashi K, Shibahara S. Microsatellite polymorphism in the human heme oxygenase-1 gene promoter and its application in association studies with Alzheimer and Parkinson disease. Human Genetic, 1997; 100(1), 145-147.

[93] Kishimoto Y, Murakami Y, Hayashi K, Takahara S, Sugimura T, Sekiya T. Detectionof a common mutation of the catalase gene in Japanese acatalasemic patients. Human Genetic, 1992; 88(5), 487-490.

[94] Kohno T, Shinmura K, Tosaka M, Tani M, Kim SR, Sugimura H, Nohmi T, Kasai H, Yokota J. Genetic polymorphisms and alternative splicing of the hOGG1 gene, that is involved in the repair of 8-hydroxyguanine in damaged DNA, Oncogene, 1998; 16, 3219–3225.

[95] Kovtun IV, Liu Y, Bjoras M, Klungland A, Wilson SH, McMurray CT. OGG1 initiates age-dependent CAG trinucleotide expansion in somatic cells. Nature, 2007; 447(7143), 447–452.

[96] Kremer B, Goldberg P, Andrew SE, Theilmann J, Telenius H, Zeisler J, Squitieri F et al.: A worldwide study of the Huntington’s disease mutation. The sensitivity and specificity of measuring CAG repeats. The New England Journal of Medicine, 1994; 330, 1401–1406.

[97] Kuhl DE, Phelps ME, Markham CH, Metter EJ, Riege WH, Winter J. Cerebral metabolism and atrophy in Huntington's disease determined by 18FDG and computed tomographic scan. Annals of Neurology, 1982; 12(5), 425–434.

[98] Lamperti C, Zeviani M. Encephalomyopathies caused by abnormal nuclear-mitochondrial intergenomic cross-talk. Acta Myologica, 2009; 28(1), 2-11.

[99] Lee VM, Balin BJ, Otvos L Jr., Trojanowski JQ. A68: a major subunit of paired helical filaments and derivazed forms of normal Tau. Science, 1991; 251(4994), 675-678.

[100] [100] Li R, Lindholm K, Yang LB, Yue X, Citron M, Yan R, Beach T, Sue L, Sabbagh M, Cai H, Wong P, Price D, Shen Y. Amyloid beta peptide load is correlated with increased beta-secretase activity in sporadic Alzheimer's disease patients. Proceedings of the National Acadademy of the Sciences of the United States of America, 2004; 101(10), 3632-3637.

[101] Linnane AW, Marzuki S, Ozawa T, Tanaka M. Mitochondrial DNA mutations as an important contributor to ageing and degenerative diseases. Lancet, 1989; 1(1), 642-645.

[102] Liu CY, Lee CF, Wei YH. Role of reactive oxygen species-elicited apoptosis in the pathophysiology of mitochondrial and neurodegenerative diseases associated with mitochondrial DNA mutations. Journal of the Formosan Medical Association, 2009; 108(8), 599-611.

[103] Mann VM, Cooper JM, Javoy-Agid F, Agid Y, Jenner P, Schapira AH. Mitochondrial function and parental sex effect in Huntington's disease. Lancet , 1990; 336(8717), 749.

[104] Mao G, Pan X, Zhu BB, Zhang Y, Yuan F, Huang J, Lovell MA, Lee MP, Markesbery WR, Li GM, Gu L. (2007). Identification and characterization of OGG1 mutations in patients with Alzheimer's disease. Nucleic Acids Research, 2007; 35(8):2759-2766.

[105] Margaglione M, Garofano R, Cirillo F, Ruocco A, Grandone E, Vecchione G, Mila, G, Di Minno G, De Blasi A, Postiglione A. Cu/Zn superoxide dismutase in patients with non-familial Alzheimer's disease. Aging (Milano), 1995; 7(1), 49-54.

[106] Mehta PD, Prittila T. Biological markers of Alzheimer s disease. Drug Development Research, 2002; 56(2), 74-84.

[107] Morovvati S, Nakagawa M, Osame M, Karami A. Analysis of CCG repeats in Huntingtin gene among HD patients and normal populations in Japan. Archives of Medical Research, 2008; 39(1), 131–133.

[108] Mythri RB, Venkateshappa C, Harish G, Mahadevan A, Muthane UB, Yasha TC, Barath MMS, Shankar SK. Evaluation of markers of oxidative stress, antioxidant function and astrocyte proliferation in the striatum and frontal cortex of Parkinson's disease brains. Neurochemical Research, 2011; 36(8), 1452-1463.

[109] Nath KA, Grande JP, Haggard JJ, Croatt AJ, Katusic ZS, Solovey A, Hebbel RP. Oxidative stress and induction of heme oxygenase-1 in the kidney in sickle cell disease. The American Journal of Pathology, 2001; 158(3), 892-903.

[110] Oldfors A, Tulinius M. Mitochondrial encephalomyophaties. The Journal of Neuropathology and Experimental Neurology, 2003; 62(3), 217-227.

[111] Otterbein LE, Choi AM. Heme oxygenase: colors of defence against cellular stress. American Journal of Physiology. Lung Cellular and Molecular Physiology, 2000; 279(6), L1029-L1037.

[112] Panov AV, Gutekunst CA, Leavitt BR, Hayden MR, Burke JR, Strittmatter WJ, Greenamyre JT. Early mitochondrial calcium defects in Huntington's disease are a direct effect of polyglutamines. Nature Neuroscience, 2002; 5(8), 731–736.

[113] Parboosingh JS, Rousseau M, Rogan F, Amit Z, Chertkow H, Johnson WG, Manganaro F, Schipper HN, Curran TJ, Stoessl J. Absence of mutations in superoxide dismutase and catalase genes in patients with Parkinson's disease. Archives of Neurology, 1995; 52(12), 1160-1163.

[114] Paredi P, Leckie MJ, Horvath I, Allegra L, Kharitonov SA, Barnes PJ. Changes in exhaled carbone monoxide and nitric oxide levels following allergen challenge in patients with asthma. The European Respiratory Journal, 1999; 13(1), 48-52.

[115] Parildar-Karpuzoğlu H, Doğru-Abbasoğlu S, Hanagasi HA, Karadağ B, Gürvit H, Emre M, Uysal M. Single nucleotide polymorphisms in base-excisionn repair genes hOGG1, APE1 and XRCC1 do not alter risk of Alzheimer's disease. Neuroscience Letters, 2008; 442(3), 287-291.

[116] Parker WD, Boyson SJ, Parks JK. Abnormalities of the electron transport chain in idiopathic Parkinson´s disease. Annals of Neurology, 1989; 26(6), 719-723.

[117] Parks JK, Smith TS, Trimmer PA, Bennett JP Jr., Parker WD Jr. Neurotoxic Abeta peptides increase oxidative stress in vivo through NMDA-receptor and nitric-oxide-synthase mecanism, and inhibit complex IV activity and induce a mitochondrial permeability transition in vitro. Journal of Neurochemistry, 2001; 76(4), 1050-1056.

[118] Paz-y-Miño C, Muñoz MJ, López-Cortés A, Cabrera A, Palacios A, Castro B, Paz-y-Miño N, Sánchez ME. (2010).Frequency of polymorphisms pro198leu in GPX-1 gene and ile58thr in MnSOD gene in the altitude Ecuadorian population with bladder cancer. Oncological Research, 2010; 18(8), 395-400.

[119] Pearce RKB, Owen A, Daniel S, Jenner P, Marsden CD. Alterations in the distribution of glutathione in substantia nigra in Parkinson´s disease. Journal of Neural Transmission, 1997; 104(6-7), 661-677.

[120] Perez-Pastene C, Graumann R, Diaz-Grez F, Miranda M, Venegas P, Godoy OT, Layson L, Villagra R, Matala JM, Herrera L, Segura-Aguilar J. Association of GST M1

null polymorphism with Parkinson's disease in a Chilean population with strong Amerindian genetic component. Neuroscience Letters, 2007; 418(2), 181-185.

[121] Perry T, Godin DV, Hansen S. Parkinson´s disease: a disorder due to nigral glutathione deficiency? Neuroscience Letters, 1982; 33(3), 305-310.

[122] Perry G, Taddeo MA, Nunomura A, Zhu X, Zenteno-Savin T, Drew KL, Shimohama S, Avila J, Castellani RJ, Smith MA. Comparative biology and pathology of oxidative stress in Alzheimer and other neurodegenerative diseases: beyond damage and response. Comparative Biochemistry and Physiology C, 2002; 133(4), 507-513.

[123] Peterson LJ, Flood PM. Oxidative stress and microglial cells in Parkinson´s disease. Mediators of inflammation, 2012; 401264.

[124] Pimentel C, Batista-Nascimento L, Rodrigues-Pousada C, Menezes RA. Oxidative stress in Alzheimer´s and Parkinson´s disease: Insights from the yeast Saccharomyces cerevisiae. Oxidative Medicine and Cellular Longevity 2012; 132146.

[125] Pinhel MA, Nakazone MA, Cação JC, Piteri RC, Dantas RT, Godoy MF, Godoy MR, Tognola WA, Conforti-Froes ND, Souza D. Glutathione S-transferase variants increase susceptibility for late-onset Alzheimer`s disease: association study and relationship with apolipoprotein E epsilon 4 allele. Clinical Chemistry and Laboratory Medicine, 2008; 46(4), 439-445.

[126] Pluta R, Barcikowska M, Januszewski S, Misicka A, Lipkowski AW. Evidence of blood-brain barrier permeability/leakage for circulationg human Alzheimer`s β-amyloid-(1-42)-peptide. NeuroReport, 1996; 7(7), 1261-1265

[127] Pluta R, Oseka M, Januszewski S, Misicka A, Barcikowska M, Lipkowski AW, Kozniewska E. Circulating human β-amyloid-(1-42)-peptide increases cerebral blood flow in anesthetized rats. Alzheimer`s Research, 1996; 2, 233-236.

[128] Polidori MC, Mecocci P, Browne SE, Senin U, Beal MF. Oxidative damage to mitochondrial DNA in Huntington's disease parietal cortex. Neuroscience Letters, 1999; 272(1), 53–56.

[129] Pollack M, Leeuwenburgh Ch. Molecular mechanisms of oxidative stress in aging: free radicals, aging, antioxidants and disease. In Handbook of Oxidants and Antioxidants in exercise. 1999. p881-923.

[130] Qian Y, Chen W, Wu J, Tao T, Bi L, Xu W, Qi H, Wang Y, Guo L. (2010). Association of polymorphism of DNA repair gene XRCC1 with sporadic late-onset Alzheimer's disease and age of onset elderly Han Chinese. Journal of the Neurological Sciences, 2010; 295(1-2), 62-65.

[131] Rebbeck TR. Molecular epidemiology of the human glutathione S-transferase genotypes GSTM1 and GSTT1 in cancer susceptibility. Cancer Epidemiology, Biomarkers, and Preventions, 1997; 6(9), 733-743.

[132] Reddy PH, Beal MF. Are mitochondria critical in the pathogenesis of Alzheimer's disease? Brain Research. Brain Research Reviews, 2005; 49(3), 618-632.

[133] Reddy PH. Amyloid precursor protein-mediated free radicals and oxidative damage: implications for the development and progression of Alzheimer`s disease. Journal of Neurochemistry, 2006; 96(1), 1-13.

[134] Robert M, Mathuranath PS. Tau and tauopathies. Neurology India, 2007; 55(1), 11-16.

[135] Sardana MK, Drummond GS, Sassa S, Kappas A. The potent heme oxygenase inducing action of arsenic and parasiticidal arsenicals. Pharmacology, 1981; 23(5), 247-253.

[136] Sawada M, Carson CJ. Changes in superoxide radical and lipid peroxide formation in the brain, heart, and liver during the lifetime of the rat. Mechanisms of Ageing and Development, 1987; 41(1-2), 125-137.

[137] Schapira AH, Cooper JM, Dexter D, Clark JB, Jenner P, Marsden CD. Mitochondrial complex I deficiency in Parkinson´s disease. Journal of Neurochemistry 1990; 54(6), 823-827.

[138] Schoneich C. Reactive oxygen species and biological aging: a mechanistic approach. Experimental Gerontology, 1999; 34(1), 9-34.

[139] Seet RCS, Lee CH-YJ, Lim ECH, Tan JJH, Quek AML, Chong W-L, Looi W-F, Huang S-H, Wang H., Chan Y-H, Halliwell B. Oxidative damage in Parkinson disease: Measurement using accurate biomarkers. Free Radical Biology and Medicine, 2010; 48(4), 560-566.

[140] Selkoe DJ. Presenilin, Notch, and the genesis and treatment of Alzheimer`s disease. Proceedings of the National Acadademy of the Sciences of the United States of America, 2001; 98(20), 11039-11041.

[141] Shacter E. Protein oxidative damage. Methods Enzymology, 2000; 319, 428-436.

[142] Shapira AH. Mitochondria in the etiology and pathogenesis of Parkinson´s disease. Lancet Neurology, 2008; 7(1), 97-109.

[143] Shibata N, Ohnuma T, Baba H, Arai H. No genetic association between polymorphisms of heme oxygenase 1 and 2 and Alzheimer`s disease in a Japanese population. Dementia and Geriatric Cognitive Disorders, 2009; 27(3), 273-277.

[144] Shringarpure R, Davies KJ. Protein turnover by the proteasome in aging and disease. Free Radical Biology and Medicine, 2002; 32(11), 1084-1089.

[145] Sian J, Dexter DT, Lees AJ, Daniel S, Agid Y, Javoy-Agid F, Jenner P, Marsden DC. Alteration in glutathione levels in Parkinson's disease and other neurodegenerative disorders affecting basal ganglia. Annals of neurology, 1994; 36(3), 348-355.

[146] Singh M, Khan AJ, Shah PP, Shukla VK, Khanna VK, Parmar D. Polymorphism in environment responsive genes and association with Parkinson disease. Molecular and Cellular Biochemistry, 2008; 312(1-2), 131-138.

[147] Smith CD, Carney JM, Starke-Red PE, Oliver CN, Stadtman ER, Floyd RA, Markesbery WR. Excess brain protein oxidation and enzyme dysfunction in normal and Alzheimer`s disease. Proceedings of the National Acadademy of the Sciences of the United States of America, 1991; 88(23), 10540-10543.

[148] Smith MA, Sayre LM, Anderson VE, Harris PLR, Beal MF, Kowall N, Perry G. Cytochemical demonstration of oxidative damage in Alzheimer disease by immunochemical enhancement of the carbonyl reaction with 2,4,-dinitrophenylhydrazine. The Journal of Histochemistry and Cytochemistry, 1998; 46(6), 731-735.

[149] Sofic E, Riederer P, Heinsen H, Beckmann H, Reynolds GP, Hebenstreit G, Youdim MB. Increased iron (III) and total iron ciontent in post mortem substantia nigra of parkinsonian brain. Journal of Neural Transmission 1998; 74(3), 199-205.

[150] Sohal RS, Agarwal S, Sohal BH. Oxidative stress and aging in the Molgolian gerbil (Meriones nguiculatus). Mechanisms of Ageing and Development, 1995; 81(1), 15-25.

[151] Spalletta G, Bernardini S, Bellincampi L, Federici G, Trequattrini A, Ciappi F, Bria P, Caltagirone C, Bossù P. Glutathione S-transferase P1 and T1 gene polymorphisms predict longitudinal course and age at onset of Alzheimer disease. The American Journal of Geriatriatric Psychiatry, 2007; 15(10), 879-887.

[152] Sprenger R, Schlagenhaufer R, Kerb R, Bruhn C, Brockmöller J, Roots I, Brinkmann U. Characterization of the glutathione S-transferase GSTT1 deletion: discrimination of all genotypes by polymerase chain reaction indicate a trimodular genotype-phenotype correlation. Pharmacogenetics, 2000; 10(6), 557-565.

[153] Stadtman ER. Protein oxidation and aging. Science, 1992; 257(5074), 1220-1224.

[154] Stadtman ER. Oxidation of free amino acids and amino acids residues in proteins by radiolysis and by metal-catalyzed reaction. Annual Review of Biochemistry, 1993; 62, 797-821.

[155] Stoy N, Mackay GM, Forrest CM, Christofides J, Egerton M, Stone TW, Darlington LG. Tryptophan metabolism and oxidative stress in patients with Huntington's disease, Journal of Neurochemistry, 2005; 93(3), 611–623.

[156] Squitier F, Andrew SE, Goldberg YP, Kremer B, Spence N, Zeisler J, Nichol K, Theilmann J, Greenberg J, Goto J. DNA haplotype analysis of Huntington disease reveals clues to the origins and mechanisms of CAG expansion and reasons for geographic variations of prevalence. Human Molecular Genetics, 1994; 3(12), 2103–2114.

[157] Stroombergen MC, Waring RH. (1990). Determination of glutathione S-transferase mu and theta polymorphisms in neurological disease. Human and Experimental Toxicology, 1999; 18(3), 141-145.

[158] Swerdlow RH, Khan SM. A „mitochondrial cascade hypothesis" for sporadic Alzheimer's disease. Medical Hypotheses, 2004; 63(1), 8-20.

[159] Szebenyi G, Morfini GA, Babcock A. Neuropathogenic forms of huntingtin and androgen receptor inhibit fast axonal transport. Neuron, 2003; 40 (1), 41–52.

[160] Tanzi RE, Bertram L. Twenty years of the Alzheimer`s disease amyloid hypothesis: a genetic perspective. Cell 2005; 120, 545-555.

[161] Tappel AL. Selenium-glutathione peroxidase: properties and synthesis. Current Topics in Cellular Regulation, 1984; 24, 87-97.

[162] Thomas T, Thomas G, McLendon C, Sutton T, Mullan M. Beta-Amyloid-mediated vasoactivity and vascular endothelial damage. Nature 1996; 380, 168-177.

[163] Tyler SJ, Dawbarn D, Wilcock GK, Allen SJ. (2002). Alpha- and beta-secretase: profound changes in Alzheimer's disease. Biochemical Biophysical Research Communications, 2002; 299(3):, 373-376.

[164] Ukkola O, Erkkilä PH, Savolainen MJ, Kesäniemi YA. Lack of association between polymorphisms of catalase, copper-zinc superoxide dismutase (SOD), extracellular SOD and endothelial nitric oxide synthase genes and macroangiopathy in patients with type 2 diabetes mellitus. Journal of Internal Medicine, 2001; 249(5), 451-459.

[165] Van der Walt JM, Nicodemus KK, Martin ER, Scott WK, Nance MA, Watts RL, Hubble JP, Haines JL, Koller WC, Lyons K, Pahwa R, Stern MB, Colcher A, Hiner BC, Jankovic J, Ondo WG, Allen Jr. FH, Goetz CG, Small GW, Mastaglia F, Stajich JM, McLaurin AC, Middleton LT, Scott BL, Perikan-Vance MA, Vance JM. Mitochondrial polymorphisms significantly reduce the risk of Parkinson disease. American Journal of Human Genetic, 2003; 72(4), 804-811.

[166] Van Remmen H, Richardson A. Oxidative damage to mitochondria and aging. Experimental Gerontology, 2001; 36(7), 957-968.

[167] Veal EA, Toone WM, Jones N, Morgan BA. Distinct roles for glutathione S-transferases in the oxidative stress response in Schizosaccharomyces pombe. The Journal of Biological Chemistry, 2002; 277(38), 35523-35531.

[168] Venkateshappa C, Harish G, Mythri RB, Mahadevran A, Barath MMS, Shankar SK. Increased oxidative damage and decreased antioxidant function in aging human sustantia nigra compared to striatum: Implication for Parkinson′ disease. Neurochemical Research, 2012; 37(2), 358-369.

[169] Von Sonntag C, Schuchmann HP. Suppression of hydroxyl radical reactions in biological systems: considerqations based on competition kinetics. Methods Enzymology, 1994; 233, 47-56.

[170] Vonsattel JP, Myers RH, Stevens TJ, Ferrante RJ, Bird ED, Richardson EP Jr.. Neuropathological classification of Huntington'sdisease. Journal of Neuropathology and Experimental Neurology, 1985; 44(6), 559–577.

[171] Wahner AD, Glatt ChE, Bronstein JM, Ritz B. Glutathione S-transferase mu, omega, pi and theta class variants and smoking in Parkinson's disease. Neuroscience letters 2007; 413(3), 274-278.

[172] Wang V, Chen SY, Chuang TC, Shan DE, Soong BW, Kao MC. Val-9-Ala and Ile +58Thr polymorphism of MnSOD in Parkinson's disease. Clinical Biochemistry 2010; 43(12), 979-982.

[173] Wiener HW, Perry RT, Chen Z, Harrell LE, Go RC. A polymorphism in SOD2 is associated with development of Alzheimer's disease. Genes Brain Behaviour, 2007; 6(8), 770-775.

[174] Xiong K, Cai H, Luo XG, Struble RG, Clough RW, Yan XX. Mitochondrial respiratory inhibition and oxidative stress elevated beta-secretase (BACE1) proteins and activity in vivo in the rat ratina. Experimental Brain Research, 2007; 181(3), 435-446.

[175] Xu S, Wang Y, Roe B, Pearson WR. Characterization of the human class Mu glutathione S-transferase gene cluster and the GSTM1 deletion. The Journal of Biological Chemistry, 1998; 273(6), 3517-3527.

[176] Yu BP, Yang R. Critical evaluation of the free radical theory of aging. A proposal for the oxidative stress hypothesis. Annals of New Yourk Academy of Science, 1996; 786, 1-11.

[177] Zeevalk GD, Razmpour R, Bernard LP. Gluthatione and Parkinson´s disease: Is this the elephant in the room? Biomedicine and Pharmacotherapy 2008; 62(4), 236-249.

[178] Zhang BR, Tian J, Yan YP, Yin XZ, Zhao GH, Wu ZY, Gu WH, Xia K, Tang BS. CCG polymorphisms in the huntingtin gene have no effect on the pathogenesis of patients with Huntington's disease in mainland Chinese families. Journal of the Neurological Sciences, 2012; 312(1-2), 92–96.

[179] Zhao J, Fu Y, Yasvoina M, Shao P, Hitt B, O'Connor T, Logan S, Maus E, Citron M, Berry R, Binder L, Vassar R. (2007). Beta-site amyloid recursor protein cleaving enzyme 1 levels become elevated in neurons around amyloid plaques: implications for Alzheimer's disease pathogenesis. The Journal of Neuroscience, 2007; 27(14), 3639-3649.

[180] Zhou XF, Cui J, DeStefano AL, Chazaro I, Farrer LA, Manolis AJ, Gavras H, Baldwin CT. Polymorphisms in the promoter region of catalase gene and essential hypertension. Disease Markers, 2005; 21(1), 3-7.

[181] Zhu X, Smith MA, Perry G, Aliev G. Mitochondrial failures in Alzheimer`s disease. American Journal of Alzheimers Disease and Other Dementias, 2004; 19(6), 345-352.

[182] Zlokovic BV. Clearing amyloid through the blood-brain barrier. Journal of Neurochemistry, 2004; 89(4), 807-811.

Chapter 19

Intermediate Filaments in Neurodegenerative Diseases

Rodolphe Perrot and Joel Eyer

Additional information is available at the end of the chapter

http://dx.doi.org/10.5772/54676

1. Introduction

In adult central (CNS) and peripheral nervous system (PNS), intermediate filaments (IFs) are the most abundant cytoskeletal components [1]. Neurons express differentially several IF proteins depending on their developing stage or their localization in the nervous system. In CNS, IFs are principally composed of the neurofilament (NF) triplet proteins (called NFL (light, 68 kDa), NFM (medium, 160 kDa) and NFH (heavy, 205 kDa); type IV) and α-internexin (66 kDa; type IV), while in the PNS, NFs are made up of NFL, NFM, NFH and peripherin (57 kDa; type III) [2, 3]. Neurons may also express other IF proteins, including nestin (200 kDa; type IV), vimentin (57 kDa, type III) syncoilin isoforms (Sync1 (64 kDa), Sync2 (64 kDa); type III) and synemin isoforms (Low synemin (41 kDa), Middle or beta synemin (150 kDa), High or alpha synemin (180 kDa); type IV). While present in perikarya and dendrites, IFs are particularly abundant in large myelinated axons, where they are essential for axon radial growth during development and axon caliber maintenance [4]. Consequently they are crucial to optimize the conduction velocity of the nerve impulse. They also contribute to the dynamic properties of the axonal cytoskeleton during neuronal differentiation, axon outgrowth, regeneration and guidance [5]. The IF proteins share a common tripartite structure with a globular head, a central α-helical rod domain and variable tail domains that differ in length and amino acids composition. The central rod domain of approximately 310 amino acids contains four α-helical regions and is involved in the assembly of 10 nm filaments [6]. NFM and NFH subunits differ from other neuronal IF proteins by their long tail domains containing numerous repeats of Lys-Ser-Pro (KSP) phosphorylation sites [4].

An increasing body of evidence supports the view that the most common mechanism of chronic neurodegenerative disorders involves abnormal protein production, processing or misfolding and subsequent accumulation in nervous system. Alterations in the metabolism and/or organization of neuronal IFs are frequently associated, directly or indirectly, with various neurodegenerative diseases, including amyotrophic lateral sclerosis (ALS), Charcot-Marie-Tooth (CMT) disease, giant axonal neuropathy (GAN), neuronal intermediate filament inclusion disease (NIFID), Parkinson disease (PD), diabetic neuropathy, dementia with Lewy bodies and spinal muscular atrophy [7]. While IF abnormalities in neurodegenerative disorders could simply reflect a pathological consequence of neuronal dysfunction, recent studies using transgenic mouse models suggested that IF disorganization itself can also produce deleterious effects and therefore could contribute to the neurodegeneration process. Glial IF, and more particularly GFAP in astrocytes, is also the target of mutations leading to neurodegenerative diseases. Astrocytes express various IF proteins, including nestin, vimentin and synemin, but GFAP is the most abundant. GFAP is a type III IF protein existing under different spliced forms. The relative abundance of these GFAP transcripts is variable and can be dependent upon astrocyte location or pathological states [8]. *GFAP* mutations lead to accumulations of GFAP protein and cause Alexander disease (AXD), a rare leukodystrophy. Here, we tempted to cover the current knowledge related to neuronal and glial IF involvement in human neurodegenerative diseases (Table 1).

Disease	Mutations in IF genes	Accumulation of IFs	Possible causes of IF accumulation	Possible roles of IF in disease pathogenesis
ALS	- Only 3 variants identified in *NEFH* gene. - Peripherin mutations identified in 3 sporadic ALS patients.	Accumulation of peripherin and extensively phosphorylated NFs in the perikaryon of motor neurons and in axonal spheroids.	- Defect of axonal transport caused by abnormal phosphorylation of NFs and/or alteration of the molecular motors. - Modification of NF stoichiometry. - Alteration of post-translational IF proteins modifications.	Paradoxically, perikaryal NF aggregates appeared protective in mouse models of ALS, slowing disease progression in these animals. - NFs may act as calcium chelators or phosphorylation sink. - Removal of NFs from the axonal compartment could enhance axonal transport.
CMT	20 mutations in the *NEFL* gene have been linked to CMT2E and CMT1F (represent ≈ 2% of CMT cases).	- Axonal swellings containing disorganized NFs. - *In vitro*, co-expression of most NFL mutants with Wt NFM or NFH results in the formation of aggregates within the cell body.	- Most mutated NFL proteins fail to self-assemble or co-assemble with Wt subunits, and affect axonal transport of Wt and mutant NFs. - Mutations of heat-shock protein can also cause NFL aggregate.	- Perturbation of the axonal transport by trapping molecular motors and organelles in the cell body. - Alteration of mitochondrial morphology and dynamic.
GAN	No	- Enlarged axons filled with abnormally packed NFs.	- An acceleration of NF transport concomitant with a normal rate of NF protein synthesis and insertion into transport system would lead	- Perturbation of the axonal transport.

Disease	Mutations in IF genes	Accumulation of IFs	Possible causes of IF accumulation	Possible roles of IF in disease pathogenesis
		- Generalized aggregation of other neuronal and non-neuronal IFs.	to the formation of distal axonal swelling with packed NFs. - Disturbed cytoskeleton regulation and modulation.	
NIFID	No	Neuronal cytoplasmic inclusions containing all type IV neuronal IFs, and especially α-internexin.	Not determined.	Not determined. Abnormal accumulation of IFs may only be a secondary phenomenon.
PD	A point mutation in the *NEFM* gene was reported in only one case of PD with early onset.	Cytoplasmic inclusion bodies (Lewy bodies) composed of α-synuclein, NF proteins, ubiquitin and proteasome subunits. Inappropriate phosphorylation and proteolysis of NFs occur in Lewy bodies.	Not determined.	Data suggest no direct implication of IFs in pathogenesis of PD.
AXD	≈ 100 mutations in the *GFAP* gene were identified in AXD patients. ≈ 95% of AXD cases are due to GFAP mutation.	Presence of protein aggregates (Rosenthal fibers) composed of GFAP, αB-crystallin, HSP27 and ubiquitin within the cytoplasm of astrocytes throughout the CNS.	-Decreased degradation of GFAP. - Up-regulation of αB-crystallin and HSP27 are associated to the aggregation of GFAP. - Some mutations could impair interaction of GFAP with partners which normally prevent its assembly, resulting in the accumulation of GFAP polymers. - Insufficient amount of plectin seems promote GFAP aggregates.	The specific aspects of astrocytes functions that are compromised by the mutations of GFAP have not yet been discovered, but inhibited proteasome activity and activated stress pathways seemed to be important consequences of GFAP accumulation.

Table 1. IFs in neurodegenerative diseases.

2. Neuronal intermediate filaments and neurodegenerative diseases

2.1. Amyotrophic lateral sclerosis

ALS, also referred to as Lou Gehrig's disease, is a neurodegenerative disease which, by affecting the motor neurons in the motor cortex, brain stem and spinal cord, causes progressive physical impairment, together with worsening limitations in the functions of breathing, swallowing and communication. The disease has an incidence rate of 1-2 per 100,000, with a higher occurrence in men than in women. There is no cure and death usually occurs within 3 to 5 years from symptom onset. Only 10% of cases are inherited in an autosomal dominant pattern with the remaining 90% sporadic. 20% of all the familial cases are due to mutations in Cu/Zn superoxide dismutase 1 (SOD1), the most abundant cytosolic enzyme.

One common pathological finding of both sporadic and familial ALS is the accumulation of NFs and/or peripherin in the perikaryon of motor neurons and in axonal spheroids [9]. Because of the presence of IF proteins in these aggregates, several studies have searched for mutations in genes coding for NF proteins and peripherin. The discovery of a small number of NF gene variants in ALS patients suggested the involvement of NFs in the pathogenesis of the disease. Indeed, codon deletions or insertions in the KSP repeat motifs of NFH have been identified in patients with sporadic ALS [10-12]. However, two others studies failed to identify such variants in the NF genes linked to sporadic and familial ALS [13, 14], suggesting that mutations in the NF genes are not a systematic common cause of ALS but could be a risk factor for sporadic ALS. Peripherin mutations have also been identified in three sporadic ALS patients [15-17], including a frameshift mutation in the *PRPH* gene able to disrupt the NF network assembly *in vitro*, reinforcing the view that NF disorganization may contribute to pathogenesis. These results suggest that peripherin mutations may be responsible for a small percentage of ALS cases. Two peripherin isoforms have been linked to ALS: aggregate-inducing Per28 is upregulated in patients with ALS, at both the mRNA and protein levels, and an antibody specific for Per28 stained the filamentous inclusions [18]. The Per61 splice variant is neurotoxic and has been observed in ALS mouse models and human patients [19]. These observations raise the possibility that missplicing of peripherin could lead to disease. It is also of interest to note the presence of high NFL and NFH levels and auto-antibodies against NFL in cerebrospinal fluid of ALS patients [20-22]. Furthermore, plasma NFH levels closely reflect later stages of disease progression and therapeutic response in a mouse model of ALS [23]. In the same way, a significant relation exists between cerebrospinal fluid NFL levels and disease progression in ALS patients [24]. Accordingly, it seems that NFs levels may be valuable biomarkers of later disease progression in ALS.

NFs found in perikaryal aggregates are extensively phosphorylated, a process that occurs normally only within the axon [25]. The mechanisms governing the formation of IF aggregates are still not clearly established but defects of axonal transport or abnormal stoichiometry of IF proteins could be involved. Perturbations of the axonal transport of NFs and organelles are one of the earliest pathological changes seen in several transgenic mouse models of ALS [26-29]. The premature phosphorylation of NF tail-domains in motor neurons cell bodies could directly mediate their accumulation in this region. Glutamate excitotoxicity, another pathogenic process in ALS, may induce this abnormal phosphorylation of NFs. Treatment of primary neurons with glutamate activates members of the mitogen-activated protein kinase family which phosphorylate NFs with ensuing slowing of their axonal transport [30]. In addition, glutamate leads to caspase cleavage and activation of protein kinase N1 (PKN1), a NF head-rod domain kinase [31]. This cleaved form of PKN1 disrupts NF organization and axonal transport. Excitotoxicity mediated by non-N-methyl-D-aspartic acid (NMDA) receptor is also associated with the aberrant colocalization of phosphorylated and dephosphorylated NF proteins [32]. Inhibition of Pin1, a prolyl isomerase, was suggested as a possible therapeutic target to reduce pathological accumulation of phosphorylated NFs. Pin1 associates with phosphorylated NFH in neurons and is found in aggregates in spinal cord from ALS patients [33]. Its inhibition by inhibitor or down-regulating Pin1 levels reduces glutamate-induced perikaryal accumulation of phosphorylated NFH. Finally, riluzole protects against glutamate-induced slowing of NF axonal transport by decreasing perikaryal NF side-arm phosphorylation [34], probably via the inhibition of ERK and p38 activities, two NF kinases activated in ALS.

Alterations of the anterograde or retrograde molecular motors may also be responsible for aggregation of IFs. Mutation of dynein or $p150^{glued}$ [35], overexpression of dynamitin [36] and absence of kinesin heavy chain isoform 5A (KIF5A) [37] induce NF accumulations in mice. Recent studies suggest that inhibition of retrograde transport is more susceptible to cause accumulation of NFs than inhibition of anterograde transport. The inhibition of dynein by increasing the level of dynamitin induces aberrant focal accumulation of NFs within axonal neurites whereas inhibition of kinesin inhibits anterograde transport but does not induce similar focal aggregations [38]. Similarly, the neuron-specific expression of Bicaudal D2 N-terminus (BICD2-N), a motor-adaptor protein, impairs dynein-dynactin function, causing the appearance of giant NF swellings in the proximal axons [39]. However these mice did not develop signs of motor neuron degeneration and motor abnormalities.

Modification in NF stoichiometry was also proposed to induce accumulation of NFs. Singly overexpressing any of the NF subunit in transgenic mice led to prominent motor neuropathy characterized by the presence of abnormal NF accumulations resembling those found in ALS [40-42]. Remarkably, the motor neuron disease caused by excess human NFH (hNFH) can be rescued by restoring a correct stoichiometry of NF subunits via the overexpression of hNFL in a dosage-dependent fashion [43]. Overexpression of peripherin in mice also provokes the formation of cytoplasmic protein aggregates and the subsequent selective loss of motor neurons during ageing [44, 45]. This loss is preceded by axonal transport defects and formation of axonal spheroids [46]. Because NFL mRNA levels are reduced in cases of ALS, Beaulieu et al. [45] generated double transgenic mice overexpressing peripherin and deficient for NFL (Per;NFL-/- mice). Here, the onset of peripherin-mediated disease is accelerated by the deficiency of NFL. Without NFL, peripherin interacts with NFM and NFH to form disorganized IF structures. This could explain why the number of IF inclusion bodies is increased in Per;NFL-/- mice, leading to an earlier neuronal death and to defects of fast axonal transport in cultured Per;NFL-/- neurons [47]. In contrast, peripherin toxicity can be attenuated by coexpression of NFL or NFH [48, 49], illustrating once again the importance of IF protein stoichiometry. NFH overexpression shifted the intracellular localization of inclusion bodies from the axonal to the perikaryal compartment of motor neurons, suggesting that the toxicity of peripherin inclusions may be related to their axonal localization, possibly by altering the axonal transport. However, it should be noted that peripherin is not a key contributing factor to the neuronal death in disease caused by SOD1 mutations because absence or overexpression of peripherin in $SOD1^{G37R}$ mice do not affect the onset and progression of motor neuron disease [50].

Changes in stoichiometry were reported in ALS motor neurons as the levels of NFL, α-internexin and peripherin mRNA are decreased, while in familial ALS the levels of peripherin mRNA appear to be abnormally elevated [51-53]. This suggests a change in the stoichiometry of cytoskeletal protein expression which could be conducive to the formation of neurofilamentous aggregates in ALS. This decrease of IF mRNA could be due in part to modification in their stability. Several NFL mRNA binding proteins have been identified in human, including 14-3-3 proteins [54], TAR (trans-active regulatory) DNA-binding protein (TDP43) [55], both mutant and wild-type SOD1 [56] and Rho guanine nucleotide exchange factor (RGNEF) [57]. These proteins are incorporated in ALS intraneuronal aggregates and affect the stability of NFL mRNA. Mice expressing human TDP-43 displayed reduced NF mRNAs and proteins contents, inducing a decrease of caliber of their motor axons [58]. The involvement of TDP-43 in ALS pathogenesis was reinforced by the recent discovery of several mutant forms of this protein in familial and sporadic ALS [59]. Motor neurons from mice expressing such mutated TDP-43 displayed peripherin and NFs (NFM and NFH) aggregates, concomitant with a down-regulation of NFL and an overexpression of peripherin [60]. In addition, they detected in these mice the presence of abnormal splicing variants of peripherin, such as Per61, that can contribute to formation of IF aggregates. RGNEF is another RNA binding protein that acts as an NFL mRNA stability factor via 3′ untranslated region destabilization and reduces NFL protein levels when overexpressed in a stable cell line. Furthermore, RGNEF cytoplasmic inclusions were detected in ALS spinal motor neurons that colocalized with ubiquitin, p62/sequestosome-1, and TDP-43 [61]. These observations provide a possible mechanism for NF aggregate formation together with a link between ALS and Rho signaling pathways.

Neuronal IF abnormalities in ALS may also occur as a result of post-translational protein modifications. Indeed, advanced glycation endproducts were detected in NF aggregates of motor neurons in familial and sporadic ALS [62]. *O*-glycosylation of NFM is strongly decreased in spinal cord of different models for ALS, whereas phosphorylation is increased relative to total NFM [63, 64], suggesting competition of the binding sites of these two modifications and a potential mechanism for the formation of NF protein accumulations in ALS. Interestingly, inhibition of *O*-GlcNAcase (OGA), the enzyme catalyzing removal of *O*-GlcNAc, increased levels of *O*-GlcNAc modified NFM in spinal cords of control mice, but not in mutant SOD1 mice. Moreover, phosphorylation state of NFM appeared unchanged in these mutant mice [64]. The authors speculate that this lack of difference in NFM phosphorylation in mutant SOD1 mice may arise from the aggregation of hyperphosphorylated NFs, which may prevent dephosphorylation and subsequent *O*-GlcNAc modification. It was also showed that SOD1 can catalyze nitration of tyrosines by peroxynitrite in the rod and head domains of NFL [65]. However, no significant changes were detected in the nitration of NFL isolated from cervical spinal cord tissue of sporadic ALS cases [66].

Finally, it seems that non-neuronal cells could be directly involved in the formation of cytoskeletal aggregates within proximal axon from motor neurons. Indeed, cultured mouse spinal motor neurons in contact with non-neuronal cells displayed swellings that were morphologically and neurochemically comparable to axonal spheroids that develop *in vivo* in ALS transgenic mouse models [67]. These swellings contained NFL, NFM,

NFH, α-internexin and peripherin, and induced the accumulation of mitochondria and vesicle-like structures, suggesting a disruption of the axonal transport. Moreover, the severity of this axonopathy correlated with the phenotype of the glial cells, with a significant increase being induced by a glial feeder layer expressing mutant SOD1 or that was pre-aged prior to plating the motor neurons [67].

To further determine whether NFs are directly involved in SOD1-mediated disease, mice expressing mutant SOD1 were mated with transgenic mice deficient for axonal NFs. The withdrawal of NFs from the axonal compartment and their perikaryal accumulation induced by the expression of NFH-β-galactosidase fusion protein conferred no beneficial effect to $SOD1^{G37R}$ mice [68], indicating that axonal NFs are not necessary for SOD1-mediated disease. This was also observed in $SOD1^{G85R}$ mice deprived of NFL, but the absence of axonal NFs in these animals prolongs their life span by approximately 15% [69]. Surprisingly, overexpression of mouse NFL or mouse NFH in $SOD1^{G93A}$ mice [70], and overexpression of hNFH in $SOD1^{G37R}$ mice [71], also increase their life span by respectively 15% and 65%. This suggests a protective effect of NF perikaryal accumulation in motor neuron disease caused by mutant SOD1. While the mechanism of protection is unclear, it seems that perikaryal accumulation of NFs rather than their axonal deficiency is responsible for slowing disease in these models. Indeed, the formation of large perikaryal aggregates and a massive depletion of axonal NFs due to the expression of the human NFH43 allele cause more positive effects than human NFH44 allele which induces smaller aggregates and more axonal NFs [71]. Moreover, the disruption of one allele for each NF gene induces a 40% decrease of axonal NF proteins content and an important axonal atrophy without perikaryal accumulation of NFs in $SOD1^{G37R}$ mice, but it does not extend their life span nor does it alleviate the loss of motor axons [72]. Several hypotheses were proposed to explain this protective effect of perikaryal aggregates in SOD1-mediated disease. Through their multiple calcium-binding sites NFs may act as calcium chelators. Supporting this hypothesis, a significant neuroprotection was obtained by overexpressing the calcium-binding protein calbindin-D28k in cultured motor neurons [73]. It was also proposed that perikaryal accumulations of NFs in motor neurons may alleviate ALS pathogenesis by acting as a phosphorylation sink for cyclin-dependent kinase 5 dysregulation induced by mutant SOD1, thereby reducing the excessive phosphorylation of tau and other neuronal substrates [72]. This was supported by the fact that NF accumulations contain hyperphosphorylated NFM and NFH subunits in ALS patients [25] and in SOD1 mutant mice [74]. However, removal of NFM and NFH sidearms led to a delay of disease in SOD1 mutant mice rather than the acceleration predicted by a kinase dysregulation model [75], indicating that perikaryal phosphorylation of NFs is not an essential contributor to reduced toxicity of SOD1 mutants and that abnormal phosphorylation of NF proteins may be a detrimental factor. Alternatively, axonal removal of NFs could enhance axonal transport, which is impaired in SOD1 mice, by providing a more flexible axoplasm.

Finally, it was shown that NFs are involved in the localization of NMDA receptors in the neuronal plasma membrane by interacting with the NMDA NR1 subunit [76]. Thus, accumulation of NFs could interfere with glutamate receptor function and prevent glutamate excitotoxicity. However, NF aggregate-bearing neurons demonstrate increased intracellular calcium levels and enhanced cell death in response to NMDA receptor activation without increased NMDA receptor expression. These results suggest that the presence of NF aggregates renders motor neurons more susceptible to NMDA-mediated excitotoxicity [77].

2.2. Charcot-Marie-Tooth disease

CMT represents a heterogeneous group of inherited peripheral neuropathies affecting both motor and sensory neurons to the muscles. CMT is the most common inherited disorder of the PNS, with approximately 1 per 2,500 people affected. Patients slowly lose function of their feet/legs and hand/arms as nerves to the extremities degenerate. First signs typically appear in the first or second decade of life, although it may be detected in infancy. This disease shows a high degree of heterogeneity, both in the clinical presentation and at the genetic level. CMT was originally subclassified into CMT1 and CMT2 on the basis of electrophysiological properties and histopathology. CMT1 is a demyelinating disease with reduced nerve conduction velocity whereas CMT2 is an axonal neuropathy with relatively normal nerve conduction velocity. CMT patients show a high degree of heterogeneity, due to mutations in multiple genes. This led to the distinction of other subtypes of CMT, including CMT3 (or Dejerine-Sottas disease, a particularly severe demyelinating form of CMT), CMT4 (autosomal recessive form of demyelinating CMT) and CMTX (X-linked form of CMT with both demyelinating and axonal features). Moreover, each type of CMT has several subtypes.

Vogel et al. [78] reported the presence of NF accumulations in CMT. Evidence for the involvement of IFs in the pathogenesis of CMT was provided by the identification of 20 mutations of the *NEFL* gene on chromosome 8 in patients with CMT1F and CMT2E. Mutations in *NEFL* gene are responsible for approximately 2% of CMT cases and a high percentage of CMT2 cases. These mutations are located throughout the three functional domains of this protein (head, rod and tail) and consist of substitutions, deletions and frame-shift mutations. Co-expression of most NFL mutants with wild-type NFM or NFH subunits disrupted the NF cytoskeleton *in vitro*, resulting in the formation of aggregates within the cell body [79, 80]. The first two CMT-associated *NEFL* mutations, NFL^{P8R} and NFL^{Q333P}, were identified in respectively a Belgian and a Russian family. In addition to disturb the assembly of NFs, these mutations affect the axonal transport of wild-type and mutant NFs, but also the transport of mitochondria and human amyloid β protein precursor, resulting in alterations of retrograde axonal transport, fragmentation of the Golgi apparatus and increased neuritic degeneration [79, 80]. The effect of these mutant proteins on filament assembly was dominant, since wild-type NFL could not rescue the assembly defect. Filament formation was also abolished in SW13 cells by the rod domain A148V mutation [81]. These data provide possible mechanisms by which these mutants could be involved in axonal degeneration and CMT pathogenesis.

The Pro-22 residue of NFL is also the target of several mutations: P22R, P22S and P22T. The P22R mutation, identified in a Korean family, is associated with demyelinating neuropathy features of CMT1F [82]. The P22S substitution was first described in a Slovenian CMT2 family [83], then in an Italian family developing a primary axonopathy characterized by giant axons with swellings composed essentially of aggregated NFs [84]. Interestingly, clinical and electrophysiological studies from patients with P22S mutation revealed a mixed axonal and demyelinating neuropathy [85], emphasizing the complexity of genotype-phenotype correlations in CMT. Finally, the P22T mutation was detected in unrelated Japanese patients with CMT disease [86]. The formation of NF aggregates in patients expressing NFL^{P22S} and NFL^{P22T} mutant proteins could be explain by the ability of these mutations to abolish the phosphorylation of the adjacent Thr21 by cyclin-dependent kinase 5, which normally inhibits filament assembly [87]. The phosphorylation of NFL head domain by PKA alleviated aggregates in cortical neurons, providing a potential therapeutic approach to dissociate NF aggregates in CMT disease [87].

The screening of 323 patients with CMT or related peripheral neuropathies allowed the identification of six disease-associated missense mutations and one 3-bp in-frame deletion in the *NEFL* gene [88]. Other mutations were also detected in Korean CMT patients [89], in a German family [90], and four mutations in the head and rod domains of NFL, including a L268P substitution and a del322Cys_326 Asn deletion, were identified by the screening of 177 patients [91]. Most of these mutated proteins (except E7K and D469N) form aggregates, and thus could alter the axonal transport following their abnormal aggregation in cell bodies and axons. A duplication-insertion mutation of NFL in a patient with CMT was also reported [92], which probably provoked neuronal degeneration through both aggregation and destabilization of the IF network. Finally, new mutations in the *NEFL* gene were identified following the screening of 223 Japanese CMT patients [93]. Four heterozygous missense mutations (P8L, E90K, N98S and E396K) were detected in five unrelated patients as well as a homozygous nonsense mutation (E140Stop) in one patient. All these patients displayed moderate delayed nerve conduction velocities, possibly caused by a loss of large diameter fibers. This study suggested that nonsense *NEFL* mutations probably cause a recessive phenotype, while missense mutations cause a dominant phenotype [93]. The majority of NFL mutations are linked to axonal forms of CMT but their implication in demyelinating CMT cannot be excluded since nerves from patients expressing NFL^{L268P} or NFL^{E90K} showed evidence of Schwann cell abnormalities [88, 91].

The first mouse model of the CMT2E disease expressed the $hNFL^{P22S}$ mutant protein specifically in the nervous system and recapitulate many of the overt phenotypes observed in CMT2E patients, including aberrant hind limb posture, motor deficits, hypertrophy of muscle fibres and loss of muscle innervation without neuronal loss [94]. To address whether CMT2E disease is potentially reversible, this mouse model was based on the tetracycline-responsive gene system that allows the suppression of mutant $hNFL^{P22S}$ expression in mature neurons through administration of doxycycline. Remarkably, a 3-month treatment of these mice with doxycycline after disease onset efficiently down-regulated expression of $hNFL^{P22S}$ and reversed the neurological phenotype [94], providing hope that future therapeutic strategies might not only stop progress of CMT2E disease but also reverse it. A novel line of CMT2E mice that constitutively express $hNFL^{E397K}$ was recently generated [95]. As with the $hNFL^{P22S}$ mice, these mice developed as early as 4 months signs consistent with CMT2E patients, such as aberrant hind limb posture, digit deformities, reduced locomotor activity and reduced motor nerve conduction velocities. However, some aspects differed between the two lines of CMT2E mice. Indeed, $hNFL^{E397K}$ mice showed no significant denervation and their muscles were atrophied. Moreover, they showed only relatively mild signs of nerve pathology, including ectopic accumulations of phosphorylated NFs in motor neuron cell bodies, NF disorganization in motor and sensory roots, and reduced axonal caliber [95]. The divergence in cellular pathology between the two animal models may suggests that overt CMT2E phenotypes may arise through different cellular mechanisms.

Mutations of myotubularin-related protein 2 (MTMR2) (CMT4B), heat-shock protein B1 (HSPB1) (CMT2F) or HSPB8 (CMT2L) can also cause NFL aggregation [96-99], indicating that mutation of NFs is not the only mechanism inducing their accumulation in CMT. Co-expression of Wt HSPB1 with P8R or Q333P CMT mutant NFL reduced their aggregation, induced reversal of mutant NFL aggregates and decreased mutant NFL-induced loss of motor neuron viability [100]. On the opposite, mutant HSPB1 was found to have an inhibitory effect on the assembly of NFL in transfected cells. Zhai et al. [100] showed that deletion of NFL markedly reduces degeneration and loss of motor neurons induced by mutant HSPB1. Finally, mice expressing mutant HSPB1 throughout the nervous system showed axonal pathology in spinal cord and peripheral nerve that was age-dependent, with evidence of impaired NF cytoskeleton, associated with organelle accumulation. These data suggest that overexpression of mutant HSPB1 in neurons is sufficient to cause pathological changes in mice that are seen in patients with CMT. Mutant MTMR2 also induces abnormal NFL assembly in transfected cells [98] and mice lacking MTMR2 develop a CMT-like neuropathy, including several characteristics of dysmyelination [101]. A similar phenotype was observed following Schwann cell-specific *MTMR2* inactivation, whereas neuron-specific inactivation did not provoke myelin outfoldings nor axonal defects, suggesting that loss of MTMR2 in Schwann cells, but not in motor neurons, is both sufficient and necessary to cause CMT4B neuropathy [102]. In addition to disrupt the NF network, recent studies showed that expression of NFL^{P8R} or NFL^{Q333P} in cultured motor neurons caused the rounding of mitochondria and decreased their rate of fusion concomitant with increased motility [103, 104], indicating an important function of NFs in mitochondrial dynamics. Cotransfection of HSPB1 helped to maintain normal NF network, axonal caliber and mitochondrial morphology. On the other hand, the cotransfection of HSPA1 was effective in neurons expressing NFL^{Q333P}, but not NFL^{P8R}, suggesting that chaperone-based therapies have potential for the treatment of CMT2E but their efficacy would depend on the profile of HSPs induced and the type of *NEFL* mutation.

2.3. Giant axonal neuropathy

GAN is a rare progressive neurodegenerative disorder with early onset affecting both PNS and CNS. Phenotypic variability has been reported but typical clinical features include distal limb weakness, areflexia and a marked gait disturbance. The motor deficits encompass amyotrophy, muscle weakness and evolve with skeletal deformations and loss of ambulation by the adolescence. As the disorder progresses, CNS involvement includes electroencephalographic abnormalities, mental retardation, speech defect, seizures and defective upper motor neuron function. GAN is caused by mutations in the *GAN* gene encoding the ubiquitously expressed protein gigaxonin. Gigaxonin belongs to a protein family that is characterized by an N-terminal BTB (broad-complex, Tramtrack, and Bric a brac) domain and six kelch repeats [105]. BTB/

kelch proteins are organizers of the cytoskeletal network and closely linked to the ubiquitin degradation pathway. More than 45 distinct mutations of the gigaxonin have been identified to date along the entire *GAN* gene in patients. By revealing a high instability of gigaxonin in multiple lymphoblasts cell lines from unrelated patients, Cleveland et al. [106] showed that GAN is caused by a loss of function of gigaxonin.

The major cytopathological hallmark of GAN is the presence of distal enlarged axons, also called giant axons, filled with abnormally packed IFs associated with a reduced number of MTs [107]. In contrast, axonal segments proximal to the swellings exhibit a reduced number of NFs [108]. Disorganization and accumulation of other types of IFs are also found in skin fibroblasts, Schwann cells and muscle fibers [109-111], suggesting a critical role of gigaxonin in maintaining cytoskeletal architecture. A decreased inter-NF distance was observed in sural nerve axons of a GAN patient and, more surprisingly, the mean diameter of NFs was increased (12.4 nm in GAN compared with 10.1 nm in controls) [112]. Although the mechanism leading to the distal axonal accumulation of NFs is still unclear, an acceleration of their axonal transport was observed in optic nerve from experimentally induced GAN rat model, concomitant with a proximal decreased content of NFs and their distal accumulation [113]. The authors proposed that acceleration of NF transport in the presence of a normal rate of NF protein synthesis and insertion into transport system would lead to the formation of distal axonal swellings with packed NFs.

In order to determine how loss of gigaxonin's function leads to GAN, mice deleted in exons 3-5 of the *GAN* gene ($GAN^{\Delta 3\text{-}5}$ mice) were produced [114]. These mice develop strong motor deficits as early as 6 months of age, including reduction of spontaneous movement, bizarre limb posture and overall weakness. However, they displayed normal life span and fertility, and giant axons were never seen. Nevertheless these mice exhibited enlarged axons with densely packed NF, leading to the segregation of axonal organelles, a feature characteristic of human GAN pathology. This was accompanied by an axonal loss at the age of 9-12 months. However, it should be noted that some null mice showed no overt neurological phenotypes, suggesting that some genetic modifiers may exist [115]. Another mouse model with deletion of exon 1 of the *GAN* gene was generated [116] which exhibited no overt phenotype over 15 months in contrast to $GAN^{\Delta 3\text{-}5}$ mice. Nevertheless, they developed aggregates composed of non-phosphorylated NFH and α-internexin in cerebral cortex and thalamus. Small aggregates of NFL and peripherin also formed in cell bodies of dorsal root ganglion neurons. Moreover, increased levels of neuronal IF proteins were detected in various regions of the nervous system, confirming the importance of gigaxonin in modulating the levels and organization of IF proteins. Given the very different phenotypes between these two GAN models, Ganay et al. [117] conducted a behavioral analysis over a 72-week period in their own $GAN^{\Delta 3\text{-}5}$ mice as well as in $GAN^{\Delta 3\text{-}5}$ mice developed by Ding et al [114]. Analysis performed on their own model revealed difference depending on the genetic background. Indeed, a mild but persistent motor impairment was reported in the 129/SvJ genetic background, while C57BL/6 animals displayed rather a deterioration of sensory functions. Despite the modest phenotypic manifestation and no pronounced signs of neurodegeneration, these mice exhibited severe cytoskeletal alterations, including an increase in the diameter of NFs, an overt impairment in their orientation and a strikingly increased abundance of the three NF subunits. Finally, they tested motor deficits in GAN$^{\Delta3\text{-}5}$ mice produced by Ding et al [114] and detected no clinical signs within the first year. This is consistent with a mild progression of the disease in mice and suggests that the three existing models probably display a phenotype of similar intensity. Altogether, these data shown that the absence of gigaxonin results in a milder version of the GAN disease in mice at the behavioral level, associated with a severe disorganization of the NF network that recapitulates what is observed in patients [117].

Gigaxonin was shown to be a direct key player in the Ubiquitin Proteasome System (UPS). Indeed, BTB-containing proteins, including gigaxonin have been found to be the substrate adaptors of Cul3-dependant E3 ubiquitin ligases, interacting with Cul3 and the substrates through the BTB and the C-terminal domains, respectively [118-120]. Gigaxonin was shown to promote the ubiquitin-mediated degradation of its three known substrates, the microtubule-associated protein 1B (MAP1B) [121], tubulin folding cofactor B (TBCB) [122] and MAP1S (also called MAP8) [114]. Disease associated gigaxonin mutations perturb its association with these partners while gigaxonin ablation results in their accumulation [114, 122, 123]. This raised the possibility that IF accumulation in GAN results from a MT reorganization/destabilization. However, it is intriguing to note that these proteins have opposite effects on MT network: MAP1B is a MT-stabilizing phosphoprotein, whereas overexpression of TBCB depolymerizes MTs. Using primary fibroblasts derived from skin biopsies of multiple GAN patients with aberrant aggregates of vimentin, Cleveland et al. [106] demonstrated that vimentin aggregation is greatly enhanced in conditions driving quiescence and is not caused by an abnormal accumulation of the tubulin chaperone TBCB and its effect on MT stability. Moreover, the prolonged depletion of the MT network did not induce GAN-like aggregates of vimentin in normal fibroblasts. These results indicated that the generalized disorganization of IFs in GAN patients may not involve TBCB-mediated MT disassembly and must be regulated by a yet unidentified mechanism [106]. Recently, proteomic analysis performed in fibroblasts from four GAN patients provided new insights into disease mechanisms [124]. Although the major role of gigaxonin is reported to be degradation of cytoskeleton-associated proteins, the amount of 76 structural cytoskeletal proteins was unaltered. However, several proteins linked to regulation of the cytoskeleton network were found to be upregulated or downregulated. The authors speculated that in GAN, dysregulation of the cytoskeletal network is responsible for formation of aggregates of IFs. In the case of fibroblasts, disturbed cytoskeletal regulation could lead to a hyperphosphorylation state of vimentin that results in massive depolymerization of vimentin filaments and finally in collapse of the vimentin network. The unpolymerized filaments are collected in the aggresome near the nucleus where they form the typical aggregates [124].

2.4. Neuronal intermediate filament inclusion disease

NIFID is a recently described uncommon neurological disorder of early onset with a heterogeneous clinical phenotype, including sporadic fronto-temporal dementia associated with a pyramidal and/or extrapyramidal movement disorder. The symptoms comprise behavioural

http://dx.doi.org/10.5772/54676

and personality changes, which can be associated to memory loss, cognitive impairment, language impairment, hyperreflexia and motor weakness. Neuropathologically, NIFID is characterized by widespread degeneration of the frontal and temporal lobes. The cytopathological characteristics consist of neuronal loss, gliosis, swollen neurons and presence of large inclusions in the cell body of many neurons that are immunoreactive for all of the class IV neuronal IFs and especially in α-internexin [125, 126]. These inclusions of α-internexin but negative for tau or synuclein distinguish NIFID from other disease that involve IF inclusions, such as synucleinopathies (e.g., PD), tauopathies (e.g., AD and frontotemporal dementia), and motor neuron disease. Although α-internexin has been observed in neuronal inclusions in other neurodegenerative disorders, it is generally a relatively minor component. This raises the question whether α-internexin-positive neuronal inclusions in NIFID reflect any selective neuronal dysfunction, and as such if they are associated with some specific clinical symptoms. Genetic screening revealed no pathogenic variants for all type IV neuronal IFs, SOD1, NUDEL and gigaxonin [127, 128]. To date, no genetic mutations leading to NIFID have been described.

Interestingly, the number of IFs aggregates is high in areas with reduced neuronal loss, and low in sites of intense neuronal degeneration. Cairns et al. [125] proposed that the formation of these inclusions is an early event in the pathogenesis of NIFID, and these aggregates are then released and degraded into the extracellular space following degeneration of the neuron. The mechanism of IF aggregation and the role they play in neuronal dysfunction and cell death are still unclear. Although immunoreactivity for IFs was initially described as the defining pathological feature of NIFID, not all the inclusions in NIFID are IF-positive. It now appears that aggregates of FUS (fused in sarcoma) protein, is a more consistent feature of NIFID. Indeed, intracellular accumulations of FUS are more often encountered than IF inclusions and all neurons that contained abnormal IF aggregates also contained FUS inclusions [129]. It should also be noted that clusters of FUS-immunoreactive inclusions are larger than those revealed by NFH or α-internexin [130]. The authors interpreted this finding as suggesting that FUS plays a more central role in the pathogenesis of NIFID and that the abnormal accumulation of IFs is likely a secondary phenomenon. It now remains to determine the exact implication of FUS in the pathogenesis of NIFID.

2.5. Diabetic neuropathy

Diabetes is the leading cause of peripheral neuropathy worldwide. About 60 to 70 percent of people with diabetes have some form of neuropathy. People with diabetes can develop nerve problems at any time, but risk rises with age and longer duration of diabetes. Diabetic neuropathies are complex, heterogeneous disorders that affect dorsal root ganglia and sensory axons more so than motor fibers. Nerve damage is likely due to a combination of factors, including metabolic factors (e.g., high blood glucose, abnormal blood fat levels), neurovascular factors leading to damage to the blood vessels, autoimmune factors, lifestyle factors and inherited traits that increase susceptibility to nerve disease. Although its pathogenesis has not been fully elucidated, diabetic neuropathy is characterized by slower conduction velocity, impairment of axonal transport, axonal atrophy and reduced capacity for nerve regeneration. All these features of nerve function depend on the integrity of the axonal cytoskeleton and particularly on NFs. In agreement with this, multiple abnormalities of NF biology were identified in models of diabetes. An impairment of the axonal transport of NFs, actin and tubulin concomitant with a proximal increase and a distal decrease of axonal calibers were observed in rats with streptozotocin-induced diabetes and in BioBreeding rats (a model of spontaneous type I diabetes) [131, 132]. The distal axonal atrophy is accompanied by a concomitant NF loss in this region [133], and accumulations of highly phosphorylated NF epitopes are present in proximal axonal segments of dorsal root ganglia sensory neurons from diabetic patients [134]. An increase of NF phosphorylation, correlated with activation of JNK, was also detected in lumbar dorsal root ganglia from rat models [135]. Finally, there were a substantial decline in the mRNA levels of all three NF subunits as well as reduced NF numbers and densities within large myelinated sensory of long-term diabetic models [136]. All these results suggest that NF abnormalities may contribute to the development of diabetic neuropathy, or may be affected by this disease. However, slowing of conduction velocity in diabetic models occurs much earlier than loss of NF investment or axonal atrophy [136]. To further elucidate the contribution of NFs to diabetic neuropathy pathogenesis, the effect of streptozotocin-induced diabetes was analyzed in NFH-LacZ transgenic mice characterized by axons completely lacking NFs [137]. Interestingly, diabetic mice lacking NFs developed progressive slowing of conduction velocity in their motor and sensory fibres and displayed decreased nerve action potential amplitudes earlier than diabetic mice with normal IF cytoskeleton. Moreover, superimposing diabetes on axons without NFs also accentuated axonal atrophy. Administration of insulin that restored normoglycemia reversed conduction slowing and restored sensory axon caliber. These findings indicate that changes in NF expression, transport or post-translational modifications cannot account alone for neurological features of diabetic neuropathy, but these IFs may help axons to better resist the negative effects of diabetes [137].

2.6. Parkinson disease

Parkinson's disease (PD) is the second most common neurodegenerative disorder after AD, with a prevalence of about 2% among people over the age of 65 years. This disease is marked by the depletion of dopaminergic melanin-containing neurons in the substantia nigra pars compacta and a consequent loss of dopamine in the striatum. Another important pathological feature is the presence, especially in substantia nigra pars compacta neurons, of eosinophilic cytoplasmic inclusion bodies named Lewy bodies, composed of α-synuclein, NF proteins, ubiquitin and proteasome subunits. Various features distinguish NFs in PD, including inappropriate phosphorylation and proteolysis in Lewy bodies [138, 139], decreased NFL and NFH mRNA levels [140], and reduced protein level of NFL and NFM [141]. A point mutation in the *NEFM* gene was reported in a case of PD with early onset [142]. This mutation consisted in a substitution of Ser for Gly at residue 336, a highly conserved region in the rod domain 2B of NFM, and was argued to disrupt NF assembly. Although three other unaffected family members also carried this mutation, the authors had then proposed that aberrations in neuronal IFs could lead to the development of the pathology seen in PD. However, the G336S mutation does not disrupt the assembly and the distribution of NFs *in vitro* [143] and the screenings of PD patients of similar or different ethnic background failed to identify this mutations [144,

145], arguing against the implication of this *NEFM* mutation in pathogenesis of PD. Interestingly, research has shown that changes in the levels of NFL in the cerebrospinal fluid may be used as a biomarker for the identification of PD [146] and that the serum levels of anti-NF protein antibodies increase significantly in patients with PD [147]. Finally, it seemed that the serum level of NFs in patients with PD was significantly correlated with duration of the disease and age [148]. These findings support the idea that axonal injury causes the release of cytoskeleton proteins, and changes in the concentrations of serum NFs are probably related to the severity of axonal injuries.

3. Glial intermediate filament GFAP and Alexander disease

Neuronal IFs are not the only class of IF to be responsible for the development of neurological disorders. Glial IF can also be the primary cause of a CNS disorder. Indeed, GFAP, the major constituent of astrocytic IFs, is directly involved in the development of the AXD. This disease is a fatal, progressive white matter disorder that has been classified into three types based on the age of onset: infantile, juvenile and adult. The infantile type, with onset between birth and about two years of age, is the most frequent form of the disease and is fatal either within that period or by around the age of 10 years. Clinical symptoms comprise progressive megalencephaly, seizures and impaired cognitive function, which may be associated with ataxia and hydrocephalus. Such phenotypes become progressively less common for the juvenile and adult forms (for recent reviews, see [149, 150]). Both the infantile and juvenile forms usually appear to be sporadic while the adult form is often familial.

AXD is a primary astrocytic disease and its manifestations are the result of astrocyte dysfunctions leading to both myelin damage and neuron dysfunction. Neuronal loss is often reported but axons are relatively well preserved in demyelinated areas. The pathological hallmark of AXD is the presence of protein aggregates known as Rosenthal fibers within the cytoplasm of astrocytes throughout the CNS, but especially those located in the subpial, periventricular and subependymal zones. Different constituents were identified in Rosenthal fibers: GFAP, αB-crystallin, HSP27 and ubiquitin [151-153]. Although GFAP is also expressed in glial cells of the PNS and in several other organs, Rosenthal fibers were not reported outside the CNS of AXD patients.

To examine the function of GFAP *in vivo*, GFAP knock-out mice were generated [154-157]. These studies showed that mice lacking GFAP displayed astrocytes devoid of the IF, but still developed and reproduced normally. Only subtle phenotypes emerged with age, arguing for a role of GFAP in the white matter architecture, blood-brain barrier integrity, astrocyte-neuronal interactions and in modulating synaptic efficacy in the CNS [156, 157]. This is consistent with the known roles of astrocytes that help to form blood brain barrier, promote synaptic plasticity and coordinate neuronal activity. To determine the influence of increased GFAP expression on astrocyte function, mice overexpressing the human *GFAP* gene were produced [158]. Mice in the highest expressing lines developed a phenotype close to that observed in AXD. Indeed, their brains contain many inclusion bodies indistinguishable from human

Rosenthal fibers, astrocytes are hypertrophic and these animals died from an encephalopathy at an age that is inversely correlated with the level of expression of the transgene. However, no myelin abnormalities were observed. Microarray analysis performed on olfactory bulbs of these animals recently highlighted the appearance of an initial stress response by astrocytes which results in the activation of microglia and compromised neuronal function [159]. All these results suggested that a primary alteration in GFAP may be responsible for AXD.

Sequence analysis of DNA samples from AXD patients was thus performed and revealed that most cases are associated with mutations in the *GFAP* gene [160]. Since then, numerous mutations of this gene were identified; many of them being located in highly conserved domains of the encoded protein that play specific roles in the assembly of IF network [8, 150]. It was estimated that more than 95% of AXD cases are due to *GFAP* mutation. To date, all the identified mutations are heterozygous and nearly all of them involve amino acid substitutions, but several insertion or deletion/insertion alterations have also been reported (a continually updated list of all published mutations is maintained at the Waisman Center of the University of Wisconsin-Madison; www.waisman.wisc.edu/alexander). Numerous mutations cluster in the coils 1A and 2B of GFAP and two sites (R79 and R239) account for approximately half of all patients affected. The comparison of mutations occurring in the various IF proteins revealed that frequent mutations lying in the 2A segment seem to be unique to GFAP. It is possible that molecular partners specifically interact with this region of GFAP but not with the equivalent region of other IFs. The calcium-binding protein S100B binds to the N-terminal part of GFAP-coil 2A [161]. As S100B prevents GFAP assembly [162], mutations in this domain could impair GFAP-S100B interactions, resulting in the accumulation of GFAP polymers and possibly aggregates. It seems that a correlation exists between the different mutations and the severity of the disease. However, there also exists significant phenotypic variability and age of onset for the same mutation [163], suggesting that epigenetic and environmental factors influence the appearance and timing of disease symptoms. It should also be noted that in rare cases of AXD, no mutations in the *GFAP* gene has been found [164], indicating that there may be additional causes of the disease.

The discovery of GFAP mutations led to the generation of knock-in mice with missense mutations homologous to those found in humans (R76H and R236H, which correspond to the R79H and R239H mutations in human) [165, 166]. If the presence of mutant GFAP *per se* seemed insufficient for aggregate formation, a 30% increase in GFAP content over that in wild-type induced the formation of Rosenthal fibers in multiples sites throughout the CNS [166]. These animals were also more susceptible to kainate-induced seizures. Nevertheless, they had a normal lifespan, showed no overt behavioral defects and general white matter architecture and myelination appeared normal. These features resemble those found in the adult form of AXD rather than in the infantile form. This indicates that the presence of GFAP aggregates containing mutant GFAP is not sufficient to induce a major phenotype of AXD, even though it causes some abnormalities in the mouse. Interestingly, further elevation of GFAP via crosses to GFAP transgenic animals led to a shift in GFAP solubility, an increased stress response, and ultimately death [165]. This correlates GFAP protein levels to the severity of the disease.

http://dx.doi.org/10.5772/54676

While the genetic basis for AXD is now firmly recognized, there is little information concerning the mechanisms by which GFAP mutations lead to disease. Several study showed that mutations of GFAP alters the normal solubility and organization of GFAP networks [163, 167]. When expressed alone, these mutant proteins lost their ability to form filament *in vitro*. But in presence of assembly partners, such as wild-type GFAP or vimentin, they were still capable of incorporation into filament networks in transfected cells. If wild-type GFAP is prone to aggregate, mutations of GFAP exacerbates this accumulation [168]. Insufficient amounts of plectin, due to R239C GFAP expression, were also proposed to promote GFAP aggregation and Rosenthal fibers formation in AXD [169]. Both inhibited proteasome activity and activated stress pathways seemed to be important consequences of GFAP accumulation [168]. As a positive feedback response, both the proteasome hypofunction and JNK activation exacerbated GFAP accumulation, increasing susceptibility of the cell to stressful stimuli. It thus appeared that accumulations of GFAP protein would be more deleterious to the astrocytes than the mutant protein itself. However, as a positive consequence, up-regulation of αB-crystallin and HSP27 were also associated to the aggregation of GFAP in AXD patients [153, 170] as well as in cell and animal models [159, 165, 168]. Increased αB-crystallin levels would contribute to the disaggregation of GFAP aggregates and could protect cells from apoptotic events [171]. Moreover, a recent study demonstrated that AXD mutant GFAP accumulation stimulates autophagy which in turn contributes to decrease GFAP levels [172]. The balance between the positive and negative effects of GFAP accumulation might define the survival or death of the cell. Compounds known to reduce GFAP expression *in vitro*, such as quercetin, might be useful as therapeutics. For instance, treatment with the antibiotic ceftriaxone alleviates intracytoplasmic aggregates of mutant GFAP by inducing the up-regulation of HSP27 and αB-crystallin, poly-ubiquitination and autophagy, and by reducing the *GFAP* promoter transcriptional regulation [173]. Curcumin was also reported to have beneficial effects in an *in vitro* model of AXD. Indeed, curcumin is able to induce both HSP27 and αB-crystallin, to reduce expression of both RNA and protein of endogenous GFAP, to induce autophagy and, finally, to rescue the filamentous organization of the GFAP mutant protein, thus suggesting a role of this spice in counteracting the pathogenic effects of *GFAP* mutations [174].

The *GFAP* gene is known to generate different splice variants, including the most abundant isoform GFAP-α, and seven other differentially expressed transcripts including GFAP-δ (human homologous GFAP-ε). GFAP-δ is incapable of self-assembly into IF *per se*, but can incorporate a filament network composed of GFAP-α if the proportion of GFAP-δ to GFAP-α remains <10% [175]. However, elevating the proportion of GFAP-δ perturbs association of αB-crystallin with the IF fraction and induced IF bundling and aggregation in transiently transfected cells. Interestingly, GFAP-δ isoform is preferentially expressed in the same populations of astrocytes that contain the most Rosenthal fibers in AXD. This raises the possibility that GFAP-δ may play a key role in aggregate formation in combination with mutated GFAP. It remains to determine whether GFAP-α:GFAP-δ ratio is perturbed in AXD tissues.

4. Conclusion

IFs abnormalities are reminiscent in multiple human neurodegenerative disorders. Despite extensive efforts over the past 40 years, processes leading to these abnormalities as well as their precise contribution to disease pathogenesis often remain poorly understood. For instance, if it is clearly established that mutation in IF genes can be a primary cause of neurodegenerative disorders, the question as to how they induce neurodegeneration frequently remain unsolved. Although transgenic mouse models have been somewhat helpful in understanding some mechanisms, most of these animals displayed a much less severe phenotype than patients and results have not always been completely clear-cut. A growing body of evidence suggests that perturbation of IF axonal transport and/or stoichiometry are directly involved in the formation of intracellular IF aggregates. Destabilization of IF mRNA could be responsible for alteration in IF stoichiometry whereas aberrant post-translational modifications could affect their transport. More investigations are also necessary to identify IF partners. The importance of IF-associated proteins in the development of neurodegenerative disorders was also highlighted by the identification of mutations in genes encoding IF partners that mimic IF-related disease. This is particularly the case of gigaxonin in GAN. A particular attention should also be paid to elucidate the role that IF proteins may play in signaling. Finally, it will be important to elucidate why certain types of IF accumulations appear more toxic than others. While perikaryal accumulations are generally well tolerated, axonal inclusions are often noxious. The more deleterious effect of axonal aggregates on axonal transport could be a promising avenue to explore in the future and the identification of compounds able to remove these IF aggregates is crucial to the development of new therapeutic approaches.

Author details

Rodolphe Perrot[1] and Joel Eyer[2]

1 Service Commun d'Imageries et d'Analyses Microscopiques, Université d'Angers, Institut de Biologie en Santé – IRIS, CHU, France

2 Laboratoire de Neurobiologie & Transgenese, UPRES-EA3143, Institut de Biologie en Santé – IRIS, CHU, France

References

[1] Julien JP and Mushynski WE. Neurofilaments in health and disease. Prog Nucleic Acid Res Mol Biol 1998;61 1-23

[2] Yuan A, Rao MV, Sasaki T, Chen Y, Kumar A, Veeranna, Liem RK, Eyer J, Peterson AC, Julien JP and Nixon RA. Alpha-internexin is structurally and functionally associ-

ated with the neurofilament triplet proteins in the mature CNS. J Neurosci 2006;26 (39) 10006-19

[3] Yan Y, Jensen K and Brown A. The polypeptide composition of moving and stationary neurofilaments in cultured sympathetic neurons. Cell Motil Cytoskeleton 2007;64 (4) 299-309

[4] Perrot R, Berges R, Bocquet A and Eyer J. Review of the multiple aspects of neurofilament functions, and their possible contribution to neurodegeneration. Mol Neurobiol 2008;38 (1) 27-65

[5] Nixon RA and Shea TB. Dynamics of neuronal intermediate filaments: a developmental perspective. Cell Motil Cytoskeleton 1992;22 (2) 81-91

[6] Fuchs E and Weber K. Intermediate filaments: structure, dynamics, function, and disease. Annu Rev Biochem 1994;63 345-82

[7] Perrot R and Eyer J. Neuronal intermediate filaments and neurodegenerative disorders. Brain Res Bull 2009;80 (4-5) 282-95

[8] Quinlan RA, Brenner M, Goldman JE and Messing A. GFAP and its role in Alexander disease. Exp Cell Res 2007;313 (10) 2077-87

[9] Corbo M and Hays AP. Peripherin and neurofilament protein coexist in spinal spheroids of motor neuron disease. J Neuropathol Exp Neurol 1992;51 (5) 531-7

[10] Figlewicz DA, Krizus A, Martinoli MG, Meininger V, Dib M, Rouleau GA and Julien JP. Variants of the Heavy Neurofilament Subunit Are Associated with the Development of Amyotrophic-Lateral-Sclerosis. Human Molecular Genetics 1994;3 (10) 1757-1761

[11] Tomkins J, Usher P, Slade JY, Ince PG, Curtis A, Bushby K and Shaw PJ. Novel insertion in the KSP region of the neurofilament heavy gene in amyotrophic lateral sclerosis (ALS). Neuroreport 1998;9 (17) 3967-3970

[12] Al-Chalabi A, Andersen PM, Nilsson P, Chioza B, Andersson JL, Russ C, Shaw CE, Powell JF and Leigh PN. Deletions of the heavy neurofilament subunit tail in amyotrophic lateral sclerosis. Human Molecular Genetics 1999;8 (2) 157-164

[13] Rooke K, Figlewicz DA, Han FY and Rouleau GA. Analysis of the KSP repeat of the neurofilament heavy subunit in familial amyotrophic lateral sclerosis. Neurology 1996;46 (3) 789-790

[14] Vechio JD, Bruijn LI, Xu ZS, Brown RH and Cleveland DW. Sequence variants in human neurofilament proteins: Absence of linkage to familial amyotrophic lateral sclerosis. Annals of Neurology 1996;40 (4) 603-610

[15] Gros-Louis F, Lariviere R, Gowing G, Laurent S, Camu W, Bouchard JP, Meininger V, Rouleau GA and Julien JP. A frameshift deletion in peripherin gene associated

with amyotrophic lateral sclerosis. Journal of Biological Chemistry 2004;279 (44) 45951-45956

[16] Leung CL, He CZ, Kaufmann P, Chin SS, Naini A, Liem RKH, Mitsumoto H and Hays AP. A pathogenic peripherin gene mutation in a patient with amyotrophic lateral sclerosis. Brain Pathology 2004;14 (3) 290-296

[17] Corrado L, Carlomagno Y, Falasco L, Mellone S, Godi M, Cova E, Cereda C, Testa L, Mazzini L and D'Alfonso S. A novel peripherin gene (PRPH) mutation identified in one sporadic amyotrophic lateral sclerosis patient. Neurobiol Aging

[18] Xiao S, Tjostheim S, Sanelli T, McLean JR, Horne P, Fan Y, Ravits J, Strong MJ and Robertson J. An aggregate-inducing peripherin isoform generated through intron retention is upregulated in amyotrophic lateral sclerosis and associated with disease pathology. Journal of Neuroscience 2008;28 (8) 1833-1840

[19] Robertson J, Doroudchi MM, Nguyen MD, Durham HD, Strong MJ, Shaw G, Julien JP and Mushynski WE. A neurotoxic peripherin splice variant in a mouse model of ALS. Journal of Cell Biology 2003;160 (6) 939-949

[20] Niebroj-Dobosz I, Dziewulska D and Janik P. Auto-antibodies against proteins of spinal cord cells in cerebrospinal fluid of patients with amyotrophic lateral sclerosis (ALS). Folia Neuropathol 2006;44 (3) 191-6

[21] Zetterberg H, Jacobsson J, Rosengren L, Blennow K and Andersen PM. Cerebrospinal fluid neurofilament light levels in amyotrophic lateral sclerosis: impact of SOD1 genotype. Eur J Neurol 2007;14 (12) 1329-33

[22] Brettschneider J, Petzold A, Sussmuth SD, Ludolph AC and Tumani H. Axonal damage markers in cerebrospinal fluid are increased in ALS. Neurology 2006;66 (6) 852-6

[23] Lu CH, Petzold A, Kalmar B, Dick J, Malaspina A and Greensmith L. Plasma Neurofilament Heavy Chain Levels Correlate to Markers of Late Stage Disease Progression and Treatment Response in SOD1(G93A) Mice that Model ALS. PLoS One 2012;7 (7) e40998

[24] Tortelli R, Ruggieri M, Cortese R, D'Errico E, Capozzo R, Leo A, Mastrapasqua M, Zoccolella S, Leante R, Livrea P, Logroscino G and Simone IL. Elevated cerebrospinal fluid neurofilament light levels in patients with amyotrophic lateral sclerosis: a possible marker of disease severity and progression. Eur J Neurol 2012;

[25] Manetto V, Sternberger NH, Perry G, Sternberger LA and Gambetti P. Phosphorylation of neurofilaments is altered in amyotrophic lateral sclerosis. J Neuropathol Exp Neurol 1988;47 (6) 642-53

[26] Collard JF, Cote F and Julien JP. Defective axonal transport in a transgenic mouse model of amyotrophic lateral sclerosis. Nature 1995;375 (6526) 61-4

[27] Williamson TL and Cleveland DW. Slowing of axonal transport is a very early event in the toxicity of ALS-linked SOD1 mutants to motor neurons. Nat Neurosci 1999;2 (1) 50-6

[28] Zhang B, Tu P, Abtahian F, Trojanowski JQ and Lee VM. Neurofilaments and orthograde transport are reduced in ventral root axons of transgenic mice that express human SOD1 with a G93A mutation. J Cell Biol 1997;139 (5) 1307-15

[29] Bilsland LG, Sahai E, Kelly G, Golding M, Greensmith L and Schiavo G. Deficits in axonal transport precede ALS symptoms in vivo. Proc Natl Acad Sci U S A

[30] Ackerley S, Grierson AJ, Brownlees J, Thornhill P, Anderton BH, Leigh PN, Shaw CE and Miller CC. Glutamate slows axonal transport of neurofilaments in transfected neurons. J Cell Biol 2000;150 (1) 165-76

[31] Manser C, Stevenson A, Banner S, Davies J, Tudor EL, Ono Y, Leigh PN, McLoughlin DM, Shaw CE and Miller CC. Deregulation of PKN1 activity disrupts neurofilament organisation and axonal transport. FEBS Lett 2008;582 (15) 2303-8

[32] King AE, Dickson TC, Blizzard CA, Foster SS, Chung RS, West AK, Chuah MI and Vickers JC. Excitotoxicity mediated by non-NMDA receptors causes distal axonopathy in long-term cultured spinal motor neurons. Eur J Neurosci 2007;26 (8) 2151-9

[33] Kesavapany S, Patel V, Zheng YL, Pareek TK, Bjelogrlic M, Albers W, Amin N, Jaffe H, Gutkind JS, Strong MJ, Grant P and Pant HC. Inhibition of Pin1 reduces glutamate-induced perikaryal accumulation of phosphorylated neurofilament-H in neurons. Mol Biol Cell 2007;18 (9) 3645-55

[34] Stevenson A, Yates DM, Manser C, De Vos KJ, Vagnoni A, Leigh PN, McLoughlin DM and Miller CC. Riluzole protects against glutamate-induced slowing of neurofilament axonal transport. Neurosci Lett 2009;454 (2) 161-4

[35] Hafezparast M, Klocke R, Ruhrberg C, Marquardt A, Ahmad-Annuar A, Bowen S, Lalli G, Witherden AS, Hummerich H, Nicholson S, Morgan PJ, Oozageer R, Priestley JV, Averill S, King VR, Ball S, Peters J, Toda T, Yamamoto A, Hiraoka Y, Augustin M, Korthaus D, Wattler S, Wabnitz P, Dickneite C, Lampel S, Boehme F, Peraus G, Popp A, Rudelius M, Schlegel J, Fuchs H, Hrabe de Angelis M, Schiavo G, Shima DT, Russ AP, Stumm G, Martin JE and Fisher EM. Mutations in dynein link motor neuron degeneration to defects in retrograde transport. Science 2003;300 (5620) 808-12

[36] LaMonte BH, Wallace KE, Holloway BA, Shelly SS, Ascano J, Tokito M, Van Winkle T, Howland DS and Holzbaur EL. Disruption of dynein/dynactin inhibits axonal transport in motor neurons causing late-onset progressive degeneration. Neuron 2002;34 (5) 715-27

[37] Xia CH, Roberts EA, Her LS, Liu X, Williams DS, Cleveland DW and Goldstein LS. Abnormal neurofilament transport caused by targeted disruption of neuronal kinesin heavy chain KIF5A. J Cell Biol 2003;161 (1) 55-66

[38] Motil J, Dubey M, Chan WK and Shea TB. Inhibition of dynein but not kinesin induces aberrant focal accumulation of neurofilaments within axonal neurites. Brain Res 2007;1164 125-31

[39] Teuling E, van Dis V, Wulf PS, Haasdijk ED, Akhmanova A, Hoogenraad CC and Jaarsma D. A novel mouse model with impaired dynein/dynactin function develops amyotrophic lateral sclerosis (ALS)-like features in motor neurons and improves lifespan in SOD1-ALS mice. Hum Mol Genet 2008;17 (18) 2849-62

[40] Cote F, Collard JF and Julien JP. Progressive neuronopathy in transgenic mice expressing the human neurofilament heavy gene: a mouse model of amyotrophic lateral sclerosis. Cell 1993;73 (1) 35-46

[41] Gama Sosa MA, Friedrich VL, Jr., DeGasperi R, Kelley K, Wen PH, Senturk E, Lazzarini RA and Elder GA. Human midsized neurofilament subunit induces motor neuron disease in transgenic mice. Exp Neurol 2003;184 (1) 408-19

[42] Xu Z, Cork LC, Griffin JW and Cleveland DW. Increased expression of neurofilament subunit NF-L produces morphological alterations that resemble the pathology of human motor neuron disease. Cell 1993;73 (1) 23-33

[43] Meier J, Couillard-Despres S, Jacomy H, Gravel C and Julien JP. Extra neurofilament NF-L subunits rescue motor neuron disease caused by overexpression of the human NF-H gene in mice. J Neuropathol Exp Neurol 1999;58 (10) 1099-110

[44] Beaulieu JM, Nguyen MD and Julien JP. Late onset of motor neurons in mice overexpressing wild-type peripherin. J Cell Biol 1999;147 (3) 531-44

[45] Beaulieu JM, Jacomy H and Julien JP. Formation of intermediate filament protein aggregates with disparate effects in two transgenic mouse models lacking the neurofilament light subunit. J Neurosci 2000;20 (14) 5321-8

[46] Millecamps S, Robertson J, Lariviere R, Mallet J and Julien JP. Defective axonal transport of neurofilament proteins in neurons overexpressing peripherin. J Neurochem 2006;98 (3) 926-38

[47] Perrot R and Julien JP. Real-time imaging reveals defects of fast axonal transport induced by disorganization of intermediate filaments. Faseb J 2009;23 (9) 3213-25

[48] Robertson J, Beaulieu JM, Doroudchi MM, Durham HD, Julien JP and Mushynski WE. Apoptotic death of neurons exhibiting peripherin aggregates is mediated by the proinflammatory cytokine tumor necrosis factor-alpha. J Cell Biol 2001;155 (2) 217-26

[49] Beaulieu JM and Julien JP. Peripherin-mediated death of motor neurons rescued by overexpression of neurofilament NF-H proteins. J Neurochem 2003;85 (1) 248-56

[50] Lariviere RC, Beaulieu JM, Nguyen MD and Julien JP. Peripherin is not a contributing factor to motor neuron disease in a mouse model of amyotrophic lateral sclerosis caused by mutant superoxide dismutase. Neurobiol Dis 2003;13 (2) 158-66

[51] Bergeron C, Beric-Maskarel K, Muntasser S, Weyer L, Somerville MJ and Percy ME. Neurofilament light and polyadenylated mRNA levels are decreased in amyotrophic lateral sclerosis motor neurons. J Neuropathol Exp Neurol 1994;53 (3) 221-30

[52] Strong MJ, Leystra-Lantz C and Ge WW. Intermediate filament steady-state mRNA levels in amyotrophic lateral sclerosis. Biochem Biophys Res Commun 2004;316 (2) 317-22

[53] Wong NK, He BP and Strong MJ. Characterization of neuronal intermediate filament protein expression in cervical spinal motor neurons in sporadic amyotrophic lateral sclerosis (ALS). J Neuropathol Exp Neurol 2000;59 (11) 972-82

[54] Ge WW, Volkening K, Leystra-Lantz C, Jaffe H and Strong MJ. 14-3-3 protein binds to the low molecular weight neurofilament (NFL) mRNA 3' UTR. Mol Cell Neurosci 2007;34 (1) 80-7

[55] Strong MJ, Volkening K, Hammond R, Yang W, Strong W, Leystra-Lantz C and Shoesmith C. TDP43 is a human low molecular weight neurofilament (hNFL) mRNA-binding protein. Mol Cell Neurosci 2007;35 (2) 320-7

[56] Ge WW, Wen W, Strong W, Leystra-Lantz C and Strong MJ. Mutant copper-zinc superoxide dismutase binds to and destabilizes human low molecular weight neurofilament mRNA. J Biol Chem 2005;280 (1) 118-24

[57] Volkening K, Leystra-Lantz C and Strong MJ. Human low molecular weight neurofilament (NFL) mRNA interacts with a predicted p190RhoGEF homologue (RGNEF) in humans. Amyotroph Lateral Scler 11 (1-2) 97-103

[58] Shan X, Chiang PM, Price DL and Wong PC. Altered distributions of Gemini of coiled bodies and mitochondria in motor neurons of TDP-43 transgenic mice. Proc Natl Acad Sci U S A 107 (37) 16325-30

[59] Swarup V and Julien JP. ALS pathogenesis: Recent insights from genetics and mouse models. Prog Neuropsychopharmacol Biol Psychiatry

[60] Swarup V, Phaneuf D, Bareil C, Robertson J, Rouleau GA, Kriz J and Julien JP. Pathological hallmarks of amyotrophic lateral sclerosis/frontotemporal lobar degeneration in transgenic mice produced with TDP-43 genomic fragments. Brain 2011;134 (Pt 9) 2610-26

[61] Droppelmann CA, Keller BA, Campos-Melo D, Volkening K and Strong MJ. Rho guanine nucleotide exchange factor is an NFL mRNA destabilizing factor that forms cytoplasmic inclusions in amyotrophic lateral sclerosis. Neurobiol Aging 2012;

[62] Chou SM, Wang HS, Taniguchi A and Bucala R. Advanced glycation endproducts in neurofilament conglomeration of motoneurons in familial and sporadic amyotrophic lateral sclerosis. Molecular Medicine 1998;4 (5) 324-332

[63] Ludemann N, Clement A, Hans VH, Leschik J, Behl C and Brandt R. O-glycosylation of the tail domain of neurofilament protein M in human neurons and in spinal cord

tissue of a rat model of amyotrophic lateral sclerosis (ALS). J Biol Chem 2005;280 (36) 31648-58

[64] Shan X, Vocadlo DJ and Krieger C. Reduced protein O-glycosylation in the nervous system of the mutant SOD1 transgenic mouse model of amyotrophic lateral sclerosis. Neurosci Lett 2012;516 (2) 296-301

[65] Crow JP, Ye YZ, Strong M, Kirk M, Barnes S and Beckman JS. Superoxide dismutase catalyzes nitration of tyrosines by peroxynitrite in the rod and head domains of neurofilament-L. Journal of Neurochemistry 1997;69 (5) 1945-1953

[66] Strong MJ, Sopper MM, Crow JP, Strong WL and Beckman JS. Nitration of the low molecular weight neurofilament is equivalent in sporadic amyotrophic lateral sclerosis and control cervical spinal cord. Biochemical and Biophysical Research Communications 1998;248 (1) 157-164

[67] King AE, Dickson TC, Blizzard CA, Woodhouse A, Foster SS, Chung RS and Vickers JC. Neuron-glia interactions underlie ALS-like axonal cytoskeletal pathology. Neurobiol Aging 2009;

[68] Eyer J, Cleveland DW, Wong PC and Peterson AC. Pathogenesis of two axonopathies does not require axonal neurofilaments. Nature 1998;391 (6667) 584-7

[69] Williamson TL, Bruijn LI, Zhu Q, Anderson KL, Anderson SD, Julien JP and Cleveland DW. Absence of neurofilaments reduces the selective vulnerability of motor neurons and slows disease caused by a familial amyotrophic lateral sclerosis-linked superoxide dismutase 1 mutant. Proc Natl Acad Sci U S A 1998;95 (16) 9631-6

[70] Kong J and Xu Z. Overexpression of neurofilament subunit NF-L and NF-H extends survival of a mouse model for amyotrophic lateral sclerosis. Neurosci Lett 2000;281 (1) 72-4

[71] Couillard-Despres S, Zhu Q, Wong PC, Price DL, Cleveland DW and Julien JP. Protective effect of neurofilament heavy gene overexpression in motor neuron disease induced by mutant superoxide dismutase. Proc Natl Acad Sci U S A 1998;95 (16) 9626-30

[72] Nguyen MD, Lariviere RC and Julien JP. Reduction of axonal caliber does not alleviate motor neuron disease caused by mutant superoxide dismutase 1. Proc Natl Acad Sci U S A 2000;97 (22) 12306-11

[73] Roy J, Minotti S, Dong L, Figlewicz DA and Durham HD. Glutamate potentiates the toxicity of mutant Cu/Zn-superoxide dismutase in motor neurons by postsynaptic calcium-dependent mechanisms. J Neurosci 1998;18 (23) 9673-84

[74] Tu PH, Raju P, Robinson KA, Gurney ME, Trojanowski JQ and Lee VM. Transgenic mice carrying a human mutant superoxide dismutase transgene develop neuronal cytoskeletal pathology resembling human amyotrophic lateral sclerosis lesions. Proc Natl Acad Sci U S A 1996;93 (7) 3155-60

[75] Lobsiger CS, Garcia ML, Ward CM and Cleveland DW. Altered axonal architecture by removal of the heavily phosphorylated neurofilament tail domains strongly slows superoxide dismutase 1 mutant-mediated ALS. Proc Natl Acad Sci U S A 2005;102 (29) 10351-6

[76] Ehlers MD, Fung ET, O'Brien RJ and Huganir RL. Splice variant-specific interaction of the NMDA receptor subunit NR1 with neuronal intermediate filaments. J Neurosci 1998;18 (2) 720-30

[77] Sanelli T, Ge W, Leystra-Lantz C and Strong MJ. Calcium mediated excitotoxicity in neurofilament aggregate-bearing neurons in vitro is NMDA receptor dependant. J Neurol Sci 2007;256 (1-2) 39-51

[78] Vogel P, Gabriel M, Goebel HH and Dyck PJ. Hereditary motor sensory neuropathy type II with neurofilament accumulation: new finding or new disorder? Ann Neurol 1985;17 (5) 455-61

[79] Brownlees J, Ackerley S, Grierson AJ, Jacobsen NJ, Shea K, Anderton BH, Leigh PN, Shaw CE and Miller CC. Charcot-Marie-Tooth disease neurofilament mutations disrupt neurofilament assembly and axonal transport. Hum Mol Genet 2002;11 (23) 2837-44

[80] Perez-Olle R, Lopez-Toledano MA, Goryunov D, Cabrera-Poch N, Stefanis L, Brown K and Liem RK. Mutations in the neurofilament light gene linked to Charcot-Marie-Tooth disease cause defects in transport. J Neurochem 2005;93 (4) 861-74

[81] Lee IB, Kim SK, Chung SH, Kim H, Kwon TK, Min do S and Chang JS. The effect of rod domain A148V mutation of neurofilament light chain on filament formation. BMB Rep 2008;41 (12) 868-74

[82] Shin JS, Chung KW, Cho SY, Yun J, Hwang SJ, Kang SH, Cho EM, Kim SM and Choi BO. NEFL Pro22Arg mutation in Charcot-Marie-Tooth disease type 1. J Hum Genet 2008;53 (10) 936-40

[83] Georgiou DM, Zidar J, Korosec M, Middleton LT, Kyriakides T and Christodoulou K. A novel NF-L mutation Pro22Ser is associated with CMT2 in a large Slovenian family. Neurogenetics 2002;4 (2) 93-6

[84] Fabrizi GM, Cavallaro T, Angiari C, Bertolasi L, Cabrini I, Ferrarini M and Rizzuto N. Giant axon and neurofilament accumulation in Charcot-Marie-Tooth disease type 2E. Neurology 2004;62 (8) 1429-31

[85] Bhagavati S, Maccabee PJ and Xu W. The neurofilament light chain gene (NEFL) mutation Pro22Ser can be associated with mixed axonal and demyelinating neuropathy. J Clin Neurosci 2009;16 (6) 830-1

[86] Yoshihara T, Yamamoto M, Hattori N, Misu K, Mori K, Koike H and Sobue G. Identification of novel sequence variants in the neurofilament-light gene in a Japanese pop-

ulation: analysis of Charcot-Marie-Tooth disease patients and normal individuals. J Peripher Nerv Syst 2002;7 (4) 221-4

[87] Sasaki T, Gotow T, Shiozaki M, Sakaue F, Saito T, Julien JP, Uchiyama Y and Hisanaga S. Aggregate formation and phosphorylation of neurofilament-L Pro22 Charcot-Marie-Tooth disease mutants. Hum Mol Genet 2006;15 (6) 943-52

[88] Jordanova A, De Jonghe P, Boerkoel CF, Takashima H, De Vriendt E, Ceuterick C, Martin JJ, Butler IJ, Mancias P, Papasozomenos S, Terespolsky D, Potocki L, Brown CW, Shy M, Rita DA, Tournev I, Kremensky I, Lupski JR and Timmerman V. Mutations in the neurofilament light chain gene (NEFL) cause early onset severe Charcot-Marie-Tooth disease. Brain 2003;126 (Pt 3) 590-7

[89] Choi BO, Lee MS, Shin SH, Hwang JH, Choi KG, Kim WK, Sunwoo IN, Kim NK and Chung KW. Mutational analysis of PMP22, MPZ, GJB1, EGR2 and NEFL in Korean Charcot-Marie-Tooth neuropathy patients. Hum Mutat 2004;24 (2) 185-6

[90] Zuchner S, Vorgerd M, Sindern E and Schroder JM. The novel neurofilament light (NEFL) mutation Glu397Lys is associated with a clinically and morphologically heterogeneous type of Charcot-Marie-Tooth neuropathy. Neuromuscul Disord 2004;14 (2) 147-57

[91] Fabrizi GM, Cavallaro T, Angiari C, Cabrini I, Taioli F, Malerba G, Bertolasi L and Rizzuto N. Charcot-Marie-Tooth disease type 2E, a disorder of the cytoskeleton. Brain 2007;130 (Pt 2) 394-403

[92] Leung CL, Nagan N, Graham TH and Liem RK. A novel duplication/insertion mutation of NEFL in a patient with Charcot-Marie-Tooth disease. Am J Med Genet A 2006;140 (9) 1021-5

[93] Abe A, Numakura C, Saito K, Koide H, Oka N, Honma A, Kishikawa Y and Hayasaka K. Neurofilament light chain polypeptide gene mutations in Charcot-Marie-Tooth disease: nonsense mutation probably causes a recessive phenotype. J Hum Genet 2009;54 (2) 94-7

[94] Dequen F, Filali M, Lariviere RC, Perrot R, Hisanaga S and Julien JP. Reversal of neuropathy phenotypes in conditional mouse model of Charcot-Marie-Tooth disease type 2E. Hum Mol Genet 19 (13) 2616-29

[95] Shen H, Barry DM, Dale JM, Garcia VB, Calcutt NA and Garcia ML. Muscle pathology without severe nerve pathology in a new mouse model of Charcot-Marie-Tooth disease type 2E. Hum Mol Genet 2011;20 (13) 2535-48

[96] Ackerley S, James PA, Kalli A, French S, Davies KE and Talbot K. A mutation in the small heat-shock protein HSPB1 leading to distal hereditary motor neuronopathy disrupts neurofilament assembly and the axonal transport of specific cellular cargoes. Hum Mol Genet 2006;15 (2) 347-54

[97] Evgrafov OV, Mersiyanova I, Irobi J, Van Den Bosch L, Dierick I, Leung CL, Schagina O, Verpoorten N, Van Impe K, Fedotov V, Dadali E, Auer-Grumbach M, Windpas-

singer C, Wagner K, Mitrovic Z, Hilton-Jones D, Talbot K, Martin JJ, Vasserman N, Tverskaya S, Polyakov A, Liem RK, Gettemans J, Robberecht W, De Jonghe P and Timmerman V. Mutant small heat-shock protein 27 causes axonal Charcot-Marie-Tooth disease and distal hereditary motor neuropathy. Nat Genet 2004;36 (6) 602-6

[98] Goryunov D, Nightingale A, Bornfleth L, Leung C and Liem RK. Multiple disease-linked myotubularin mutations cause NFL assembly defects in cultured cells and disrupt myotubularin dimerization. J Neurochem 2008;104 (6) 1536-52

[99] Irobi J, Van Impe K, Seeman P, Jordanova A, Dierick I, Verpoorten N, Michalik A, De Vriendt E, Jacobs A, Van Gerwen V, Vennekens K, Mazanec R, Tournev I, Hilton-Jones D, Talbot K, Kremensky I, Van Den Bosch L, Robberecht W, Van Vandekerckhove J, Van Broeckhoven C, Gettemans J, De Jonghe P and Timmerman V. Hot-spot residue in small heat-shock protein 22 causes distal motor neuropathy. Nat Genet 2004;36 (6) 597-601

[100] Zhai J, Lin H, Julien JP and Schlaepfer WW. Disruption of neurofilament network with aggregation of light neurofilament protein: a common pathway leading to motor neuron degeneration due to Charcot-Marie-Tooth disease-linked mutations in NFL and HSPB1. Hum Mol Genet 2007;16 (24) 3103-16

[101] Bolino A, Bolis A, Previtali SC, Dina G, Bussini S, Dati G, Amadio S, Del Carro U, Mruk DD, Feltri ML, Cheng CY, Quattrini A and Wrabetz L. Disruption of Mtmr2 produces CMT4B1-like neuropathy with myelin outfolding and impaired spermatogenesis. J Cell Biol 2004;167 (4) 711-21

[102] Bolis A, Coviello S, Bussini S, Dina G, Pardini C, Previtali SC, Malaguti M, Morana P, Del Carro U, Feltri ML, Quattrini A, Wrabetz L and Bolino A. Loss of Mtmr2 phosphatase in Schwann cells but not in motor neurons causes Charcot-Marie-Tooth type 4B1 neuropathy with myelin outfoldings. J Neurosci 2005;25 (37) 8567-77

[103] Tradewell ML, Durham HD, Mushynski WE and Gentil BJ. Mitochondrial and axonal abnormalities precede disruption of the neurofilament network in a model of charcot-marie-tooth disease type 2E and are prevented by heat shock proteins in a mutant-specific fashion. J Neuropathol Exp Neurol 2009;68 (6) 642-52

[104] Gentil BJ, Minotti S, Beange M, Baloh RH, Julien JP and Durham HD. Normal role of the low-molecular-weight neurofilament protein in mitochondrial dynamics and disruption in Charcot-Marie-Tooth disease. Faseb J 2012;26 (3) 1194-203

[105] Bomont P, Cavalier L, Blondeau F, Ben Hamida C, Belal S, Tazir M, Demir E, Topaloglu H, Korinthenberg R, Tuysuz B, Landrieu P, Hentati F and Koenig M. The gene encoding gigaxonin, a new member of the cytoskeletal BTB/kelch repeat family, is mutated in giant axonal neuropathy. Nat Genet 2000;26 (3) 370-4

[106] Cleveland DW, Yamanaka K and Bomont P. Gigaxonin controls vimentin organization through a tubulin chaperone-independent pathway. Hum Mol Genet 2009;18 (8) 1384-94

[107] Peiffer J, Schlote W, Bischoff A, Boltshauser E and Muller G. Generalized giant axonal neuropathy: a filament-forming disease of neuronal, endothelial, glial, and schwann cells in a patient without kinky hair. Acta Neuropathol 1977;40 (3) 213-8

[108] Asbury AK, Gale MK, Cox SC, Baringer JR and Berg BO. Giant axonal neuropathy--a unique case with segmental neurofilamentous masses. Acta Neuropathol 1972;20 (3) 237-47

[109] Fois A, Balestri P, Farnetani MA, Berardi R, Mattei R, Laurenzi E, Alessandrini C, Gerli R, Ribuffo A and Calvieri S. Giant axonal neuropathy. Endocrinological and histological studies. Eur J Pediatr 1985;144 (3) 274-80

[110] Mohri I, Taniike M, Yoshikawa H, Higashiyama M, Itami S and Okada S. A case of giant axonal neuropathy showing focal aggregation and hypophosphorylation of intermediate filaments. Brain Dev 1998;20 (8) 594-7

[111] Treiber-Held S, Budjarjo-Welim H, Reimann D, Richter J, Kretzschmar HA and Hanefeld F. Giant axonal neuropathy: a generalized disorder of intermediate filaments with longitudinal grooves in the hair. Neuropediatrics 1994;25 (2) 89-93

[112] Donaghy M, King RH, Thomas PK and Workman JM. Abnormalities of the axonal cytoskeleton in giant axonal neuropathy. J Neurocytol 1988;17 (2) 197-208

[113] Monaco S, Autilio-Gambetti L, Zabel D and Gambetti P. Giant axonal neuropathy: acceleration of neurofilament transport in optic axons. Proc Natl Acad Sci U S A 1985;82 (3) 920-4

[114] Ding J, Allen E, Wang W, Valle A, Wu C, Nardine T, Cui B, Yi J, Taylor A, Jeon NL, Chu S, So Y, Vogel H, Tolwani R, Mobley W and Yang Y. Gene targeting of GAN in mouse causes a toxic accumulation of microtubule-associated protein 8 and impaired retrograde axonal transport. Hum Mol Genet 2006;15 (9) 1451-63

[115] Yang Y, Allen E, Ding J and Wang W. Giant axonal neuropathy. Cell Mol Life Sci 2007;64 (5) 601-9

[116] Dequen F, Bomont P, Gowing G, Cleveland DW and Julien JP. Modest loss of peripheral axons, muscle atrophy and formation of brain inclusions in mice with targeted deletion of gigaxonin exon 1. J Neurochem 2008;107 (1) 253-64

[117] Ganay T, Boizot A, Burrer R, Chauvin JP and Bomont P. Sensory-motor deficits and neurofilament disorganization in gigaxonin-null mice. Mol Neurodegener 2011;6 25

[118] Furukawa M, He YJ, Borchers C and Xiong Y. Targeting of protein ubiquitination by BTB-Cullin 3-Roc1 ubiquitin ligases. Nat Cell Biol 2003;5 (11) 1001-7

[119] Pintard L, Willis JH, Willems A, Johnson JL, Srayko M, Kurz T, Glaser S, Mains PE, Tyers M, Bowerman B and Peter M. The BTB protein MEL-26 is a substrate-specific adaptor of the CUL-3 ubiquitin-ligase. Nature 2003;425 (6955) 311-6

[120] Xu L, Wei Y, Reboul J, Vaglio P, Shin TH, Vidal M, Elledge SJ and Harper JW. BTB proteins are substrate-specific adaptors in an SCF-like modular ubiquitin ligase containing CUL-3. Nature 2003;425 (6955) 316-21

[121] Ding J, Liu JJ, Kowal AS, Nardine T, Bhattacharya P, Lee A and Yang Y. Microtubule-associated protein 1B: a neuronal binding partner for gigaxonin. J Cell Biol 2002;158 (3) 427-33

[122] Wang W, Ding J, Allen E, Zhu P, Zhang L, Vogel H and Yang Y. Gigaxonin interacts with tubulin folding cofactor B and controls its degradation through the ubiquitin-proteasome pathway. Curr Biol 2005;15 (22) 2050-5

[123] Allen E, Ding J, Wang W, Pramanik S, Chou J, Yau V and Yang Y. Gigaxonin-controlled degradation of MAP1B light chain is critical to neuronal survival. Nature 2005;438 (7065) 224-8

[124] Mussche S, De Paepe B, Smet J, Devreese K, Lissens W, Rasic VM, Murnane M, Devreese B and Van Coster R. Proteomic analysis in giant axonal neuropathy: New insights into disease mechanisms. Muscle Nerve 2012;46 (2) 246-56

[125] Cairns NJ, Zhukareva V, Uryu K, Zhang B, Bigio E, Mackenzie IR, Gearing M, Duyckaerts C, Yokoo H, Nakazato Y, Jaros E, Perry RH, Lee VM and Trojanowski JQ. alpha-internexin is present in the pathological inclusions of neuronal intermediate filament inclusion disease. Am J Pathol 2004;164 (6) 2153-61

[126] Uchikado H, Shaw G, Wang DS and Dickson DW. Screening for neurofilament inclusion disease using alpha-internexin immunohistochemistry. Neurology 2005;64 (9) 1658-9

[127] Momeni P, Cairns NJ, Perry RH, Bigio EH, Gearing M, Singleton AB and Hardy J. Mutation analysis of patients with neuronal intermediate filament inclusion disease (NIFID). Neurobiol Aging 2006;27 (5) 778 e1-778 e6

[128] Dequen F, Cairns NJ, Bigio EH and Julien JP. Gigaxonin mutation analysis in patients with NIFID. Neurobiol Aging 2009;

[129] Neumann M, Roeber S, Kretzschmar HA, Rademakers R, Baker M and Mackenzie IR. Abundant FUS-immunoreactive pathology in neuronal intermediate filament inclusion disease. Acta Neuropathol 2009;118 (5) 605-16

[130] Armstrong RA, Gearing M, Bigio EH, Cruz-Sanchez FF, Duyckaerts C, Mackenzie IR, Perry RH, Skullerud K, Yokoo H and Cairns NJ. Spatial patterns of FUS-immunoreactive neuronal cytoplasmic inclusions (NCI) in neuronal intermediate filament inclusion disease (NIFID). J Neural Transm 2011;118 (11) 1651-7

[131] Medori R, Autilio-Gambetti L, Monaco S and Gambetti P. Experimental diabetic neuropathy: impairment of slow transport with changes in axon cross-sectional area. Proc Natl Acad Sci U S A 1985;82 (22) 7716-20

[132] Medori R, Jenich H, Autilio-Gambetti L and Gambetti P. Experimental diabetic neuropathy: similar changes of slow axonal transport and axonal size in different animal models. J Neurosci 1988;8 (5) 1814-21

[133] Yagihashi S, Kamijo M and Watanabe K. Reduced myelinated fiber size correlates with loss of axonal neurofilaments in peripheral nerve of chronically streptozotocin diabetic rats. Am J Pathol 1990;136 (6) 1365-73

[134] Schmidt RE, Beaudet LN, Plurad SB and Dorsey DA. Axonal cytoskeletal pathology in aged and diabetic human sympathetic autonomic ganglia. Brain Res 1997;769 (2) 375-83

[135] Fernyhough P, Gallagher A, Averill SA, Priestley JV, Hounsom L, Patel J and Tomlinson DR. Aberrant neurofilament phosphorylation in sensory neurons of rats with diabetic neuropathy. Diabetes 1999;48 (4) 881-9

[136] Scott JN, Clark AW and Zochodne DW. Neurofilament and tubulin gene expression in progressive experimental diabetes: failure of synthesis and export by sensory neurons. Brain 1999;122 (Pt 11) 2109-18

[137] Zochodne DW, Sun HS, Cheng C and Eyer J. Accelerated diabetic neuropathy in axons without neurofilaments. Brain 2004;127 (Pt 10) 2193-200

[138] Forno LS, Sternberger LA, Sternberger NH, Strefling AM, Swanson K and Eng LF. Reaction of Lewy bodies with antibodies to phosphorylated and non-phosphorylated neurofilaments. Neurosci Lett 1986;64 (3) 253-8

[139] Pappolla MA. Lewy bodies of Parkinson's disease. Immune electron microscopic demonstration of neurofilament antigens in constituent filaments. Arch Pathol Lab Med 1986;110 (12) 1160-3

[140] Hill WD, Arai M, Cohen JA and Trojanowski JQ. Neurofilament mRNA is reduced in Parkinson's disease substantia nigra pars compacta neurons. J Comp Neurol 1993;329 (3) 328-36

[141] Basso M, Giraudo S, Corpillo D, Bergamasco B, Lopiano L and Fasano M. Proteome analysis of human substantia nigra in Parkinson's disease. Proteomics 2004;4 (12) 3943-52

[142] Lavedan C, Buchholtz S, Nussbaum RL, Albin RL and Polymeropoulos MH. A mutation in the human neurofilament M gene in Parkinson's disease that suggests a role for the cytoskeleton in neuronal degeneration. Neurosci Lett 2002;322 (1) 57-61

[143] Perez-Olle R, Lopez-Toledano MA and Liem RK. The G336S variant in the human neurofilament-M gene does not affect its assembly or distribution: importance of the functional analysis of neurofilament variants. J Neuropathol Exp Neurol 2004;63 (7) 759-74

[144] Han F, Bulman DE, Panisset M and Grimes DA. Neurofilament M gene in a French-Canadian population with Parkinson's disease. Can J Neurol Sci 2005;32 (1) 68-70

[145] Kruger R, Fischer C, Schulte T, Strauss KM, Muller T, Woitalla D, Berg D, Hungs M, Gobbele R, Berger K, Epplen JT, Riess O and Schols L. Mutation analysis of the neurofilament M gene in Parkinson's disease. Neurosci Lett 2003;351 (2) 125-9

[146] Abdo WF, Bloem BR, Van Geel WJ, Esselink RA and Verbeek MM. CSF neurofilament light chain and tau differentiate multiple system atrophy from Parkinson's disease. Neurobiol Aging 2007;28 (5) 742-7

[147] Karcher D, Federsppiel BS, Lowenthal FD, Frank F and Lowenthal A. Anti-neurofilament antibodies in blood of patients with neurological diseases. Acta Neuropathol 1986;72 (1) 82-5

[148] Su W, Chen HB, Li SH and Wu DY. Correlational study of the serum levels of the glial fibrillary acidic protein and neurofilament proteins in Parkinson's disease patients. Clin Neurol Neurosurg 2012;114 (4) 372-5

[149] Liem RK and Messing A. Dysfunctions of neuronal and glial intermediate filaments in disease. J Clin Invest 2009;119 (7) 1814-24

[150] Sawaishi Y. Review of Alexander disease: beyond the classical concept of leukodystrophy. Brain Dev 2009;31 (7) 493-8

[151] Bettica A and Johnson AB. Ultrastructural immunogold labeling of glial filaments in osmicated and unosmicated epoxy-embedded tissue. J Histochem Cytochem 1990;38 (1) 103-9

[152] Tomokane N, Iwaki T, Tateishi J, Iwaki A and Goldman JE. Rosenthal fibers share epitopes with alpha B-crystallin, glial fibrillary acidic protein, and ubiquitin, but not with vimentin. Immunoelectron microscopy with colloidal gold. Am J Pathol 1991;138 (4) 875-85

[153] Head MW, Corbin E and Goldman JE. Overexpression and abnormal modification of the stress proteins alpha B-crystallin and HSP27 in Alexander disease. Am J Pathol 1993;143 (6) 1743-53

[154] Gomi H, Yokoyama T, Fujimoto K, Ikeda T, Katoh A, Itoh T and Itohara S. Mice devoid of the glial fibrillary acidic protein develop normally and are susceptible to scrapie prions. Neuron 1995;14 (1) 29-41

[155] Pekny M, Leveen P, Pekna M, Eliasson C, Berthold CH, Westermark B and Betsholtz C. Mice lacking glial fibrillary acidic protein display astrocytes devoid of intermediate filaments but develop and reproduce normally. Embo J 1995;14 (8) 1590-8

[156] Liedtke W, Edelmann W, Bieri PL, Chiu FC, Cowan NJ, Kucherlapati R and Raine CS. GFAP is necessary for the integrity of CNS white matter architecture and long-term maintenance of myelination. Neuron 1996;17 (4) 607-15

[157] McCall MA, Gregg RG, Behringer RR, Brenner M, Delaney CL, Galbreath EJ, Zhang CL, Pearce RA, Chiu SY and Messing A. Targeted deletion in astrocyte intermediate filament (Gfap) alters neuronal physiology. Proc Natl Acad Sci U S A 1996;93 (13) 6361-6

[158] Messing A, Head MW, Galles K, Galbreath EJ, Goldman JE and Brenner M. Fatal encephalopathy with astrocyte inclusions in GFAP transgenic mice. Am J Pathol 1998;152 (2) 391-8

[159] Hagemann TL, Gaeta SA, Smith MA, Johnson DA, Johnson JA and Messing A. Gene expression analysis in mice with elevated glial fibrillary acidic protein and Rosenthal fibers reveals a stress response followed by glial activation and neuronal dysfunction. Hum Mol Genet 2005;14 (16) 2443-58

[160] Brenner M, Johnson AB, Boespflug-Tanguy O, Rodriguez D, Goldman JE and Messing A. Mutations in GFAP, encoding glial fibrillary acidic protein, are associated with Alexander disease. Nat Genet 2001;27 (1) 117-20

[161] McClintock KA and Shaw GS. A logical sequence search for S100B target proteins. Protein Sci 2000;9 (10) 2043-6

[162] Donato R. Functional roles of S100 proteins, calcium-binding proteins of the EF-hand type. Biochim Biophys Acta 1999;1450 (3) 191-231

[163] Li R, Johnson AB, Salomons G, Goldman JE, Naidu S, Quinlan R, Cree B, Ruyle SZ, Banwell B, D'Hooghe M, Siebert JR, Rolf CM, Cox H, Reddy A, Gutierrez-Solana LG, Collins A, Weller RO, Messing A, van der Knaap MS and Brenner M. Glial fibrillary acidic protein mutations in infantile, juvenile, and adult forms of Alexander disease. Ann Neurol 2005;57 (3) 310-26

[164] Gorospe JR, Naidu S, Johnson AB, Puri V, Raymond GV, Jenkins SD, Pedersen RC, Lewis D, Knowles P, Fernandez R, De Vivo D, van der Knaap MS, Messing A, Brenner M and Hoffman EP. Molecular findings in symptomatic and pre-symptomatic Alexander disease patients. Neurology 2002;58 (10) 1494-500

[165] Hagemann TL, Connor JX and Messing A. Alexander disease-associated glial fibrillary acidic protein mutations in mice induce Rosenthal fiber formation and a white matter stress response. J Neurosci 2006;26 (43) 11162-73

[166] Tanaka KF, Takebayashi H, Yamazaki Y, Ono K, Naruse M, Iwasato T, Itohara S, Kato H and Ikenaka K. Murine model of Alexander disease: analysis of GFAP aggregate formation and its pathological significance. Glia 2007;55 (6) 617-31

[167] Hsiao VC, Tian R, Long H, Der Perng M, Brenner M, Quinlan RA and Goldman JE. Alexander-disease mutation of GFAP causes filament disorganization and decreased solubility of GFAP. J Cell Sci 2005;118 (Pt 9) 2057-65

[168] Tang G, Xu Z and Goldman JE. Synergistic effects of the SAPK/JNK and the proteasome pathway on glial fibrillary acidic protein (GFAP) accumulation in Alexander disease. J Biol Chem 2006;281 (50) 38634-43

[169] Tian R, Gregor M, Wiche G and Goldman JE. Plectin regulates the organization of glial fibrillary acidic protein in Alexander disease. Am J Pathol 2006;168 (3) 888-97

[170] Iwaki T, Kume-Iwaki A, Liem RK and Goldman JE. Alpha B-crystallin is expressed in non-lenticular tissues and accumulates in Alexander's disease brain. Cell 1989;57 (1) 71-8

[171] Koyama Y and Goldman JE. Formation of GFAP cytoplasmic inclusions in astrocytes and their disaggregation by alphaB-crystallin. Am J Pathol 1999;154 (5) 1563-72

[172] Tang G, Yue Z, Talloczy Z, Hagemann T, Cho W, Messing A, Sulzer DL and Goldman JE. Autophagy induced by Alexander disease-mutant GFAP accumulation is regulated by p38/MAPK and mTOR signaling pathways. Hum Mol Genet 2008;17 (11) 1540-55

[173] Bachetti T, Di Zanni E, Balbi P, Bocca P, Prigione I, Deiana GA, Rezzani A, Ceccherini I and Sechi G. In vitro treatments with ceftriaxone promote elimination of mutant glial fibrillary acidic protein and transcription down-regulation. Exp Cell Res 2010;316 (13) 2152-65

[174] Bachetti T, Di Zanni E, Balbi P, Ravazzolo R, Sechi G and Ceccherini I. Beneficial effects of curcumin on GFAP filament organization and down-regulation of GFAP expression in an in vitro model of Alexander disease. Exp Cell Res 2012;318 (15) 1844-54

[175] Perng MD, Wen SF, Gibbon T, Middeldorp J, Sluijs J, Hol EM and Quinlan RA. Glial fibrillary acidic protein filaments can tolerate the incorporation of assembly-compromised GFAP-delta, but with consequences for filament organization and alphaB-crystallin association. Mol Biol Cell 2008;19 (10) 4521-33

Chapter 20

Astrocytes Role in Parkinson: A Double-Edged Sword

Ricardo Cabezas, Marco Fidel Avila, Daniel Torrente,
Ramon Santos El-Bachá, Ludis Morales,
Janneth Gonzalez and George E. Barreto

Additional information is available at the end of the chapter

http://dx.doi.org/10.5772/54305

1. Introduction

Parkinson Disease (PD) is the second most chronic neurodegenerative disorder in the world, after Alzheimer´s Disease (AD), and is estimated to affect about 1% of the population over 60 years of age. PD is caused by the disruption of dopaminergic neurotransmission in the basal ganglia, which causes a reduction in the numbers of dopaminergic neurons in the substantia nigra and formation of cytoplasmic inclusions called Lewy bodies [1].

Both in normal and pathological circumstances, astrocytes are critical supporters of neuronal function in processes such as antioxidant protection, glutamate clearance, the development and/or maintenance of blood brain barrier characteristics, the release of gliotransmitters and cytokines [2-4]. In recent years, much research on PD has focused on the astrocytic-neuronal crosstalk, suggesting that this interaction is important for future therapies against neurodegenerative processes. During brain damage events, astrocytes become transiently or permanently impaired, and the subsequent impact on neuronal cells may lead to pathological conditions such as PD [5-7].

In the present chapter, we provide a brief overview of the astrocytic functions and the pathophysiological events elicited during PD. Additionally, we explore the beneficial and damaging consequences of reactive astrogliosis in dopaminergic neurons during PD, particularly on oxidative damage, which is a main component of numerous neuropathological conditions, and that may have a damaging effect in astrocytic functions. We also highlight some of the cellular and animal models currently used in Parkinson research, such rotenone, 1-methyl-4-phenyl-1,2,3,6-tetrahydropyridine (MPTP) and paraquat as inducers, which have many similar features with this disease. Finally, a brief overview of the future perspectives in astrocytic protection during Parkinson development is discussed.

2. Parkinson′s disease

PD is a progressive neurodegenerative disorder caused by the neuronal death in the substantia nigra (SN), degeneration of dopaminergic neurotransmission, and the presence of α-synuclein and protein inclusions in neuronal cell bodies (Lewy bodies) [4-5,7]. Main symptoms of Parkinson are asymmetrical bradikinesia, rigidity, resting tremor and postural instability. Other non-motor symptoms that generate serious disability problems have also been noted, including fatigue, pain, Lewy Body dementia, psychosis, depression, and apathy [1]. Although there is not a cure for the disease, the most used and cheaper treatment for PD continues to be Levodopa [1,8]. However, about 40% of patients developed motor fluctuations and dyskinesias after 4 to 6 years of treatment [1], demonstrating that further pharmacological research is needed in order to counterbalance side effects. In this aspect, treatments using long-acting dopaminergic agents or a continuous dopaminergic effect in the striatum have been associated with less severe motor complications, given alone or in combination with L-dopa [9]. Some pharmacological agents that have shown promising applications, include dopamine agonist like apomorphine and ropinirole, and catechol-O-methyltransferase (COMT; EC 2.1.1.6) inhibitors [9].

Numerous reviews and articles agree that the exact cause of PD remains unknown [1,9-10]. Mutations in various proteins such as leucine-rich repeat kinase 2 (LRRK2; EC 2.7.11.1), Parkinson protein 2 (PARK2), probable cation-transporting ATPase type 13A2 (ATP13A2; EC 3.6.3-), phosphatase and tensin homolog (PTEN)-induced putative kinase 1 (PINK1; EC 2.7.11.1), and Parkinson disease (autosomal recessive, early onset) 7 protein (DJ-1) have been observed in familiar cases of Parkinson, which only accounts for 10-15% of diagnosed cases [6,11-12]. Interestingly, LRRK2, PINK1, and DJ-1, which are present in mitochondrial membranes, have been suggested to play a role in reactive oxygen species (ROS) production by a defective maintenance of the mitochondrial membrane potential [12-13].

A number of environmental factors have been found to induce PD-like symptoms, and are currently used in animal and cellular models of the disease. Environmental factors include vascular insults to the brain, oxidative stress, neuroleptic drugs and repeated head trauma. [6,14]. Additionally, the exposure to pesticides like rotenone or 1-methyl-4-phenylpyridinium (MPP^+) and heavy metals (manganese) increases the risk of PD development [6, 10, 14-15]. In this aspect, numerous epidemiologic and toxicologic studies have examined pesticides as a risk factor for PD and parkinsonism and the possible mechanisms by which pesticides may act [14-17].

Initiation and progression of PD is dependent upon cellular events, including failures in the protein degradation machinery, oxidative stress, mitochondrial dysfunction, defects in mitochondrial autophagy (mitophagy) and the continuous accumulation of α-synuclein, driven through cell to cell interactions between glial cells and neurons that ultimately lead to apoptosis [7,10,18]. Previous studies pointed that astrocytic α-synuclein deposition initiates the recruitment of phagocyte microglia that attacks and kills neurons in restricted brain regions [7,19], correlating this α-synuclein accumulation with nigral neuronal cell death [20], and suggest the importance of astrocytes in the initiation of the disease. Conversely, astrocytes also have beneficial roles during PD progression [21-22]. For example, astrocytes express different antioxidant molecules such as glutathione peroxidase (EC 1.11.1.9), which have been inversely correlated with the severity of dopaminergic cell loss in the respective cell groups in patients with PD [4].

3. Astrocytes in PD

3.1. Astrocytic functions

Astrocytes are the most common cell type in the mammalian brain, conforming the glia with oligodendrocytes and microglia [23]. They are characterized by the expression of the intermediate filaments glial fibrillary acidic protein (GFAP) and vimentin (Vim). Astrocytes are essential for the metabolism of the brain, transporting multiple nutrients and metabolic precursors to the neurons by the malate-asparte shuttle and other transporters [24]. There are two main types of astrocytes in the SNC: Protoplasmic astrocytes, which envelope neuronal bodies and synapses and fibrous astrocytes which interact with the nodes of Ranvier and oligodendroglia [7]. Current research has shown that only protoplasmic astrocytes have an increase in the accumulation of α-synuclein, whereas fibrous astrocytes do not [7,19].

Current knowledge indicates that astrocytes are critical for some cellular processes, such as the development and/or maintenance of blood–brain barrier characteristics, the promotion of neurovascular coupling, the attraction of cells through the release of chemokines, K^+ buffering, release of gliotransmitters, release of glutamate by calcium signaling, maintenance of general metabolism, control of the brain pH, metabolization of dopamine and other substrates by monoamine oxidases (MAOs; EC 1.4.3.4), uptake of glutamate and γ-aminobutyric acid (GABA) by specific transporters and production of antioxidants [2-3,25-27] (Figure 1). Recent evidence has shown that astrocytes are arranged in non-overlapping domains forming a syncytial network that may contact approximately 160.000 synapses, thus integrating neural activity with the vascular network [4,28]. In this aspect, astrocytic terminal processes, known as endfeet, contact the brain vasculature and enwrap the neuronal synapses, enabling the modulation of both neuronal activity and cerebral blood flow, following an elevation in intracellular Ca^{2+} levels in the endfeets [24,29].

During brain damage (including diseases, brain injury and oxidative stress), these astrocytic functions become transiently or permanently impaired, and the subsequent impact on neuronal cells may lead to pathological conditions and neurodegenerative diseases [3,26]. Neurons are more susceptible to injury than astrocytes, as they have limited antioxidant capacity, and rely heavily on their metabolic coupling with astrocytes to combat oxidative stress [3]. However, severe brain damage also results in astrocyte dysfunction, leading to increased neuronal death [30].

As previously stated, astrocytes exert both neuroprotective and neurodegenerative roles, depending on the molecules released by them, and the pathological or normal circumstances of their microenvironment [6]. For example, astrocytes release antioxidant molecules like glutathione (GSH) and superoxide dismutases (SODs; EC 1.15.1.1), and supply neurons with neurotrophic factors, such as nerve growth factor (NGF), basic fibroblast growth factor (bFG), that constitute an important attempt to protect neurons during brain damaging processes, including PD [6, 31-32]. On the other hand, during the process of reactive astrogliosis, astrocytes release inflammatory cytokines that may affect the surrounding neurons, both by the induced production of ROS and lipid peroxidation, and by the activation of apoptotic mechanisms that induce neuronal dopaminergic death [6,10]. These unusual, and sometimes contradictory, features of astrocytes in PD will be further explored in this chapter.

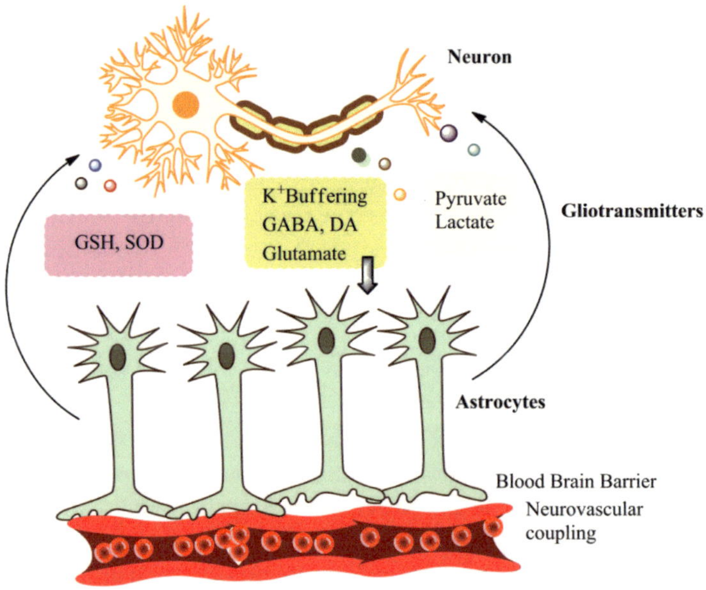

Figure 1. Astrocytes support neuronal function by multiple ways, including the development and maintenance of blood–brain barrier and promoting the neurovascular coupling. Astrocytes regulate the levels of ions, neurotransmitters and fueling molecules such as K^+, glutamate, GABA, dopamine, lactate and piruvate. Furthermore, astrocytes promote the attraction of cells through the release of chemokines, and produce beneficial antioxidants, including glutathione, superoxide dismutases (SODs 1, 2 and 3), and ascorbate.

3.2. Astrogliosis and parkinson

Reactive astrogliosis is the main reaction of astrocytes following brain insults such as infection, trauma [33-34], α-synuclein accumulation [35], ischemia [36-37] and neurodegenerative diseases [3]. This process involves both molecular and morphological changes in the astrocytes, including increased expression of GFAP, vimentin and nestin, uptake of excitotoxic glutamate, protection from oxidative stress by the production of GSH, neuroprotection by release of adenosine, degradation of amyloid-beta peptides, facilitation of blood-brain barrier, increased formation of gap junctions between astrocytes, formation of scars and, in some cases release of inflammatory cytokines, including tumor necrosis factor-α (TNF-α), and production of ROS [3,35,38-40].

Astrogliosis and microgliosis in the SN of Parkinson patients are key features of the disease, which is a nonspecific consequence of neuronal degeneration [10]. Cellular and animal models using environmental and biological toxins, especially lipopolysaccharides (LPS), herbicides and pesticides like rotenone or MPTP (1-methyl-4-phenyl-1,2,3,6-tetrahydropyridine), can induce both astrogliosis and microgliosis, which is accompanied by neuronal death, mitochondrial dysfunction and nuclear fragmentation [41-45]. Additionally, it was previously shown that the injection of LPS in rat brains was followed by an increase in the inducible nitric oxide synthase (iNOS; EC 1.14.13.39), suggesting that chronic glial activation can cause oxidative stress in the brain, similarly to that seen in neurodegenerative processes like AD and Parkinson [10, 39, 45]. A previous report showed that activated glial cells can participate in the death of dopaminergic neurons, probably by the activation of apoptosis by cytokines like TNF-α, IL-1B, IL-6 and interferon-γ and the subsequent production of nitric oxide (NO) by the iNOS that may diffuse toward the neurons and induce lipid peroxidation, DNA strands breaks and inhibition of mitochondrial metabolism [6,10]. Furthermore, cytokines released by astrocytes may bind to their specific receptors in the dopaminergic neurons, such as TNFR1 and 2, and activate proapoptotic mechanisms through the activation of caspase 3, caspase 8, and cytochrome c [10]. Interestingly, the excessive uptake of neuronal α-synuclein by astrocytes can lead to accumulation of aggregates of this protein in astrocytes, and cause an upregulation of IL-1 α, IL-1β and IL-6, followed by the release of TNF-α and IL-6 [6]. These results suggest that the inhibition of glial reaction to damage and further inflammatory processes could be considered as a promising therapy to reduce neuronal damage during PD [10].

3.3. Oxidative stress and Parkinson: Role of astrocytes

In the brain, oxidative stress and other toxic insults can trigger the overexpression and activation of neuronal nitric oxide synthase that increases NO production and may cause apoptotic cell death by inducing the release of cytochrome c from mitochondrial impairment, loss of membrane potential, the opening of permeability transition pores, and the release of proapoptotic molecules [46,47]. After brain damaging processes, neurons experience greater metabolic deterioration than glial cells. For instance, astrocytes contain glycogen stores that allow them to maintain ATP production through glycolysis and mitochondrial membrane potential by reversal of the F0-F1-ATPase (EC 3.6.3.14) [48]. For example, cultured astrocytes subjected to oxygen and glucose deprivation showed a decrease in mitochondrial membrane potential, possibly caused by the mitochondrial permeability transition pore (mtPTP) opening, which leads to a loss of intramitochondrial contents, mitochondrial respiration and ATP production [48].

Nowadays there is much evidence of the role of oxidative stress in the development of neurodegenerative diseases, such as AD, PD, Amyotrophic Lateral Sclerosis (ALS) and Huntington's disease (HD). Much of these oxidative damaging processes are associated with an imbalance on the production of ROS that leads to mitochondrial stress and impairment in energy production [47,49]. ROS, such as superoxide ($O^{\bullet}2^{-}$), can be produced in mitochondrial complexes I and III in components of the tricarboxylic-acid cycle, including α-ketoglutarate dehydrogenase (EC 1.2.4.2), and in the outter mitochondrial membrane, damaging cell components such as lipids, proteins and DNA [25, 47]. In PD, oxidative damage is a common feature, as demonstrated by increased levels of ROS in post-mortem PD brain samples [25]. Oxidative stress seems to affect various brain regions, including the SN and caudate nucleus, and it is accompanied by an increase in GFAP and astrocytic proliferation [50]. Additionally, PD patients present deficiencies in mitochondrial complex I in the SN, suggesting that a defect in this complex could contribute to neuronal degeneration in PD [25]. However, it is not clear whether the damage induced by ROS is a cause or a consequence of other cellular dysfunctions [25]. For example, a previous study on PD brains showed an increase in lipid peroxidation products, such as 4-hydroxinonenal, and in protein crosslinking and fragmentation [51], suggesting that oxidative stress may affect other brain regions apart from the SN.

Astrocytes produce numerous antioxidant molecules, such as GSH, catalase (EC 1.11.1.6) and SODs, providing further antioxidant protection to neurons. Unfortunately, it is known that the astrocytic protection afforded to neurons is limited, possibly due to a decline in GSH trafficking by chronic iNOS induction [52]. This depletion of GSH may facilitate the production of ROS and reactive nitrogen species (RNS) by astrocytes, causing alterations in neuronal proteins such as α-synuclein [25]. Furthermore, the nitration of α-synuclein by RNS can significantly enhance the synuclein fibril formation *in vitro*, similarly to what happens in PD brains [25]. In sum, the antioxidant properties of astrocytes have a fundamental role in the development of neurodegenerative diseases, and are considered as promising therapeutically targets.

4. Experimental models in Parkinson

Various pesticides, herbicides and drugs have been used in animal and *in vitro* models of Parkinson, as their effects mimic similar features of that seen in PD. Different epidemiological studies have shown a correlation between the exposure of these substances (especially in the case of pesticides) and appearance of PD [14-15, 17, 53]. A common feature of many of these neurotoxic compounds, such as rotenone, paraquat, or MPTP, is the inhibition of mitochondrial complex I, followed by the overproduction of ROS, ATP exhaustion, and induction of a wide range of abnormalities that can elicit neuronal and astrocytic cell death [54]. Additionally, neurotoxins induce nuclear fragmentation, endoplasmic reticulum (ER) stress and unfolded protein response in catecholaminergic cells, which are associated with changes in proteasomal and chaperone activities, similar to those observed in PD [45,55]. Other molecules used in PD models include the fungicide maneb, cyclodienes, organophosphates such as deltamethrin, DDT (dichlorodiphenyltrichloroethane), 2,4-dichlorophenoxyacetic acid, dieldrin, deguelin, diethyldithiocarbamate, paraquat, maneb, trifluralin and parathion (Figure 2) [15,56].

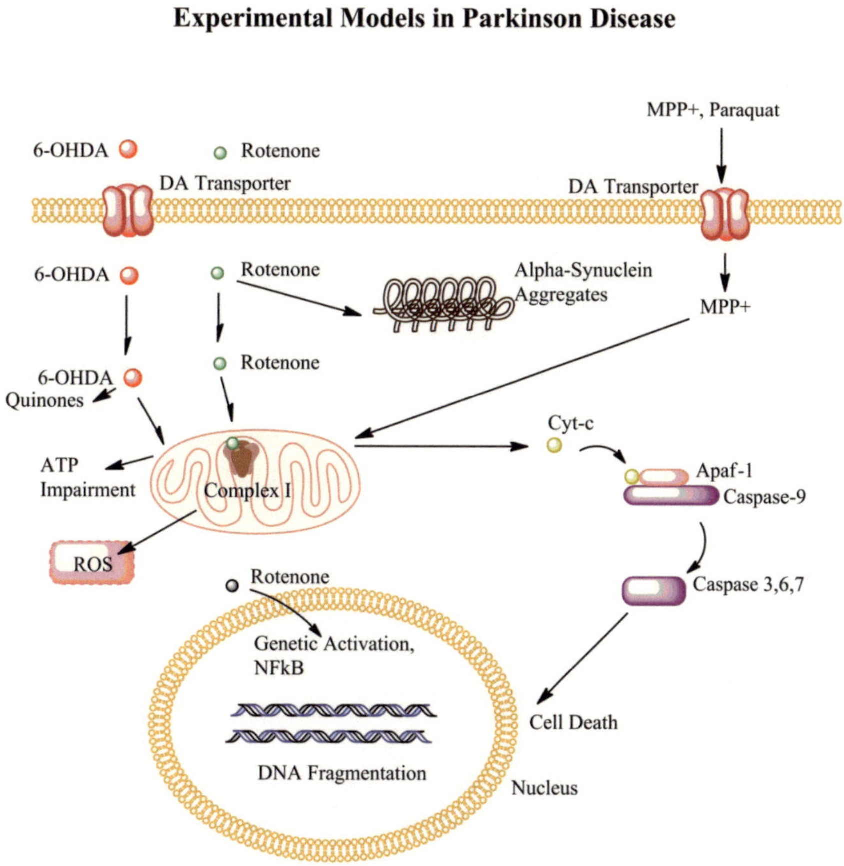

Figure 2. Experimental models in PD. Many molecules are currently used in cellular and animal models of PD, including pesticides as paraquat or rotenone and neurotoxins such as 6-OHDA and MPP^+. Paraquat, 6-hydroxydopamine (6-OHDA) and MPP^+ easily cross cell membrane through the dopamine transporter (DA) thus inducing the formation of α-synuclein aggregates and mitochondrial impairment with the subsequent production of ROS and quinones. Compounds, as rotenone, are extremely hydrophobic and penetrate easily the cellular membrane of neurons and astrocytes. Rotenone may promote processes such as the formation of α-synuclein aggregates, and the genetic activation through the nuclear translocation of NF-κB. Additionally, as an inhibitor of mitochondrial complex I, rotenone causes the impairment of ATP, the generation of ROS and the release of proapoptotic molecules, such as cytochrome c that activate caspase 9, which trigger caspases 3, 6 and 7, and induce apoptosis.

4.1. Rotenone as a Parkinson model

Rotenone is one of the most studied neurotoxic substances used as a model for PD features and oxidative stress events in cellular and animal models [14,57]. Rotenone is a naturally occurring isoflavonoid produced in the leaves, roots and rhizomes of the tropical legumes from the genres *Derris, Lonchocarpus,* and *Tephrosia*. It is extremely hydrophobic and crosses biological membranes and serves as a high-affinity noncompetitive inhibitor of complex I, thus affecting ATP generation [58]. Rotenone is commonly used in solution as a pesticide, insecticide, or in emulsified liquid form as a piscicide [59,60].

Rotenone, and other complex I inhibitors, such as MPTP, paraquat and maneb, are used as models for assessing the environmental causes of PD [12]. Previous epidemiological studies have supported the hypothesis that a prolonged exposure to pesticides is a risk factor for PD [17, 57,61]. Furthermore, a recent case-control study from the NIH, which reviewed 110 PD cases and 358 controls, and observed that PD incidence was increased 2.5 times in individuals who reported use of rotenone compared with nonusers [17]. Another study in agricultural workers from East Texas identified a significant increased risk (OR = 10.9) of PD with the continuous use of rotenone [53]. Although these reports raised important concerns on the use of rotenone, further studies are needed to assess the detailed global epidemiology of PD by this pesticide.

Much of the research on rotenone has used animal models and different routes of administration for evaluating its effects in the Central Nervous System (CNS), especially in neurons [14,57]. Several groups have demonstrated that continuous systemic administration of rotenone to rats and mice reproduces key features of PD, including selective degeneration of the nigrostriatal dopaminergic system, activation of astroglia and microglia, formation of cytoplasmic inclusions in neurons, movement disorders, and defects in mitochondrial complex I [11, 14, 57, 62-64]. Previous studies have shown that intracerebral administration of rotenone damages the nigrostriatal dopaminergic pathway in rats, including the striatum fibers and neurons [14,57]. However, the doses employed in those experiments were much higher than the standard IC_{50} for rotenone. For example, doses of 2-3 mg/kg/day, similar to that reported in platelets from PD patients, produced complex I inhibition with selective nigrostriatal degeneration and astrocyte activation [14,65]. In this matter, neuronal death is thought to be a consequence of the inhibition of mitochondrial complex I, which leads to a reduction in the energy supply and subsequent collapse of the mitochondrial membrane potential [66]. A recent study suggests that rotenone administration activates caspase-2 in mice neurons inducing the activation of downstream apoptotic effectors such as Bid, Bax, caspase 3 and 9, thus initiating apoptosis [67]. Similarly, the exposure of human dopaminergic SH- SY5Y cells to rotenone caused the nuclear translocation of nuclear factor κB (NF-κB) and the activation of caspase-3, suggesting that complex I deficiency induced by rotenone can induce NF-κB-mediated apoptosis (Figure 3) [68].

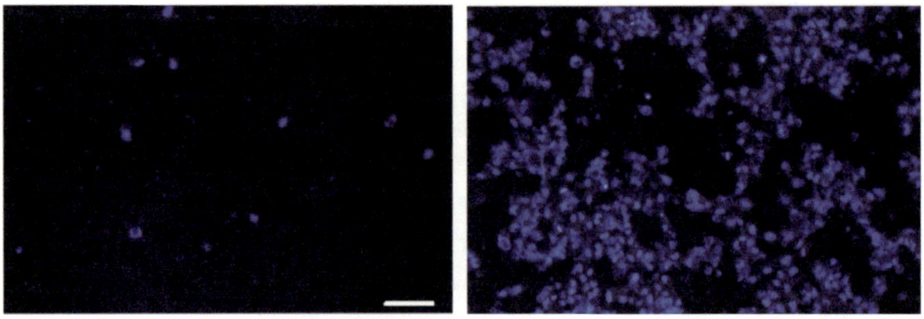

Figure 3. Rotenone-induced cell death. Astrocytic cell line ESP12 cells were treated with 30 nM of rotenone (right) or control (right), and stained for Hoetsch 33258 to assess nuclear fragmentation. Rotenone-treated cells showed increased nuclear damage compared to controls. Scale bar, 50 μm.

http://dx.doi.org/10.5772/54305

Alternatively, it has been postulated that rotenone-induced dopaminergic neuronal death could be dependent on the inflammatory process associated with microglial activation [64] thus indicating that rotenone differentially affects various types of CNS cells. Other previous experiments have shown that subcutaneous administration of rotenone resulted in a highly selective dopaminergic damage in neurons and α-synuclein aggregation, similar to the Lewy bodies of PD [63,65]. The mechanisms by which rotenone upregulates α-synuclein and causes its aggregation, are not well understood. A possible hypothesis is that aggregation is probably a consequence of oxidative modifications of α-synuclein [69]. For instance, neurons and astrocytes treated with rotenone (25 to 50 nM) showed an altered expression of g-tubulin and a disorganization of the centrosome with aggregates of α-synuclein [70]. Similarly, other studies suggest that inhibition of mitochondrial complex I activity and facilitation of α-synuclein aggregation may be closely associated with rotenone's selective dopaminergic toxicity in neurons [14,65]. Furthermore, a different approach using intragastrically administered rotenone (5 mg/Kg) in mice showed that the accumulation and aggregation of α-synuclein in neurons of the dorsal motor nucleus of the vagus (DMV) and the intermediolateral nucleus (IML) in the spinal cord was accompanied by the selective loss of dopaminergic neurons and astrogliosis, suggesting that the gastric administration of rotenone through the connection of the enteric nervous system (ENS) with anatomical structures of the CNS also induces PD-like features [11,19]. Rotenone has also been shown to cause increased expression of connexin43 (Cx43), which forms gap junctions, and P2X7 receptors that modulate cytokine secretion and gamma tubulin; these are important for the adequate function of the cytoskeleton and organelles such as the Golgi apparatus [70-73]. Moreover, rotenone induces astrogliosis and alterations in the expression of g-tubulin, signal transducer and activator of transcription 3 (STAT3), and connexin 43 in astrocytes [70, 72, 74].

In sum, the *in vitro* and *in vivo* evidences presented here show that dopaminergic neurons are more sensitive to rotenone toxicity than non-dopaminergic neurons, amacrine cells of retina and astrocytes [55, 75-77], possibly due to their lesser effective oxidative mechanisms and reduced supply of antioxidants [30,78]. However, astrocytes are more resilient to rotenone treatment than neurons, being its mitochondrial dysfunction tightly associated with increased neuronal death [2-4,74].

4.2. MPTP and Parkinson

MPTP is a widely used neurotoxicant, known for the induction of Parkinson-like symptoms such as bradikinesia, movement disorders, α-synuclein bodies, mitochondrial abnormalities, sustained inflammation in the substantia nigra and activation of the microglia [6,10,15, 79-80]. It was initially shown that in drug addicts, who were accidentally exposed to MPTP, there was a depletion of pigmented nerve cells in the substantia nigra, accompanied by astrogliosis and clustering of microgliosis around nerve cells [41], thus presenting some PD-like features.

MPTP is an alipophilic prototoxin that rapidly crosses the blood-brain barrier and damage dopaminergic neurons due to the selective uptake of the active metabolite MPP^+ via the dopamine transporter [80]. Similarly to rotenone, its neurotoxicity is induced by the inhibition of mitochondrial complex I, and subsequent energy depletion [80-81]. Additionally, MPP^+ has high affinity for noradrenergic and serotonergic uptake transporters [6,82], and its precursor, MPTP, has been mainly used in neuronal models with dopaminergic characteristics, such as the dopaminergic neuroblastoma cell line SH-SY5Y [83]. In astrocytes, MPTP has shown different (and sometimes contradictory) effects according to the experimental evidence collected in cellular and animal models. For instance, Rappold and Tieu (2010) showed that MPTP is metabolized by the astrocytic monoamineoxidase-B (MAO-B) and converted to the toxic cation MPP^+, which is extruded to the extracellular space through the organic cation transporter 3 (oct3) [6, 84]. Afterwards, MPP^+ is taken by neighboring dopaminergic neurons, thus inducing neuronal death [84]. Interestingly, silencing of oct 3 transporter in mice attenuates both the MPP^+ release from astrocytes and the subsequent impairment of dopaminergic neurons, in which makes oct3 as an important molecular target for dopaminergic related pathologies [6,84]. On the other hand, other authors have shown that MPP^+ induces negative effects in astrocytes, such as loss of viability, impairment of energetic metabolism of mitochondria, ROS generation and decrease in the glutamate clearance by astrocytes [81,85,86]. Taking into account the importance of MPTP, as a model for PD, it seems that further epidemiological research is needed to address more thoroughly the role of MPTP in astrocytic damage and PD development.

4.3. Other toxic compounds involved in Parkinson development: Paraquat and 6-OHDA

The pesticide *N,N′*-dimethyl-4,4′-bipyridinium dichloride (paraquat), which shares similar structure with MPP^+, impairs mitochondrial functions by inducing an augmented production of oxidative stress and 4-hydroxynenal *in vivo* [87]. Although paraquat may not be an efficient inhibitor of mitochondrial complex I, and so does not affect dopamine uptake [87,88], it does cause α-synuclein aggregation in C57Bl/6 mice, and alters Parkin solubility, decreasing proteasome activity and causing cellular damage [87].

Paraquat has been previously shown to induce PD-like neuronal dopaminergic lesions in animal models and neuronal cell lines (Brown et al., 2006; Berry et al., 2010). Additionally, epidemiological studies suggest that long-term exposure to paraquat is associated with PD development [15,89]. To counteract this oxidative damage induced by paraquat, and MPTP, astrocytes seem to protect dopaminergic neurons by increasing expression of antioxidant molecules, such as heme oxigenase1 (EC 1.14.99.3), glutathione S-transferase P (EC 2.5.1.18) and glutathione [90,91]. Although this protective role of astrocytes on neuronal death by paraquat is quite promising, only few studies address this interaction and further research is needed in order to establish the precise effect of paraquat in astrocytes metabolism and neuroprotection.

Similarly to paraquat, 6-Hydroxydopamine (6-OHDA) is another widely used for *in vivo* and *in vitro* animal models of PD [92]. This compound has a structure similar to dopamine and norepinephrine and exhibits a high affinity for catecholaminergic transporters such as dopamine DAT (Dopamine transporter). 6-OHDA induces dopaminergic neuronal death by the increased generation of H_2O_2 and quinones [92]. Additionally, it causes both microgliosis and astrogliosis, which is characterized by increased astrocytic proliferation in rat cortex and striatum accompanied by a marked expression of GFAP [92,93]. Taking into account that reactive astrocytes may produce various neurotrophic factors and antioxidant molecules targeting neuronal survival, it is possible that genetic manipulation of these functions in astrocytes may represent a promising strategy to improve dopaminergic neurons or neural progenitor cells survival [4,23]. These neuroprotective features of astrocyte in Parkinson are further explored in the following topic.

5. Astrocytic neuroprotection in Parkinson

Over the last years, much research has focused on specific molecules produced by astrocytes that exert neuroprotection during brain injuries and diseases including PD, both through the reuptake of glutamate, or by producing gliotransmitters, antioxidant enzimes such as SODs, growth factors, peptide hormones and heat shock proteins [4,94-98]. Many of them have shown protective effects both in dopaminergic neurons and glial cells, and have been used in animal models and clinical trials with remarkable results (Figure 4) [31,32].

5.1. Glutathione and Parkinson

Astrocytes produce beneficial antioxidants, including glutathione, superoxide dismutases (SODs 1, 2 and 3), and ascorbate, which are important for neuronal survival during neurodegenerative processes [95,99-101].

The tripeptid glutathione, as the main antioxidant in the brain, is needed for the conversion of methylglyoxal, a toxic by-product of metabolism, into d-lactate by glyoxalase 1 (EC 4.4.1.5) [94,95]. GSH is also important in limiting and repairing the deleterious actions of NO, but unfortunately GSH levels can be depleted by extremely high concentrations of NO [23]. For example, glutathione becomes rapidly oxidized to glutathione disulfide either by glutathione peroxidase (GPx) or by enzyme-independent chemical reactions [102]. This is an important effect against ROS formation in PD, as it helps reducing the inhibition of complex I by NO [103]. Astrocytes possess a greater concentration of glutathione (3,8 mmol/L) than neurons (2.5 mmol), probably due to a higher content of the astrocytic enzyme y-glutamylcysteine synthethase (EC 6.3.2.2) [6]. For example, neurons co-cultured with astrocytes exhibit higher levels of glutathione compared to neurons cultured alone, demonstrating that astrocytes provide additional antioxidant defenses to neurons [104-106]. Additionally, an increase in glutathione peroxidase-containing cells shows to be inversely correlated with the severity of dopaminergic cell loss in cell populations from patients with PD, suggesting that the quantity of glutathione peroxidase in cells might be critical for a protective effect against oxidative stress during PD [107].

The greater production of GSH by astrocytes seems to be dependent on the preferential activation of transcription factor Nrf2 in astrocytes, which leads to a more efficient GSH synthesis and higher GSH content in astrocytes than in neurons [108]. Interestingly, Nrf2 is known to regulate the expression of cytoprotective genes, and factors essential to neuronal survival [6,108]. Additionally, Nrf2 knockout mice are more sensitive to mitochondrial complex inhibitors such as MPTP and 3-nitropropionic acid [108], suggesting an important role of this transcription factor in scavenging free radicals. On the other hand, decrease in glutathione is one of the earliest biochemical changes in PD and incidental Lewy body disease [109]. Additionally, the GSH content was significantly reduced in the substantia nigra of PD patients, suggesting that GSH depletion enhances neuronal death under certain pathological conditions [6]. Interestingly, this evidence is consistent with the data in PD patients, in which glutathione-containing cells are in regions with preserved dopaminergic neurons [52].

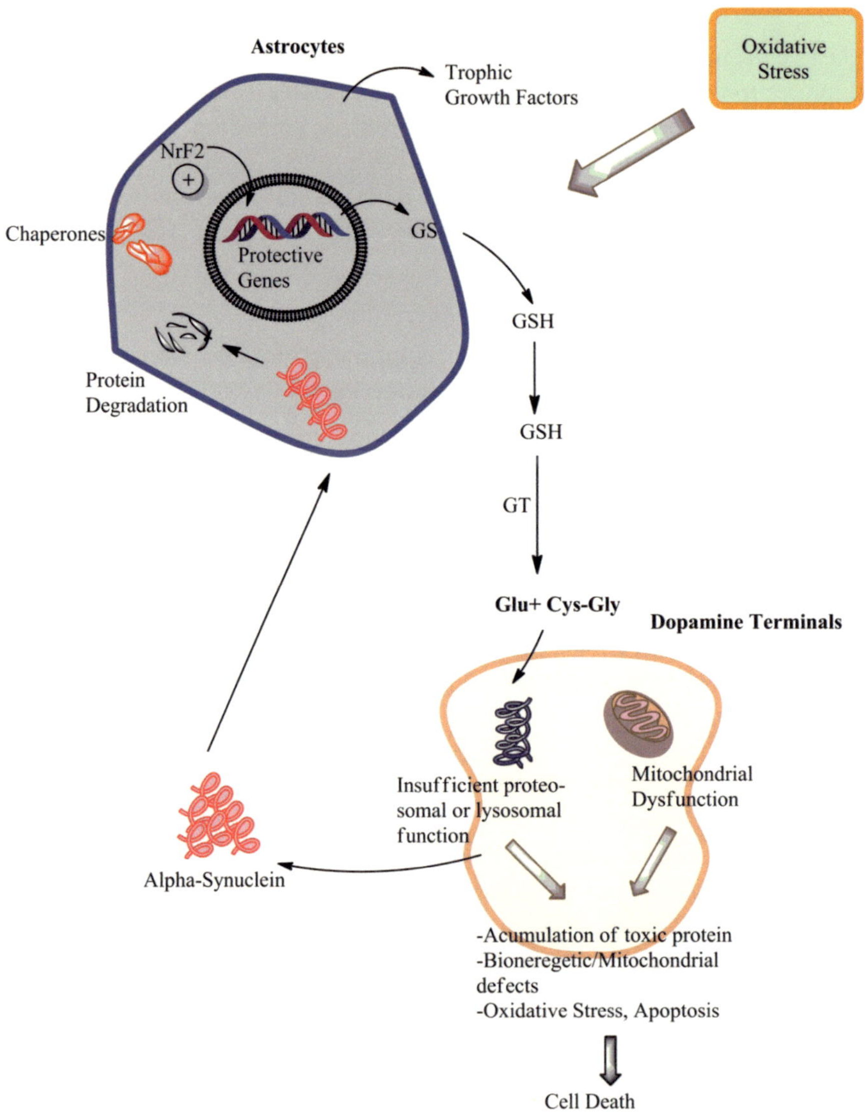

Figure 4. Astrocytes-mediate neuroprotection through multiple signaling pathways Astrocytes release glutathione, which serves as precursors for neuronal GSH synthesis, and trophic growth factors such as bFGF, GDNF, and MANF. Activation of the transcription factor Nrf2 leads to the expression of antioxidant genes, including γ-glutamylcysteine synthetase (GS), which is involved in GSH synthesis and removal or degradation of cytotoxic molecules, such as α-synuclein.

It is possible that the recovery of glutathione levels may enhance the survival of affected neurons, either by increasing synthesis of GSH or by slowing its degradation [25]. However, the GSH blood-brain barrier permeability is low, and clinical trials using injections of GSH have shown little benefits [6,25,110]. Alternatively, it has been demonstrated that the use of GSH precursors, such as glutamyl cysteine ethyl ester (GCEE) and gluthathione ethyl ester (GEE), increases significantly the intracellular glutathione levels in neuronal cells, protecting dopaminergic neurons against oxidative an nitrosative stress, both in animal and cellular models [25,109]. Finally, the modulation of Nrf2 downstream signaling may be considered as a promising strategy for enhancing the astrocytic production of GSH [108], which may counteract the oxidative imbalance that likely affects neurons in neurodegenerative processes such as PD.

5.2. Superoxide dismutases and Parkinson

Superoxide dismutases catalyze the dismutation of superoxide ions into oxygen and hydrogen peroxide [23]. As such, they are an important antioxidant defense in nearly all cells exposed to oxygen. In most mammalian cells, SOD is present in three isoforms: a cytosolic copper, zinc superoxide dismutase (SOD1); a mitochondrial manganese superoxide dismutase (SOD2); and an extracellular copper, zinc superoxide dismutase (SOD3) [23, 112]. Given its importance in neuroprotection, SODs and other antioxidant molecules released by astrocytes are highly studied in neurodegenerative diseases like PD and in other oxidative-related events. Evidence that SODs defend against oxidative stress *in situ* has been obtained using transgenic mutants that either overexpress or lack these antioxidant enzymes [111]. For example, the overexpression of Cu/Zn SOD was able to rescue dopaminergic neurons and diminishes locomotor disabilities in a *Drosophila* mutant model for α-synuclein overexpression [112]. Interestingly in PD patients, it has been shown, an specific increase in SOD levels in the substantia nigra, with no changes in activities of glutathione peroxidase, catalase and glutathione reductase (EC 1.8.1.7) [25]. A similar increase was observed in the mitochondrial isoform of SOD in the motor cortex from PD patients [113], suggesting that SODs have a greater importance than other antioxidant enzymes during PD development. Further research is needed in order to address the therapeutic application of SOD in PD and other diseases.

5.3. Astrocytic chaperones and Parkinson

Chaperones belonging to the conserved family of Heat shock proteins (Hsps) are proteins involved in the regulation of protein folding, translocation of proteins across membranes, regulation of cell death and assembling of protein [114]. Interestingly, protein aggregates, and misfolded proteins have been found in AD, Huntington, PD, prion disease, ALS and other neurological injuries [115-117]. Furthermore, previous evidence suggests that formation of unfolded proteins in astrocytes could induce the inflammatory responses previously mentioned [117].

Many Hsps are currently being considered for the potential treatment of diseases involving protein aggregation and misfolding such as the case of PD [116,118]. These include the chaperones, DJ-1, Hsp70, Hsp9- and the co-chaperone Hsp40, and members from the Bag family, such as Bag 5, CHIP and suppression of tumorigenicity 13 (ST13) [118]. Several of these chaperones are colocalized or associated with the PD related proteins, E3-ubiquitin ligase (E 6.3.2.19), parkin, α-synuclein and the dopamine transporter (DAT) [119].

DJ-1, also known as PARK7, is upregulated in reactive astrocytes and serves as a redox-sensitive chaperone with antiapoptotic properties [119]. DJ-1, both in normal and mutant forms, colocalizes with Hsp70 and CHIP in the cytosol. Following oxidative stress, this molecule is translocated to the mitochondria, where it becames associated with the chaperone GRP75 [119,120]. It has been previously shown that DJ-1 can suppress the aggregation and oligomerization of α-synuclein, thus promoting its degradation, which is dependent on the redox state of the cell environment [119,121]. Additionally, DJ-1 regulates signaling pathways such P38 mitogen-activated protein kinases (MAPK; EC 2.7.11.24), apoptosis signal-regulating kinase 1 (ASK1; EC 2.7.11.25) and protein kinase B (AKT) following cellular production of ROS, suggesting that this chaperone is an important redox-reactive molecule during oxidative stress in PD and other age-related disorders [120].

Hsp70 family of chaperones are thought to be critical in the regulation of protein oligomerization and aggregation, which are believed to be central in the molecular pathogenesis of PD and other neurodegenerative diseases [118]. For example, the overexpression of Hsp70 has been found to protect PC12 cells, and dopaminergic neurons against MPTP toxicity [118,119]. Additionally, the overexpression of Hsp70 in mice has been shown to reduce the amount of misfolded and aggregated α-synuclein species, suggesting a protection of this chaperone against α-synuclein-dependent toxicity [122]. It seems that α-synuclein degradation mediated by Hsp70 occurs in the proteasome or in the lisosomes by a selective process called chaperone-mediated autophagy (CMA) [114]. The wild type, but not a mutant form of α-synuclein is degradated by CMA, suggesting that this mechanism is important in the formation of α-synuclein aggregates during PD [114]. Importantly, the astrocytic clearance of α-synuclein by chaperones, like Hsp70, may confer additional neuroprotection to dopaminergic neurons [6,114].

Chaperones located in other organelles, such as the ER, have also been studied in the development of neurodegenerative processes. For example, homocysteine-induced endoplasmic reticulum protein, which is located in the ER membrane of neurons and astrocytes in the Central Nervous System (SNC), is found accumulated in Lewy bodies, suggesting a role in their formation and further development of PD [117]. In sum, given the central importance of chaperones in protein homeostasis, or proteostasis, they may serve as rational targets for the design of therapeutic strategies in neurodegenerative diseases associated with aberrant protein folding including PD.

5.4. Growth factors and Parkinson

Several neurotrophic and growth factors have been shown to protect dopaminergic neurons and glial cells against induced excitotoxicity by the activation of specific signaling pathways that are responsible for cell survival and axonal sprouting [31,32]. Some of them have also been tested in PD clinical trials with some promising results [31,32]. For example, brain derived neurotrophic factor (BDNF) and TNF protect neurons against excitotoxicity through activation of the transcription factor NF-kB, which induces the expression of antioxidant enzymes such as Mn-SOD and the anti-apoptotic proteins, Bcl-2 and inhibitor of apoptosis proteins IAPs [123,124]. Additionally, the endogenous administration of BDNF was shown to protect neurons within the substantia nigra from 6-OHDA and MPTP toxicity, both in rat and primate Parkinson models [31].

The family of glial cell line-derived neurotrophic factor (GDNF) comprises ligands such as GDNF, neurturin (NRTN), artemin (ARTN) and persephin. GDNF, secreted by astrocytes, is essential for the survival of dopaminergic neurons [32]. It has been shown that GDNF administration by catheter increases dopaminergic neuronal resistance against 6-OHDA toxicity, but with preservation of motor functions in rat and rhesus monkey models [96]. However, clinical trials in patients that were administered GDNF in different regions of the brain have shown mixed results and further research is needed [31, 125-127].

Insulin-like growth factors (IGFs) signaling through the phosphatidylinositol 3-kinase (PI3K/Akt) downstream pathway can protect neurons against LPS excitotoxicity in cell culture and *in vivo* [124, 128,129]. Furthermore, the activation of this signaling pathway by IGF-I can suppress α-synuclein aggregation and toxicity, suggesting a possible therapeutically strategy in PD [130]. Similarly to IGF-I, vascular endothelial growth factor (VEGF) affects the survival and proliferation of endothelial cells, neurons and astrocytes in the brain, suggesting a potential therapeutic application in PD [32]. Additionally, VEGF-B (isorform B) was found activated in a rat brain model following treatment with 40 nM rotenone, and showed neuroprotective actions by improving neuronal survival (Falk et al., 2009). Some studies suggest that VEGF promotes neuroprotection by signaling through the neuropilin receptor expressed in DA neurons, and indirectly by activating the proliferation of astroglia and by promoting angiogenesis [32,131,132]. Furthermore, the striatal injection of an adeno-associated virus (AAV)-mediated VEGF expression provided neuroprotection and behavioral improvement in rats treated with 6-OHDA [133].

Basic fibroblast growth factor (bFGF) protects hippocampal and cortical neurons against glutamate toxicity by changing the expression of *N*-methyl-D-aspartic acid (NMDA) receptors and antioxidant enzymes like superoxide dismutases and glutathione reductase [124]. Furthermore, a coculture of transgenic overexpressing FGF-2 Schwann cells with dopaminergic neurons improved the survival of dopaminergic neurons and the behavioral outcome in a parkinsonian rat model lesioned with 6-OHDA [134]. Finally, there are other neurotrophic factors that have shown dopaminergical neuronal protection in Parkinson-like models, including hepatocyte growth factor (HGF), mesencephalic astrocyte-derived neurotrophic factor (MANF), cerebral dopaminergic neurotrophic factor (CDNF), granulocyte colony-stimulating factor (G-CSF), and platelet derived growth factor (PDGF-CC) [31-32, 135-136].

6. Conclusions and future perspectives

In recent years a growing body of evidence has demonstrated that the malfunctioning of astrocytes may contribute to various neurodegenerative diseases, including Alzheimer, ALS, multiple sclerosis, and Parkinson. Importantly, astrocytes are involved in both exacerbation of damage and in neuroprotective mechanisms that are crucial for neuronal survival. In this matter, astrocytes are essential for the regulation of oxidative stress and ROS production, both in normal and in pathological circumstances.

The overexpression of antioxidant molecules such as GSH and SOD2, or chaperones such as Hsp70 has proved to be a successful experimental approach in brain diseases, including PD. The use of growth factors, both in animal models and in clinical trials, has shown promising effects in protecting dopaminergic neurons and astrocytes in damaged regions by the activation of different signaling pathways important in neuronal survival and regeneration. It is important to mention that mitochondrial protection in astrocytes is an important asset to maintain the energetic balance of the brain and the antioxidant production that contribute to neuronal protection. Therefore future efforts in neuroprotective strategies should emphasize the mitochondrial protection in astrocytes. Finally, the combination of novel drug therapies, a better understanding of the α-synuclein clearance by astrocytes, the use of neurotoxic models, growth factors use and other therapies that increase astrocyte survival and its antioxidant function may shed light on a prospective cure of PD in the near future.

Acknowledgements

This work was supported in part by grants PUJ IDs 4509 and 4327 to GEB.

Author details

Ricardo Cabezas[1], Marco Fidel Avila[1], Daniel Torrente[1], Ramon Santos El-Bachá[2], Ludis Morales[1], Janneth Gonzalez[1] and George E. Barreto[1]

*Address all correspondence to: gsampaio@javeriana.edu.co

1 Departamento de Nutrición y Bioquímica, Facultad de Ciencias, Pontificia Universidad Javeriana, Bogotá D.C., Colombia

2 Laboratorio de Neuroquímica e Biologia Celular, Universidade Federal da Bahía, Salvador, Bahia, Brazil

References

[1] Fernandez HH. Updates in the medical management of Parkinson disease. Cleveland Clinic Journal of Medicine 2012; 79(1) 28-35.

[2] Volterra A, Meldolesi J. Astrocytes, from brain glue to communication elements: the revolution continues. Nature Reviews Neuroscience 2005; 6(8) 626-640.

[3] Hamby ME, Sofroniew MV. Reactive astrocytes as therapeutic targets for CNS disorders. Neurotherapeutics 2010; 7(4) 494-506.

[4] Barreto GE, Gonzalez J, Capani F, Morales L. Role of Astrocytes in Neurodegenerative Diseases. In: Raymond Chuen-Chung Chang. (ed.) Neurodegenerative Diseases - Processes, Prevention, Protection and Monitoring. InTech; 2011. p257-272.

[5] Nutt JG, Wooten GF. Clinical practice. Diagnosis and initial management of Parkinson's disease. The New England Journal of Medicine 2005; 353(10) 1021-1027.

[6] Rappold PM, Tieu K. Astrocytes and therapeutics for Parkinson´s disease. Neurotherapeutics 2010; 7(4) 413–423.

[7] Halliday GM, Stevens CH. Glia: initiators and progressors of pathology in Parkinson's disease. Movement Disorders 2011; 26(1) 6-17.

[8] Singer C. Managing the patient with newly diagnosed Parkinson disease. Cleveland Clinic Journal of Medicine 2012; 79(Suppl 2) S3-S7.

[9] Schwartz MD, Sabetay MD. An Approach to the continuous Dopaminergic Stimulation in Parkinson´s Disease. The Israel Medical Association Journal 2012; 14(3) 175-179

[10] Hirsch EC, Breidert T, Rousselet E, Hunot S, Hartmann A, Michel PP. The role of glial reaction and inflammation in Parkinson's disease. Annals of the New York Academy of Sciences 2003; 991 214-228.

[11] Pan-Montojo F, Anichtchik O, Dening Y, Knels L, Pursche S, Jung R, et al. Progression of Parkinson´s disease pathology is reproduced by intragastric administration of rotenone in mice. PLoS One 2010; 5 (1) e8762

[12] Wang HL, Chou AH, Wu AS, Chen SY, Weng YH, Kao YC, et al. PARK6 PINK1 mutants are defective in maintaining mitochondrial membrane potential and inhibiting ROS formation of substantia nigra dopaminergic neurons. Biochimica et Biophysica Acta 2011; 1812(6) 674-684.

[13] Knott AB, Bossy-Wetzel E. Impairing the mitochondrial fission and fusion balance: a new mechanism of neurodegeneration. Annals of the New York Academy of Sciences 2008; 1147 283-292.

[14] Betarbet R, Sherer TB, MacKenzie G, Garcia-Osuna M, Panov, AV, Greenamyre, JT. Chronic systemic pesticide exposure reproduces features of Parkinson's disease. Nature Neuroscience 2000; 3(12) 1301-1306.

[15] Brown TP, Rumsby PC, Capleton AC, Rushton L, Levy LS. Pesticides and Parkinson's disease -- is there a link? Environmental Health Perspectives 2006; 114(2) 156-64.

[16] Greenamyre JT, Betarbet R, Sherer TB. The rotenone model of Parkinson's disease: genes, environment and mitochondria. Parkinsonism & Related Disorders 2003; 9 (Suppl 2) S59-S64.

[17] Tanner CM, Kamel F, Ross GW, Hoppin JA, Goldman SM, Korell M, et al. Rotenone, paraquat, and Parkinson's disease. Environmental Health Perspective 2011; 119(6) 866-872.

[18] Vives-Bauza C, Przedborski S. Mitophagy: the latest problem for Parkinson's disease. Trends in Molecular Medicine 2011; 17(3) 158-165.

[19] Braak H, de Vos RA, Bohl J, Del Tredici K. Gastric alpha-synuclein immunoreactive inclusions in Meissner's and Auerbach's plexuses in cases staged for Parkinson's disease-related brain pathology. Neuroscience Letters 2006; 396(1) 67-72.

[20] Wakabayashi K, Hayashi S, Yoshimoto M, Kudo H, Takahashi H. NACP/alpha-synuclein-positive filamentous inclusions in astrocytes and oligodendrocytes of Parkinson's disease brains. Acta Neuropathologica 2000; 99(1) 14-20.

[21] Ciesielska A, Joniec I, Kurkowska-Jastrzebska I, Cudna A, Przybylkowski A, Czlonkowska A, et al. The impact of age and gender on the striatal astrocytes activation in murine model of Parkinson's disease. Inflammation Research 2009; 58(11) 747-753.

[22] Muramatsu Y, Kurosaki R, Watanabe H, Michimata M, Matsubara M, Imai Y, et al. Cerebral alterations in a MPTP-mouse model of Parkinson's disease--an immunocytochemical study. The Journal of Neural Transmission 2003; 110(10) 1129-1144.

[23] Chen Y, Swanson RA. Astrocytes and brain injury. Journal of Cerebral Blood Flow & Metabolism 2003; 23(2) 137-149.

[24] Maragakis NJ, Rothstein JD. Mechanisms of Disease: astrocytes in neurodegenerative disease. Nature Clinical Practice Neurology 2006; 2(12) 679-689.

[25] Chinta S, Andersen J. Redox imbalance in Parkinson. Biochimica et Biophysica Acta 2008; 1780(11) 1362–1367.

[26] Kimelberg HK, Nedergaard M. Functions of astrocytes and their potential as therapeutic targets. Neurotherapeutics 2010; 7(4) 338-353.

[27] Parpura V, Grubisic V, Verkhratsky A. Ca(2+) sources for the exocytotic release of glutamate from astrocytes. Biochimica et Biophysica Acta 2011; 1813(5) 984-991.

[28] Bushong EA, Martone ME, Jones YZ, Ellisman MH. Protoplasmic astrocytes in CA1 stratum radiatum occupy separate anatomical domains. The Journal of Neuroscience 2002; 22(1) 183-192.

[29] Zonta M, Angulo MC, Gobbo S, Rosengarten B, Hossmann KA, Pozzan T, et al. Neuron-to-astrocyte signaling is central to the dynamic control of brain microcirculation. Nature Neuroscience 2003; 6(1) 43-50.

[30] Greve MW, Zink BJ. Pathophysiology of traumatic brain injury. *Mount Sinai Journal* of Medicine 2009; 76(2) 97-104.

[31] Ramaswamy S, Kordower JH. 2009. Are growth factors the answer? Parkinsonism and Related Disorders 2009; 15(Suppl 3) S176-S180.

[32] Yasuda T, Mochizuki H. Use of growth factors for the treatment of Parkinson's disease. Expert Review of Neurotherapeutics 2010; 10(6) 915-924.

[33] Barreto G, Veiga S, Azcoitia I, Garcia-Segura LM, Garcia-Ovejero D. Testosterone decreases reactive astroglia and reactive microglia after brain injury in male rats: role of its metabolites, oestradiol and dihydrotestosterone. European Journal of Neuroscience 2007; 25(10) 3039-3046.

[34] Barreto G, Santos-Galindo M, Diz-Chaves Y, Pernía O, Carrero P, Azcoitia I, Garcia-Segura LM. Selective estrogen receptor modulators decrease reactive astrogliosis in the injured brain: effects of aging and prolonged depletion of ovarian hormones. Endocrinology 2009; 150(11) 5010-5015.

[35] Gu XL, Long CX, Sun L, Xie C, Lin X, Cai H. Astrocytic expression of Parkinson's disease-related A53T alpha-synuclein causes neurodegeneration in mice. Molecular Brain 2010; 21(3) 12.

[36] Xiong X, Barreto GE, Xu L, Ouyang YB, Xie X, Giffard RG. Increased brain injury and worsened neurological outcome in interleukin-4 knockout mice after transient focal cerebral ischemia. Stroke 2011; 42(7) 2026-2032.

[37] Adelson JD, Barreto GE, Xu L, Kim T, Brott BK, Ouyang YB, et al. Neuroprotection from stroke in the absence of MHCI or PirB. Neuron 2012; 73(6) 1100-1107.

[38] Ridet, JL, Malhotra SK, Privat A, Gage FH. Reactive astrocytes: cellular and molecular cues to biological function. Trends in Neurosciences 1997; 20(12) 570-577.

[39] Sugaya K, Chou S, Xu SJ, McKinney M. Indicators of glial activation and brain oxidative stress after intraventricular infusion of endotoxin. Brain Research Molecular Brain Research 1998; 58(1-2) 1-9.

[40] Kang W, Hebert JM. Signaling pathways in reactive astrocytes, a genetic perspective. Molecular Neurobiology 2011; 43(3) 147-154.

[41] Langston JW, Forno LS, Tetrud J, Reeves AG, Kaplan JA, Karluk D. Evidence of active nerve cell degeneration in the substantia nigra of humans years after 1-methyl-4-phenyl-1,2,3,6-tetrahydropyridine exposure. Annals of Neurology 1999; 46(4) 598-605.

[42] Herrera AJ, Castaño A, Venero JL, Cano J, Machado A. The single intranigral injection of LPS as a new model for studying the selective effects of inflammatory reactions on dopaminergic system. Neurobiology of Disease 2000; 7(4) 429-447.

[43] Niranjan R, Nath C, Shukla R. The mechanism of action of MPTP-induced neuroinflammation and its modulation by melatonin in rat astrocytoma cells, C6. Free Radical Research 2010; 44(11) 1304-1316.

[44] Samantaray S, Knaryan VH, Guyton MK, Matzelle DD, Ray SK, Banik NL. The parkinsonian neurotoxin rotenone activates calpain and caspase-3 leading to motoneuron degeneration in spinal cord of Lewis rats. Neuroscience 2007; 146(2) 741-755.

[45] de Oliveira DM, Barreto G, Galeano P, Romero JI, Holubiec MI, Badorrey MS, et al. Paullinia cupana Mart. var. Sorbilis protects human dopaminergic neuroblastoma SH-SY5Y cell line against rotenone-induced cytotoxicity. Human & Experimental Toxicology 2011; 30(9) 1382-1391.

[46] Cherian L, Goodman JC, Robertson CS. Brain nitric oxide changes after controlled cortical impact injury in rats. Journal of Neurophysiology 2000; 83(4) 2171-2178.

[47] LeDoux SP, Druzhyna NM, Hollensworth SB, Harrison JF, Wilson GL. Mitochondrial DNA repair: a critical player in the response of cells of the CNS to genotoxic insults. Neuroscience 2007; 145(4) 1249-1259.

[48] Dugan LL, Kim-Han JS. Astrocyte mitochondria in in vitro models of ischemia. Journal of Bioenergetics and Biomembranes 2004; 36(4) 317-321.

[49] Patel VP, Chu CT. Nuclear transport, oxidative stress, and neurodegeneration. International Journal of Clinical and Experimental Pathology 2011; 4(3) 215-229.

[50] Mythri RB, Venkateshappa C, Harish G, Mahadevan A, Muthane UB, Yasha TC, et al. Evaluation of markers of oxidative stress, antioxidant function and astrocytic proliferation in the striatum and frontal cortex of Parkinson's disease brains. Neurochemical Research 2011; 36(8) 1452-1463.

[51] Jenner P. Oxidative stress in Parkinson's disease. Annals of Neurology 2003; 53 S26–S36.

[52] Heales SJ, Lam AA, Duncan AJ, Land JM. Neurodegeneration or neuroprotection: the pivotal role of astrocytes. Neurochemical Research 2004; 29(3) 513-519.

[53] Dhillon AS, Tarbutton GL, Levin JL, Plotkin GM, Lowry LK, Nalbone JT, et al. Pesticide/environmental exposures and Parkinson's disease in East Texas. Journal of Agromedicine 2008; 13(1) 37-48.

[54] Dick FD. Parkinson's disease and pesticide exposures. British Medical Bulletin 2006; 79-80 219-231.

[55] Nagel F, Bahr M, Dietz GP. Tyrosine hydroxylase-positive amacrine interneurons in the mouse retina are resistant against the application of various parkinsonian toxins. Brain Research Bulletin 2009; 79(5) 303-309.

[56] Caboni P, Sherer TB, Zhang N, Taylor G, Na HM, Greenamyre JT, et al. Rotenone, deguelin, their metabolites, and the rat model of Parkinson's disease. Chemical Research in Toxicology 2004; 17(11) 1540-1548.

[57] Liu B, Gao HM, Hong JS. Parkinson's disease and exposure to infectious agents and pesticides and the occurrence of brain injuries: role of neuroinflammation. Environmental Health Perspectives 2003; 111(8) 1065-1073.

[58] Greenamyre JT, MacKenzie G, Peng TI, Stephans SE. Mitochondrial dysfunction in Parkinson's disease. Biochemical Society Symposia 1999; 66 85-97

[59] Isman MB. Botanical insecticides, deterrents, and repellents in modern agriculture and an increasingly regulated world. Annual Review of Entomology 2006; 51 45-66.

[60] Patel F. Pesticidal suicide: adult fatal rotenone poisoning. Journal of Forensic and Legal Medicine 2011; 18(7) 340-342.

[61] Tuchsen F, Jensen AA. Agricultural work and the risk of Parkinson's disease in Denmark, 1981-1993. Scandinavian Journal of Work, Environment & Health 2000; 26(4) 359-362.

[62] Greenamyre JT, Cannon JR, Drolet R, Mastroberardino PG. Lessons from the rotenone model of Parkinson's disease. Trends in Pharmacological Science 2010; 31(4) 141-142.

[63] Hoglinger GU, Lannuzel A, Khondiker ME, Michel PP, Duyckaerts C, Feger J, et al. The mitochondrial complex I inhibitor rotenone triggers a cerebral tauopathy. Journal of Neurochemistry 2005; 95(4) 930-939.

[64] Ogawa N, Asanuma M, Miyazaki I, Diaz-Corrales FJ, Miyoshi K. L-DOPA treatment from the viewpoint of neuroprotection. Possible mechanism of specific and progressive dopaminergic neuronal death in Parkinson's disease. Journal of Neurology 2005; 252 (Suppl 4) IV23-IV31.

[65] Sherer TB, Betarbet R, Kim JH, Greenamyre JT. Selective microglial activation in the rat rotenone model of Parkinson's disease. Neuroscience Letters 2003; 341(2) 87-90.

[66] Gyulkhandanyan AV, Feeney CJ, Pennefather PS. Modulation of mitochondrial membrane potential and reactive oxygen species production by copper in astrocytes. Journal of Neurochemistry 2003; 87(2) 448-460.

[67] Tiwari M, Lopez-Cruzan M, Morgan WW, Herman B. Loss of caspase-2-dependent apoptosis induces autophagy after mitochondrial oxidative stress in primary cultures of young adult cortical neurons. The Journal of Biological Chemistry 2011; 286(10) 8493-8506.

[68] Wang HL, Chou AH, Wu AS, Chen SY, Weng YH, Kao YC, et al. PARK6 PINK1 mutants are defective in maintaining mitochondrial membrane potential and inhibiting

ROS formation of substantia nigra dopaminergic neurons. Biochimica et Biophysica Acta 2011; 1812(6) 674-684.

[69] Greenamyre JT, Betarbet R, Sherer TB. The rotenone model of Parkinson's disease: genes, environment and mitochondria. Parkinsonism & Related Disorders 2003; 9 (Suppl 2) S59-S64.

[70] Diaz-Corrales FJ, Asanuma M, Miyazaki I, Miyoshi K, Ogawa N. Rotenone induces aggregation of gamma-tubulin protein and subsequent disorganization of the centrosome: relevance to formation of inclusion bodies and neurodegeneration. Neuroscience 2005; 133(1) 117-135.

[71] Kawasaki A, Hayashi T, Nakachi K, Trosko JE, Sugihara K, Kotake Y, et al. Modulation of connexin 43 in rotenone-induced model of Parkinson's disease. Neuroscience 2009; 160(1) 61-68.

[72] Zhang S, Liang R, Zhou F, Huang X, Ding JH, Hu, G. Reversal of rotenone-induced dysfunction of astrocytic connexin43 by opening mitochondrial ATP-sensitive potassium channels. Cellular and Molecular Neurobiology 2010; 31(1) 111-117.

[73] Gao XF, Wang W, Yu Q, Burnstock G, Xiang ZH. He C. Astroglial P2X7 receptor current density increased following long-term exposure to rotenone. Purinergic Signalling 2011; 7(1) 65-72.

[74] Sarafian TA, Montes C, Imura T, Qi J, Coppola G, Geschwind DH, et al. Disruption of astrocyte STAT3 signaling decreases mitochondrial function and increases oxidative stress in vitro. PloS One 2010; 5(3) e9532.

[75] Ahmadi FA, Grammatopoulos TN, Poczobutt AM, Jones SM, Snell LD, Das M, et al. 2008. Dopamine selectively sensitizes dopaminergic neurons to rotenone-induced apoptosis. Neurochemical Research 2008; 33(5) 886-901.

[76] Norazit A, Meedeniya AC, Nguyen MN, Mackay-Sim A. Progressive loss of dopaminergic neurons induced by unilateral rotenone infusion into the medial forebrain bundle. Brain Research 2010; 1360, 119-129.

[77] Radad K, Gille G, Rausch WD. Dopaminergic neurons are preferentially sensitive to long-term rotenone toxicity in primary cell culture. Toxicology In Vitro 2008; 22(1) 68-74.

[78] Verkhratsky A, Rodriguez JJ, Parpura V. Calcium signalling in astroglia. Molecular and Cellular Endocrinology 2012; 353(1-2) 45-56.

[79] McGeer PL, McGeer EG. Glial reactions in Parkinson's disease. Movement Disorders 2008; 23(4) 474-83.

[80] Sonsalla PK, Zeevalk GD, German DC. Chronic intraventricular administration of 1-methyl-4-phenylpyridinium as a progressive model of Parkinson's disease. Parkinsonism & Related Disorders 2008; 14(Suppl 2): S116-S118.

[81] Di Monte, DA, Tokar I, Langston JW, Impaired glutamate clearance as a consequence of energy failure caused by MPP(+) in astrocytic cultures. Toxicology and Applied Pharmacology 1999; 158(3) 296-302.

[82] Javitch JA, D'Amato RJ, Strittmatter SM, Snyder SH. Parkinsonism-inducing neurotoxin, *N*-methyl-4-phenyl-1,2,3,6-tetrahydropyridine:uptake of the metabolite *N*-methyl-4-phenylpyridine by dopamine neurons explain selective toxicity. Proceedings of the National Academy of Sciences of the United States of America 1985; 82(7) 2173–2177.

[83] Xie HR, Hu LS, Li GY. SH-SY5Y human neuroblastoma cell line: in vitro cell model of dopaminergic neurons in Parkinson's disease. Chinese Medical Journal 2010; 123(8) 1086-1092.

[84] Cui M, Aras R, Christian WV, Rappold PM, Hatwar M, Panza J, et al. The organic cation transporter-3 is a pivotal modulator of neurodegeneration in the nigrostriatal dopaminergic pathway. Proceedings of the National Academy of Sciences of the United States of America 2009; 106(19) 8043– 8048.

[85] Di Monte DA, Wu EY, Delanney LE, Irwin I, Langston JW. Toxicity of 1-methyl-4-phenyl-1,2,3,6-tetrahydropyridine in primary cultures of mouse astrocytes. The Journal of Pharmacology and Experimental Therapeutics 1992; 261(1) 44-49.

[86] Bi J, Wang XB, Chen L, Hao S, An LJ, Jiang B, et al. Catalpol protects mesencephalic neurons against MPTP induced neurotoxicity via attenuation of mitochondrial dysfunction and MAO-B activity. Toxicology in Vitro 2008; 22(8) 1883-1889.

[87] Berry C, La Vecchia C, Nicotera P. Paraquat and Parkinson's disease. Cell Death and Differentiation 2010; 17(7) 1115-1125.

[88] Richardson JR, Quan Y, Sherer TB, Greenamyre JT, Miller GW. Paraquat neurotoxicity is distinct from that of MPTP and rotenone. Toxicological Sciences 2005; 88(1) 193–201.

[89] Liou HH, Tsai MC, Chen CJ, Jeng JS, Chang YC, Chen SY, et al. Environmental risk factors and Parkinson's disease: a case-control study in Taiwan. Neurology 1997; 48(6) 1583–1588.

[90] Olesen BT, Clausen J, Vang O. Characterization of the transcriptional profile in primary astrocytes after oxidative stress induced by Paraquat. Neurotoxicology 2008; 29(1) 13-21.

[91] Rathinam ML, Watts LT, Narasimhan M, Riar AK, Mahimainathan L, Henderson GI. Astrocyte mediated protection of fetal cerebral cortical neurons from rotenone and paraquat. Environmental toxicology and pharmacology 2012; 33(2) 353-60.

[92] Bové J, Prou D, Perier C, Przedborski S Toxin-induced models of Parkinson′s disease. NeuroRX: the journal of the American society for experimental Neurotherapeutics 2005; 2(3) 484–494.

[93] Wachter B, Schurger S, Rolinger J, von Ameln-Mayerhofer A, Berg D, Wagner HJ, et al. Effect of 6-hydroxydopamine (6-OHDA) on proliferation of glial cells in the rat cortex and striatum: evidence for de-differentiation of resident astrocytes. Cell and Tissue Research 2010; 342(2) 147-60.

[94] Bambrick L, Kristian T, Fiskum G. Astrocyte mitochondrial mechanisms of ischemic brain injury and neuroprotection. Neurochemical Research 2004; 29(3) 601-608.

[95] Dringen R. Metabolism and functions of glutathione in brain. Progress in Neurobiology 2000; 62(6) 649-671.

[96] Safi R, Gardaneh M, Panahi Y, Maghsoudi N, Zaefizadeh M, Gharib E. Optimized quantities of GDNF overexpressed by engineered astrocytes are critical for protection of neuroblastoma cells against 6-OHDA toxicity. The Journal of Molecular Neuroscience 2011; 46(3) 654-665.

[97] Zheng L, Ishii Y, Tokunaga A, Hamashima T, Shen J, Zhao QL, et al. Neuroprotective effects of PDGF against oxidative stress and the signaling pathway involved. The Journal of Neuroscience Research 2010; 88(6) 1273-1284.

[98] Ouyang YB, Xu LJ, Emery JF, Lee, AS, Giffard RG. Overexpressing GRP78 influences Ca2+ handling and function of mitochondria in astrocytes after ischemia-like stress. Mitochondrion 2011; 11(2) 279-286.

[99] Anderson CM, Swanson RA. Astrocyte glutamate transport: review of properties, regulation, and physiological functions. Glia 2000; 32(1) 1-14.

[100] Sims NR, Nilsson M, Muyderman H. Mitochondrial glutathione: a modulator of brain cell death. Journal of Bioenergetics and Biomembranes 2004; 36(4) 329-333.

[101] Lindenau J, Noack H, Possel H, Asayama K, Wolf G. Cellular distribution of superoxide dismutases in the rat CNS. Glia 2000; 29(1) 25-34.

[102] Hirrlinger J, Dringen R The cytosolic redox state of astrocytes: Maintenance, regulation and functional implications for metabolite trafficking. Brain Research Review 2010; 63(1-2) 177-188.

[103] Duncan AJ, Heales SJ. Nitric oxide and neurological disorders. Molecular Aspects of Medicine 2005; 26(1-2) 67-96.

[104] Giordano G, Kavanagh TJ, Costa LG. Mouse cerebellar astrocytes protect cerebellar granule neurons against toxicity of the polybrominated diphenyl ether (PBDE) mixture DE-71. Neurotoxicology 2009; 30(2) 326-329.

[105] Maier CM, Chan PH. Role of superoxide dismutases in oxidative damage and neurodegenerative disorders. Neuroscientist 2002; 8(4) 323-334.

[106] Slemmer JE, Shacka JJ, Sweeney MI, Weber JT. Antioxidants and free radical scavengers for the treatment of stroke, traumatic brain injury and aging. *Current Medicinal Chemistry 2008;* 15(4) 404-414.

[107] Damier P, Hirsch EC, Zhang P, Agid Y, Javoy-Agid F. Glutathione peroxidase, glial cells and Parkinson's disease. Neuroscience 1993; 52(1) 1-6.

[108] Johnson JA, Johnson DA, Kraft AD, Calkins MJ, Jakel RJ, Vargas MR, et al. The Nrf2-ARE pathway: an indicator and modulator of oxidative stress in neurodegeneration. Annals of the New York Academy of Sciences 2008; 1147 61-69.

[109] Martin HL, Teismann P. Glutathione—a review on its role and significance in Parkinson's disease. The FASEB Journal 2009; 23(10) 3263-3272

[110] Hauser RA, Lyons KE, McClain T, Carter S, Perlmutter D. Randomized, double-blind, pilot evaluation of intravenous glutathione in Parkinson's disease. Movement Disorders 2009; 24(7) 979-83

[111] Chan PH. Role of oxidants in ischemic brain damage. Stroke 1996; 27(6) 1124-1129.

[112] Botella JA, Bayersdorfer F, Schneuwly S. Superoxide dismutase overexpression protects dopaminergic neurons in a Drosophila model of Parkinson's disease. Neurobiology of Disease 2008; 30(1) 65-73.

[113] Radunović A, Porto WG, Zeman S, Leigh PN. Increased mitochondrial superoxide dismutase activity in Parkinson's disease but not amyotrophic lateral sclerosis motor cortex. Neuroscience Letters 1997; 239(2-3) 105-108.

[114] Witt SN. Hsp70 molecular chaperones and Parkinson's disease. Biopolymers 2010; 93(3) 218-28.

[115] Kakizuka, A. Protein precipitation: a common etiology in neurodegenerative disorders? Trends in Genetics 1998; 14(10) 396-402.

[116] Giffard RG, Xu L, Zhao H, Carrico W, Ouyang Y, Qiao Y, et al. Chaperones, protein aggregation, and brain protection from hypoxic/ischemic injury. Journal of Experimental Biology 2004; 207(Pt 18) 3213-3220.

[117] Slodzinski H, Moran LB, Michael GJ, Wang B, Novoselov S, Cheetham ME, et al. Homocysteine-induced endoplasmic reticulum protein (herp) is up-regulated in parkinsonian substantia nigra and present in the core of Lewy bodies. Clinical Neuropathology 2009; 28(5) 333-43.

[118] Kalia SK, Kalia LV, McLean PJ. Molecular chaperones as rational drug targets for Parkinson's disease therapeutics. CNS & Neurological Disorders-Drug Targets 2010; 9(6) 741-53.

[119] Bandopadhyay R, de Belleroche J. Pathogenesis of Parkinson's disease: emerging role of molecular chaperones. Trends in Molecular Medicine 2010; 16(1) 27-36.

[120] Kahle PJ, Waak J, Gasser T. DJ1 and prevention of oxidative stress in Parkinson's disease and other age related disorders. Free Radical Biology and Medicine 2009; 47(10) 1354-61.

[121] Shendelman S, Jonason A, Martinat C, Leete T, Abeliovich A. DJ-1 is a redox-dependent molecular chaperone that inhibits alpha-synuclein aggregate formation. PLoS Biol 2004; 2(11) e362.

[122] Klucken J, Shin Y, Masliah E, Hyman BT, McLean PJ. Hsp70 Reduces alpha-synuclein aggregation and Toxicity. The Journal of Biological Chemistry 2004; 279(24) 25497-25502.

[123] Lee J, Giordano S, Zhang J. Autophagy, mitochondria and oxidative stress: cross-talk and redox signalling. The Biochemical Journal 2012; 441(2) 523-540.

[124] Mattson MP. Glutamate and neurotrophic factors in neuronal plasticity and disease. Annals of the New York Academy of Sciences 2008; 1144 97-112.

[125] Nutt JG, Burchiel KJ, Comella CL, Jankovic J, Lang AE, Laws ER, Jr., et al. Randomized, double-blind trial of glial cell line-derived neurotrophic factor (GDNF) in PD. Neurology 2003; 60(1) 69–73.

[126] Gill SS, Patel NK, Hotton GR, O'Sullivan K, McCarter R, Bunnage M, et al. Direct brain infusion of glial cell line-derived neurotrophic factor in Parkinson disease. Nature Medicine 2003; 9(5) 589–95.

[127] Patel NK, Bunnage M, Plaha P, Svendsen CN, Heywood P, Gill SS. Intraputamenal infusion of glial cell line-derived neurotrophic factor in PD: a two-year outcome study. Annals of Neurology 2005; 57(2) 298–302.

[128] Aberg ND, Brywe KG, Isgaard J. Aspects of growth hormone and insulin-like growth factor-I related to neuroprotection, regeneration, and functional plasticity in the adult brain. Scientific World Journal 2006; 6, 53-80.

[129] Pang, Y., Zheng, B., Campbell, L.R., Fan, L.W., Cai, Z., Rhodes, P.G. IGF-1 can either protect against or increase LPS-induced damage in the developing rat brain. Pediatric Research 2010; 67(6) 579-584.

[130] Kao SY. Rescue of alpha-synuclein cytotoxicity by insulin-like growth factors. Biochemical and Biophysical Research Communications 2009; 385(3) 434-438.

[131] Yasuhara T, Shingo T, Kobayashi K, Takeuchi A, Yano A, Muraoka K, et al. Neuroprotective effects of vascular endothelial growth factor (VEGF) upon dopaminergic neurons in a rat model of Parkinson's disease. European Journal of Neuroscience 2004; 19(6) 1494-1504.

[132] Yasuhara T, Shingo T, Muraoka K, wen Ji Y, Kameda M, Takeuchi A, et al. The differences between high and low-dose administration of VEGF to dopaminergic neurons of *in vitro* and *in vivo* Parkinson's disease model. Brain Research 2005; 1038(1) 1-10.

[133] Tian YY, Tang CJ, Wang JN, Feng Y, Chen XW, Wang L, et al. Favorable effects of VEGF gene transfer on a rat model of Parkinson disease using adeno-associated viral vectors. Neuroscience Letters 2007; 421(3) 239-244.

[134] Timmer M, Muller-Ostermeyer F, Kloth V, Winkler C, Grothe C, Nikkhah G. Enhanced survival, reinervation, and functional recovery of intrastriatal dopamine grafts co-transplanted with Schwann cells overexpressing high molecular weight FGF-2 isoforms. Experimental Neurology 2004; 187(1) 118-136.

[135] Tang Z, Arjunan P, Lee C, Li Y, Kumar A, Hou X, et al. Survival effect of PDGF-CC rescues neurons from apoptosis in both brain and retina by regulating GSK3beta phosphorylation. Journal of Experimental Medicine 2010; 207(4) 867-880.

[136] Sullivan AM, Toulouse A. Neurotrophic factors for the treatment of Parkinson's disease. Cytokine & Growth Factor Reviews 2011; 22(3) 157-65.

Chapter 21

Zinc and Neurodegenerative Diseases

Masahiro Kawahara, Keiko Konoha,
Hironari Koyama, Susumu Ohkawara and
Yutaka Sadakane

Additional information is available at the end of the chapter

http://dx.doi.org/10.5772/54489

1. Introduction

Zinc (Zn) is an essential trace element for most organisms. It plays important roles in various physiological functions such as the mitotic cell division, the immune system, the synthesis of proteins and DNA as a co-factor of more than 300 enzymes or metalloproteins [1]. Recent studies revealed that Zn signaling plays crucial roles in various biological systems of humans [2]. Zn deficiency in human childhood is known to cause the dwarfism, the retardation of mental and physical development, the immune dysfunction, and the learning disabilities [3]. In adults, Zn deficiency causes the taste and odor disorders.

The human body contains approximately 2 g of Zn, mostly in the testes, muscle, liver, and brain tissues. In the brain, Zn is found at the highest concentrations in the hippocampus, amygdala, cerebral cortex, thalamus, and olfactory cortex [4]. The total Zn content of the hippocampus is estimated to be 70–90 ppm (dry weight). Although some Zn in the brain binds firmly to metalloproteins or enzymes, a substantial fraction (approximately 10% or more) either forms free Zn ions (Zn^{2+}) or is loosely bound, and is histochemically detectable by staining using chelating reagents. This chelatable Zn is stored in presynaptic vesicles of specific excitatory glutamatergic neurons and is secreted from these vesicles into synaptic clefts along with glutamate during neuronal excitation. Recent studies have suggested that this secreted Zn^{2+} plays crucial roles in information processing, synaptic plasticity, learning, and memory (Fig. 1A). Indeed, Zn^{2+} in the hippocampus is essential for the induction of long-term potentiation (LTP), a form of synaptic information storage that has become a well-known paradigm for the mechanisms underlying memory formation [5].

However, despite its importance, excess Zn is neurotoxic and implicated in neurodegenerative diseases. In this chapter, we review the current understanding about the link between the disruption of Zn homeostasis and the pathogenesis of various neurodegenerative diseases including senile dementia.

2. Zinc and vascular type of dementia

2.1. Zn-induced neurodegeneration after ischemia

Senile dementia is a serious problem in a rapidly aging world. Its prevalence increases with age. Approximately 25% of elderly individuals are affected by the diseases. In Japan, 3 million people have been estimated to be affected by senile dementia by 2025, and the number continues to grow annually. Senile dementia is mainly divided to Alzheimer's disease (AD) and vascular-type dementia (VD). VD is a degenerative cerebrovascular disease, and its risk factors include aging, sex difference (male), diabetes, and high blood pressure. The most common type of VD is caused by a series of small strokes or ischemia [6]. Following transient global ischemia or stroke, the interruption of blood flow and the resulting oxygen-glucose deprivation induce long-lasting membrane depolarization and cause an excessive release of glutamate into synaptic clefts. Thereafter, the excess glutamate causes over-stimulation of its receptors, namely, *N*-methyl-D-aspartate (NMDA)-type receptors, amino-3-hydroxy-5-methyl-4-isoxazolepropionic acid (AMPA)-type receptors, and kainite-type receptors. Finally, Ca^{2+} dyshomeostasis, *i.e.*, the entry of large quantities of Ca^{2+} occurring in glutamate-responsive neurons, triggers the delayed death of vulnerable populations of neurons such as pyramidal neurons in the hippocampus —an area associated with learning and memory. Thereafter, the development of an infarct and the subsequent cognitive dysfunction mark the pathogenesis of VD in elderly people. Approximately 30% of stroke patients show symptoms of dementia within 3 months of the initial stroke [7].

Increasing evidence suggests that Zn is central to ischemia-induced neuronal death and finally the pathogenesis of VD [8]. In ischemic conditions, a considerable amount of Zn (up to 300μM) is co-released with glutamate into synaptic clefts by membrane depolarization. Zn caused the apoptotic death of primary cultured cortical neurons. Furthermore, the chelatable Zn reportedly moved from presynaptic terminals into postsynaptic neuronal cell bodies. The increase in intracellular Zn^{2+} levels ($[Zn^{2+}]_i$), namely, "Zn translocation," occurs in vulnerable neurons in the CA1 or CA3 regions of the hippocampus prior to the onset of the delayed neuronal death after transient global ischemia [9]. This Zn translocation is reported to enhance the appearance of the infarct. Administration of calcium EDTA (Ca EDTA), a membrane-impermeable chelator that chelates cations except for calcium, blocked the translocation of Zn, protected the hippocampal neurons after transient global ischemia, and reduced the infarct volume [10]. Thus, Zn translocation is recognized to be the primary event in the pathway of Zn-induced neuronal death. Sensi *et al.* observed a temporal change of $[Zn^{2+}]_i$ in cultured cortical neurons using a zinc-sensitive fluorescent dye; those results revealed that at least three major routes of Zn^{2+} entry have been identified; voltage-gated Ca^{2+} channels (VGLC), NMDA-type glutamate receptors (NMDA-R), and AMPA/kainite-type glutamate receptors (A/K-R). Although the NMDA-type glutamate receptors are present in most neu-

http://dx.doi.org/10.5772/54489

rons, the permeablity of Zn^{2+} and Ca^{2+} through AMPA/kainate channels is greater than NMDA-receptor channels [11].

In a normal condition, most hippocampal neurons express AMPA receptors with subunit GluR2, which are poorly permeable to divalent cations including Ca^{2+} and Zn^{2+}(A/K-R). However, after ischemia, the acute reduction in the expression of GluR2 subunit occurs, and neurons possess specific type of AMPA receptors which channels are directly Ca^{2+} permeable (Ca-AMPA/kainate channels; Ca-A/K-R)) [12]. The appearance of Ca-AMPA/kainate channels causes the increased permeability of Ca^{2+} and enhances the toxicity. Therefore, the expression of Zn^{2+}-permeable Ca-AMPA/kainite channels and the entry of Ca^{2+} and/or Zn^{2+} through the channels are mediators of the delayed neuronal death after ischemia. Considering that Ca EDTA, a zinc chelator, attenuates the ischemia-induced down-regulation of GluR2 gene [10], Zn is also implicated in the transcriptional regulation in Ca-AMPA/kainite channels.

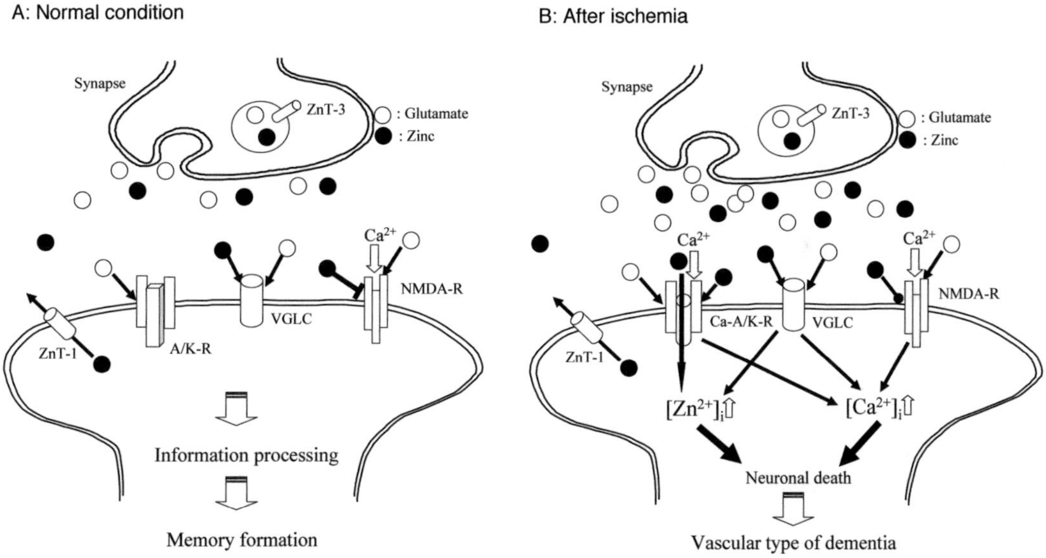

Figure 1. Zinc in normal or pathological conditions in the brain. Under normal conditions (A), neuronal excitation causes the release of glutamate and Zn. Zn regulates the postsynaptic excitability by binding to NMDA-type glutamate receptors (NMDA-R). However, under pathological conditions such as ischemia (B), oxygen-glucose deprivation induces the release of excess glutamate as well as Zn into the synaptic clefts. Excess Zn enhances the expression of Ca-AMPA/kainite channels (Ca-A/K-R), and is translocated through the Ca-A/K-R or through other pathways such as voltage-gated L-type Ca^{2+} channels (VGLC) into the target neuron, where Zn acts to inhibit various enzymes, inhibit mitochondrial respiration, cause energy depletion, and produce reactive reactive oxygen species (ROS). Excess glutamate induces elevation of intracellular Ca^{2+} levels in the target neuron. Elevated levels of intracellular Ca^{2+} then trigger various apoptotic pathways such as the activation of calpain, caspases or other enzymatic pathways related to apoptosis; ultimately this leads to neuronal death.

Zn-specific membrane transporter proteins (Zn transporters) also control Zn homeostasis; they facilitate zinc influx in deficiency and efflux during zinc excess. Recent genetic and molecular approaches revealed the implications of abnormalities in Zn transporters in various human diseases [13]. Zn transporter 1 (ZnT-1), a membrane protein with six transmembrane domains, is widely distributed in mammalian cells, and is co-localized with chelatable Zn in the brain. ZnT-1 is activated by excess Zn and the expression of ZnT-1 is induced after transient global ischemia. On the contrary, dietary Zn deficiency decreases expression of ZnT-1. Consequently, it is provable that ZnT-1 plays a pivotal role in efflux of Zn and in protection from Zn toxicity. Another important Zn transporter in the brain is ZnT-3, which localizes in the membranes of presynaptic vesicles, transports Zn into synaptic vesicles, and maintains high Zn concentrations in the vesicles. Although the physiological role of ZnT-3 and vesicular zinc remain elusive, recent studies have suggested the implication of ZnT-3 or other Zn transporters in the pathogenesis of AD and other neurodegenerative diseases [14].

2.2. Molecular mechanism of Zn-induced neurotoxicity: GT1-7 cells as an *in vitro* model system

Understanding the molecular mechanism of Zn-induced neuronal death is of great importance for the treatment of VD. Numerous studies have been undertaken to elucidate the mechanism of Zn-induced neuronal death. To this end, many researchers have investigated Zn neurotoxicity *in vitro* mainly using primary cultured neurons from rat cerebral cortex or hippocampus [15] or PC-12 cells, a pheochromocytoma cell line [16]. However, the roles of Zn are highly complex. For example, Zn reportedly inhibits NMDA-type glutamate receptors and regulates the excitability of glutamatergic neurons, which are toxic to neurons. Therefore, distinguishing of the effects of Zn and glutamate by using neuronal cells which possess glutamate receptors has proved difficult.

We found that GT1-7 cells, immortalized hypothalamic neurons, are much more sensitive to Zn than other neuronal cells are [17,18] (Fig. 2A). Zn caused the apoptotic death of GT1-7 cells in a dose-dependent and time-dependent manner. The degenerated GT1-7 cells were terminal deoxynucleotidyl transferase-mediated biotinylated UTP nick-end labeling (TUNEL) positive and exhibited the DNA fragmentation.

The GT1-7 cells were originally developed by Mellon *et al.* by genetically targeting tumorigenesis of mouse hypothalamic neurons [19]. The cells possess neuronal characteristics such as the extension of neurites, secretion of gonadotropin-releasing hormone (GnRH), and expression of neuron-specific proteins or receptors including microtubule-associated protein 2 (MAP2), tau protein, neurofilament, synaptophysin, $GABA_A$ receptors, dopamine receptors, and L-type Ca^{2+} channels. Additionally, the GT1-7 cells either lack or possess low levels of ionotropic glutamate receptors and do not exhibit glutamate toxicity [20]. These properties make the GT1-7 cell line an excellent model system for the investigation of Zn-induced neurotoxicity.

We investigated the detailed characteristics of Zn-induced death in GT1-7 cells and its mechanisms. First, we tested the effects of various pharmacological agents prior to Zn treatment of GT1-7 cells. Neither antagonists nor agonists of excitatory neurotransmitters (D-APV, glutamate, and CNQX), or those of inhibitory neurotransmitters (bicuculline, muscimol, baclofen, and GABA) attenuated the viability of GT1-7 cells after Zn exposure. Our findings in GT1-7 cells, which lack such glutamate receptors, are inconsistent with previous studies that agonists of glutamate receptors, such as NMDA or AMPA, enhance Zn-induced neurotoxicity in cultured cortical neurons [21].

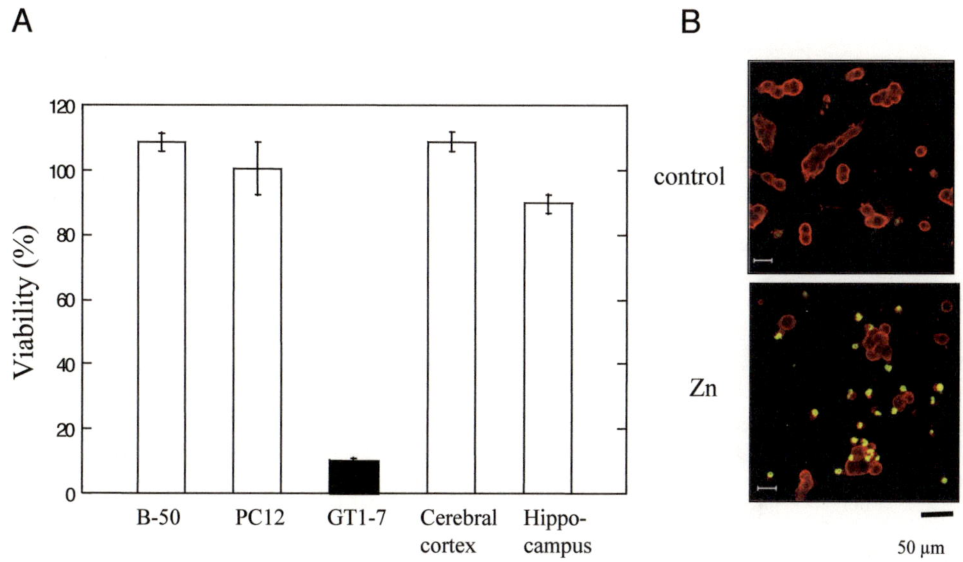

Figure 2. Apoptotic death of GT1-7 cells after exposure to Zn. A: Viability of various neuronal cells after exposure to Zn. Cultured neuronal cells (GT1-7 cells, PC-12 cells, B-50 cells (a neuroblastoma cell line), primary cultured neurons of the rat cerebral cortex, and primary cultured neurons of the rat hippocampus) were administered to 50 µM of Zn. After 24h, cell viability was analyzed by WST-1 method. B: TUNEL staining of Zn intoxicated GT1-7 cells GT1-7 cells were exposed to 50 µM Zn, and were observed with TUNEL staining after 24h.

To evaluate the involvement of other metal ions in Zn neurotoxicity, we investigated the viability of GT1-7 cells with or without various metal ions after exposure to Zn [22]. The equimolar addition of Al^{3+} and Gd^{3+} significantly inhibited Zn-induced neurotoxicity. Moreover, overloading of Ca^{2+} and Mg^{2+} inhibited the Zn-induced death of GT1-7 cells; Zn protected GT1-7 cells from neurotoxicity induced by Ca^{2+} overload, and *vice versa* (Fig. 3B). Furthermore, Kim *et al.* reported that Zn neurotoxicity in PC-12 cells was attenuated by an L-type Ca^{2+} channel blocker, nimodipine, and enhanced by the L-type Ca^{2+} channel activator, S(-)-Bay K 8644 [16]. Additionally, Zn neurotoxicity was attenuated by aspirin, which prevents Zn^{2+} entry through voltage-gated Ca^{2+} channels. These pharamacological evidence suggests that Ca dyshomeostasis is involved in the mechanism of Zn-induced neurotoxicity.

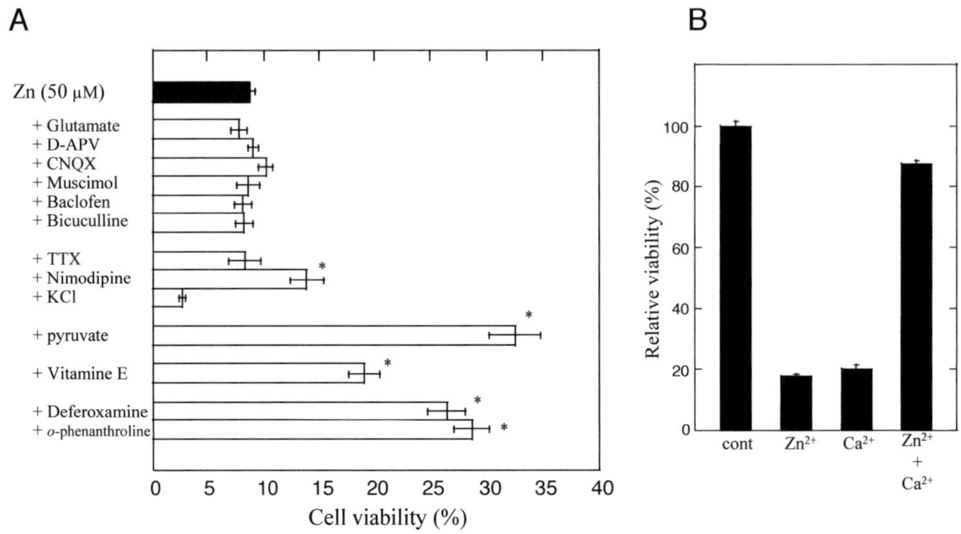

Figure 3. Effects of various pharmacological substances on Zn-induced death of GT1-7 cells. A: GT1-7 cells were exposed to 50μM of Zn^{2+} with agonists or antagonisits of neurotransmitters (D-APV (D-2-amino-5-phosphonovalerate), glutamate, CNQX (6-cyano-7-nitroquinoxaline-2,3-dione), bicuculline, muscimol, baclofen, GABA (gamma-aminobutyric acid)), channel blockers (TTX(tetrodotoxin), nimodipine), etc. B: GT1-7 cells were exposed to Zn^{2+} with or without Ca^{2+}.

2.3. Implication of Ca dyshomeostasis in Zn-induced neuronal death

To address this issue, we employed a high-resolution multi-site video imaging system with fura-2 as the cytosolic free calcium reporter fluorescent probe for the observation of temporal changes in $[Ca^{2+}]_i$ after exposure to Zn (Fig. 4). This multisite fluorometry system enables the simultaneous long-term observation of temporal changes in $[Ca^{2+}]_i$ of more than 50 neurons. The elevations in $[Ca^{2+}]_i$ were observed among GT1-7 cells after 3-30 min of the exposure to Zn [18]. Detailed analysis of Zn-induced $[Ca^{2+}]_i$ revealed that pretreatment of Al^{3+} significantly blocked the Zn-induced $[Ca^{2+}]_i$ elevations. Thus, it is possible that Al^{3+}, a known blocker of various types of Ca^{2+} channels, attenuate Zn-induced neurotoxicity by blocking Zn-induced elevations in $[Ca^{2+}]_i$.

We also showed that the administration of sodium pyruvate, an energy substrate, significantly inhibited the Zn-induced death of GT1-7 cells [17]. The results are consistent with findings of other studies using primary cultured cortical neurons, oligodendrocyte progenitor cells, or retinal cells. Furthermore, the administration of pyruvate attenuated the neuronal death after ischemia *in vivo* [23]. Shelline and his colleagues reported that Zn exposure decreased the levels of NAD^+ and ATP in cultured cortical neurons, and that treatment with pyruvate restored the NAD^+ level [24]. An imaging study using a Zn-sensitive fluorescent dye and a mitochondrial marker revealed that Zn is localized within mitochondria. Zn is reported to inhibit various mitochondrial enzymes and the intracellular trafficking of mitochondria. It has also been reported that Zn produced ROS and caused oxidative damage resulting from mitochondrial impairments. Therefore, energy failure and the inhibition of glycolysis in mitochondria may be involved in Zn neurotoxicity [25].

2.4. Carnosine as an endogenous protective substance against Zn neurotoxicity

Considering the implication of Zn in transient global ischemia, substances that protect against Zn-induced neuronal death could be potential candidates for the prevention or treatment of neurodegeneration following ischemia, and ultimately provide a lead to treatments for VD. With the aim of exploring this idea, we developed a rapid, sensitive, and convenient assay system for the mass-screening of such substances by using GT1-7 cells. We examined the potential inhibitory effects of various agricultural products such as vegetable extracts, fruits extracts, and fish extracts, and found that extracts from eel muscles significantly protected against Zn-induced neurotoxicity [26]. Finally, we demonstrated that carnosine (ß-alanyl histidine), a small hydrophilic peptide abundant in eel muscles, protected GT1-7 cells from Zn-induced neurotoxicity in a dose-dependent manner. Therefore, we applied for the patent on carnosine as a drug for the treatment of VD or for slowing the progress of cognitive decline after ischemia (the application No. 2006-145857; the publication No. 2007-314467 in Japan) [27]. Carnosine is a naturally occurring dipeptide and is commonly present in vertebrate tissues, particularly within the skeletal muscles and nervous tissues [28]. It is found at high concentrations in the muscles of animals or fish which exhibit high levels of exercise, such as horses, chickens, and whales. The concentration of carnosine in the muscles of such animals is estimated to be 50–200 mM, and carnosine is believed to play important roles in the buffering capacities of muscle tissue. During high-intensity anaerobic exercise, proton accumulation causes a decrease in intracellular pH, which influences various metabolic functions. The p*K*a value of carnosine is 7.01, close to intracellular pH.

Therefore, carnosine contributes to physicochemical non-bicarbonate buffering in skeletal muscles, and the administration of carnosine has been reported to induce hyperactivity in animals.

Carnosine reportedly has various functions including anti oxidant, anti glycation, anti crosslink, and considered to be an endogenous neuroprotective, anti-aging substances. Considering the advantegeous properties of carnosine Considering the advantegeous properties of carnosine (relatively non-toxic, heat-stable, and water-soluble), the dietary supplementation of carnosine might be an effective strategy for the prevention or treatment of neurodegenerative diseases such as ischemia, VD, AD, and prion diseases. Corona et al. reported that supplementation of carnosine improved learning abilities of Alzheimer's model mice [29]. We demonstrated that neurotoxicity of prion protein fragment was attenuated by Zn and carnosine [30].

3. Zn and Alzheimer's disease diseases

3.1. Amyloid cascade hypothesis and Zn

AD is a severe senile type of dementia first reported in 1906. The pathological hallmarks of AD are the deposition of extracellular senile plaques, intracellular neurofibrillary tangles (NFTs), and the selective loss of synapses and neurons in the hippocampal and cerebral cortical regions. The major component of NFTs is the phosphorylated tau protein. Senile plaques are largely comprised of ß-amyloid protein (AßP) [31]. Numerous biochemical, toxicological, cell biological, and genetic studies have supported the idea termed "amyloid cascade hypothesis" which suggests that the neurotoxicity caused by AßP play a central role in AD [32,33]. AβP is a small peptide with 39–43 amino acid residues. It is derived from the proteolytic cleavage of a large precursor protein (amyloid precursor protein; APP). AβP has an intrinsic tendency to self-assemble to form sodium dodecyl sulfate (SDS)-stable oligomers. Moreover, oligomerization and conformational changes in AßP are important for its neurodegeneration process. In an aqueous solution, freshly prepared and dissolved AβP exists as a monomeric protein with a random coil structure. However, following incubation at 37°C for several days (*aging*), AβPs form aggregates (oligomers) with β-pleated sheet structures, and finally form insoluble aggregates, termed amyloid fibrils (Fig. 5). The *aged* AβP peptides were considerably more toxic to cultured neurons than *fresh* (freshly prepared just before the experiment) AβP. AßP is secreted in the cerebrospinal fluid (CSF) of young individuals as well as in aged or dementia patients [34]. Therefore, factors that accelerate or inhibit the oligomerization may play essential roles in the pathogenesis of AD. Several factors such as the concentration of peptides, pH, composition of solvents, temperature, oxidations, mutations, and racemization of AßP can influence the oligomerization processes [35].

Interestingly, rodent AßP exhibits less tendency to oligomerization than human AßP *in vitro* and the accumulation of AßP is rarely observed in the brains of rodents (rats or mice) as compared to primates (humans or monkeys). As shown in Fig. 5, the amino acid sequences of human and rodent AßP are similar, but rodent AßP differs from primate only 3 amino acids (Arg^5, Tyr^{10}, and His^{13}) from primate AßP. All three amino acids have the ability to bind metals. Therefore, trace elements including Al, Zn, Cu, Fe as the accelerating factor of AßP are of particularly interest.

We have investigated the metal-induced oligomerization of AßP and found that the metals including Al, Zn, Fe, Cu, and Cd enhanced the oligomerization. However, the oligomerization induced by Al is more marked than that induced by other metals [36,37]. Furthermore, while Zn-aggregated AßPs are rarely observed on the surface of cultured neurons several days after its exposure, Al-aggregated AßPs bind tightly to the surface of cultured neurons and form fibrillar deposits. Bush et al. reported the Zn- or Cu- induced oligomerization of AßP [38,39], and have developed the chelation therapy for AD treatment [40]. Clioquinol (quinoform), a chelator of Cu^{2+} or Zn^{2+}, inhibits oligomerization of AßP and attenuates the accumulation of amyloid in the brains of experimental animals. Clinical trials using its analogue PBT2 are under investigation. However, considering that the morphology of AßP oligomers treated with metals including Al, Cu, Fe, Zn are quite different [41] and that re-

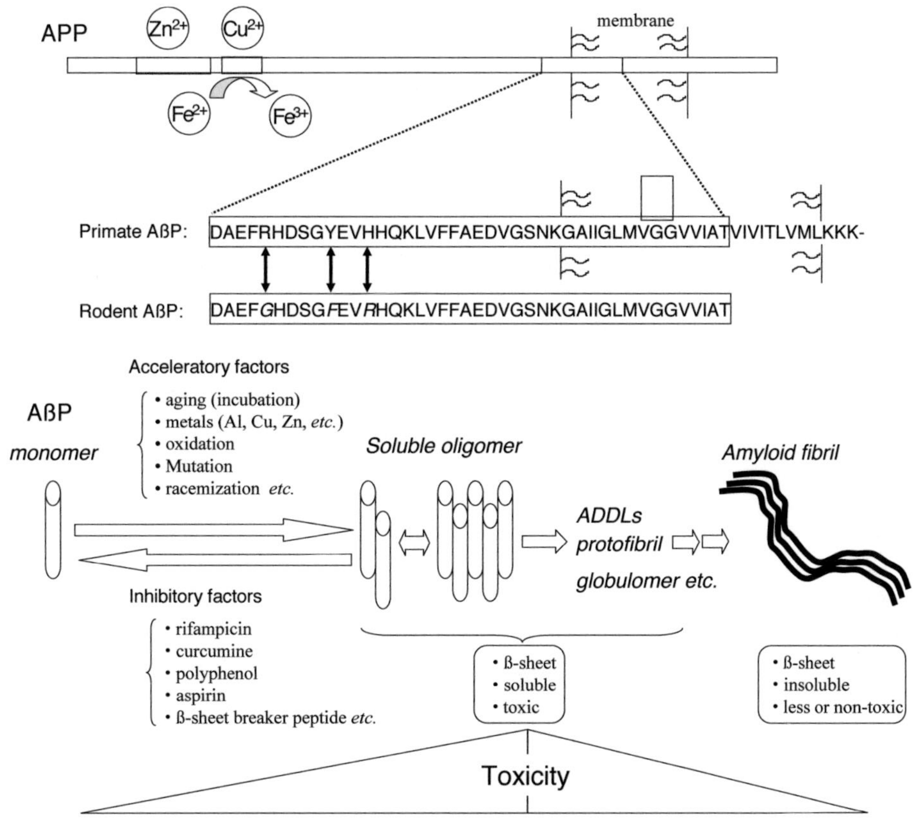

Figure 5. Amyloid cascade hypothesis and the implications of Zn and other metals. AßP is secreted from its precursor APP, a Zn- or Cu- binding protein. AßP monomers exhibit random-coil structures. However, during aging or in the presence of some acceleratory factors, AßP self-aggregates and forms several types of oligomers (SDS-soluble oligomers, ADDLS, globulomers, protofibrils, etc.) and finally forms insoluble aggregates, which are termed amyloid fibrils. Oligomeric soluble AßP s are toxic, although monomers and fibrils are rather nontoxic.

cent approaches using size-exclusion chromatography, gel electrophoresis, and atomic force microscopy have demonstrated that identified soluble oligomers are neurotoxic, further studies about metal-induced oligomerization are necessary.

APP also possesses copper/zinc binding sites in its amino-terminal domain and in the AßP domain and may be involved in homeostasis of these metals [42]. Duce *et al.* demonstrated that APP has ferroxidase activity, which converts Fe^{2+} to Fe^{3+} and regulates free pro-oxidant Fe^{2+} concentrations. They also found that Zn^{2+} inhibits the ferroxidase activity of APP [43]. Thus, the interaction with Zn and other metals in the functions of APP are of great interst.

3.2. AßP -induced neuronal death and Zn

Zn is involved in the mechanism of AßP-induced neurotoxicity. There is considerable interest regarding the mechanism by which AßPs cause neuronal death. In 1993, Arispe *et al.* first demonstrated that AßP directly incorporates into artificial lipid bilayer membranes and forms cation-selective (including Ca^{2+}) ion channels [44,45]. We revealed that AßP formed amyloid channels on the GT1-7 cell membranes and their characteristics were considerably similar to those observed on artificial lipid bilayers; cation-selective, multilevel [46]., and that AßP causes the increase of intracellular Ca^{2+} in GT1-7 cells and degeneration [47]. These results strongly support the hypothetical idea termed 'amyloid channel hypothesis', namely, that the direct incorporation of AßPs and the subsequent imbalances of Ca^{2+} and other ions through amyloid channels may be the primary event in AßP neurotoxicity [48].

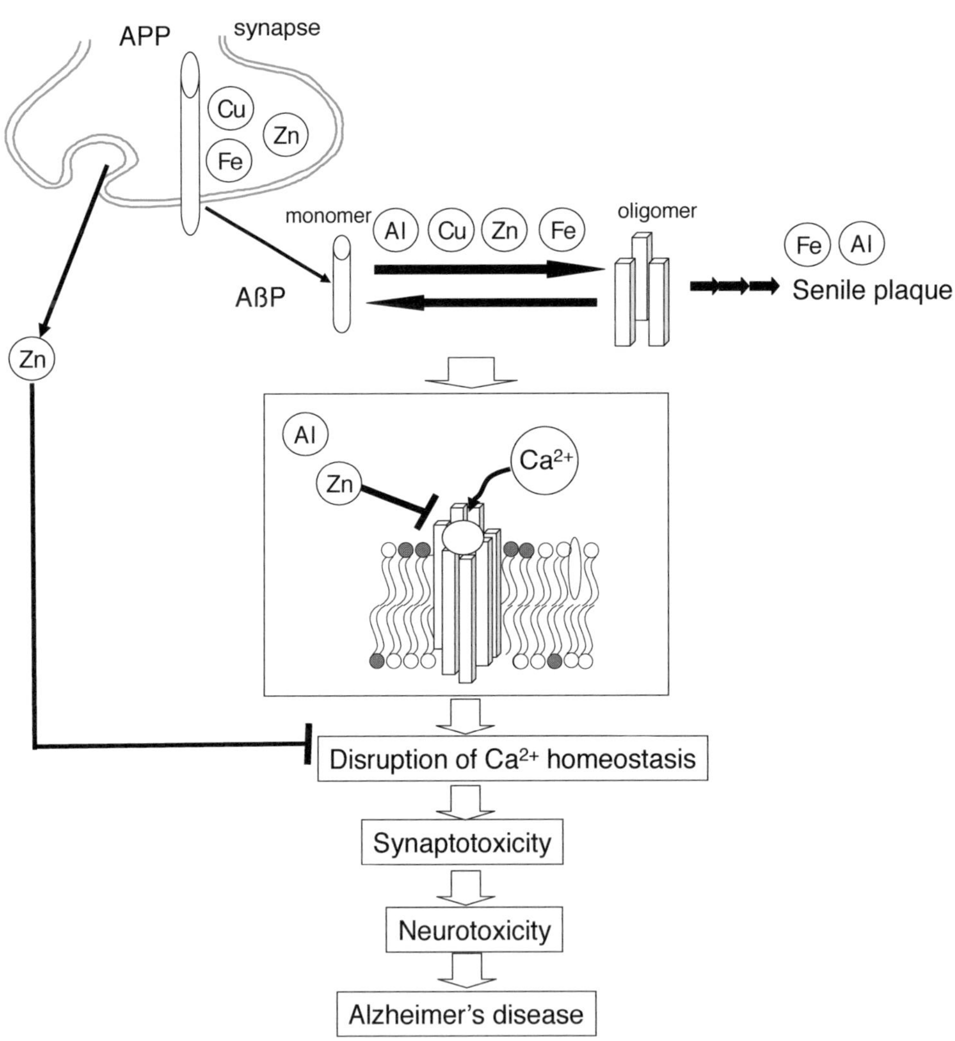

Figure 6. Zn and other metals in the pathogenesis of Alzheimer's disease. Details are shown in the text.

Inorganic cations such as Al^{3+} or Zn^{2+} inhibit current induced by amyloid channels [44,45]. Zn reportedly inhibited AßP-induced Ca^{2+} increase. We have revealed that the amyloid channel activity formed on membranes of GT1-7 cells was inhibited by addition of Zn^{2+}, and recovered by Zn chelator, *o*-phenanthroline [47]. Considering that Zn binds to His residues of AßP, Arispe *et al.* found that histidine-related peptide derivatives such as His-His are effective in the inhibition of amyloid channels, the attenuation of AßP-induced $[Ca^{2+}]_i$ changes, and the protection of neurons from AßP toxicity. Among various compounds tested, small amphiphilic pyridinium salts were revealed to block the amyloid channel and protect neurons [49].

Based on our and other findings about the link between Zn and the pathogenesis of AD, we made a hypothetical scheme about the link between AD pathogenesis and Zn (Fig. 6). AßPs are normally secreted from APP, which exists in the synapse. Secreted AßPs are usually degraded proteolytically by proteases within a short period. However, Zn or other metals enhance the oligomerization and accumulation of AßP. After incorporation into the membrane, the conformation of AßPs change and the accumulated AßPs aggregate on the membranes.. Finally, aggregated AßP oligomers form ion channels leading to the various neurodegenerative processes.Unlike endogenous Ca^{2+} channels, these AßP channels are not regulated by usual blockers. Thus, once formed on membranes, a continuous flow of $[Ca^{2+}]_i$ is initiated. Disruption of calcium homeostasis triggers several apoptotic pathways and promotes numerous degenerative processes, including free radical formation and tau phosphorylation, thereby accelerating neuronal death. Meanwhile, Zn^{2+}, which are secreted into synaptic clefts in a neuronal activity-dependent manner, inhibit AßP-induced Ca^{2+} entry, and thus have a protective function in AD.

4. Conclusion

Based on results of our own and other numerous studies, the disruption of Zn homeostasis, namely both zinc depletion and excess zinc, cause severe damage to neurons and linked with various neurodegenerative diseases including VD and AD. Increasing evidence suggests the implications of Zn in the pathogenesis of other neurodegenerative disease including prion diseases, Parkinson disease, ALS etc. Zn acts as a contributor of the disease in one part, and as a protector in another part. Thus, Zn might play a role like that of Janus, an ancient Roman god of doorways with two different faces, in the brain (Fig. 7).

Our new approach to ischemia-induced neurodegeneration from the perspective of the Zn hypothesis will lead to new therapeutic tools for the treatment and/or prevention of VD. Further research about the role of Zn in neuronal injury and the significance of Zn homeostasis might give rise to the development of new treatments for neurodegenerative diseases. In this context, the advantegeous properties of carnosine (relatively non-toxic, heat-stable, and water-soluble) as a possible candidate for the prevention or treatment of neurodegenerative diseases such as ischemia, VD, AD, and prion diseases are important.

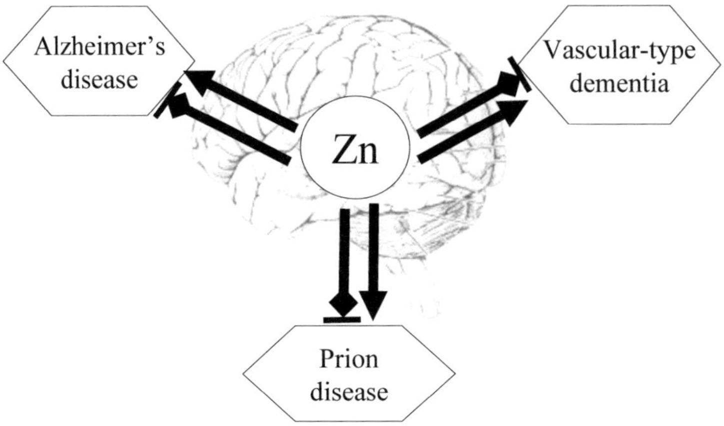

Figure 7. Zn as Janus in brain

As described here, Zn plays important roles in memory formation, and protects neurons from various neurodegenerative diseases. Meanwhile, excess Zn is neurotoxic and may enhance the pathogenesis of the diseases.

Author details

Masahiro Kawahara[1], Keiko Konoha[2], Hironari Koyama[2], Susumu Ohkawara[2] and Yutaka Sadakane[3]

1 Department of Bio-Analytical Chemistry, Musashino University, Research Institute of Pharmaceutical Sciences, Musashino University, Nishitokyo-shi, Tokyo, Japan

2 Department of Analytical Chemistry, School of Pharmaceutical Sciences, Kyushu University of Health and Welfare, Miyazaki, Japan

3 Faculty of Pharmaceutical Sciences, Suzuka University of Medical Science, Mie, Japan

References

[1] Hambidge M. Human zinc deficiency. J Nutr 2000; 130: 1344S-9S.

[2] Hirano T, Murakami M, Fukada T, et al. Roles of zinc and zinc signaling in immunity: zinc as an intracellular signaling molecule. Adv Immunol 2008; 97: 149-76.

[3] Prasad AS. Impact of the discovery of human zinc deficiency on health. J Am Coll Nutr 2009; 28: 257-65.

[4] Frederickson CJ et al. Importance of zinc in the central nervous system: the zinc-containing neuron. J Nutr 2000; 130: 1471S-83S.

[5] Tamano H and Takeda A. Dynamic action of neurometals at the synapse. Metallomics 2011; 3(7):656-61..

[6] Lee JM et al. Brain tissue responses to ischemia. J Clin Invest 2000; 106: 723-31.

[7] de Haan EH et al. Cognitive function following stroke and vascular cognitive impairment. Curr Opin Neurol 2006; 19: 559-64.

[8] Weiss JH, Sensi SL, Koh JY. Zn^{2+}: a novel ionic mediator of neural injury in brain disease. Trends Pharmacol Sci 2000; 21: 395-401.

[9] Koh JY et al. The role of zinc in selective neuronal death after transient global cerebral ischemia. Science 1996; 272: 1013-6.

[10] Calderone A et al. Late calcium EDTA rescues hippocampal CA1 neurons from global ischemia-induced death. J Neurosci 2004; 24: 9903-13.

[11] Sensi SL et al. Measurement of intracellular free zinc in living cortical neurons: routes of entry. J Neurosci 1997;17: 9554-64.

[12] Pellegrini-Giampietro DE et al. The GluR2 (GluR-B) hypothesis: Ca^{2+}-permeable AMPA receptors in neurological disorders. Trends Neurosci 1997; 20: 464-70.

[13] Fukada T and Kambe T. Molecular and genetic features of zinc transporters in physiology and pathogenesis. Metallomics 2011; 3: 662-74.

[14] Lovell MA. A potential role for alterations of zinc and zinc transport proteins in the progression of Alzheimer's disease. J Alzheimers Dis. 2009; 16(3): 471-83.

[15] Koh JY and Choi DW. Zinc toxicity of cultured cortical neurons: involvement of N-methyl-D-asparatate receptors. Neuroscience 1994; 4: 1049-1057.

[16] Kim AH. L-type Ca^{2+} channel-mediated Zn^{2+} toxicity and modulation by ZnT-1 in PC12 cells. Brain Res 2000; 886: 99-107.

[17] Kawahara M et al. Pyruvate blocks zinc-induced neurotoxicity in immortalized hypothalamic neurons. Cellular and Molecular Neurobiology 2002; 22: 87-93.

[18] Koyama H et al. Zinc neurotoxicity and the pathogenesis of vascular-type dementia: Involvement of calcium dyshomeostasis and carnosine. J Clin Toxicol 2012 S3: 002. doi:10.4172/2161-0495.S3-002.

[19] Mellon PL et al. Immortalization of hypothalamic GnRH neurons by genetically targeted tumorigenesis. Neuron 1990; 5: 1-10.

[20] Mahesh VB et al. Characterization of ionotropic glutamate receptors in rat hypothalamus, pituitary and immortalized gonadotropin-releasing hormone (GnRH) neurons (GT1-7 cells). Neuroendocrinology 1999; 69: 397-407.

[21] Kawahara M et al. Characterization of zinc-induced apoptosis of GT1-7 cells. Biomed Res Trace Elements 2002; 13: 280-281.

[22] Konoha K, Sadakane Y, Kawahara M. Effects of gadolinium and other metal on the neurotoxicity of immortalized hypothalamic neurons induced by zinc. Biomed Res Trace Elements 2004; 15: 275-277.

[23] Lee JY et al. Protection by pyruvate against transient forebrain ischemia in rats. J Neurosci 2001; 21: RC171.

[24] Sheline CT et al. Zinc-induced cortical neuronal death: contribution of energy failure attributable to loss of NAD(+) and inhibition of glycolysis. J Neurosci 2000; 20: 3139-3146.

[25] Sensi SL et al. Modulation of mitochondrial function by endogenous Zn^{2+} pools. Proc Natl Acad Sci U S A 2003; 100: 6157-62.

[26] Konoha K, Sadakane Y, Kawahara M. Carnosine protects GT1-7 cells against zinc-induced neurotoxicity: a possible candidate for treatment for vascular type of dementia. Trace Nutrient Res 2006; 23:1-8.

[27] Kawahara M et al. Protective substances against zinc-induced neuronal death after ischemia: carnosine a target for drug of vascular type of dementia. Recent Patents on CNS Drug Discovery 2007; 2: 145-149.

[28] Hipkiss AR. Carnosine and its possible roles in nutrition and health. Adv Food Nutr Res 2009; 57: 87-154.

[29] Corona C et al. Effects of dietary supplementation of carnosine on mitochondrial dysfunction, amyloid pathology, and cognitive deficits in 3xTg-AD mice. PLoS One 2011; 6(3):e17971.

[30] Kawahara M et al. Zinc, copper, and carnosine attenuate neurotoxicity of prion fragment PrP106-126. Metallomics 2011; 3: 726-734.

[31] Selkoe DJ. The molecular pathology of Alzheimer's disease. Neuron 1991; 6: 487-98.

[32] Hardy J and Selkoe DJ. The amyloid hypothesis of Alzheimer's disease: progress and problems on the road to therapeutics. Science 2002; 297: 353-6.

[33] Kawahara M et al. Calcium dyshomeostasis and neurotoxicity of Alzheimer's beta-amyloid protein. Expert Rev Neurother 2009; 9: 681-93.

[34] Fukuyama R et al. Age-dependent change in the levels of Aß40 and Aß42 in cerebrospinal fluid from control subjects, and a decrease in the ratio of Aß42 to Aß40 level in cerebrospinal fluid from Alzheimer's disease patients. Eur Neurol 2000; 43:155-60.

[35] Kawahara M. Role of calcium dyshomeostasis via amyloid channels in the pathogenesis of Alzheimer’s disease. Current Pharmaceutical Design 2010; 16: 2779-2789.

[36] Kawahara M et al. Aluminum promotes the aggregation of Alzheimer's amyroid ß-protein in vitro, Biochem. Biophys. Res. Commun. 198: 531-535 (1994).

[37] Kawahara M et al. Effects of aluminum on the neurotoxicity of primary cultured neurons and on the aggregation of ß-amyloid protein. Brain Res. Bull 2001; 55: 211-217.

[38] Bush AI et al. Rapid induction of Alzheimer Aß amyloid formation by zinc. Science 1994; 265: 1464-1467.

[39] Atwood CS et al. Dramatic aggregation of Alzheimer aß by Cu(II) is induced by conditions representing physiological acidosis. J Biol Chem 1998; 273: 12817-26.

[40] Kenche VB and Barnham KJ. Alzheimer's disease & metals: therapeutic opportunities. Br J Pharmacol 2011; 163(2):211-9.

[41] Chen WT et al. Distinct effects of Zn^{2+}, Cu^{2+}, Fe^{3+}, and Al^{3+} on amyloid-beta stability, oligomerization, and aggregation: amyloid-beta destabilization promotes annular protofibril formation. J Biol Chem 2011; 286(11): 9646-56.

[42] Bush AI et al. A novel zinc(II) binding site modulates the function of the beta A4 amyloid protein precursor of Alzheimer's disease. J Biol Chem 1993; 268(22): 16109-12.

[43] Duce JA et al. Iron-export ferroxidase activity of β-amyloid precursor protein is inhibited by zinc in Alzheimer's disease. Cell 2010;142(6):857-67.

[44] Arispe N et al. Alzheimer disease amyloid ß protein forms calcium channels in bilayer membranes: Blockade by tromethamine and aluminum. Proc Natl Acad Sci USA 1993; 90: 567-571.

[45] Arispe N et al. Zn^{2+} interactions with Alzheimer's amyloid ß protein calcium channels. Proc Natl Acad Sci USA 1996; 93: 1710-1715.

[46] Kawahara M et al. Alzheimer's disease amyloid ß-protein forms Zn^{2+}-sensitive, cation-selective channels across excised membrane patches from hypothalamic neurons. Biophys J 1997; 73: 67-75.

[47] Kawahara M et al. Alzheimer's ß-amyloid, human islet amylin and prion protein fragment evoke intracellular free-calcium elevations by a common mechanism in a hypothalamic GnRH neuronal cell-line. J Biol Chem 2000; 275: 14077-14083.

[48] Kawahara M et al. Membrane incorporation, channel formation, and disruption of calcium homeostasis by Alzheimer's ß-amyloid protein, Int J Alzheimer Dis 2011; doi 304583.

[49] Diaz JC et al. Small molecule blockers of the Alzheimer Aß calcium channel potently protect neurons from Aß cytotoxicity. Proc Natl Acad Sci USA 2009;106(9):3348-53.

Chapter 22

Oligodendrocyte Metabolic Stress in Neurodegeneration

Daniel Radecki and Alexander Gow

Additional information is available at the end of the chapter

http://dx.doi.org/10.5772/54461

1. Introduction

Neurodegeneration can be viewed in general terms as a common endpoint for a large and diverse group of nervous system diseases that arise in patients with disparate clinical symptoms. As such, neurodegeneration is a convergent pathology wherein clinical signs are largely dependent on the location and identity of the degenerating cells. For example, in patients for whom substantia nigra neurons are degenerating, the accompanying symptoms reflect Parkinson disease (PD). Many of the symptoms are unique to PD, thereby enabling diagnosis, and would rarely be confused with those of patients suffering from amyotrophic lateral sclerosis (ALS), for whom ventral horn motor neurons in the spinal cord are lost. In the same vein, disease in patients with Alzheimer disease (AD) or multiple sclerosis (MS) stem from the loss of distinct cell populations which confer unique phenotypes.

Despite these disease specific phenotypes, recent evidence indicates that their underlying pathophysiology, and that of many others, involves activation of a signaling pathway known as the unfolded protein response (UPR). This suggests the exciting possibility of a shared disease mechanism and, potentially, a common treatment strategy such as the use of a single class of drugs.

Research efforts from many laboratories have begun to elucidate the importance of the UPR to disease etiology. For example, causative mutations in familial forms of PD and AD are found in genes that encode components of protein aggregation and degradation pathways such as the ubiquitin-proteasome pathway, which strongly suggests that sporadic forms of these diseases also arise from perturbed protein folding or degradation [1-3]. In addition, the etiology of MS, which was once understood to be entirely caused by autoimmune attacks on the central nervous system (CNS), is becoming increasingly unclear because of new evidence pointing to an underlying degenerative pathology in oligodendrocytes that involves UPR induction and secondary activation of the immune system. Finally, the etiology of oligodendrocyte metabolic diseases including at least two of the leukodystrophies, vanishing white matter disease (VWM) and Pelizaeus-Merzbacher disease (PMD), is known to involve UPR activation.

In this review, we begin with a general definition of normal versus disease states in terms of cell homeostasis and its relation to UPR signaling, metabolic stress and neurodegeneration. Next, we examine essential aspects of the UPR signaling cascade, as well as emerging concepts about UPR activation and function, and conclude with an examination of MS as a primary UPR disease rather than its typical consideration as a primary autoimmune disease.

2. Metabolic stress and the concept of homeostasis

An increasing awareness of the pathophysiology of neurodegeneration has led to the realization that metabolic stress is a major contributor to disease etiology. This novel view can be conceptualized as follows. Cells under normal metabolic conditions are described as maintaining homeostasis. Metabolic stress is viewed as a loss of homeostasis, defined as any pathological process that impedes cell function.

Intracellular signaling pathways have evolved to detect and counteract many forms of metabolic stress. These pathways modify cell activity and impart significant protection under pathological conditions, thereby maintaining homeostasis. However, when metabolic stress disrupts homeostasis, cells become vulnerable to apoptosis leading to brain atrophy and disease. These concepts have been principally developed to account for the pathophysiology and disease severity that we observe in animal models of PMD [4-7]. However, they are also relevant to other oligodendrocyte diseases as well as major neurological diseases like AD, PD and ALS.

3. Misfolded proteins trigger UPR signaling

Two of the most important homeostatic features of normal cell function are the consistent and efficient translation of proteins and the post-translational folding and processing of those proteins into their stable higher-ordered conformations. However, not all protein molecules achieve native conformations after translation even in normal cells, and particularly in genetic diseases when missense or nonsense mutations in coding exons of genes confer distinct misfolded conformations on the translated products [8, 9].

In cases of transmembrane or secreted proteins that are synthesized on the ER (endoplasmic reticulum) in eukaryotes, misfolded or abnormal folding intermediates are prevented from being transported beyond this compartment by the quality control machinery of the cell. These nascent polypeptide chains are either removed from the ER and degraded via the ubiquitin-proteasome system or are shunted into the lysosome by autophagy [10, 11]. However, if the synthesis of these polypeptides surpasses the rate of degradation, they accumulate in the ER, causing metabolic stress and induction of the UPR [12].

The importance of UPR signaling to cell homeostasis and survival is highlighted by the degree of conservation of this pathway in prokaryotes and in eukaryotes from yeast to mammals. Significant increases in signaling complexity in higher eukaryotes also indicates the growing importance of this pathway in multicellular organisms through evolution [13]. In most cases for eukaryotes, activation of the UPR by misfolded proteins causes rapid shutdown of global protein translation, expansion of intracellular membrane-bound compartments, induction of molecular chaperone expression and increased degradation of misfolded proteins.

In the event that such comprehensive changes in cell structure, reprogramming and metabolism are ineffective at curbing UPR signaling and reestablishing homeostasis, cells will inevitably undergo apoptosis in a manner that limits damage to neighboring cells and the survival of the organism [14]. Surprisingly, the nature of the trigger that induces apoptosis appears to be divergent in different cell types, and several hypotheses have been developed to explain the bulk of published studies as detailed below.

3.1. UPR signaling in mammals

In general terms, the UPR signaling cascade maintains cell homeostasis, metabolism and cell survival [13, 15, 16]. In higher eukaryotes, the UPR can be divided into three pathways named for the proteins that initiate signaling: IRE1α (inositol requiring protein 1α), ATF6 (activating transcription factor 6) and PERK (pancreatic endoplasmic reticulum kinase). Together, these pathways increase expression of molecular chaperone proteins, protein degradation and decrease global translation to alleviate misfolding and restore homeostasis. [12, 17].

3.1.1. The IRE1 pathway

The IRE1α receptor is a transmembrane protein that is localized to the ER and detects the accumulation of misfolded proteins or, in more general terms, serves as a sensor of changes in secretory pathway protein flux. IRE1α was the first component of the UPR cascade to be identified in any eukaryote and is the only UPR sensor present in yeast [14, 18]. The ER luminal domain is topographically similar to the Major Histocompatibility Class (MHC) proteins of the immune system and appears to bind to the molecular chaperone protein, BiP, which maintains IRE1α as a monomer and prevents its activation. However, misfolded protein accumulation in the ER lumen sequesters BiP from IRE1α and allows this receptor to homodimerize leading to transautophosphorylation and activation of its cytoplasmic endoribonuclease P domain [19].

A major downstream target of the IRE1α nuclease domain is an mRNA that encodes the bzip transcription factor, X-box Binding Protein 1 (XBP1) [20]. Processing of this mRNA removes a short internal 26 base intron and completes the major open reading frame that encodes functional XBP1. The major target genes of XBP1 include molecular chaperones which are ER-resident proteins that bind to unfolded or misfolded polypeptides [14]. Accordingly, the IRE1α pathway detects changes in protein flux and acts to increase the folding capacity of the ER, ultimately completing a negative feedback loop on the UPR.

3.1.2. The ATF6 pathway

A second UPR pathway is initiated through activation of the membrane-tethered ATF6 protein and converges with IRE1α signaling. ATF6 interacts with BiP, similar to IRE1α. Misfolded proteins displace BiP from the ATF6 luminal domain and enable the protein to traffic from the ER to the Golgi apparatus where it is cleaved by the site 1 and site 2 proteases (S1P and S2P, respectively). The resulting cytosolic N-terminal fragment of ATF6 is the functional bzip transcription factor that heterodimerizes with XBP1 and induces expression of molecular chaperone genes including BiP, glucose-regulated protein 94 (GRP94) and other genes encoding protein folding pathway proteins [15, 19]. ATF6 also upregulates proteins associated with the ER Associated Degradation (ERAD) pathway, which is a checkpoint in the ER that ubiquitinates proteins and shuttles them into the cytoplasm for proteasome-mediated degradation [21]. Thus, ATF6 helps to upregulate chaperones to relieve mild protein misfolding, but can also activate degradation of proteins that are severely misfolded and cannot be rescued by chaperones.

3.1.3. The PERK pathway

A third UPR pathway is regulated by an ER-resident receptor known as PERK. The luminal domain of PERK functions analogously to that of IRE1α in binding BiP, and is also activated by dimerization and transautophosphorylation. The cytoplasmic domain of PERK is a protein kinase, a major target of which is the alpha subunit of eukaryotic initiation factor 2 (eIF2α). eIF2α is a critical component in ribosome assembly and can be inactivated by phosphorylation, which leads to the shut down of global protein synthesis [17].

Despite global translation arrest, a small number of proteins that are critical to the UPR signaling are actively translated, including the bzip transcription factors, activating transcription factor 4 (ATF4), ATF3 and the CCAAT-enhancer-binding protein homologous protein (CHOP) as well as the regulatory subunit of protein phosphatase 1 (PP1), known as growth-arrest and DNA damage protein 34 (GADD34) [17, 22]. The GADD34-PP1 complex is targeted to the ER membrane to dephosphorylate p-eIF2α and reinitiate protein translation. Thus, the PERK pathway temporarily halts protein synthesis to suppress additional accumulation of misfolded proteins in the ER. The pathway subsequently reactivates protein synthesis by opposing the phosphorylation activity of PERK. Thus, because of the time that is necessary to complete each of the steps downstream of eIF2α phosphorylation, the PERK pathway can be considered to be a time-delay circuit that forms a negative feedback loop to regulate UPR signaling.

3.2. Adaptive and maladaptive facets of UPR signaling

A common theme among the three branches of the UPR cascade is the similar activation of the ER-resident receptors by changes in protein flux leading to transcriptional or translational changes that reduce the accumulation of misfolded polypeptides and ultimately negatively feedback to switch off the UPR. Collectively, these activities comprise the adaptive arm of the UPR cascade, which adjusts cell metabolism to maintain homeostasis and promote cell survival. However, the UPR cascade also appears to include a maladaptive arm, the major function of which is to trigger apoptosis in the event that cells fail to maintain homeostasis.

Although the maladaptive arm of the UPR is widely known and discussed in published studies, the molecular mechanisms underlying its activation are poorly understood. Many studies identify CHOP or a decoy kinase known as Tribbles3 (Trib3) as major components of the maladaptive trigger for apoptosis [23, 24]; however, this view reveals a significant conundrum. Thus, if PERK signaling requires CHOP expression to complete the negative feedback loop that dephosphorylates eIF2α as part of the adaptive response, why would CHOP expression trigger apoptosis as part of the maladaptive response?

There are three principal hypotheses that address this issue. The first proposes that CHOP is a molecular rheostat that drives distinct downstream pathways as a function of expression level [25, 26]. The second suggests that the IRE1 and PERK pathways act in concert to effect cell survival but drive apoptosis when the activities of these pathways are unbalanced [20]. The third hypothesizes that apoptosis is triggered stochastically at a restriction point in the PERK pathway, which is more-or-less coincident with the reinitiation of protein translation upon eIF2α dephosphorylation [17, 27].

3.2.1. CHOP as a rheostat

Studies in human embryonic kidney 293 (HEK293) cells utilizing genetic and chemical induction of the UPR have led to the hypothesis of graded activation, mediated by CHOP, with apoptosis resulting from the highest levels of expression [25, 26]. Transient ER stress requires a UPR; however, the response itself would be modulated so that mild stress generates tapered transient CHOP induction, and severe prolonged stress causes sustained CHOP expression. Indeed, a modulated CHOP response has been observed during molecular and mechanical stress in vitro that activates PERK in the ER, with sustained PERK activation causing sustained CHOP expression and increased apoptosis. In contrast, oligodendrocytes undergoing severe metabolic stress and widespread apoptosis do not express CHOP, suggesting that its induction is transient even during severe stress [4, 6, 28].

3.2.2. Balanced IRE1 and PERK signaling

From their in vitro manipulation of the IRE1 and PERK pathways in HEK293 cells, Walter and colleagues [29] identified disparate roles for each pathway that could account for divergent UPR phenotypes in animal models of disease. The results showed that activating the PERK pathway alone decreased cell proliferation in vitro and triggered a morphological dedifferentiation characterized by a loss of cell processes. In contrast, unilateral IRE1 activation increased cell numbers. Because activation of the PERK and IRE1 pathways stem from the accumulation of misfolded proteins, it is likely that the relative activation levels of these pathways generates a balance between proliferation and differentiation that determines the fate of the cells.

3.2.3. Stochastic apoptosis

The third hypothesis stems from the results of several in vivo studies involving CNS and PNS myelin mutant mice [17]. In contrast to in vitro studies in many cell types where CHOP expression drives apoptosis and CHOP loss-of-function promotes cell survival, ablation of the *Chop* gene in oligodendrocytes renders them much more susceptible to apoptosis under UPR conditions [6, 30]. Thus, CHOP promotes cell survival. In addition, induction of CHOP in Schwann cells does not induce cell death but, rather, causes dedifferentiation of these cells to promote their survival [27]. A similar mechanism is also observed in osteoblasts [31]. Together, these and other studies [29, 32] indicate that PERK signaling protects myelinating cells from apoptosis. If so, how do these cells undergo apoptosis?

One possibility is that myelinating cells become vulnerable to apoptosis at a restriction point in the PERK pathway as protein translation is restarted. At this restriction, the PP1-GADD34 complex dephosphorylates eIF2α and demand for ATP, GTP, NADH and other high-energy intermediates would dramatically increase. Sub-threshold levels of these critical molecules, perhaps also exacerbated by dissipation of the mitochondrial membrane potential, would occur stochastically in individual cells during translation-suppression and cause a loss of homeostasis leading to cell death. Under mild metabolic stress conditions, most cells would maintain supra-threshold levels of critical molecules and survive beyond the restriction point. Some of these cells would undergo apoptosis during subsequent UPR-induction cycles. Ultimately, the stronger the stress, the greater the number of UPR cycles, and the higher the likelihood that cells would undergo apoptosis.

4. Oligodendrocyte metabolic stress and neurodegenerative disease

Oligodendrocytes play a critical role in the CNS by myelinating axons to ensure efficient saltatory conduction and reliable communication between neurons over long distances as well as to promote neuronal survival [33]. The surface area of myelin membrane that is synthesized by each oligodendrocyte within a few days during development exceeds that of the cell body by several hundred fold, which makes oligodendrocytes one of the most metabolically active cell types [34]. Thus, it is not surprising that these cells are vulnerable to metabolic stress and undergo apoptosis associated with protein misfolding [4, 33, 35]. Genetic diseases that disrupt oligodendrocyte metabolism are associated with UPR signaling and are well characterized at the molecular level. It is also becoming increasingly clear that other diseases of oligodendrocytes, such as MS, involve this signaling pathway.

http://dx.doi.org/10.5772/54461

4.1. Leukodystrophy and metabolic stress as a model of neurodegenerative disease etiology

The leukodystrophies are a group of diseases characterized by a systemic absence of white matter in the CNS resulting in sensorimotor deficits, ataxia, hypotonia and eventual decline in cognitive function [36]. Although leukodystrophies affect all white matter tracts to varying extents, they differ in their primary causes. For example, in the case of PMD the absence of white matter stems from mutations in the gene encoding the most abundant myelin protein, proteolipid protein-1 (PLP1) [37-39], while VWM disease is caused by mutations in genes that encode subunits of the eIF2 complex [40]. In many cases, metabolic stress is severe enough that the disease develops in childhood and dramatically affects the life span of the patient [6, 38, 39, 41, 42]. The common mechanism between these leukodystrophies is the failure to manage and remove misfolded proteins, some of which rapidly activate the UPR leading to metabolic stress and apoptosis [38, 39]. Importantly, metabolic stress in oligodendrocytes also leads to secondary neuron loss [43], which demonstrates the potentially severe consequences of this disease mechanism beyond the primary cell type involved.

4.1.1. Pelizaeus-Merzbacher disease

Arguably, PMD is one of the most extensively characterized neurodegenerative UPR disease in terms of molecular and cellular etiology. In virtually all patients, disease stems from genetic lesions in the *X*-linked *Plp1* gene [44]. The gene products are polytopic membrane proteins that constitute approximately 50% of the total protein in the CNS myelin sheath and the developmental expression levels of this gene are among the most abundantly expressed in mammals.

Mutations in the *Plp1* gene arises from three types of genetic lesions: duplications, deletions and missense/nonsense mutations. These lesions confer disease symptoms with a wide range of clinical severity that are mild in the case of deletions, severe in the case of duplications and mild or severe for coding region mutations. In general, mild phenotypes are associated with reduced oligodendrocyte function but relatively little cell death while severe forms cause widespread apoptosis and a virtual absence of white matter [45, 46].

4.1.1.1. Gene duplications and deletions in PMD

Mild forms of disease caused by deletion of the entire *Plp1* gene or nonsense mutations in exon 1 are characterized by clinical presentation in middle age patients, often in the form of cognitive decline [43, 44] and a length-dependent dying back neuropathology. Although the absence of *Plp1* expression in patients does not significantly reduce oligodendrocyte function and the amount of myelin formed during development, the absence of this protein reduces the long-term stability of long myelinated tracts such as the corticospinal tract, which degenerate in later life. Importantly, the stability of the CNS specifically requires the PLP1 protein, and cannot be conferred by the alternatively-spliced PLP1 isoform, called DM-20, which lacks a 35 amino acid segment in the cytoplasmic domain of the protein [47].

In contrast, *Plp1* duplications cause severe phenotypes perinatally or within the first year of life. Children and adolescents with duplications exhibit severe cognitive decline in conjunction with physical disabilities including loss of motor function and coordination [6, 48]. Because of extremely high PLP1 expression levels during normal development, duplications may effectively overwhelm the secretory pathway in oligodendrocytes and disrupt cell function or survival. Whether this disruption involves defective cholesterol trafficking [49] or immune activation [50] is currently unclear.

4.1.1.2. Plp1 mutations in PMD

Approximately 30% of PMD patients harbor mutations in the *Plp1* coding region that cause missense or nonsense changes in the protein primary structure. These changes arise throughout the coding region and cause a spectrum of disease severities in patients [43, 44]. Although there does not appear to be a correlation between the location of a mutation and disease severity, most mutations in the transmembrane domains cause severe disease. This is a general feature of membrane domain mutations in many secretory pathway proteins. Accordingly, the underlying cell biology of coding region mutations is proposed to stem from a failure of protein folding and trafficking through the secretory pathway, leading to metabolic stress and activation of the UPR [6, 12, 43, 44, 51]. Two missense mutations in PMD patients have also been identified in mice. Although similarities of disease symptoms and pathology conferred by each mutation might be anticipated because the PLP1 primary structure is identical in rodents and humans, the robustness of these findings provides a strong basis for using the animal models to model PMD [4, 52-55].

4.1.2. Animal models of PMD

A common goal in the analysis and development of therapeutic strategies to treat many neurodegenerative diseases is the generation of animal models, particularly in rodents which are amenable to genetic manipulation. Naturally-occurring animal models of PMD have been described in multiple species including dog, rabbit, rat and mouse [56-59], and engineered mutations have been generated in rats and mice [47, 52, 58, 60, 61].

The *jimpy* mouse, which exhibits a severe behavioral phenotype, is the original *Plp1* allele identified and has been characterized in greatest detail [57]. More recently, the *rumpshaker* (*rsh*) and *myelin synthesis-deficient* (*msd*) alleles have become popular not only because they exhibit mild and severe phenotypes, respectively, but also because the specific single amino acid changes harbored by these strains are also found in humans [54, 62].

4.1.2.1. Mild disease in rsh mice

This allele was originally described by Griffiths and colleagues and harbors an isoleucine to threonine mutation at codon 187 (I187T) in the second extracellular domain of PLP1 [54, 63]. These mice are fertile and exhibit a normal life span with behavioral changes becoming evident between 13 – 19 days after birth (P13 – 19), depending on the background strain of the colony. The total myelin content of the brain is reduced to 40–50%. PLP1 is virtually absent from *rsh* myelin sheaths, but DM-20 is present at normal levels[54]. This selective trafficking defect is consistent with the protein misfolding hypothesis [4, 5, 7, 51]. Oligodendrocyte metabolic stress leading to apoptosis is observed to occur at a moderate level in this strain [6, 28] despite early claims to the contrary [64].

4.1.2.2. Severe disease in msd mice

The *msd* mutation was originally described by Baumann and colleagues [65] and is characterized by an alanine to valine substitution at codon 243 (A243V) in PLP1 [66]. Mice harboring this mutation exhibit severe symptoms, with behavioral changes evident by P13 and a short life span of 3 - 4 weeks. The amount of myelin in the *msd* CNS is severely reduced to approximately 5% of normal and the phenotype is very similar to that of *jimpy* mice on the same genetic background [62, 67]. Oligodendrocyte apoptosis is widespread in these mice and, similar to *rsh* mice, involves metabolic stress and activation of the UPR [4, 6, 12]. PMD patients with the corresponding mutation have a severe form of the disease with systemic demyelination and widespread oligodendrocyte death.

Importantly, some patients with severe forms of PMD such as those corresponding to the *msd* mutation also show signs of neuron loss as a consequence of profound hypomyelination. These observations establish the principle that the survival of each of the major neural cell types is interdependent; thus, a primary insult in oligodendrocytes in the form of metabolic stress has secondary consequences for neurons [4, 6, 37]. Furthermore, symptoms in PMD can include autoimmune disease [68], which has major significance for the classification of MS as a neurodegenerative disease and suggests that the etiology may arise, at least in some instances, from primary metabolic stress in oligodendrocytes leading to secondary immune activation.

4.2. Is MS a neurodegenerative metabolic stress disease of oligodendrocytes?

Multiple sclerosis is the most common neurological disease in young adults worldwide and is typically described as an autoimmune attack on CNS white matter tracts resulting in focal lesions and degeneration of myelin throughout the CNS [69]. There are three major forms of this disease, relapse remitting MS (RRMS), secondary progressive MS (SPMS) and primary progressive MS (PPMS). RRMS is the most prevalent form and is characterized by patients for which lesions develop spontaneously and cause transient loss of neurological function (also known as a relapse) followed by essentially full recovery (known as remission). Disease in RRMS patients eventually transitions from these transient symptoms to SPMS, when patients do not fully recover neurological function after relapses and sensorimotor deficits become more continuous and progressive. PPMS defines the third category, which is clinically similar to SPMS but without a preceding RRMS phase. Thus, patients experience rapid severe degeneration [69-71].

Results from recent long-term clinical trials in RRMS patients that were medicated with any of several new immune suppressant therapies demonstrate that dramatic reductions in the number of new demyelinating lesions is accompanied by only modest amelioration of clinical symptoms [72-75]. Moreover, patients continue to experience disease progression. These data indicate that the number of autoimmune attacks on the CNS is not strongly correlated with increasing disease severity and that there may be additional unknown mechanisms involved in the pathogenesis. If so, then immune attacks may actually be secondary to an underlying primary etiology.

Clues about the nature of such an unknown etiology in MS are scarce, but may be found in the clinical literature. For example, a few case reports detailing the misdiagnosis of PMD as childhood MS indicate that the symptoms of these two diseases overlap significantly. Indeed, the responsiveness of one of these patients to steroids suggests that PMD symptoms can be exacerbated by immune system activation at some level and perhaps similar to MS. Together, these reports provide tantalizing, if anecdotal, evidence that metabolic stress in oligodendrocytes could be one form of a primary etiology that secondarily activates the immune system [76-78].

4.2.1. Neurodegeneration in MS

The immune demyelinating lesion in white matter is an important component of MS pathology that has been studied extensively [76, 79-81]. However, a plethora of the clinical symptoms, particularly those affecting the daily activities of patients and significantly reducing their quality of life, stem from axonal transection and loss of neurons in gray matter regions [82]. The significance of this degenerative feature is that emergent immune suppressive therapies might not be expected to have a major impact in halting symptom progression [81, 83, 84]. Cognitive decline, memory loss, partial paralysis, and optic neuritis are caused by the loss of neurons in different brain regions that are spared from direct immune attacks but still contribute to disease, especially for the more severe SPMS and PPMS forms [78, 85].

Gray matter cortical atrophy may constitute the majority of the total tissue atrophy observed in MS patients, especially those with SPMS and PPMS [86-88]. Although this pathological feature has been known for decades, one of the most important advances contributing to our understanding and acceptance of neuron loss as a major, if not the principal, symptom of MS is the increasing sensitivity for detecting gray matter lesions using clinical diagnostic MRIs. Thus, with renewed interest and appreciation for this issue, there is an urgent need to understand the underlying pathogenesis. In this regard, the development of novel animal models will lead to new hypotheses and the development of novel therapeutic strategies.

4.2.2. Current and future MS models

Because of the characterization of MS as a primary autoimmune disease, a large proportion of animal model studies, particularly in mice, have focused on developing and characterizing immune models such as experimental autoimmune encephalomyelitis (EAE) [79, 81, 89, 90]. These models rely on priming the peripheral immune system with injected peptides from various myelin proteins to stimulate the immune system to attack and demyelinate white matter tracts. Damage is largely confined to spinal cord and is characterized by immune cell profiles of $CD4^+$, $CD8^+$ T-cells and $CD68^+$ macrophages as well as proinflammatory cytokine release [79, 91-93]. However, these models have significant shortcomings in modeling MS pathology. For example, the neurological phenotypes in affected mice largely stems from tissue edema rather than demyelination. Although some models generate immune mediated demyelination, symptoms are monophasic rather than multiphasic and relapsing-remitting, in contrast to the most common form of MS [94]. Finally, in the absence of gray matter lesions and subsequent neuronal degeneration, these models fail to recapitulate the most debilitating features of MS that contribute to the declining quality of life for patients [77].

To overcome such shortcomings, we have developed a novel genetic mouse model of MS pathology that is based on primary metabolic stress in oligodendrocytes [95]. The etiology of disease in these mice has been characterized in mechanistic detail [4-7, 51] and we are currently determining if we can recapitulate the degenerative white and gray matter lesions that arise in MS patients without specifically provoking the immune system to attack the CNS. Furthermore, we are determining if our primary insult in oligodendrocytes can secondarily induce a relapsing-remitting or progressive autoimmune phenotype in the mice that would account for the pathophysiology observed in MS patients in terms of metabolic stress rather than primary autoimmune activation.

5. Identifying metabolic stress for the diagnosis of neurodegenerative diseases

For many neurodegenerative diseases, progress toward finding treatments and cures is painstakingly slow. This is in part limited by current capabilities for real-time imaging of the CNS as well as by ethical constraints that protect the health of patients and often exclude invasive procedures such as biopsies. These limitations largely confine research studies to post-mortem tissue, or generating in vitro and in vivo animal models, to develop treatments for disease. In many cases, these approaches have proved only partially effective for the study of neurodegenerative diseases [79, 94, 96, 97].

Recently, several imaging technologies have advanced significantly and become sufficiently widespread in hospitals for routine application to neurodegenerative diseases like AD and MS, including magnetic resonance imaging (MRI), magnetic resonance spectroscopy (MRS), and positron emission tomography (PET) [98-100].

5.1. Magnetic resonance imaging

Magnetic resonance techniques are widely used in clinical diagnostics of many diseases since their development approximately 40 years ago [86, 101]. Nevertheless, there are significant drawbacks for their use in neurodegenerative diseases, particularly with respect to early disease detection [69, 102]. MRI is the most common technique used, and is particularly important for identifying white matter pathology such as hypomyelination or demyelinating lesions, as well as gray matter degeneration, because it can easily detect differences in tissue structure or composition between normal and diseased regions. Applications to expand the utility of this technique beyond the structural realm include injectable biomarkers to detect subclinical disease or to follow the evolution of lesions in real time, but these are currently nonexistent except for animal studies [103].

The imaging of metabolic changes in structurally normal regions of the CNS can be achieved using MRS [100, 104], but this technology is currently limited to a few major neurochemicals at low resolution. MRS can be used to detect neuron cell loss by monitoring levels of the neurochemical, N-acetyl aspartate (NAA), which is specific to this cell type [99]. However, the time, expense and difficulty of scanning more than one region of the CNS at a time severely limits the use of MRS for early disease detection when clinicians are uncertain about the specific location of lesions.

5.2. Positron emission tomography

Positron emission tomography involves the incorporation of radioactive molecules into metabolites that are selectively taken up by defined cell populations so that their location and metabolic activity can be analyzed [105]. This technique has the potential to generate detailed information about the molecular basis of neurodegeneration because the metabolism of affected cells changes dramatically as they lose homeostasis. PET has been used successfully in diseases such as AD and PD where degeneration of specific neuronal populations can be monitored *in vivo* even before patients experience significant symptoms [106]. However, a significant drawback with this technique is its low resolution, which renders the technique very limited for small animal model studies.

6. Treatments for metabolic stress in neurodegenerative diseases

Increasing awareness and more sophisticated technologies have enabled earlier detection of neurodegenerative processes. However, the development of treatment strategies often has been hampered, in large measure because of the enormous plasticity of the CNS which enables neuronal circuits to compensate for ongoing damage and cell loss. Thus, these diseases only become clinically apparent at advanced stages when damage is widespread and irreparable.

The treatment of neurodegenerative diseases is also hampered by the fact that a number of these diseases stem from toxic gain-of-function, rather than loss-of-function, phenotypes. For example, deletion of the *Plp1* gene is the most mild form of PMD; thus, the loss of the protein in myelin does not confer a strong phenotype. However, mutations that cause PLP1 to misfold are toxic to oligodendrocytes because of the extremely rapid accumulation of the intermediates in the ER, which overwhelm the capacity of the UPR to eliminate them through the ubiquitin-proteasome system [107]. Therapeutic strategies to insert a wild type *Plp1* allele into these patients would fail unless the toxic protein from the mutant allele were also eliminated.

The lessons learned from PMD and other neurodegenerative diseases could be relevant to MS and may help to explain why this disease is recalcitrant to treatments that only target the immunological aspects of the pathophysiology. Thus, considering MS as a gain-of-function disease with an underlying condition of unknown etiology that is exacerbated by autoimmune activation may shed new light on the pathophysiology and lead to novel therapeutic strategies to ameliorate the symptoms [70, 108, 109].

7. Conclusion

Although neurodegenerative diseases have typically been defined as a disparate group of diseases involving neurons, there is clear evidence in the clinical and basic science literature against such a narrow viewpoint. For example, diseases of the white matter such as PMD and MS arise from primary insults to oligodendrocytes and cause neuron loss in gray matter and lead to behavioral changes and memory loss. This reflects a broader consideration that all major cell types of the CNS are interdependent and degenerative changes in one of these will lead to loss of at least some of the other cell types.

In similar vein, the fundamental belief by immunologists that MS is a primary autoimmune disease is no longer tenable. Clear evidence from large clinical trials demonstrates that the elimination of adaptive immune cells from the CNS by various forms of immune suppression does not halt the progression of disease at early or late stages. The simplest interpretation of these data is that there is an underlying etiology that is poorly understood and must be recognized. In light of overlapping symptoms between PMD and MS, it is plausible that metabolic stress could play a primary role in oligodendrocyte degeneration with secondary activation of immune cells. Indeed, several studies have demonstrated induction of the UPR in MS tissue.

Nomenclature

UPR (unfolded protein response), IRE (inositol requiring protein), PERK (pancreatic endoplasmic reticulum kinase), ATF (activating transcription factor), XBP (X-box binding protein), CHOP (CCAAT/-enhancer binding protein homologous protein), PLP1 (proteolipid protein-1), GADD34 (growth arrest and DNA damage protein 34), BiP (chaperone protein), eIF2α (eukaryotic initiation factor 2 α), PP1 (protein phosphatase 1), GRP94 (glucose-regulated protein 94), S1P (site 1 protease), S2P (site 2 protease), ERAD (endoplasmic reticulum associated degradation), ataxia (lack of voluntary muscle coordination), hypotonia (low muscle tone), RRMS (relapse-remitting Multiple Sclerosis), SPMS (secondary progressive Multiple Sclerosis), PPMS (primary progressive Multiple Sclerosis), CD4,8,68 (cluster of differentiation, immune cell specific glycoproteins), *rumpshaker* mutation (*rsh*), *myelin-synthesis deficient* mutation (*msd*), MRI (magnetic resonance imaging), MRS (magnetic resonance spectroscopy), PET (positron emission tomography).

Acknowledgements

This work was supported by grants to A.G. from the National Institutes of Health, NINDS, NS067157 and the National Multiple Sclerosis Society, RG4078 and RG4639.

Author details

Daniel Radecki[1] and Alexander Gow[1,2,3*]

*Address all correspondence to: agow@med.wayne.edu

1 Center for Molecular Medicine and Genetics, Wayne State University School of Medicine, Detroit, MI, USA

2 Carman and Ann Adams Department of Pediatrics, Wayne State University School of Medicine, Detroit, MI, USA

3 Department of Neurology, Wayne State University School of Medicine, Detroit, MI, USA

References

[1] Coppede F. Genetics and Epigenetics of Parkinson's Disease. The Scientific World Journal 2012;2012: 12.

[2] Chen W-T, Hong C-J, Lin Y-T, Chang W-H, Huang H-T, Liao J-Y, Chang Y-J, Hsieh Y-F, Cheng C-Y, Liu H-C, Chen Y-R, Cheng IH. Amyloid-Beta (Aβ) D7H Mutation Increases Oligomeric Aβ42 and Alters Properties of Aβ-Zinc/Copper Assemblies. PLoS ONE 2012;7(4): e35807.

[3] Inayathullah M, Teplow DB. Structural dynamics of the ΔE22 (Osaka) familial Alzheimer's disease-linked amyloid β-protein. Amyloid 2011;18(3): 98-107.

[4] Gow A, Southwood CM, Lazzarini RA. Disrupted Proteolipid Protein Trafficking Results in Oligodendrocyte Apoptosis in an Animal Model of Pelizaeus-Merzbacher Disease. The Journal of Cell Biology 1998;140(4): 925-934.

[5] Southwood C, Gow A. Molecular pathways of oligodendrocyte apoptosis revealed by mutations in the proteolipid protein gene. Microscopy Research and Technique 2001;52(6): 700-708.

[6] Southwood CM, Garbern J, Jiang W, Gow A. The unfolded protein response modulates disease severity in Pelizaeus-Merzbacher disease. Neuron 2002;36(4): 585-96.

[7] Gow A, Lazzarini R. A cellular mechanism governing the severity of Pelizaeus –Merzbacher disease. Nature Genetics 1996;13: 422-428.

[8] Doyle KM, Kennedy D, Gorman AM, Gupta S, Healy SJM, Samali A. Unfolded proteins and endoplasmic reticulum stress in neurodegenerative disorders. Journal of Cellular and Molecular Medicine 2011;15(10): 2025-2039.

[9] Tosic M, Matthey B, Gow A, Lazzarini RA, Matthieu JM. Intracellular transport of the DM-20 bearing shaking pup (shp) mutation and its possible phenotypic consequences. Journal of Neuroscience Research 1997;50(5): 844-852.

[10] Scheper W, Nijholt DAT, Hoozemans JJM. The unfolded protein response and proteostasis in Alzheimer disease: Preferential activation of autophagy by endoplasmic reticulum stress. Autophagy 2011;7(8): 910-911.

[11] Yu Z, Wang AM, Adachi H, Katsuno M, Sobue G, Yue Z, Robins DM, Lieberman AP. Macroautophagy Is Regulated by the UPR–Mediator CHOP and Accentuates the Phenotype of SBMA Mice. PLoS Genet 2011;7(10): e1002321.

[12] Gow A, Sharma R. The unfolded protein response in protein aggregating diseases. NeuroMolecular Medicine 2003;4(1): 73-94.

[13] Mori K. Signalling Pathways in the Unfolded Protein Response: Development from Yeast to Mammals. Journal of Biochemistry 2009;146(6): 743-750.

[14] Zhang K, Kaufman RJ. The unfolded protein response. Neurology 2006;66(1 suppl 1): S102-S109.

[15] Walter P, Ron D. The Unfolded Protein Response: From Stress Pathway to Homeostatic Regulation. Science 2011;334(6059): 1081-1086.

[16] Ye C, Verchot J. Role of unfolded protein response in plant virus infection. Plant Signaling & Behavior 2011;6(8): 1212-1215.

[17] Gow A, Wrabetz L. CHOP and the endoplasmic reticulum stress response in myelinating glia. Current Opinion in Neurobiology 2009;19(5): 505-510.

[18] Hetz C. The unfolded protein response: controlling cell fate decisions under ER stress and beyond. Nat Rev Mol Cell Biol 2012;13(2): 89-102.

[19] Cao S, Kaufman R. Unfolded protein response. Current Biology 2012;22(16): R622-R626.

[20] Gardner BM, Walter P. Unfolded Proteins Are Ire1-Activating Ligands That Directly Induce the Unfolded Protein Response. Science 2011;333(6051): 1891-1894.

[21] Egawa N, Yamamoto K, Inoue H, Hikawa R, Nishi K, Mori K, Takahashi R. The Endoplasmic Reticulum Stress Sensor, ATF6α, Protects against Neurotoxin-induced Dopaminergic Neuronal Death. Journal of Biological Chemistry 2011;286(10): 7947-7957.

[22] Teske BF, Wek SA, Bunpo P, Cundiff JK, McClintick JN, Anthony TG, Wek RC. The eIF2 kinase PERK and the integrated stress response facilitate activation of ATF6 during endoplasmic reticulum stress. Molecular Biology of the Cell 2011;22(22): 4390-4405.

[23] Ohoka N, Yoshii S, Hattori T, Onozaki K, Hayashi H. TRB3, a novel ER stress-inducible gene, is induced via ATF4-CHOP pathway and is involved in cell death. EMBO J 2005;24(6): 1243-1255.

[24] Zou C-G, Cao X-Z, Zhao Y-S, Gao S-Y, Li S-D, Liu X-Y, Zhang Y, Zhang K-Q. The Molecular Mechanism of Endoplasmic Reticulum Stress-Induced Apoptosis in PC-12 Neuronal Cells: The Protective Effect of Insulin-Like Growth Factor I. Endocrinology 2009;150(1): 277-285.

[25] Bi M, Naczki C, Koritzinsky M, Fels D, Blais J, Hu N, Harding H, Novoa I, Varia M, Raleigh J, Scheuner D, Kaufman RJ, Bell J, Ron D, Wouters BG, Koumenis C. ER stress-regulated translation increases tolerance to extreme hypoxia and promotes tumor growth. EMBO J 2005;24(19): 3470-3481.

[26] Mak BC, Wang Q, Laschinger C, Lee W, Ron D, Harding HP, Kaufman RJ, Scheuner D, Austin RC, McCulloch CA. Novel Function of PERK as a Mediator of Force-induced Apoptosis. Journal of Biological Chemistry 2008;283(34): 23462-23472.

[27] Saporta MAC, Shy BR, Patzko A, Bai Y, Pennuto M, Ferri C, Tinelli E, Saveri P, Kirschner D, Crowther M, Southwood C, Wu X, Gow A, Feltri ML, Wrabetz L, Shy ME. MpzR98C arrests Schwann cell development in a mouse model of early-onset Charcot–Marie–Tooth disease type 1B. Brain 2012;135(7): 2032-2047.

[28] Sharma R, Gow A. Minimal role for caspase 12 in the unfolded protein response in oligodendrocytes in vivo. Journal of Neurochemistry 2007;101(4): 889-897.

[29] Lin JH, Li H, Zhang Y, Ron D, Walter P. Divergent Effects of PERK and IRE1 Signaling on Cell Viability. PLoS ONE 2009;4(1): e4170.

[30] Lin W, Kemper A, Dupree JL, Harding HP, Ron D, Popko B. Interferon-γ inhibits central nervous system remyelination through a process modulated by endoplasmic reticulum stress. Brain 2006;129(5): 1306-1318.

[31] Shirakawa K, Maeda S, Gotoh T, Hayashi M, Shinomiya K, Ehata S, Nishimura R, Mori M, Onozaki K, Hayashi H, Uematsu S, Akira S, Ogata E, Miyazono K, Imamura T. CCAAT/Enhancer-Binding Protein Homologous Protein (CHOP) Regulates Osteoblast Differentiation. Molecular and Cellular Biology 2006;26(16): 6105-6116.

[32] Lin W, Kunkler PE, Harding HP, Ron D, Kraig RP, Popko B. Enhanced Integrated Stress Response Promotes Myelinating Oligodendrocyte Survival in Response to Interferon-γ. The American Journal of Pathology 2008;173(5): 1508-1517.

[33] Bradl M, Lassmann H. Oligodendrocytes: biology and pathology. Acta Neuropathologica 2010;119(1): 37-53.

[34] Pfeiffer SE, Warrington AE, Bansal R. The oligodendrocyte and its many cellular processes. Trends in Cell Biology 1993;3(6): 191-197.

[35] D'Antonio M, Feltri ML, Wrabetz L. Myelin under stress. Journal of Neuroscience Research 2009;87(15): 3241-3249.

[36] Perlman SJ, Mar S, Leukodystrophies Neurodegenerative Diseases, editor, Editor Editors. 2012, Springer US. p. 154-171.

[37] Mar S, Noetzel M. Axonal Damage in Leukodystrophies. Pediatric Neurology 2010;42(4): 239-242.

[38] Sakai N. Pathogenesis of leukodystrophy for Krabbe disease: Molecular mechanism and clinical treatment. Brain and Development 2009;31(7): 485-487.

[39] Sawaishi Y. Review of Alexander disease: Beyond the classical concept of leukodystrophy. Brain and Development 2009;31(7): 493-498.

[40] van der Voorn J, van Kollenberg B, Bertrand G, Van Haren K, Scheper G, Powers J, van der Knaap M. The unfolded protein response in vanishing white matter disease. Journal of Neuropathology and Experimental Neurology 2005;69(5): 770-775.

[41] Castaneda J, Lim M, Cooper J, Pearce D. Immune system irregularities in lysosomal storage disorders. Acta Neuropathologica 2008;115(2): 159-174.

[42] Powers J, Liu Y, Moser A, Moser H. The inflammatory myelinopathy of adreno-leukodystrophy: cells, effector molecules, and pathogenic implications. Journal of Neuropathology and Experimental Neurology 1992;51(6): 630-643.

[43] Garbern J. Pelizaeus-Merzbacher disease: Genetic and cellular pathogenesis. Cellular and Molecular Life Sciences 2007;64(1): 50-65.

[44] Garbern J, Cambi F, Shy M, Kamholz J. THe molecular pathogenesis of pelizaeus-merzbacher disease. Archives of Neurology 1999;56(10): 1210-1214.

[45] Boison D, Stoffel W. Disruption of the compacted myelin sheath of axons of the central nervous system in proteolipid protein-deficient mice. Proceedings of the National Academy of Sciences 1994;91(24): 11709-11713.

[46] Griffiths I, Klugmann M, Thomson T, Anderson C, Vouyiouklis D, Nave K-A. Current concepts of PLP and its role in the nervous system. Microscopy Research and Technique 1998;41(5): 344-358.

[47] Stecca B, Southwood CM, Gragerov A, Kelley KA, Friedrich VL, Gow A. The Evolution of Lipophilin Genes from Invertebrates to Tetrapods: DM-20 Cannot Replace Proteolipid Protein in CNS Myelin. The Journal of Neuroscience 2000;20(11): 4002-4010.

[48] Kagawa T, Ikenaka K, Inoue Y, Kuriyama S, Tsujii T, Nakao J, Nakajima K, Aruga J, Okano H, Mikoshiba K. Glial cell degeneration and hypomyelination caused by over-expression of myelin proteolipid protein gene. Neuron 1994;13(2): 427-442.

[49] Saher G, Rudolphi F, Corthals K, Ruhwedel T, Schmidt K-F, Lowel S, Dibaj P, Barrette B, Mobius W, Nave K-A. Therapy of Pelizaeus-Merzbacher disease in mice by feeding a cholesterol-enriched diet. Nature Medicine 2012;18(7): 1130-1135.

[50] Tatar CL, Appikatla S, Bessert D, Paintlia AS, Singh I, Skoff RP. Increased Plp1 gene expression leads to massive microglial cell activation and inflammation throughout the brain. ASN Neuro 2010;2(4).

[51] Gow A, Friedrich VLJ, R.A. L. Many Naturally Ocurring Mutations of Myelin Proteolipid Protein Impair Its Intracellular Transport. Journal of Neuroscience Research 1994;37(5): 574-583.

[52] Duncan ID, Hammang JP, Trapp BD. Abnormal compact myelin in the myelin-deficient rat: absence of proteolipid protein correlates with a defect in the intraperiod line. Proceedings of the National Academy of Sciences 1987;84(17): 6287-6291.

[53] Vela JM, González B, Castellano B. Understanding glial abnormalities associated with myelin deficiency in the jimpy mutant mouse. Brain Research Reviews 1998;26(1): 29-42.

[54] Griffiths I, Scott I, McCulloch M, Barri J, McPhilemy K, Cattanach BM. Rumpshaker mouse: a new X-linked mutation affecting myelination: evidence for a defect in PLP expression. Journal of Neurocytology 1990;19(2): 273-283.

[55] Nave K, Bloom F, Milner R. A single nucleotide difference in the gene for myelin proteolipid protein defines the jimpy mutation in mouse. Journal of Neurochemistry 1987;49(6): 1873-1877.

[56] Nadon NL, Duncan ID, Hudson LD. A point mutation in the proteolipid protein gene of the 'shaking pup' interrupts oligodendrocyte development. Development 1990;110(2): 529-537.

[57] Hudson LD, Berndt JA, Puckett C, Kozak CA, Lazzarini RA. Aberrant splicing of proteolipid protein mRNA in the dysmyelinating jimpy mutant mouse. Proceedings of the National Academy of Sciences 1987;84(5): 1454-1458.

[58] Boison D, Stoffel W. Myelin-deficient rat: a point mutation in exon III (A----C, Thr75----Pro) of the myelin proteolipid protein causes dysmyelination and oligodendrocyte death. The European Molecular Biology Organization 1989;8(11): 3295-3302.

[59] Domanska-Janik K, J. S, A. T. Immunohistochemical study of myelin-specific proteins in pt rabbits. Folia Neuropathology 1997;35(1): 1-7.

[60] Kagawa T, Nakao J, Yamada M, Shimizu K, Hayakawa T, Mikoshiba K, Ikenaka K. Fate of Jimpy-Type Oligodendrocytes in Jimpy Heterozygote. Journal of Neurochemistry 1994;62(5): 1887-1893.

[61] Schneider AM, Griffiths IR, Readhead C, Nave KA. Dominant-negative action of the jimpy mutation in mice complemented with an autosomal transgene for myelin proteolipid protein. Proceedings of the National Academy of Sciences 1995;92(10): 4447-4451.

[62] Gardinier MV, Macklin MB. Myelin proteolipid protein gene expression in jimpy and jimpy(msd) mice. Journal of Neurochemistry 1988;51(2): 360-369.

[63] Jung M, Sommer I, Schachner M, Nave K-A. Monoclonal Antibody O10 Defines a Conformationally Sensitive Cell-Surface Epitope of Proteolipid Protein (PLP): Evidence that PLP Misfolding Underlies Dysmyelination in Mutant Mice. The Journal of Neuroscience 1996;16(24): 7920-7929.

[64] Schneider A, Montague P, Griffiths I, Fanarraga M, Kennedy P, Brophy P, Nave K-A. Uncoupling of hypomyelination and glial cell death by a mutation in the proteolipid protein gene. Nature 1992;358(6389): 758-761.

[65] Baumann NA, Jacque CM, Pollet SA, Harpin ML. Fatty Acid and Lipid Composition of the Brain of a Myelin Deficient Mutant, the "Quaking" Mouse. European Journal of Biochemistry 1968;4(3): 340-344.

[66] Gencic S, Hudson L. Conservative amino acid substitution in the myelin proteolipid protein of jimpymsd mice. The Journal of Neuroscience 1990;10(1): 117-124.

[67] Wolf MK, Kardon GB, Adcock LH, Billings-Gagliardi S. Hypomyelinated mutant mice. V. Relationship between jp and jpmsd re-examined on identical genetic backgrounds. Brain Res 1983;271(1): 121-129.

[68] Kassmann CM, Nave KA. Oligodendroglial impact on axonal function and survival - a hypothesis. Current Opinion in Neurology 2008;21(3): 235-241.

[69] Polman CH, Reingold SC, Banwell B, Clanet M, Cohen JA, Filippi M, Fujihara K, Havrdova E, Hutchinson M, Kappos L, Lublin FD, Montalban X, O'Connor P, Sandberg-Wollheim M, Thompson AJ, Waubant E, Weinshenker B, Wolinsky JS. Diagnostic criteria for multiple sclerosis: 2010 Revisions to the McDonald criteria. Annals of Neurology 2011;69(2): 292-302.

[70] Comabella M, Vandenbroeck K. Pharmacogenomics and Multiple Sclerosis: Moving Toward Individualized Medicine. Current Neurology and Neuroscience Reports 2011;11(5): 484-491.

[71] Hartung H-P, Lehmann HC, Kieseier BC, Hughes RAC. Novel treatment for immune neuropathies on the horizon. Journal of the Peripheral Nervous System 2011;16(2): 75-83.

[72] Kappos L, Radue E-W, O'Connor P, Polman C, Hohlfeld R, Calabresi P, Selmaj K, Agoropoulou C, Leyk M, Zhang-Auberson L, Burtin P. A Placebo-Controlled Trial of Oral Fingolimod in Relapsing Multiple Sclerosis. New England Journal of Medicine 2010;362(5): 387-401.

[73] Polman CH, O'Connor PW, Havrdova E, Hutchinson M, Kappos L, Miller DH, Phillips JT, Lublin FD, Giovannoni G, Wajgt A, Toal M, Lynn F, Panzara MA, Sandrock AW. A Randomized, Placebo-Controlled Trial of Natalizumab for Relapsing Multiple Sclerosis. New England Journal of Medicine 2006;354(9): 899-910.

[74] Comi G, Jeffery D, Kappos L, Montalban X, Boyko A, Rocca MA, Filippi M. Placebo-Controlled Trial of Oral Laquinimod for Multiple Sclerosis. New England Journal of Medicine 2012;366(11): 1000-1009.

[75] Kappos L, Li D, Calabresi PA, O'Connor P, Bar-Or A, Barkhof F, Yin M, Leppert D, Glanzman R, Tinbergen J, Hauser SL. Ocrelizumab in relapsing-remitting multiple sclerosis: a phase 2, randomised, placebo-controlled, multicentre trial. The Lancet; 378(9805): 1779-1787.

[76] Fairless R, Williams SK, Hoffmann DB, Stojic A, Hochmeister S, Schmitz F, Storch MK, Diem R. Preclinical Retinal Neurodegeneration in a Model of Multiple Sclerosis. The Journal of Neuroscience 2012;32(16): 5585-5597.

[77] Lassmann H, van Horssen J. The molecular basis of neurodegeneration in multiple sclerosis. FEBS Letters 2011;585(23): 3715-3723.

[78] Petratos S, Azari M, Ozturk E, Roula O, Papadopoulos R, Bernard C. Novel Therapeutic Targets for Axonal Degeneration in Multiple Sclerosis. Journal of Neuropathology and Experimental Neurology 2010;69(4): 323-334.

[79] Gaupp S, Pitt D, Kuziel WA, Cannella B, Raine CS. Experimental Autoimmune Encephalomyelitis (EAE) in CCR2−/− Mice: Susceptibility in Multiple Strains. The American Journal of Pathology 2003;162(1): 139-150.

[80] Bradl M, Linington C. Animal models of demyelination. Brain Pathology 1996;6(3): 303-311.

[81] Becher B, Segal B. TH17 cytokines in autoimmune neuro-inflammation. Current Opinion in Immunology 2011;23(6): 707-712.

[82] Peterson JW, Bo L, Mork S, Chang A, Trapp BD. Transected Neurites, Apoptotic Neurons, and Reduced Inflammation in Cortical Multiple Sclerosis Lesions. Annals of Neurology 2001;50(3): 389-400.

[83] Pucci E, Giuliani G, Solari A, Simi S, Minozzi S, Di Pietrantonj C, Galea I Natalizumab for relapsing remitting multiple sclerosis. Cochrane Database of Systematic Reviews, 2011. CD007621 DOI: 10.1002/14651858.CD007621.pub2.

[84] Whetten-Goldstein K, Sloan FA, Goldstein LB, Kulas ED. A comprehensive assessment of the cost of multiple sclerosis in the United States. Multiple Sclerosis 1998;4(5): 419-425.

[85] Zhang J, Kramer EG, Asp L, Dutta DJ, Navrazhina K, Pham T, Mariani JN, Argaw AT, Melendez-Vasquez CV, John GR. Promoting myelin repair and return of function in multiple sclerosis. FEBS Letters 2011;585(23): 3813-3820.

[86] Bluestein KT, Pitt D, Knopp MV, Schmalbrock P. T1 and proton density at 7 T in patients with multiple sclerosis: an initial study. Magnetic Resonance Imaging 2012;30(1): 19-25.

[87] Poloni G, Minagar A, Haacke EM, Zivadinov R. Recent developments in imaging of multiple sclerosis. Neurologist 2011;17(4): 185-204.

[88] Mainero C, Benner T, Radding A, van der Kouwe A, Jensen R, Rosen B, Kinkel R. In vivo imaging of cortical pathology in multiple sclerosis using ultra-high field MRI. Neurology 2009;73: 941-948.

[89] Ajami B, Bennett JL, Krieger C, McNagny KM, Rossi FMV. Infiltrating monocytes trigger EAE progression, but do not contribute to the resident microglia pool. Nature Neuroscience 2011;14(9): 1142-1149.

[90] Chen F, Shaw MK, Li J, Lisak RP, Tse HY. Adoptive transfer of myelin basic protein-induced experimental autoimmune encephalomyelitis between SJL and B10.S mice: Correlation of priming milieus with susceptibility and resistance phenotypes. Journal of Neuroimmunology 2006;173(1–2): 146-154.

[91] Morgan L, Shah B, Rivers LE, Barden L, Groom AJ, Chung R, Higazi D, Desmond H, Smith T, Staddon JM. Inflammation and dephosphorylation of the tight junction protein occludin in an experimental model of multiple sclerosis. Neuroscience 2007;147(3): 664-73.

[92] Shaw MK, Kim C, Ho K-L, Lisak RP, Tse HY. A combination of adoptive transfer and antigenic challenge induces consistent murine experimental autoimmune encephalomyelitis in C57BL/6 mice and other reputed resistant strains. Journal of Neuroimmunology 1992;39(1–2): 139-149.

[93] Tischner D, Weishaupt A, Brandt Jvd, Müller N, Beyersdorf N, Ip CW, Toyka KV, Hünig T, Gold R, Kerkau T, Reichardt HM. Polyclonal expansion of regulatory T cells interferes with effector cell migration in a model of multiple sclerosis. Brain 2006;129(10): 2635-2647.

[94] Gold R, Linington C, Lassmann H. Understanding pathogenesis and therapy of multiple sclerosis via animal models: 70 years of merits and culprits in experimental autoimmune encephalomyelitis research. Brain 2006;129(8): 1953-1971.

[95] Gow A, Chapter nine - Using Temporal Genetic Switches to Synchronize the Unfolded Protein Response in Cell Populations In Vivo, in Methods in Enzymology. 2011, Academic Press. p. 143-161.

[96] Abraira V, Alvarez-Cermeño JC, Arroyo R, Cámara C, Casanova B, Cubillo S, de Andrés C, Espejo C, Fernández O, Ferrer J, Figueredo MA, García-Merino A, García-Sánchez MI, García-Trujillo JA, Gómez M, González-Oria C, Gosis A, Izquierdo G, Jímenez J, López-Trascasa M, Montalbán X, Moreno MJ, Muñoz D, Nuñez V, Muriel A, Navarro J, Olascoaga J, Oreja-Guevara C, Prada A, Ramil E, Ramo-Tello C, Rodríguez C, Rodríguez E, Rodríguez-Frías F, Rodríguez-Antigüedad A, Rodríguez-Molina JJ, Ruiz E, Saiz A, Sarasola E, Simó M, Yagüe J, Villar LM. Utility of oligoclonal IgG band detection for MS diagnosis in daily clinical practice. Journal of Immunological Methods 2011;371(1–2): 170-173.

[97] Denic A, Macura S, Mishra P, Gamez J, Rodriguez M, Pirko I. MRI in Rodent Models of Brain Disorders. Neurotherapeutics 2011;8(1): 3-18.

[98] Patel NH, Vyas NS, Puri BK, Nijran KS, Al-Nahhas A. Positron Emission Tomography in Schizophrenia: A New Perspective. Journal of Nuclear Medicine 2010;51(4): 511-520.

[99] Rigotti DJ, Inglese M, Gonen O. Whole-Brain N-Acetylaspartate as a Surrogate Marker of Neuronal Damage in Diffuse Neurologic Disorders. American Journal of Neuroradiology 2007;28(10): 1843-1849.

[100] Tartaglia MC, Arnold DL. The role of MRS and fMRI in multiple sclerosis. Advanced Neurology 2006;98: 185-202.

[101] Lewellen T, Williams D, Olson D. Image quality with nuclear magnetic resonance imaging systems. American Journal of Roentgenology 1981;137(5): 1092-1093.

[102] Geurts JJG, Barkhof F. Grey matter pathology in multiple sclerosis. The Lancet Neurology 2008;7(9): 841-851.

[103] Tang KS, Shapiro EM. Enhanced magnetic cell labeling efficiency using –NH2 coated MPIOs. Magnetic Resonance in Medicine 2011;65(6): 1564-1569.

[104] De Stefano N, Filippi M, Miller D, Pouwels PJ, Rovira A, Gass A, Enzinger C, Matthews PM, Arnold DL. Guidelines for using proton MR spectroscopy in multicenter clinical MS studies. Neurology 2007;69(20): 1942-52.

[105] Kumar A, Asano E, Chugani HT. α-[11C]-methyl-L-tryptophan PET for tracer localization of epileptogenic brain regions: clinical studies. Biomarkers in Medicine 2011;5(5): 577-584.

[106] Kadir A, Nordberg A. Target-Specific PET Probes for Neurodegenerative Disorders Related to Dementia. Journal of Nuclear Medicine 2010;51(9): 1418-1430.

[107] Fonseca SG, Gromada J, Urano F. Endoplasmic reticulum stress and pancreatic β-cell death. Trends in Endocrinology and Metabolism 2011;22(7): 266-274.

[108] Gensicke H, Leppert D, Yaldizli Ö, Lindberg RLP, Mehling M, Kappos L, Kuhle J. Monoclonal Antibodies and Recombinant Immunoglobulins for the Treatment of Multiple Sclerosis. CNS Drugs 2012;26(1): 11-37.

[109] He D, Zhou H, Han W, Zhang S Rituximab for relapsing-remitting multiple sclerosis. Cochrane Database of Systematic Reviews, 2011. DOI: 10.1002/14651858.CD009130.pub2.

Section 4

Miscellaneous

Chapter 23

Spinal Muscular Atrophy: Classification, Diagnosis, Background, Molecular Mechanism and Development of Therapeutics

Faraz Tariq Farooq, Martin Holcik and
Alex MacKenzie

Additional information is available at the end of the chapter

http://dx.doi.org/10.5772/53800

1. Introduction

Spinal muscular atrophy (SMA) is an autosomal recessive neurodegenerative disease and one of the most common genetic causes of infant death. The loss or mutation of the SMN1 gene results in reduced SMN protein level leading to motor neuron death and progressive muscle atrophy. Although recent progress has been made in our understanding of the molecular mechanisms underlying the pathogenesis of the disease, there is currently no cure for SMA. In this review, we summarize the clinical manifestations, molecular pathogenesis, diagnostic strategy and development of therapeutic regimes for the better understanding and treatment of SMA.

2. Epidemiology

Spinal muscular atrophy (SMA) is an autosomal recessive neuromuscular disorder characterized by the loss of motor neurons from the anterior horn of the spinal cord which leads to muscle weakness, hypotonia and ultimately muscle atrophy [1]. With a pan ethnic incidence of 1:11,000 live births and a carrier frequency of 1:50, SMA is one of the leading genetic causes of infant death globally [1-5].

3. Clinical classification

Due to the range of clinical severity, SMA is broadly classified into four major categories characterized by the age of onset as well as severity of the disease [6-9]. SMA type I, which was originally described by Werdnig and Hoffmann in the late 18th century is the most severe and prevalent form of the disease and accounts for more than 50% of the known diagnosed cases of SMA. Type I SMA presents within the first six months after birth and although historically patients succumbed within the first 2 years of life, with better ventilatory and nutritional support, the life expectancy of children with type I SMA can be increased beyond the 5th birthday. Infants with type I SMA experience a rapid loss of skeletal muscle mass with profound hypotonia and general muscle weakness characterized by poor head control, difficulty with suckling, swallowing and an inability to sit without support. These children develop problems with breathing over time due to impaired bulbar function and respiratory muscle weakness leading to respiratory insufficiency. Respiratory failure due to aspiration pneumonia is an important cause of SMA mortality [6, 10, 11]. The intermediate form of SMA, known as type II, has an onset between 6 and 18 months of age. Patients with type II SMA can sit unaided but still develop progressive muscle weakness and can never stand or walk on their own. Other symptoms and physical signs include respiratory insufficiency due to reduced bulbar function, poor weight gain, fine hand tremors and joint contractures [6]. SMA type III has an onset between 18 months to 30 years of age. Patients are able to stand and walk unaided, however they develop variable degree of muscle weakness which leads to a broad spectrum of physical signs and symptoms. While most walk independently, some lose ambulation during early adulthood and require wheelchair assistance. Others develop cramps and joint overuse problems; some develop scoliosis [6, 12, 13]. Type IV SMA is the mildest form of the condition and is characterized by adult onset with normal mobility. They have mild muscle weakness in adulthood with normal longevity [6] (Table 1).

SMA Type	Other Names	Age of Onset	Life Span	Highest Motor Activity
Type I years (Severe)	Werdnig- Hoffmann disease	0-6 months	2-5	Never sit
Type II (Intermediate)	SMA, Dubowitz type	7-18 months	>2 years	Sit, Never stand
Type III (Mild)	Kugelberg-Welander disease	>18 months	Adult	Stand and walk (may require assistance)
Type IV (Adult)	------------	Adulthood	Normal	Walk during adulthood-unassisted (some muscle weakness)

Table 1. Classification of SMA disease

http://dx.doi.org/10.5772/53800

4. Diagnosis and treatment

The diagnosis of SMA is made by a thorough patient history and physical examination followed by genetic testing. The survival of motor neuron (SMN) -1 genotyping has to a large degree replaced electromyography (EMG) and muscle biopsies (Fig 1) [2, 14]. There is in 2012 no cure for SMA; current treatment is symptomatic and supportive. This includes clinical management through family education and counselling along with attention to pulmonary, gastrointestinal/nutrition and orthopedics/rehabilitation in an effort to managing symptoms of the patients [9].

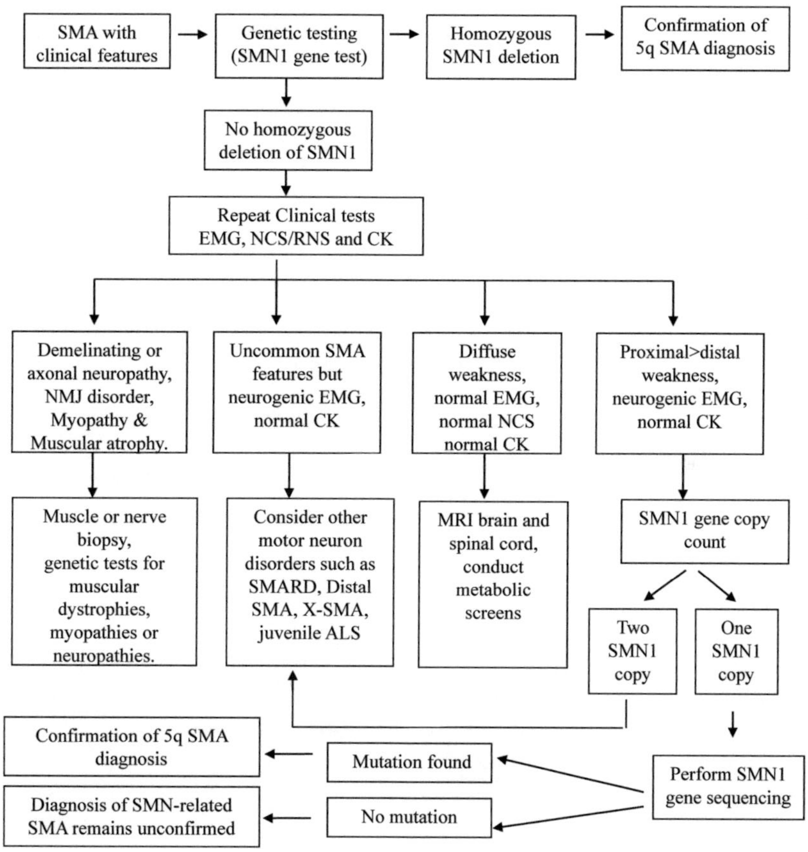

Figure 1. SMA diagnosis

5. Genetics of the disease

The SMA disease causing *SMN1* gene maps to a complex genomic region of chromosome 5q13.1. This region is characterized by an inverted duplication of the element with 4 genes

(*SMN*, neuronal apoptosis inhibitor protein *{NAIP}*, *SERF and GTFH2)* present in telomeric and centromeric copies (Fig 2a) [15, 16]. In 1995, it was reported that homozygous deletions of the *SMN1* gene were observed in and thus likely the cause of 95% of SMA patients [15]. All SMA patients have one or more copies of a nearly identical gene, *SMN2*. These two genes are distinguished by five nucleotide changes in exon 7 and 8. The critical nucleotide difference which makes *SMN2* only partially functional is a C to T transition at position 6 of exon 7. This change leads to the exclusion of exon 7 in the majority of transcripts. This mRNA is subsequently translated to form an unstable truncated non-oligomerizing isoform of SMN protein. However, *SMN2* gene still produces 5-10% functional full length SMN transcripts (Fig 1.2b) [15, 17, 18]. The *SMN2* gene is present in variable copy numbers in the population; all SMA patients have one or more copy of the *SMN2* gene which, due to its partial functionality, acts as a positive disease modifier. There is thus an inverse correlation between the number of *SMN2* gene (which can produce between 10-50% of SMN protein depending on copy number) and the severity of the disease [2]. Low levels of SMN protein allows embryonic development but is not enough, in the long term, to allow motor neurons to survive in the spinal cord [19, 20]. Type I patients usually have 2 copies whereas Type II have 3 copies of *SMN2*. Type III and IV have 3-4 copies of the *SMN2* gene. Individuals with 5 or more copies of the *SMN2* gene, despite having no functional *SMN1* gene are completely asymptomatic and are protected against the disease manifestation.

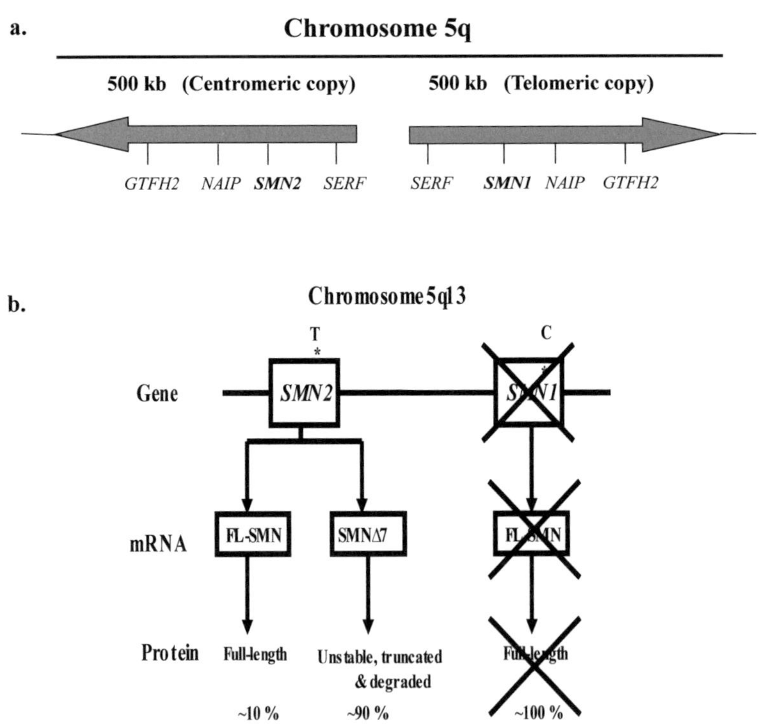

Figure 2. (a) Human SMN locus and (b) genetics of SMA patients

6. Pathology

The pathological hallmark of all forms of SMA is the loss of motor neurons from the lower brainstem and the anterior horn of the spinal cord [21]. Anterograde axonal degeneration results in denervation of the myocytes within the motor unit. This sometimes leads to reinnervation of muscle, where adjacent uninjured motor neurons sprout leads to fiber type grouping of myocytes. Histopathologic assessment of SMA muscle tissues reveals a large number of rounded atrophic fibers resulting from denervation. The widely held notion had been that SMA is primarily a neuronopathy (involving the cell body) with secondary degeneration of the axons. However, more recent observations in the field have shifted the focus of SMA pathology from the motor neuron cell body to the distal axon [22, 23] and the possibility of a synaptopathic defect [20, 24]. Specifically it has been suggested that the presynaptic transcriptome may be in some manner dysregulated; the direct inference is that SMN plays a role in the peripheral transport of critical mRNA, among which is that species encoding beta-actin. Regardless of the subcellular location of SMN mediated pathology, SMA is primarily considered as a motor neuron disease and consequently treatment strategies focus on drugs which can cross the blood brain barrier (BBB) to target the central nervous system (CNS). However, motor neuron autonomy of SMA pathogenesis has recently been called into question as multi-system involvement (including cardiovascular, peripheral necrosis and liver defects) have been reported recently in both SMA patients and SMA mice models [25-33]. In addition, one report has outlined the superiority of systemic SMN antisense oligonucleotide (ASO) therapy compared with intrathecal delivery in severe murine SMA calling into question the exclusive role of the motor neuron in disease causation [33].

7. Function of the SMN protein

SMN is a 294 amino acid long ubiquitously expressed protein with a molecular weight of 38 kilodaltons (kD). SMN is found in both the nucleus and cytoplasm. Within the nucleus, it is localized both throughout the nucleoplasm as well as in nuclear structures called Gems and Cajal bodies [34]. It is also found in abundance within the growth cones of the motor neurons [35]. SMN has been implicated in ribonucleoprotein biogenesis (e.g. assembly, metabolism and transport of various ribonucleoproteins), as well as playing a major role in the splicing machinery. It is part of a multiprotein complex comprised of Gemins [2-8], spliceosomal U-snRNPs, Sm proteins and profilins called the SMN complex. This complex is essential for the biogenesis of snRNPs [36-45]. Given the variety of roles that SMN has been implicated in, not surprisingly, the complete absence of SMN genes is embryonically lethal in virtually all metazoan life forms tested, indeed even cell cultures cannot survive without SMN [19, 20, 46].

8. Molecular mechanism: splicing defect in SMA

Splicing is mediated by a complex called the spliceosome, the activity of which depends on a number of factors. In particular, various cis- and trans-acting elements regulate the splicing of both *SMN1* and *SMN2*. The C-T transition at position 6 of exon 7 in *SMN2* gene disrupts the function of an exonic splice enhancer (ESE; recognized by SF2/ASF to promote exon 7 inclusion) and/or creates an exonic splice suppressor (ESS; recognized by hnRNP A1/A2) which results in exon 7 skipping (Fig 3) [47-53].

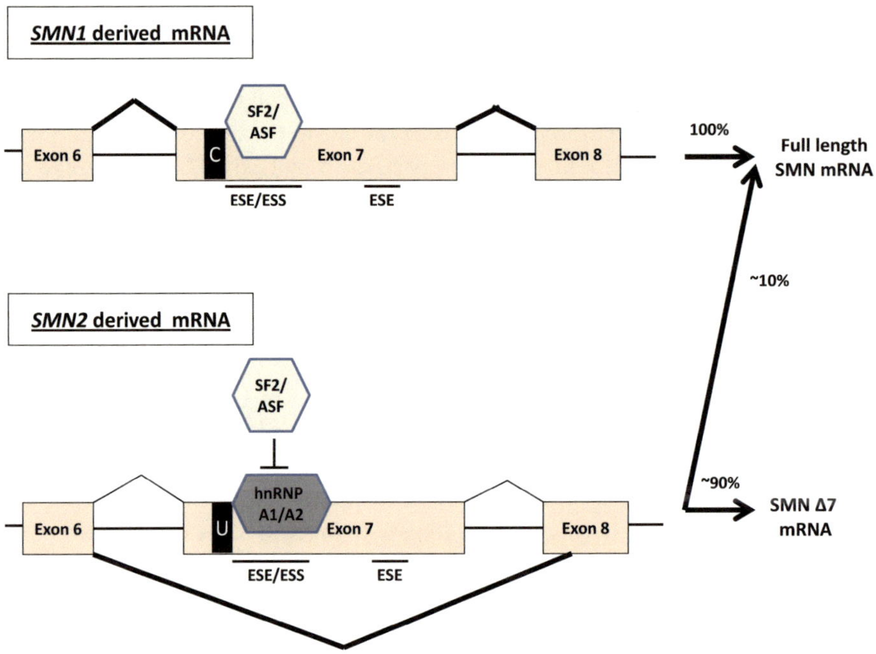

Figure 3. Splicing in SMA

9. Therapeutic strategies

Although there is no cure for SMA, the *SMN2* gene locus serves as a target for SMA treatment. The general treatment strategies for SMA are to compensate fully or in part for the absence of *SMN1* gene by increasing the levels of functional SMN protein levels though three distinct approaches: i) to induce the expression of *SMN2*, ii) to modulate splicing of *SMN2* transcript, and iii) to stabilize the full length SMN mRNA and/or protein. In addition, gene and stem cell therapies are also under development for the treatment of SMA. These and other strategies are discussed below.

1. **SMN dependent therapies**: As outlined above, there is an inverse correlation between the *SMN2* gene copy number and disease severity [54, 55] which implies that directly targeting the *SMN2* gene in SMA patients through different pathways could be one key for the development of a SMA drug treatment. Alternatively, SMN protein can also be produced through gene replacement therapy.

a. **Activation of *SMN2* promoter**: Histone deacetylases (HDACs) repress transcription of genes including *SMN2* by chromatin condensation. Thus, HDAC inhibitors can increase transcription of the *SMN2* gene and can produce more full length SMN transcripts and protein which may have a beneficial effect in patients. Various HDAC inhibitors have been analyzed in cell culture, mouse models and in clinical trials as potential therapeutic for SMA. Sodium butyrate, Valproic acid (VPA) and phenylbutyrate showed promise in cell culture and mouse models and were also well tolerated by the patients [56-63]. However, no clinical improvement was observed in SMA patients with HDAC inhibitors [61-63].

   Recent studies with other HDAC inhibitors, LBH589, Trichostatin A (TSA) and Suberoylanilide hydroxamic acid (SAHA) showed *SMN2* gene induction in culture as well as in a number of animal models of neurodegeneration [62, 64-66]. In addition to these compounds, we have shown that the lactation hormone prolactin (PRL) which can both cross the blood brain barrier and, through binding to its receptor, activate the JAK2/STAT5 pathway also upregulates *SMN2* gene transcription [68]. Interestingly the degree of induction in SMN seen with the prolactin in the genetically engineered Δ7 SMA mouse model (where *SMN2* gene is the only source of SMN protein) is significantly greater than that seen in cell culture and wild type mice. We have determined that this is because of the difference between the promoter regions in *SMN1* and *SMN2* genes, the latter uniquely having STAT5a transcription binding motifs. This might prove beneficial as all SMA patients have *SMN2* as the only source of SMN protein. Since PRL has been successfully tested and proven safe in humans for the treatment of lactation deficient mothers [67], it may bypass other compounds which are yet to be tested for clinical safety and join the short list of drugs which may have immediate potential SMA therapeutic potential [68].

b. **Correction of splicing**: The suppression of exon 7 skipping to produce more full length transcript from the *SMN2* gene is another treatment strategy being explored for SMA. HDAC inhibitors such as VPA, TSA and sodium butyrate appear to have a dual effect on SMN mRNA expression; they not only open chromatin structure and therefore increase the rate of transcription but also appear to affect the splicing process [56-58, 64]. The antibiotic aclarubicin has been shown to increase full length SMN transcript by altering the splicing process *in vitro* [69]. The most promising compounds which correct splicing by preventing *SMN2* exon 7 skipping are antisense oligos (ASOs). An ASO complementary to *SMN2* exon 7 pre-mRNA sequences has been shown to inhibit binding of negative splicing factors and increase full length SMN transcript and protein production [30, 33, 70, 71]. The major hurdle in using ASOs for SMA therapeutics, however, is their inability to cross the blood brain barrier. However, Hua et al. 2011 documented a marked improvement in motor function along with an increase in survival in SMA mice with systemic delivery of ASO which results into increase in SMN levels mostly in peripheral tissues especially in liver. Interestingly, they documented only a slight increase in SMN levels in CNS tissues [33]. However, there are a number of issues which need to be addressed before clinical introduction of ASOs for SMA treatment (clinical safety, quantity of ASO, cost, immune response etc) [72].

c. **Full length SMN transcript stabilization**: In this relatively new approach by by Singh *et al.*, decapping enzyme DcpS, an integral part of the RNA degradation machinery, was targeted by C5-substituted quinazolines which interact and open the enzyme into a catalytically inactivated conformation. Full length SMN mRNA decay is in this fashion blocked, ultimately increasing SMN protein in cell culture [73].

   In a different approach, SMN mRNA has been shown to have a specific AU rich element (ARE) region in its 3' UTR which marks the mRNA for degradation. Our laboratory has shown that activation of the p38 pathway results in the accumulation of RNA binding protein HuR in the cytoplasm which then binds to the ARE in 3'UTR region of SMN mRNA and stabilizes the transcript. Importantly, transcript stabilization is not associated with any discernible inhibition of SMN protein translation. This study provided a novel mechanism through which SMN mRNA could be stabilized using p38 activating compounds which can cross the blood brain barrier to develop new therapeutics for SMA treatment [74].

d. **Full length SMN protein stabilization**: Aminoglycosides are class of antibiotics which have been shown to mask premature stop codon mutations in some genes, allowing read through translation to occur. This moderates translation termination through an alteration in the conformation of the ribosomal reading site. Various aminoglycosides including tobramycin and amikacin have been used successfully in patient fibroblasts to increase SMN protein levels. However, their *in vivo* efficacy and safety has yet to be demonstrated [75-77].

   An alternative potential therapeutic approach involves targeting the ubiquitin-proteasome pathway which mediates intracellular protein turnover. Proteins are marked with poly ubiquitin (Ub) molecules by the action of the enzymes E1 (Ub activating enzyme), E2 (Ub conjugating enzyme) and E3 (Ub ligase). The polyubiquitin modification marks the protein for destruction by the proteasome complex. SMN is one of the many proteins degraded by the ubiquitin proteasome pathway. It has been shown that FDA approved proteasome inhibitor bortezomib increases SMN both in vitro and in vivo by blocking proteolysis of SMN protein. However, it should be noted that bortezomib cannot cross the BBB; thus, it must be used in combination with other drugs which can cross the BBB for the treatment of SMA [78].

e. **Gene therapy**: One of the most encouraging SMA therapeutic advances is the use of gene therapy which shows significant promise. In the last three years several groups have used self complementary adeno-associated virus (scAAV) 8 and 9 vectors carrying the *SMN1* cDNA to treat mice models of SMA, resulting in the most dramatic extension in the life span of mice yet observed combined with an overall amelioration of disease phenotype [79-82]. However, early pre-symptomatic intervention is necessary for the success of this therapy as is seen with other treatment strategies as well. Moreover, several challenges must be addressed for this mode of SMA treatment before bringing it to clinical application successfully. The most pressing issues are clinical safety, dealing with the cross-species barriers, the cost of virus production along with the possibility of an immune response to AAV which can neutralize its impact [83].

2. **SMN-independent strategies**: There have been some recent advances in SMN-independent strategies for the treatment of SMA. These include:

a. **Stem cell therapy**: Stem cell therapy has generated much attention as a treatment for motor neuron diseases, including SMA, through replacement of the lost motor neurons and, more realistically perhaps, supporting the existing neuron population. Primary murine neuronal stem cells as well as embryonic stem cell-derived neural stem cells injected into the spinal cord of animal models of SMA have been shown to ameliorate disease phenotype and increase survival [84, 85]. It is unclear whether this is through motor neuron and other cell replacement and/or through neuroprotection of host motor neurons by the numerous factors released from the donor cells. Although induced pluripotent stem (iPS) cells from an SMA patient have been differentiated into motor neurons [86, 87], there are several obstacles which hinder their use as a therapeutic for SMA treatment. These challenges include the production of the large number of stem cells and their successful transplantation into the patients, which could populate and cover the entire nervous system. Also, lentivirus vectors are used to deliver the cocktail of factors, required to produce iPS cells *in vitro*; these would be unsuitable for use in patients as they have the potential for insertional mutagenesis which could result into oncogenesis. Finally, even if motor neurons could develop *in situ*, the prospect that they would at a meaningful level connect with the host CNS must be viewed as highly unlikely at this time.

b. **Modifying neuromuscular junctions through actin dynamics**: The pharmacological Rho-kinase inhibitor (downstream effector of RhoA-GTP which plays role in actin dynamics) dramatically increases the life span of a mild SMA mouse model and improves disease phenotype. This improvement in the disease phenotype is independent of SMN increase, mainly through making neuromuscular junctions (NMJ) better, larger and more mature [88]. This suggests that there are novel SMN independent avenues for the development of therapeutics for SMA.

10. Future directions

Combination therapy: The impressive results seen so far with gene therapy and ASO's in the field of SMA will be difficult to equal with a monotherapy approach. However, unless and until gene therapy and ASO treatments are cleared for clinical safety as a therapeutic option for SMA treatment, combinatorial approaches for SMA shall likely be necessary to target not only CNS but also other tissues which are affected because of a lack of SMN. As outlined above, SMA can be targeted through different approaches, we can in a safe combination use compounds which are already FDA approved and can increase SMN levels through *SMN2* gene activation (such as PRL) along with *SMN2* transcript stabilizers (p38 pathway activators such as celecoxib) and/or SMN protein stabilizer (proteasome inhibitor bortezomib) [18] and/or neuroprotective compounds (Rho kinase inhibitor) [19], or a cocktail of the best suitable combination of these compounds (Fig 5.1). I believe that this approach will speed up the

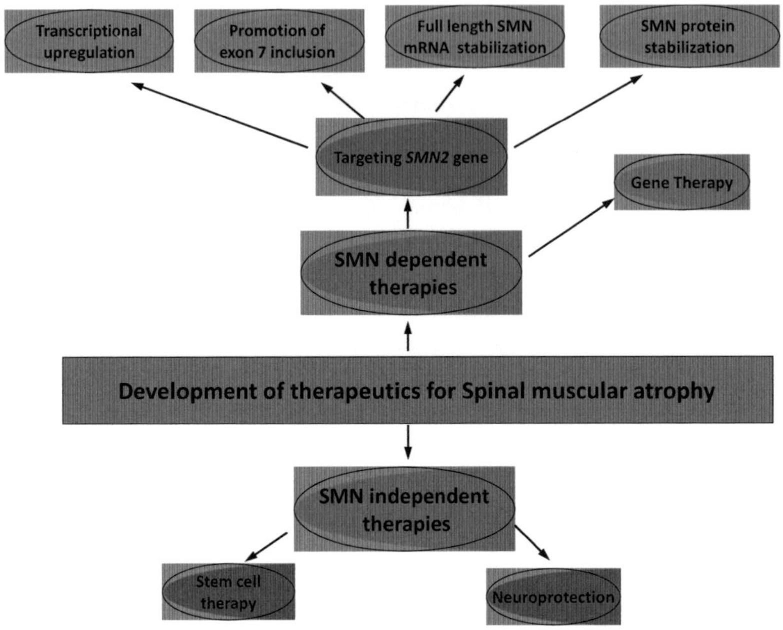

Figure 4. Development of therapeutics for SMA

process of finding the best possible and safest treatment of SMA. This approach is currently being assayed in our laboratory and others, showing some positive and promising results in the severe mouse model of the disease. More work is required to assess the potential drug interactions and their side effects in the animal models of the disease before pushing this approach for human clinical trials.

Designing clinical trials for SMA: In the last 5 years, a tremendous amount of promising translational work has been done using animal models of the SMA which is progressing rapidly towards the pre-clinical stage. However there are major challenges for designing a perfect clinical trial for SMA which includes 1) Variability of the disease phenotype, 2) lack of molecular biomarkers, 3) Accessibility of treatment centers and 4) lack of agreement for standard of care and disease management. However these issues are likely to be resolved as recently there has been a remarkable cooperation and collaboration between researchers, clinicians, industry, government and volunteer organizations which is bringing everyone on the same page to address these issues and reach a consensus for designing standard human clinical trials for SMA internationally.

Early intervention: New born screening: We and others have seen, irrespective of the modality, that early timing of the treatment is critical for maximum benefit in the mouse model of the disease. Presymptomatic identification of infants with SMA through new-born screening represents an important step in the effective treatment of SMA. In essence we shall need to intervene before the damage is done; to do so we need to rapidly identify infants with SMA, cases who will also serve as the best candidates to show the efficacy of promising therapeutic treatments in the near future. Children in which the disease has already progressed may also benefit with the use of best combinational approach, however the aim will be more towards ameliorating the disease progress and preserving the function of remaining motor neurons and other tissues rather than a complete reversal of the disease phenotype.

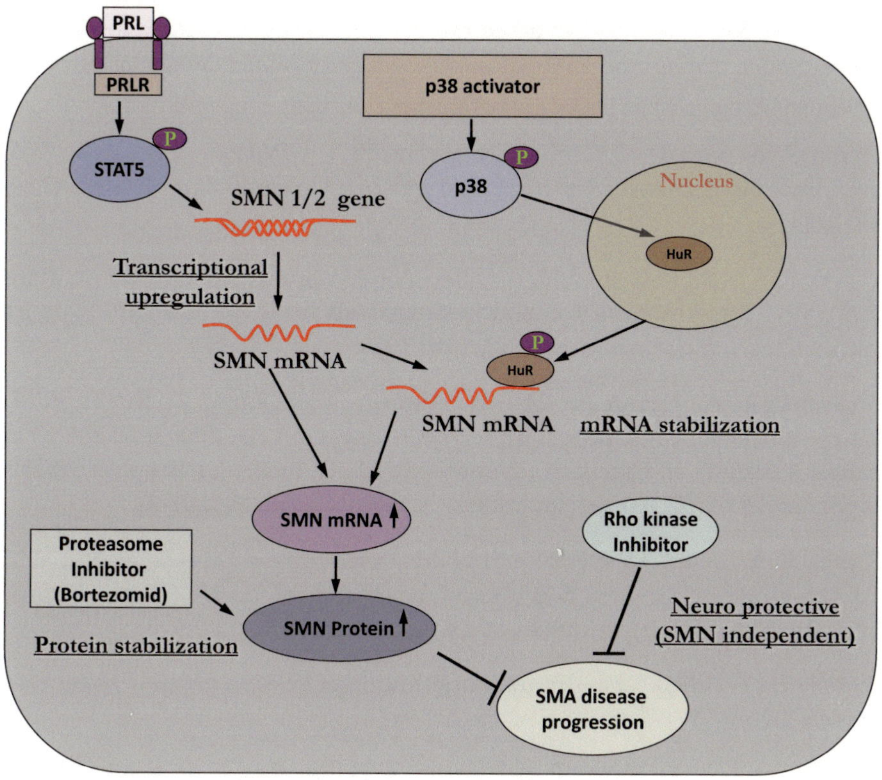

Figure 5. Proposed model of combination therapy for SMA treatment.

Author details

Faraz Tariq Farooq[1,2*], Martin Holcik[1,2] and Alex MacKenzie[1,2]

*Address all correspondence to: faraztfarooq@gmail.com

1 University of Ottawa, Ottawa, Canada

2 Apoptosis Research Center, CHEO Research Institute, CHEO, Ottawa, Canada

No conflicts of interest are reported.

References

[1] Pearn, J. (1978). Incidence, prevalence, and gene frequency studies of chronic childhood spinal muscular atrophy. J. Med. Genet. , 15, 409-413.

[2] Feldkotter, M, Schwarzer, V, Wirth, R, Wienker, T. F, & Wirth, B. (2002). Quantitative analyses of SMN1 and SMN2 based on real-time lightCycler PCR: fast and highly reliable carrier testing and prediction of severity of spinal muscular atrophy. Am. J. Hum. Genet. , 70, 358-368.

[3] Ogino, S, Leonard, D. G, Rennert, H, Ewens, W. J, & Wilson, R. B. (2002). Genetic risk assessment in carrier testing for spinal muscular atrophy. Am. J. Med. Genet. , 110, 301-307.

[4] Ogino, S, Wilson, R. B, & Gold, B. (2004). New insights on the evolution of the SMN1 and SMN2 region: simulation and meta-analysis for allele and haplotype frequency calculations. *Eur. J. Hum. Genet.* , 12, 1015-1023.

[5] Sugarman, E. A., Nagan, N., Zhu, H., Akmaev, V. R., Zhou, Z., Rohlfs, E. M., Flynn, K., Hendrickson, B. C., Scholl, T., Sirko-Osadsa, D. A., Allitto, B.A. 2012. Pan-ethnic carrier screening and prenatal diagnosis for spinal muscular atrophy: clinical laboratory analysis of >72,400 specimens. Eur. J. Hum. Genet. 20(1):27-32.

[6] Zerres, K, & Davies, K. E. (1999). th ENMC International Workshop: Spinal Muscular Atrophies: recent progress and revised diagnostic criteria 17-19 April 1998, Soestduinen, The Netherlands. *Neuromuscul. Disord.* , 9, 272-278.

[7] Dubowitz, V. (1995). Chaos in the classification of SMA: a possible resolution. *Neuromuscul. Disord.* , 5, 3-5.

[8] Iannaccone, S. T, Russman, B. S, Browne, R. H, Buncher, C. R, White, M, & Samaha, F. J. (2000). Prospective analysis of strength in spinal muscular atrophy. DCN/Spinal Muscular Atrophy Group. *J. Child Neurol.* , 15, 97-101.

[9] Wang, C. H, Finkel, R. S, Bertini, E. S, Schroth, M, Simonds, A, Wong, B, Aloysius, A, Morrison, L, Main, M, Crawford, T. O, et al. (2007). Consensus statement for standard of care in spinal muscular atrophy. *J. Child Neurol.* , 22, 1027-1049.

[10] Hagen, O, Glanzman, J. M, Mcdermott, A. M, Ryan, M. P, Flickinger, P. A, Quigley, J, Riley, J, Sanborn, S, Irvine, E, Martens, C, et al. (2007). An expanded version of the Hammersmith Functional Motor Scale for SMA II and III patients. *Neuromuscul. Disord.* , 17, 693-697.

[11] Thomas, N. H, & Dubowitz, V. (1994). The natural history of type I (severe) spinal muscular atrophy. *Neuromuscul. Disord.* , 4, 497-502.

[12] Zerres, K, Rudnik-schoneborn, S, Forrest, E, Lusakowska, A, Borkowska, J, & Hausmanowa-petrusewicz, I. (1997). A collaborative study on the natural history of child-

hood and juvenile onset proximal spinal muscular atrophy (type II and III SMA): 569 patients. *J. Neurol. Sci.* , 146, 67-72.

[13] Zerres, K, Wirth, B, & Rudnik-schoneborn, S. (1997). Spinal muscular atrophy--clinical and genetic correlations. *Neuromuscul. Disord.* , 7, 202-207.

[14] Prior, T. W, & Russman, B. S. (1993). Spinal Muscular Atrophy. In *GeneReviews.* R.A. Pagon, T.D. Bird, C.R. Dolan, and K. Stephens, editors. University of Washington, Seattle. Seattle (WA).

[15] Lefebvre, S, Burglen, L, Reboullet, S, Clermont, O, Burlet, P, Viollet, L, Benichou, B, Cruaud, C, Millasseau, P, & Zeviani, M. (1995). Identification and characterization of a spinal muscular atrophy-determining gene. *Cell* , 80, 155-165.

[16] Mahadevan, M. S, Korneluk, R. G, & Roy, N. MacKenzie, A., and Ikeda, J. (1995). SMA genes: deleted and duplicated. *Nat. Genet.* , 9, 112-113.

[17] Lorson, C. L, Hahnen, E, Androphy, E. J, & Wirth, B. (1999). A single nucleotide in the SMN gene regulates splicing and is responsible for spinal muscular atrophy. *Proc. Natl. Acad. Sci. U. S. A.* , 96, 6307-6311.

[18] Monani, U. R, Lorson, C. L, Parsons, D. W, Prior, T. W, Androphy, E. J, Burghes, A. H, & Mcpherson, J. D. (1999). A single nucleotide difference that alters splicing patterns distinguishes the SMA gene SMN1 from the copy gene SMN2. *Hum. Mol. Genet.* , 8, 1177-1183.

[19] Schrank, B, Gotz, R, Gunnersen, J. M, Ure, J. M, Toyka, K. V, Smith, A. G, & Sendtner, M. (1997). Inactivation of the survival motor neuron gene, a candidate gene for human spinal muscular atrophy, leads to massive cell death in early mouse embryos. *Proc. Natl. Acad. Sci. U. S. A.* , 94, 9920-9925.

[20] Simic, G. (2008). Pathogenesis of proximal autosomal recessive spinal muscular atrophy. *Acta Neuropathol.* , 116, 223-234.

[21] Murayama, S, Bouldin, T. W, & Suzuki, K. (1991). Immunocytochemical and ultrastructural studies of Werdnig-Hoffmann disease. *Acta Neuropathol.* , 81, 408-417.

[22] Pinter, M. J, Waldeck, R. F, Wallace, N, & Cork, L. C. (1995). Motor unit behavior in canine motor neuron disease. *J. Neurosci.* , 15, 3447-3457.

[23] Cork, L. C, Struble, R. G, & Gold, B. G. DiCarlo, C., Fahnestock, K.E., Griffin, J.W., and Price, D.L. (1989). Changes in size of motor axons in hereditary canine spinal muscular atrophy. *Lab. Invest.* , 61, 333-342.

[24] Kariya, S, Park, G. H, Maeno-hikichi, Y, Leykekhman, O, Lutz, C, Arkovitz, M. S, Landmesser, L. T, & Monani, U. R. (2008). Reduced SMN protein impairs maturation of the neuromuscular junctions in mouse models of spinal muscular atrophy. *Hum. Mol. Genet.* , 17, 2552-2569.

[25] Menke, L. A, Poll-the, B. T, Clur, S. A, Bilardo, C. M, Van Der Wal, A. C, Lemmink, H. H, & Cobben, J. M. (2008). Congenital heart defects in spinal muscular atrophy

type I: a clinical report of two siblings and a review of the literature. *Am. J. Med. Genet. A.* 146A:, 740-744.

[26] Rudnik-schoneborn, S, Heller, R, Berg, C, Betzler, C, Grimm, T, Eggermann, T, Eggermann, K, Wirth, R, Wirth, B, & Zerres, K. (2008). Congenital heart disease is a feature of severe infantile spinal muscular atrophy. *J. Med. Genet.* , 45, 635-638.

[27] Bevan, A. K, Hutchinson, K. R, Foust, K. D, Braun, L, Mcgovern, V. L, Schmelzer, L, Ward, J. G, Petruska, J. C, Lucchesi, P. A, Burghes, A. H, et al. (2010). Early heart failure in the SMNΔ7 model of spinal muscular atrophy and correction by postnatal scAAV9-SMN delivery. *Hum. Mol. Genet.* , 19, 3895-3905.

[28] Heier, C. R, Satta, R, & Lutz, C. and DiDonato, C.J. (2010). Arrhythmia and cardiac defects are a feature of spinal muscular atrophy model mice. *Hum. Mol. Genet.* , 19, 3906-3918.

[29] Shababi, M, Habibi, J, Yang, H. T, Vale, S. M, Sewell, W. A, & Lorson, C. L. (2010). Cardiac defects contribute to the pathology of spinal muscular atrophy models. *Hum. Mol. Genet.* , 19, 4059-4071.

[30] Williams, J. H, Schray, R. C, Patterson, C. A, Ayitey, S. O, Tallent, M. K, & Lutz, G. J. (2009). Oligonucleotide-mediated survival of motor neuron protein expression in CNS improves phenotype in a mouse model of spinal muscular atrophy. *J. Neurosci.* , 29, 7633-7638.

[31] Rudnik-schoneborn, S, Vogelgesang, S, Armbrust, S, Graul-neumann, L, Fusch, C, & Zerres, K. (2010). Digital necroses and vascular thrombosis in severe spinal muscular atrophy. *Muscle Nerve* , 42, 144-147.

[32] Araujo AdeQ., Araujo, M., and Swoboda, K.J. (2009). Vascular perfusion abnormalities in infants with spinal muscular atrophy. *J. Pediatr.* , 155, 292-294.

[33] Hua, Y, Sahashi, K, Rigo, F, Hung, G, Horev, G, Bennett, C. F, & Krainer, A. R. (2011). Peripheral SMN restoration is essential for long-term rescue of a severe spinal muscular atrophy mouse model. *Nature* , 478, 123-126.

[34] Liu, Q, & Dreyfuss, G. (1996). A novel nuclear structure containing the survival of motor neurons protein. *EMBO J.* , 15, 3555-3565.

[35] Zhang, H, Xing, L, Rossoll, W, Wichterle, H, Singer, R. H, & Bassell, G. J. (2006). Multiprotein complexes of the survival of motor neuron protein SMN with Gemins traffic to neuronal processes and growth cones of motor neurons. *J. Neurosci.* , 26, 8622-8632.

[36] Friesen, W. J, & Dreyfuss, G. (2000). Specific sequences of the Sm and Sm-like (Lsm) proteins mediate their interaction with the spinal muscular atrophy disease gene product (SMN). *J. Biol. Chem.* , 275, 26370-26375.

[37] Buhler, D, Raker, V, Luhrmann, R, & Fischer, U. (1999). Essential role for the tudor domain of SMN in spliceosomal U snRNP assembly: implications for spinal muscular atrophy. *Hum. Mol. Genet.* , 8, 2351-2357.

[38] Jones, K. W, Gorzynski, K, Hales, C. M, Fischer, U, Badbanchi, F, Terns, R. M, & Terns, M. P. (2001). Direct interaction of the spinal muscular atrophy disease protein SMN with the small nucleolar RNA-associated protein fibrillarin. *J. Biol. Chem.* , 276, 38645-38651.

[39] Meister, G, Buhler, D, Laggerbauer, B, Zobawa, M, Lottspeich, F, & Fischer, U. (2000). Characterization of a nuclear 20S complex containing the survival of motor neurons (SMN) protein and a specific subset of spliceosomal Sm proteins. *Hum. Mol. Genet.* , 9, 1977-1986.

[40] Mourelatos, Z, Abel, L, Yong, J, Kataoka, N, & Dreyfuss, G. (2001). SMN interacts with a novel family of hnRNP and spliceosomal proteins. *EMBO J.* , 20, 5443-5452.

[41] Narayanan, U, Achsel, T, Luhrmann, R, & Matera, A. G. (2004). Coupled in vitro import of U snRNPs and SMN, the spinal muscular atrophy protein. *Mol. Cell* , 16, 223-234.

[42] Pellizzoni, L, Baccon, J, Charroux, B, & Dreyfuss, G. (2001). The survival of motor neurons (SMN) protein interacts with the snoRNP proteins fibrillarin and GAR1. *Curr. Biol.* , 11, 1079-1088.

[43] Pellizzoni, L, Charroux, B, & Dreyfuss, G. (1999). SMN mutants of spinal muscular atrophy patients are defective in binding to snRNP proteins. *Proc. Natl. Acad. Sci. U. S. A.* , 96, 11167-11172.

[44] Pellizzoni, L, Charroux, B, Rappsilber, J, Mann, M, & Dreyfuss, G. (2001). A functional interaction between the survival motor neuron complex and RNA polymerase II. *J. Cell Biol.* , 152, 75-85.

[45] Fischer, U, Liu, Q, & Dreyfuss, G. (1997). The SMN-SIP1 complex has an essential role in spliceosomal snRNP biogenesis. *Cell* , 90, 1023-1029.

[46] Kariya, S, Mauricio, R, Dai, Y, & Monani, U. R. (2009). The neuroprotective factor Wld(s) fails to mitigate distal axonal and neuromuscular junction (NMJ) defects in mouse models of spinal muscular atrophy. *Neurosci. Lett.* , 449, 246-251.

[47] Hofmann, Y, Lorson, C. L, Stamm, S, Androphy, E. J, & Wirth, B. (2000). Htra2-beta 1 stimulates an exonic splicing enhancer and can restore full-length SMN expression to survival motor neuron 2 (SMN2). *Proc. Natl. Acad. Sci. U. S. A.* , 97, 9618-9623.

[48] Chen, H. H, Chang, J. G, Lu, R. M, Peng, T. Y, & Tarn, W. Y. (2008). The RNA binding protein hnRNP Q modulates the utilization of exon 7 in the survival motor neuron 2 (SMN2) gene. *Mol. Cell. Biol.* , 28, 6929-6938.

[49] Hofmann, Y, & Wirth, B. (2002). hnRNP-G promotes exon 7 inclusion of survival motor neuron (SMN) via direct interaction with Htra2-beta1. *Hum. Mol. Genet.* , 11, 2037-2049.

[50] Young, P. J. DiDonato, C.J., Hu, D., Kothary, R., Androphy, E.J., and Lorson, C.L. (2002). SRp30c-dependent stimulation of survival motor neuron (SMN) exon 7 inclusion is facilitated by a direct interaction with hTra2 beta 1. *Hum. Mol. Genet.* , 11, 577-587.

[51] Cartegni, L, & Krainer, A. R. (2002). Disruption of an SF2/ASF-dependent exonic splicing enhancer in SMN2 causes spinal muscular atrophy in the absence of SMN1. *Nat. Genet.* , 30, 377-384.

[52] Cartegni, L, & Krainer, A. R. (2003). Correction of disease-associated exon skipping by synthetic exon-specific activators. *Nat. Struct. Biol.* , 10, 120-125.

[53] Kashima, T, & Manley, J. L. (2003). A negative element in SMN2 exon 7 inhibits splicing in spinal muscular atrophy. *Nat. Genet.* , 34, 460-463.

[54] Mcandrew, P. E, Parsons, D. W, Simard, L. R, Rochette, C, Ray, P. N, Mendell, J. R, Prior, T. W, & Burghes, A. H. (1997). Identification of proximal spinal muscular atrophy carriers and patients by analysis of SMNT and SMNC gene copy number. *Am. J. Hum. Genet.* , 60, 1411-1422.

[55] Campbell, L, Potter, A, Ignatius, J, Dubowitz, V, & Davies, K. (1997). Genomic variation and gene conversion in spinal muscular atrophy: implications for disease process and clinical phenotype. *Am. J. Hum. Genet.* , 61, 40-50.

[56] Chang, J. G, Hsieh-li, H. M, Jong, Y. J, Wang, N. M, Tsai, C. H, & Li, H. (2001). Treatment of spinal muscular atrophy by sodium butyrate. *Proc. Natl. Acad. Sci. U. S. A.* , 98, 9808-9813.

[57] Sumner, C. J, Huynh, T. N, Markowitz, J. A, Perhac, J. S, Hill, B, Coovert, D. D, Schussler, K, Chen, X, Jarecki, J, Burghes, A. H, et al. (2003). Valproic acid increases SMN levels in spinal muscular atrophy patient cells. *Ann. Neurol.* , 54, 647-654.

[58] Brichta, L, Hofmann, Y, Hahnen, E, Siebzehnrubl, F. A, Raschke, H, Blumcke, I, Eyupoglu, I. Y, & Wirth, B. (2003). Valproic acid increases the SMN2 protein level: a well-known drug as a potential therapy for spinal muscular atrophy. *Hum. Mol. Genet.* , 12, 2481-2489.

[59] Tsai, L. K, Tsai, M. S, Ting, C. H, & Li, H. (2008). Multiple therapeutic effects of valproic acid in spinal muscular atrophy model mice. *J. Mol. Med. (Berl)* , 86, 1243-1254.

[60] Andreassi, C, Angelozzi, C, Tiziano, F. D, Vitali, T, De Vincenzi, E, Boninsegna, A, Villanova, M, Bertini, E, Pini, A, Neri, G, et al. (2004). Phenylbutyrate increases SMN expression in vitro: relevance for treatment of spinal muscular atrophy. *Eur. J. Hum. Genet.* , 12, 59-65.

[61] Swoboda, K. J, Scott, C. B, Reyna, S. P, & Prior, T. W. LaSalle, B., Sorenson, S.L., Wood, J., Acsadi, G., Crawford, T.O., Kissel, J.T. et al. (2009). Phase II open label study of valproic acid in spinal muscular atrophy. *PLoS One* 4:e5268.

[62] Garbes, L, Riessland, M, Holker, I, Heller, R, Hauke, J, Trankle, C, Coras, R, Blumcke, I, Hahnen, E, & Wirth, B. (2009). LBH589 induces up to 10-fold SMN protein levels by several independent mechanisms and is effective even in cells from SMA patients non-responsive to valproate. *Hum. Mol. Genet.* , 18, 3645-3658.

[63] Mercuri, E, Bertini, E, Messina, S, Solari, A, Amico, D, Angelozzi, A, Battini, C, Berardinelli, R, Boffi, A, Bruno, P, et al. (2007). Randomized, double-blind, placebo-controlled trial of phenylbutyrate in spinal muscular atrophy. *Neurology* , 68, 51-55.

[64] Avila, A. M, Burnett, B. G, Taye, A. A, Gabanella, F, Knight, M. A, Hartenstein, P, & Cizman, Z. Di Prospero, N.A., Pellizzoni, L., Fischbeck, K.H. et al. (2007). Trichostatin A increases SMN expression and survival in a mouse model of spinal muscular atrophy. *J. Clin. Invest.* , 117, 659-671.

[65] Narver, H. L, Kong, L, Burnett, B. G, Choe, D. W, Bosch-marce, M, Taye, A. A, Eckhaus, M. A, & Sumner, C. J. (2008). Sustained improvement of spinal muscular atrophy mice treated with trichostatin A plus nutrition. *Ann. Neurol.* , 64, 465-470.

[66] Riessland, M, Ackermann, B, Forster, A, Jakubik, M, Hauke, J, Garbes, L, Fritzsche, I, Mende, Y, Blumcke, I, Hahnen, E, et al. (2010). SAHA ameliorates the SMA phenotype in two mouse models for spinal muscular atrophy. *Hum. Mol. Genet.* , 19, 1492-1506.

[67] Powe, C. E, Allen, M, Puopolo, K. M, Merewood, A, Worden, S, Johnson, L. C, Fleischman, A, & Welt, C. K. (2010). Recombinant human prolactin for the treatment of lactation insufficiency. *Clin. Endocrinol. (Oxf)* , 73, 645-653.

[68] Farooq, F, Molina, F. A, & Hadwen, J. MacKenzie, D., Witherspoon, L., Osmond, M., Holcik, M., and MacKenzie, A. (2011). Prolactin increases SMN expression and survival in a mouse model of severe spinal muscular atrophy via the STAT5 pathway. *J. Clin. Invest.* , 121, 3042-3050.

[69] Andreassi, C, Jarecki, J, Zhou, J, Coovert, D. D, Monani, U. R, Chen, X, Whitney, M, Pollok, B, Zhang, M, Androphy, E, et al. (2001). Aclarubicin treatment restores SMN levels to cells derived from type I spinal muscular atrophy patients. *Hum. Mol. Genet.* , 10, 2841-2849.

[70] Singh, N. N, Singh, R. N, & Androphy, E. J. (2007). Modulating role of RNA structure in alternative splicing of a critical exon in the spinal muscular atrophy genes. *Nucleic Acids Res.* , 35, 371-389.

[71] Singh, N. N, Shishimorova, M, Cao, L. C, Gangwani, L, & Singh, R. N. (2009). A short antisense oligonucleotide masking a unique intronic motif prevents skipping of a critical exon in spinal muscular atrophy. *RNA Biol.* , 6, 341-350.

[72] MacKenzieA. (2012). Sense in antisense therapy for spinal muscular atrophy. *N. Engl. J. Med.* , 366, 761-763.

[73] Singh, J, Salcius, M, Liu, S. W, Staker, B. L, Mishra, R, Thurmond, J, Michaud, G, Mattoon, D. R, Printen, J, Christensen, J, et al. (2008). DcpS as a therapeutic target for spinal muscular atrophy. *ACS Chem. Biol.* , 3, 711-722.

[74] Farooq, F, Balabanian, S, Liu, X, & Holcik, M. and MacKenzie, A. (2009). Mitogen-activated protein kinase stabilizes SMN mRNA through RNA binding protein HuR. *Hum. Mol. Genet.* 18:4035-4045., 38.

[75] Heier, C. R. and DiDonato, C.J. (2009). Translational readthrough by the aminoglycoside geneticin (G418) modulates SMN stability in vitro and improves motor function in SMA mice in vivo. *Hum. Mol. Genet.* , 18, 1310-1322.

[76] Mattis, V. B, Rai, R, Wang, J, Chang, C. W, Coady, T, & Lorson, C. L. (2006). Novel aminoglycosides increase SMN levels in spinal muscular atrophy fibroblasts. *Hum. Genet.* , 120, 589-601.

[77] Wolstencroft, E. C, Mattis, V, Bajer, A. A, Young, P. J, & Lorson, C. L. specific requirement for SMN protein activity: the role of aminoglycosides in inducing elevated SMN protein levels. *Hum. Mol. Genet.* , 14, 1199-1210.

[78] Kwon, D. Y, Motley, W. W, Fischbeck, K. H, & Burnett, B. G. (2011). Increasing expression and decreasing degradation of SMN ameliorate the spinal muscular atrophy phenotype in mice. *Hum. Mol. Genet.* , 20, 3667-3677.

[79] Foust, K. D, Wang, X, Mcgovern, V. L, Braun, L, Bevan, A. K, Haidet, A. M, Le, T. T, Morales, P. R, Rich, M. M, Burghes, A. H, et al. (2010). Rescue of the spinal muscular atrophy phenotype in a mouse model by early postnatal delivery of SMN. *Nat. Biotechnol.* , 28, 271-274.

[80] Passini, M. A, Bu, J, Roskelley, E. M, Richards, A. M, Sardi, S. P, Riordan, O, Klinger, C. R, Shihabuddin, K. W, Cheng, L. S, & Cns-targeted, S. H. gene therapy improves survival and motor function in a mouse model of spinal muscular atrophy. *J. Clin. Invest.* , 120, 1253-1264.

[81] Valori, C. F, Ning, K, Wyles, M, Mead, R. J, Grierson, A. J, Shaw, P. J, & Azzouz, M. (2010). Systemic delivery of scAAV9 expressing SMN prolongs survival in a model of spinal muscular atrophy. *Sci. Transl. Med.* 2:35ra42.

[82] Dominguez, E, Marais, T, Chatauret, N, Benkhelifa-ziyyat, S, Duque, S, Ravassard, P, Carcenac, R, Astord, S, De Moura, A. P, Voit, T, et al. (2011). Intravenous scAAV9 delivery of a codon-optimized SMN1 sequence rescues SMA mice. *Hum. Mol. Genet.* , 20, 681-693.

[83] MacKenzieA. (2010). Genetic therapy for spinal muscular atrophy. *Nat. Biotechnol.* , 28, 235-237.

[84] Corti, S, Nizzardo, M, Nardini, M, Donadoni, C, & Salani, S. Del Bo, R., Papadimitriou, D., Locatelli, F., Mezzina, N., Gianni, F. et al. (2009). Motoneuron transplantation rescues the phenotype of SMARD1 (spinal muscular atrophy with respiratory distress type 1). *J. Neurosci.* , 29, 11761-11771.

[85] Corti, S, Nizzardo, M, Nardini, M, Donadoni, C, Salani, S, Ronchi, D, Simone, C, Falcone, M, Papadimitriou, D, Locatelli, F, et al. (2010). Embryonic stem cell-derived neural stem cells improve spinal muscular atrophy phenotype in mice. *Brain* , 133, 465-481.

[86] Dimos, J. T, Rodolfa, K. T, Niakan, K. K, Weisenthal, L. M, Mitsumoto, H, Chung, W, Croft, G. F, Saphier, G, Leibel, R, Goland, R, et al. (2008). Induced pluripotent stem cells generated from patients with ALS can be differentiated into motor neurons. *Science* , 321, 1218-1221.

[87] Ebert, A. D, Yu, J, & Rose, F. F. Jr, Mattis, V.B., Lorson, C.L., Thomson, J.A., and Svendsen, C.N. (2009). Induced pluripotent stem cells from a spinal muscular atrophy patient. *Nature* , 457, 277-280.

[88] Bowerman, M, Beauvais, A, Anderson, C. L, & Kothary, R. (2010). Rho-kinase inactivation prolongs survival of an intermediate SMA mouse model. *Hum. Mol. Genet.* , 19, 1468-1478.

Chapter 24

Pharmacological Treatment of Acute Ischemic Stroke

Humberto Mestre, Yael Cohen-Minian,
Daniel Zajarias-Fainsod and Antonio Ibarra

Additional information is available at the end of the chapter

http://dx.doi.org/10.5772/53774

1. Introduction

Cerebral infarction, generally referred to as stroke for practical purposes henceforth, is a medical emergency that generates severe neurological deficits while compromising cardiovascular and respiratory function. Each year approximately 795,000 people experience a new or recurrent stroke. This disease can be differentiated into two subcategories: hemorrhagic and ischemic. The ischemic subgroup is responsible for up to 87% of all strokes [1]. This pathology is of critical importance to healthcare professionals due to the fact that every 40 seconds someone in the United States suffers a stroke [2]. Moreover, it is the fourth leading cause of death in the US where 1 in every 18 deaths are stroke-related [2]. However, the mortality rate of stroke is relatively low at 8.1% according to the most recent accepted statistics [2]. In consequence, stroke is the leading cause of disability in the United States. Besides the direct effect that stroke has on the economy (US $18.8 billion), it will indirectly generate an expenditure of US $2.21 trillion from now until 2050, on account of loss of earnings resulting from the 26% of patients who suffer from a stroke that require assistance with activities in daily living or institutionalization in nursing homes [2]. The epidemiological and economic impact that stroke has on society demands the development of an effective treatment strategy during the acute ischemic phase. Current therapies have been primarily aimed at the four cornerstones of acute ischemic stroke (AIS): (1) the prevention and treatment of secondary complications; (2) reperfusion strategies directed at arterial recanalization; (3) neuroprotective strategies aimed at cellular and metabolic targets; and (4) the inhibition or modulation of the inflammatory response. To date, the mainstay of treatment is arterial recanalization with recombinant tissue plasminogen activator (rtPA), in conjunction with the early onset of an aspirin regimen. It must be noted, however, that the great majority of stroke patients are not eligible for thrombolysis with only around 5% receiving rtPA [3-5]; mainly because the use of intravenous rtPA has many contraindications, a limited time window, and a moderate success rate. Most patients presenting to hospital stroke units have either a contraindication to rtPA therapy (e.g. a bleeding diathesis, recent surgery, etc.) or, more commonly, are no longer within the time frame for thrombolytic therapy. Although many initiatives to find therapies that will target the other facets of AIS have been undertaken, most have failed. One area of particular interest is that of neuroprotection. Several attempts to generate a neuroprotective drug that will reduce ischemia-associated destruction of neuronal tissue improving the general outcome after AIS have had dismal results. These drugs display a formidable benefit during the animal model phase of research but have been unable to reproduce this effect in human clinical trials. These interventions are aimed at treating stroke in its acute phases and preventing sequels that will result in permanent disability. The ideal treatment of AIS begets a multistep approach: necessary due to the fact that the pathophysiology of stroke is multi-mechanistic. This work will present the current status of drug therapy in AIS and analyze the direction in which the field is moving. The aim of this review is to guide the reader through a general panorama of interventional pharmacological treatment of AIS.

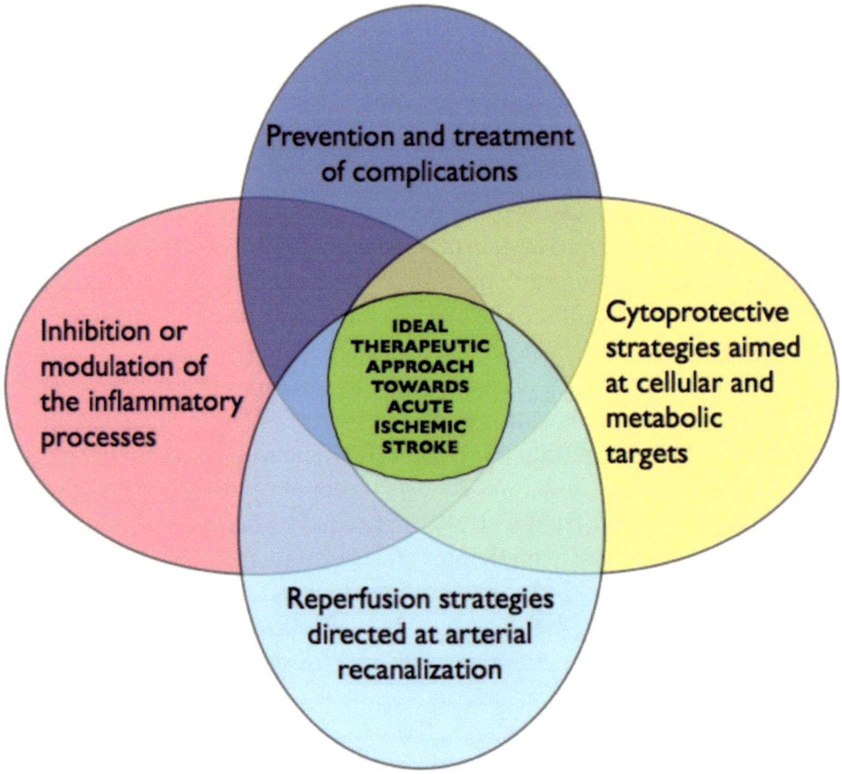

Figure 1. Schematic visualization of the ideal therapeutic approach towards AIS. Due to the notorious failure of interventional stroke research throughout the years it is essential for the field to reboot its attempts and abandon the search for dubiously named "wonder drugs". The optimal treatment for AIS will lie on effective prevention and if the pathology cannot be prevented it will depend on an integral management. This therapeutic strategy must incorporate and address all of the cornerstones of AIS.

2. Etiology

Stroke is not only a multifactorial disease but also a gamma of different pathologies with markedly varied etiology that manifest themselves in a clinically similar way. For this reason, the accurate diagnosis of the stroke patient involves not only differentiating a stroke from other diseases with comparable clinical features, but also determining the type of stroke and its etiology.

Stroke can be classified as ischemic or hemorrhagic. The latter implies the rupture of intracranial vessels leading, in a very generalized sense, to mass effect, compression, and inflammation leading to neuronal death. The present chapter will be devoted entirely to the pathology that is an acute ischemic stroke (AIS) and the treatment guidelines currently in use as well as novel science in this field. In an effort to appropriately describe the etiology of AIS it is first necessary to explain the different origins of the ischemia, namely: cardioembolic, atheroembolic, atherothrombotic and miscellaneous.

Cardioembolic stroke is the most common and is characterized by the formation of a clot within the cardiac chambers that is ejected and travels peripherally where it finally encounters and lodges in a vessel of sufficiently small caliber obstructing blood flow distally. These emboli are due to numerous pathologies however, the great majority, approximately 75%, are due to atrial fibrillation (AF) [6]. Patients with AF have increased blood residence time in the left atrium; in those who are not adequately anticoagulated, platelet aggregation and coagulation may occur within the atrium. Typically, when a patient with AF is cardioverted to sinus rhythm the ejection fraction from the atria improves substantially increasing the probability that an existing latent thrombus may be expelled into the aorta. Since the common carotid arteries—and consequently the internal carotid arteries—are the most direct path, these emboli usually travel into the cerebral vasculature where, upon obstructing irrigation to brain tissue, cause an acute ischemic stroke. Other, less typical, causes of cardioembolic stroke include emboli originating from thrombi forming on prosthetic or diseased heart valves, cardiac myxomas, vegetations secondary to infectious endocarditis, among others, as well as the direct shunting of venous thrombi to the systemic arterial vasculature by means of a patent foramen ovale.

Although, atheroembolic stroke has a clinical picture akin to that of cardioembolic stroke, the etiology is substantially different. Patients with atheromatous plaques in the ascending aorta, the arteries of the head and neck, or its tributaries, have damaged and reactive endothelial cells in these vessels with exposed tissue factor, etc. This predisposes to the formation of unstable thrombi in these regions. In certain circumstances, particularly during a valsalva maneuver—usually associated with exertion or straining—the friable thrombus fractures releasing an embolus which travels upstream and becomes embedded in the cerebral vasculature. Likewise, atheromatous plaques may rupture releasing a gelatinous cholesterol based substance, which can also cause the embolization of the smaller arteries supplying the brain. Atheroembolic stroke is particularly common in patients with dyslipidemias and is associated with low levels of high-density lipoprotein (HDL) and high levels of low-density lipoproteins (LDL).

In contrast, atherothrombotic stroke predominates in those with dyslipidemia and comorbid pathologies including systemic arterial hypertension and diabetes mellitus. In both diseases affliction of the smaller cerebral vessels beyond the first bifurcations after the circle of Willis is more common rather than before the anastomosis at the same level as is typical of dyslipidemias. Arterial hypertension causes damage to the endothelium and also hypertrophy of the medial muscular layer of the vessels leading to marked stenosis. Conversely, diabetes leads to angiopathy of both the macrovasculature and microvasculature [7]. Although the microvascular disease associated with hyperglycemia is a recognized factor in the development of generalized brain ischemia it is a chronic degenerative disease rather than a precipitant of acute ischemia. The macrovascular pathology associated with diabetes is less well understood; notwithstanding, the correlation between increased stroke risk and diabetes mellitus is quite established. The mechanism is believed to be multifactorial, probably due to the associated metabolic syndrome, which involves the triad of dyslipidemia, hyperglycemia and hypertension leading to endothelial dysfunction, hypercoagulability and atheroma: all significant stroke factors [8]. The clinical picture of atherothrombotic stroke is gradual in stark contrast to embolic-type stokes and is characterized by repeated transient ischemic attacks (TIAs). The pathogenesis involves the gradual development of atheromatous plaques in the medium calliber arteries of the cerebral vasculature, namely the anterior cerebral, the middle cerebral and the posterior cerebral arteries. Thrombus formation takes place in these dysfunctional vessel walls and the lumen becomes reduced. It is unlikely that the lumen will become completely obliterated through this process, however the unstable thrombus often shifts, briefly obstructing the irrigation upstream leading to a TIA or a stroke in progress. Eventually the obstruction is longer lasting leading to widespread or more permanent damage characteristic of a completed stroke.

It is worth mentioning a fourth miscellaneous category, which groups all other causes of ischemic stroke. Among the notable causes are dissections of neck or thoracic arteries leading to a loss of perfusion to the brain. Moreover, pulmonary thrombosis similarly obstructs blood return to the left heart and leads to brain ischemia. Non-thrombotic emboli, such as air, fat or of tumoral origin can likewise lead to an AIS. These causes are relatively rare and together account for less than 5% of AIS; nevertheless, the clinician should always consider investigating these as plausible causes when determining the origin of an atypical case [2]. The present review shall, nonetheless omit further reference to miscellaneous causes of stroke.

Due to the marked difference in etiology and pathogenesis of these first three types of AIS, it is wise to emphasize the necessity of an accurate diagnosis in order to specifically target therapy to the cause of the stroke in an effort to minimize tissue damage and reduce the risk of further strokes.

3. Risk factors

As previously mentioned AIS is a multifactorial and polycausative pathology and as such, various factors interact to increase the risk of a stroke. However, research in this field has led to the statistical determination of the influence of some of the most common risk factors in an effort to prevent this all-too-common disease. Systemic arterial hypertension (HTN) is a well-recognized factor leading to stroke and is associated with a two-fold lifetime risk of stroke. However, clarification of this statistic is necessary as HTN, although a strong risk factor for ischemic atherothrombotic stroke as mentioned above, is more often linked to hemorrhagic type strokes. Heart arrhythmias such as AF in particular, have a relative risk for stroke of 5 and thus account for the great majority of cardioembolic stroke with nearly 25% of all strokes in 80-year olds and above being attributable to AF [2]. Smoking is perhaps the most important modifiable risk factor. Smokers are two to four times more likely to suffer a stroke, not to mention have a higher morbidity and mortality rate than non-smokers after a stroke [2]. Moreover, the risk is dose dependent and upon cessation of smoking the risk rapidly falls and after 20 years the risk is nearly that of a person who has never smoked [2]. Additionally, a sedentary lifestyle is associated with a relative risk for stroke of around 3 in contrast to a relative risk of less than 1 for persons who regularly exercise [2]. Other somewhat modifiable risk factors include metabolic disorders: dyslipidemias being a major contributor to stroke risk as the promote the formation of atheroma and cause hematologic disturbances. Diabetes mellitus—with its associated complications—obviously contributes and is a major risk factor; sleep apnea has a two-fold to four-fold risk of stroke depending on the severity of the apnea [2].

Clearly, having knowledge of these risk factors is important when making an effort directed at eliminating risk factors or reducing their impact as a means of prevention

4. Pathophysiology

The core of AIS pathophysiology is the complete interruption of cerebral blood flow (CBF) leading to energy depletion and oxygen starvation with necrotic neuronal death within the first couple of minutes. Modern day therapeutic strategies are aimed at arterial recanalization in order to reestablish CBF. This rapid return to normal CBF is the turning point in salvaging the surrounding tissue of the focal necrotic core. This area lies above the threshold of cell death and below functional levels of CBF, and is commonly known as the penumbra. The penumbra is the principal target of all pharmacological treatments in AIS. The goal of AIS therapeutics is a strategy that will encompass the four cornerstones previously mentioned. The first step depends on the prompt diagnosis of AIS and the treatment aimed at preventing and treating secondary complications of the disease. The second is a fast and effective recanalization of the occluded vessel (i.e. thrombolysis) in order to ameliorate the hypoperfusion of the penumbra. Drugs that target arterial recanalization have the goal of quickly reestablishing CBF and alleviating this area of ischemia allowing the tissue to return to homeostasis. Third, are specific neuroprotective strategies that will intervene in the apoptotic cascade, excitotoxicity, reactive oxygen species (ROS) production and lipid peroxidation further protecting the ischemic tissue or reversing its damage. This branch of interventional AIS research is aimed at discovering compounds that will allow the neural tissue to better survive this period of limited oxygen and nutrients. The fourth and final step is to modulate the inflammatory response to abolish the deleterious effects of unrestrained inflammation. This section will briefly delineate the most characteristic mechanisms of AIS pathophysiology in order to allow the reader to integrate the mechanisms of action and therapeutic targets of each drug.

Immediately after CBF is interrupted, cells continue to need a constant supply of energy in the form of adenosine triphosphate (ATP). The lack of perfusion decimates the concentration of molecular oxygen forcing the cell to divert energy production from classic aerobic cellular respiration towards anaerobic ATP synthesis (Figure 2A). This alternate metabolic route poses several detriments when compared to homeostatic energy production: firstly, this pathway results in a decrease in the yield of ATP per glucose molecule and, secondly, it creates lactic acid as byproduct. The changes brought about by the energetic deficit and the shift in pH cause energy-dependent ion channels to dysfunction [9]. The loss of ionic interchange alters the cells polarity and inherently affects voltage-dependent mechanisms [10]. One such voltage-dependent process is neurotransmitter release, particularly glutamate. This excitatory neurotransmitter is highly abundant in the central nervous system and is the ligand for the *N*-methyl-D-aspartate (NMDA), 2-amino-3-(3-hydroxy-5-methyl-isoxazol-4-yl) propanoic acid (AMPA) and kainate receptors [10]. After AIS the loss in ionic regulation causes the excessive release of glutamate and impairs its reuptake: a process known as excitotoxicity [11]. The pathway through which glutamate mediates this cytotoxic effect is mediated by calcium ions. The binding of glutamate to its receptors activates the influx of calcium ions into the neuron [12]. The increasing concentration of calcium ions, act as second messengers and overloads the cell by activating intracellular phospholipases, nucleases and proteases. This battery of enzymes degrades essential structures including the cell membrane, DNA, and intracellular proteins [13]. Additionally, the disruption of the ionic gradient of extracellular sodium to intracellular potassium, which relies on ATP-dependent channels, causes changes in the osmotic potential of the cell. The influx of water causes lysis and cytotoxic edema; this reduces the size of the extracellular space and accounts for some of the edema seen after stroke [13]. This state of stress results in the overactive production of ROS which overloads the cell's antioxidant enzymes such as superoxide dismutase and the antioxidant vitamins A and E [14]. The inability to cope with the increased concentration of free radicals causes lipid peroxidation of the cell membrane [15]. The ROS-mediated destruction of the cell membrane further damages the cell and releases phospholipids into the microenvironment that act as precursors in the production of arachidonic acid, which is further transformed into a variety of signaling molecules [16]. Most notably, prostaglandins and leukotrienes are produced, which are responsible for initiating the inflammatory response. The presence of ROS within the cell also opens the mitochondrial permeability transition pore (MPTP), which allows the escape of cytochrome C, a powerful trigger of apoptosis [17]. Other clinically relevant mechanisms of degeneration are the activation of poly-ADP-ribose polymerase (PARP) [18] and cortical spreading depression (CSD) [19]. When talking about AIS, there exists a secondary cascade of degenerative effects known as reperfusion injury (Figure 2D). We recommend referring to the provided source for a complete understanding of this phenomenon as it relates to arterial recanalization [20]. The compound effect of this degenerative cascade that take place after AIS results in the necrosis or apoptosis of the neuronal population within the penumbra in addition to the already irreversably damaged necrotic core.

http://dx.doi.org/10.5772/53774

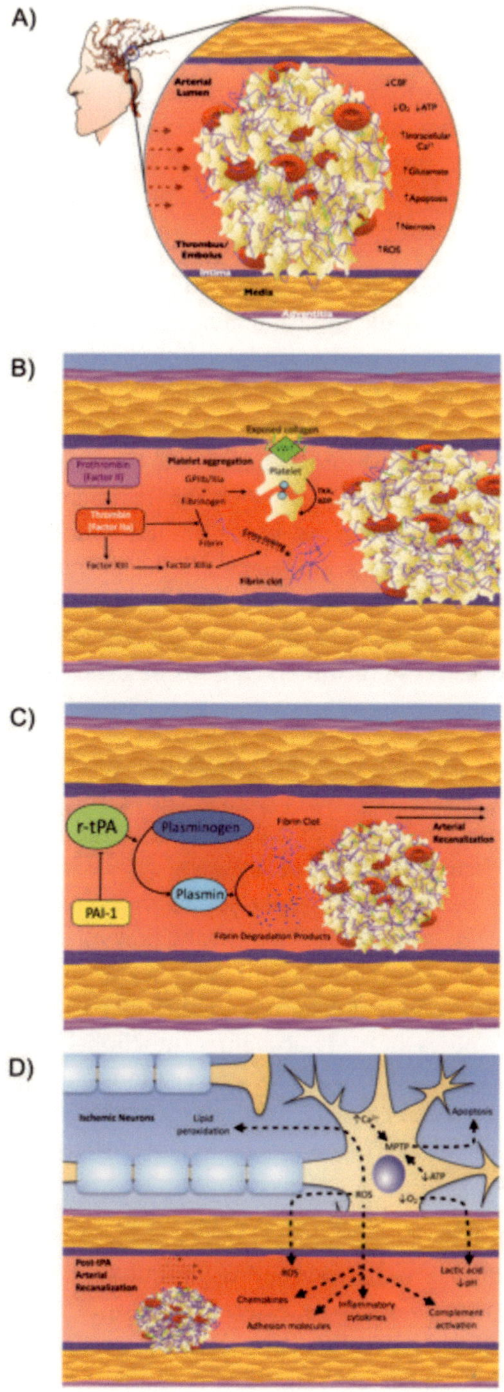

Figure 2. A) The pathophysiology of stroke; B) The formation of the thrombus/embolus; C) The mechanism of action of tPA; D) Reperfusion injury.

5. Methodology

The goal of this review is threefold: the first is to clarify for the modern day clinician the accepted stroke treatment guidelines currently in effect; the second is to analyze all clinical trials that have concluded or are still underway; and the third is to analyze animal model studies that have promising results using novel agents that have not been evaluated in a clinical setting.

The systematic review had rigorous search criteria. Firstly, a review of all the accepted guidelines was used to determine the clinical management of AIS. The latest guidelines were published in 2007-2008 and remain in effect today due to the lack of an updated revision. The guidelines that dictate the integral treatment of patients with AIS are those compiled by the American Heart Association (AHA) in 2007, the European Stroke Organisation (ESO) Executive Committee and the National Institute of Health and Clinical Excellence (NICE) of the UK completed in 2008. The latest systematic review on the treatment of AIS were published in by the American College of Chest Physicians and is limited to antiplatelet and antithrombotic management. To facilitate the readers' understanding of current drug therapy in AIS, only recommendations with a level of evidence A-B and a class of I-II were included. In no way does this study substitute the necessity to review the guidelines for the management of AIS in a clinical setting, nor should these recommendations be used in contradiction to nationally accepted practices or hospital protocol.

In order to compile all clinical trials underway, a thorough search of the U.S. National Institutes of Health clinical trial database (www.clinicaltrials.gov), the Internet Stroke Center Trial Registry (www.strokecenter.org/trials/) and the World Health Organization's International Clinical Trials Registry Platform Search Portal (www.apps.who.int/trialsearch/) was undertaken. Due to the nature of the review, only pharmacological interventional randomized controlled trials (RCT) were considered; this meant that all cell-based and physical (this includes cryotherapy and electrical stimulation) therapies were excluded. Other criteria used to refine the search were: trials that had not published preliminary results or had been prematurely terminated, studies that did not evaluate functional outcome, the lack of statistical significance against a placebo or control group, interventions outside the acute setting or those that treated complications of AIS. To aid in the usefulness of this review, the studies excluded by the previous criteria will be briefly mentioned in table format.

The third step consisted of searching for basic experimental research used in animal models of AIS. A computerized search of the National Library of Medicine and the National Institutes of Health MEDLINE database was performed using PubMed. Only published literature in English from 2008 to 2012 was taken into consideration seeing as it was deemed chronologically relevant. Since the objective of this literature revision decided to include only the most promising therapies a strict exclusion criteria was drafted. Parameters of exclusion were studies not performed in *in vivo* models, that had no functional outcome analysis, that did not achieve a $P < 0.05$, that used pre-AIS treatment strategies and that used an invasive administration route that would deem it clinically unfeasible.

http://dx.doi.org/10.5772/53774

The organizational presentation of all existing and potential AIS treatments will help the field by allowing the researcher to see what has and what hasn't been done while introducing the most cutting edge therapies already being studied.

6. Current treatment guidelines

In order to clarify this for the scientific community a systematic review of the existing literature on the pharmacological treatment of AIS is presented below and, in an effort to facilitate the application of the current guidelines in the clinical setting, a treatment algorithm summarizing these recommendations is provided (Figure 3).

Currently the medical treatment approach of AIS focuses on the treatment of the immediate acute phase in an effort to reduce the progression of the ischemia, followed simultaneously by an attempt at revascularization and reperfusion of the brain parenchyma. Further treatment includes the reduction of the damage and neuronal cell death caused by the ischemia and subsequent metabolic cascade brought about by the abrupt reperfusion. This involves the use of neuroprotective strategies and a pharmacological approach to reducing the inflammatory response. Finally, treatment focuses on rehabilitation and retarding the progression of the vascular disease as well as prevention of further strokes. To understand the medical treatment strategies described above, following is provided a detailed description of the pharmacological agents that are used in the treatment of AIS and the science behind these choices of medications.

7. Thrombolysis

The pinnacle of stroke therapy is without doubt thrombolysis and is rapidly becoming the gold-standard treatment in AIS. The NINDS rtPA Stroke Study compared the use of intravenous rtPA given within three hours after stroke onset versus placebo [21]. The rtPA-treated group showed a significant neurological improvement when compared to the untreated group. Despite a greater incidence of intracranial hemorrhage in the treatment group, both treatments exhibited similar survival at three months. This expedited the approval of this therapy by the US Food and Drug administration in 1996.

Recombinant tPA (rtPA) is a genetically synthesized tPA molecule that works in precisely the same way as endogenous tPA. It catalyzes the cleavage of the zymogen plasminogen to yield the active enzyme plasmin. Plasmin in turn is responsible for the degradation of the interlinked fibrin monomers that make up the fibrin clot into soluble products. Endogenous tPA is usually present in relatively small amounts and regulates the breakdown of fibrin plugs in vessels and keeps coagulation in check. In turn, plasminogen activator inhibitor 1 (PAI-1) regulates the activation of tPA, thus hindering the degradation of the fibrin clot. However, when rtPA is administered by infusion, there is insufficient PAI-1 to control the action of tPA, hence activated plasmin is produced in sufficient quantities to breakdown existing fibrin clots (Figure 2C). Perhaps paradoxically, rtPA has been shown to induce fibrinogen binding of platelets and platelet aggregation. Although thromboxanes were not shown to increase significantly in one study, it is logical to assume that adjunctive therapy with antiplatelet agents such as aspirin or some of the more novel drugs is a sensible approach to preventing rethrombosis after rtPA therapy [22]. Another study showed that rtPA does in fact activate platelets but then in turn is also responsible for inhibiting aggregation [23]. A more recent review on the subject concludes that therapies should consider protecting from extensive activation of platelets after tPA therapy [24].

According to all the recently published major guidelines, intravenous (IV) rtPA thrombolysis is highly recommended in all eligible patients. The criteria for eligibility are however long and strict which accounts for less than 10% of patients being eligible for IV thrombolysis with rtPA. These criteria are summarized in Table 1 in Figure 3. Treatment should be started less than 3 hours from the onset of stroke symptoms, however the guidelines provided by the American College of Chest Physicians recommend against the use of IV rtPA when infusion cannot be started before 4.5 hours have transpired since symptom onset. This left a gray zone between 3 and 4.5 hours in which the benefit of using IV rtPA may, in most cases, outweigh the risks; nevertheless, the evidence for this was not sufficiently strong for a fervent recommendation to be made. Most recently, a study by a science advisory from the American Stroke Association has declared that after reviewing the data from the ECASS-3 trial, sufficient evidence had mounted to make a full recommendation for the use of IV rtPA if therapy was started within 4.5 hours of symptom onset [25].

Therapy with rtPA is given at a dose of 0.9 mg/kg IV without exceeding a maximum dose of 90 mg with 10% given as a loading bolus over 1 minute and the remainder as an infusion over 60 minutes. During the infusion and for one hour after concluding the infusion, the patient's vital signs should be monitored and neurological assessment done every 15 minutes. Thereafter, observations should be carried out every 30 min for the next 6 hours and hourly afterward until 24 hours have transpired since treatment.

Additionally, fibrinolytic therapy can be administered by the intra-arterial (IA) route directly to the artery occluded by the thrombus. This however requires that the center have cerebral angiography equipment and highly trained interventional neuroradiologist to carry out this procedure. The use of IA rtPA therapy is recommended for patients who are no longer eligible for IV infusion of rtPA due to the time-window restraints but are still within the 6-hour cutoff time for IA treatment. Also, patients who are excluded from IV rtPA due to contraindications such as recent surgery may be eligible for IA treatment instead in the case of occlusion of the middle cerebral artery (MCA) or another proximal cerebral artery. Nevertheless, IA therapy should not be considered an alternative to IV infusion when patients are eligible for the latter [26,27]. The combination of IV/IA rtPA therapy is not recommended [25].

8. Antiplatelet therapy

Due to the thrombotic origin of AIS and the involvement of platelet aggregation in the development of said thrombus, antiplatelet drugs play an obvious and pivotal role in the medical treatment. Perhaps the most widely used antiplatelet agent is non-steroidal anti-inflammatory drugs (NSAID) acetylsalicylic acid, commonly referred to as aspirin, and its many derivatives. Although both historically and currently used as an anti-inflammatory drug, aspirin at low doses is an avid inhibitor of platelet aggregation. The mechanism of action of this medication is as dependent on its pharmacokinetics as its pharmacodynamics. As an anti-inflammatory, aspirin must become distributed within the tissues and inside intracellular compartment in order to effectively block the cyclooxygenases (COX) and thus the synthesis of prostaglandins. This necessitates higher dosages in order to achieve a sufficiently high concentration that falls within the therapeutic window. Conversely, in order to function as a platelet anti-aggregant, aspirin requires significantly lower doses as it must only become distributed within the intravascular compartment—in fact only in the portal circulation thus being independent of systemic bioavailability. Needless to say, aspirin at anti-inflammatory doses achieves a therapeutic effect on platelet binding, however, at antiplatelet doses aspirin has a minimal effect on tissue cyclooxygenase and in consequence the adverse effects of NSAID therapy on the gastric mucosa.

Aspirin binds and inhibits the platelet COX-1 irreversibly and consequently impairs the production of prostaglandins and thromboxanes, noting thromboxane A_2 (TXA_2) in particular. The absence of TXA_2 leads to the reduction in the TXA_2-mediated amplification of platelet activation and thus hinders the platelet aggregation phenotype that includes morphological changes and expression of the fibrinogen receptor necessary for platelet aggregation. Nevertheless, numerous other pathways for platelet activation exist, such as those mediated by thrombin and epinephrine that can sufficiently promote the active phenotype and lead to platelet plug formation in the vessel wall when subendothelial collagen and von Willebrand factor (vWf) are exposed (Figure 2C).

Low-dose (50 – 100 mg daily) aspirin is prescribed typically as a prophylactic in the prevention of cardiovascular and cerebrovascular disease. Taken daily, it effectively reduces platelet efficiency despite adequate platelet concentration in the full blood count. Due to the irreversible inactivation of platelet enzymes, adequate platelet function is only restored upon production of new platelets after halting aspirin treatment. Since platelets have an average lifespan of 10 days it is estimated that 10% of platelets are replaced every day; moreover for proper hematological function it is required that approximately 20% of platelets be functional. Thus, normal blood clotting is achieved two days after discontinuing a low-dose aspirin regimen. Although high-dose aspirin (above 300 mg daily) provides a similar inhibition time window of platelet function and recovery after cessation of treatment; nonetheless, the incidence of gastrointestinal adverse effects (i.e. gastritis) is much higher than on low-dose aspirin. However, if the formulation of high-dose aspirin includes an enteric coating, the therapeutic time window and recovery are significantly prolonged. This effect however is not seen with enteric-coated low-dose aspirin.

The role of aspirin in the prophylaxis of ischemic cerebrovascular events and stroke is well accepted. Numerous studies and systematic reviews have shown a highly significant risk reduction (13%) in the incidence of AIS when daily low-dose aspirin is taken without a greatly significant increase in the incidence of hemorrhagic complications including stroke [28].

Despite the well-recognized use of aspirin in prevention, its use in the initial treatment of AIS is somewhat contested. According to the AHA Guidelines for the early management of adults with ischemic stroke (2007), although aspirin therapy immediately after an AIS is not standard, starting aspirin within 48 hours of the onset of symptoms is routine in many centers and according to studies poses "a modest but statistically significant benefit" [26]. Most recently, in 2012, the American College of Chest Physician published a revised set of guidelines in which starting aspirin at doses of between 160 and 325 mg daily within 48 hours of the onset of symptoms is recommended [27]. The general consensus is that an initial 325 mg dose of aspirin should be given to most patients suffering from a stroke or TIA within 24 hours of the onset of stroke or as early as possible, but not before 24 hours have transpired since thrombolytic therapy, except when contraindicated by evidence of intracranial hemorrhage, bleeding diathesis, recent surgery and sensitivity to aspirin, among others. After the initial loading dose, subsequent daily low-dose aspirin might be more adequate than the higher dose as there is no evidence suggesting that the higher dose provides better protection from further strokes while there is an associated higher risk of intracranial bleeding with the chronic use of high-dose aspirin therapy in comparison with low-dose therapy.

The use of other antiplatelet medication such as clopidogrel, ticlopidine and dipyridamole has not been as formally evaluated in trials, as has aspirin. The routine use of these drugs is not recommended, however it is reasonable to suggest the use of, for example, clopidogrel at an initial dose of 300 mg, as it will efficiently inhibit platelet aggregation, when aspirin is not tolerated by the patient [29]. Likewise, a subsequent daily dose of 75 mg of clopidogrel will maintain platelet aggregation at bay. Furthermore, the guidelines provided by the American College of Chest Physicians recommend the use of aspirin in combination with dipyridamole or clopidogrel over aspirin therapy alone [27].

9. Anticoagulant therapy

Anticoagulants are a heterogeneous group of pharmacological agents that by interacting with the coagulation cascade disrupt the formation of the fibrin mesh that forms the scaffold of the clot. When in homeostasis, the blood elements that participate in this process are kept at check thus preventing the formation of a blood clot *in situ*, or thrombus, inside the blood vessels. Although a comprehensive review of the coagulation cascade would be beyond the scope of this text some knowledge is prerequisite in order to adequately comprehend the pharmacology of these drugs. In simplistic terms, coagulation is activated by two somewhat distinct processes that ultimately lead to a common pathway that results in the activation of prothrombin to thrombin, which in turn converts fibrinogen to fibrin and the formation of the clot thereof. The extrinsic pathway involves the rapid activation of the cascade when clotting factors are exposed to tissue factor (TF) after damage of the vessel endothelium. Alternatively, the intrinsic, or contact activation pathway is triggered by the formation of cascade complexes on collagen after tissue damage. This leads to the eventual activation of the common pathway, although experts now believe that the action of TF is required for the adequate amplification and eventual formation of the thrombus [30]. Anticoagulants interfere with the cascade in

http://dx.doi.org/10.5772/53774

distinct ways: the coumarinic anticoagulants like warfarin inhibit phylloquinone (Vitamin K) epoxide reductase and as a consequence render useless the clotting factors II, VII, IX and X that depend on Vitamin K as a cofactor. This action can be assessed by measuring the action of the extrinsic pathway by means of the time required for coagulation after addition of TF *in vitro* a test known as the prothrombin time (PT) or its normalized equivalent to normal values, the international normalized ratio (INR). Conversely, heparin, another common anticoagulant with numerous variants, activates antithrombin and hence inactivates thrombin and halts coagulation at its final stages. Similarly, this is measured *in vitro* by the activated partial thromboplastin time test, which evaluates the efficiency of the contact activation pathway. Prolongation of the normal times in both instances is interpreted as impaired coagulation.

As with antiplatelet therapy, a distinction between the use of anticoagulants for the prevention of AIS or TIA and that of anticoagulation as a means of treatment in the initial stages post-AIS must be made. Likewise, the incidence of an early recurrence of stroke is considered a complication of AIS and although technically speaking anticoagulants are prescribed prophylactically for this reason, this is considered a standard treatment in the acute phase of stroke and not actual preventive therapy. The use of anticoagulants in the prevention of AIS is beyond the scope of this review, however it must be noted that their use is widespread and is generally accepted. The use of oral coumarinics, such as warfarin, in the prevention of complications of atrial fibrillation such as AIS is common practice.

On the other hand, the use of anticoagulants in the first stages of AIS has been tried with little success. Both the International Stroke Trial and the consensus panel assembled by the National Institute of Neurological Disorders and Stroke (NINDS) recommend against the use of anticoagulants such as heparin within 24 hours of treatment with rtPA [26,27]. This is due to the marked increase in symptomatic intracranial hemorrhage seen in the trials testing anticoagulants for AIS. Additional trials testing the benefits of other anticoagulants yielded less than acceptable results for the low-molecular weight (LMW) heparins dalteparin (compared to aspirin), certoparin, nadroparin and danaparoid [31]. The outcome was particularly dire for those with moderate to severe strokes (National Institutes of Health Stroke Scale (NIHSS) scores of ≥15). One trial did however show that heparin administered with the first 3 hours after the onset of stroke improved the outcome significantly. However, since the time-window for the treatment is similar to that of rtPA it is necessary to compare these treatment options, as the concomitant use is not an option. Currently no anticoagulant is recommended in the treatment of the acute stages of AIS nevertheless, there is an interest in the development of a safe anticoagulant that can be co-administered with thrombolytics in order to reduce the risk of re-thrombosis. Additionally, coumarinics have not been tested for use in the acute treatment of stroke as these are mainly oral agents and are therefore reserved for long-term treatment such as in prophylaxis of first or subsequent events. Patients with cardioembolic stroke need to receive oral prophylactic anticoagulation particularly when associated with AF. Initiation must be delayed to avoid the risk of intracranial bleeding: patients with mild stroke or TIA (NIHSS scores of ≤10) may be started on warfarin, or newer agents such as dabigatran, titrating dose to an INR between 2.0 and 3.0 after 48 hours if there is no contraindication. Patients with moderate to severe strokes should not receive anticoagulants after 2 to 4 weeks have elapsed [32].

10. Neuroprotective therapy

Despite widespread interest in this field and the amount of published studies, none have passed clinical trials with the same observable effect seen in animal models. The AHA guideline published in 2007 deemed that at present there are no neuroprotective agents that have shown to reduce tissue damage and improve the neurological outcome of AIS. The committee determined the inexistence of a potential neuroprotective drug with a Class III, Level of Evidence A [26]. Up till now, the recommendations have not changed. Clinical and/or federal authorities have not approved the use of any neuroprotective compound in the management of AIS. The main reason for the inability of these drugs to produce a marked benefit in clinical trials when they are so successful in animal models remains elusive; however in the coming sections several limitations will be described.

11. The state of current science

Drug discovery in the area of interventional AIS research is one of the largest fields in science. Everyday thousands of papers are published trying new or old compounds with a variety of different analysis techniques. The search criteria for this review returned 20,416 papers that commented on possible therapeutic pharmacological interventions in AIS. The exclusion criterion that was employed drastically reduced the database of studies; however the result was still 213 different treatments that are currently being investigated. In order to make this review of greater value only the treatments that have been evaluated by several groups and are closer to the clinic have been included. The following are the most remarkable pharmacological agents currently being considered as treatment for AIS. However, so that the review does not lose the general panorama, several tables have been elaborated in order for the reader to have easy access to supplementary information if necessary.

12. Thrombolytics

The elevated risk of complications after administration of tPA such as hemorrhagic transformation has triggered the search for safer fibrinolytics. Desmoteplase is a plasminogen activator isolated from the saliva of bats. It is currently undergoing clinical trials because it has proven to be more fibrin-selective than recombinant tPA. The secondary effects of tPA such as neurotoxicity and inducing the dysfunction of the blood-brain barrier (BBB) are also bypassed with desmoteplase. The Desmoteplase in Acute Ischemic Stroke (DIAS) trials are now in their third and fourth session and they are ongoing (DIAS 3 and 4). Preliminary results suggest that

http://dx.doi.org/10.5772/53774

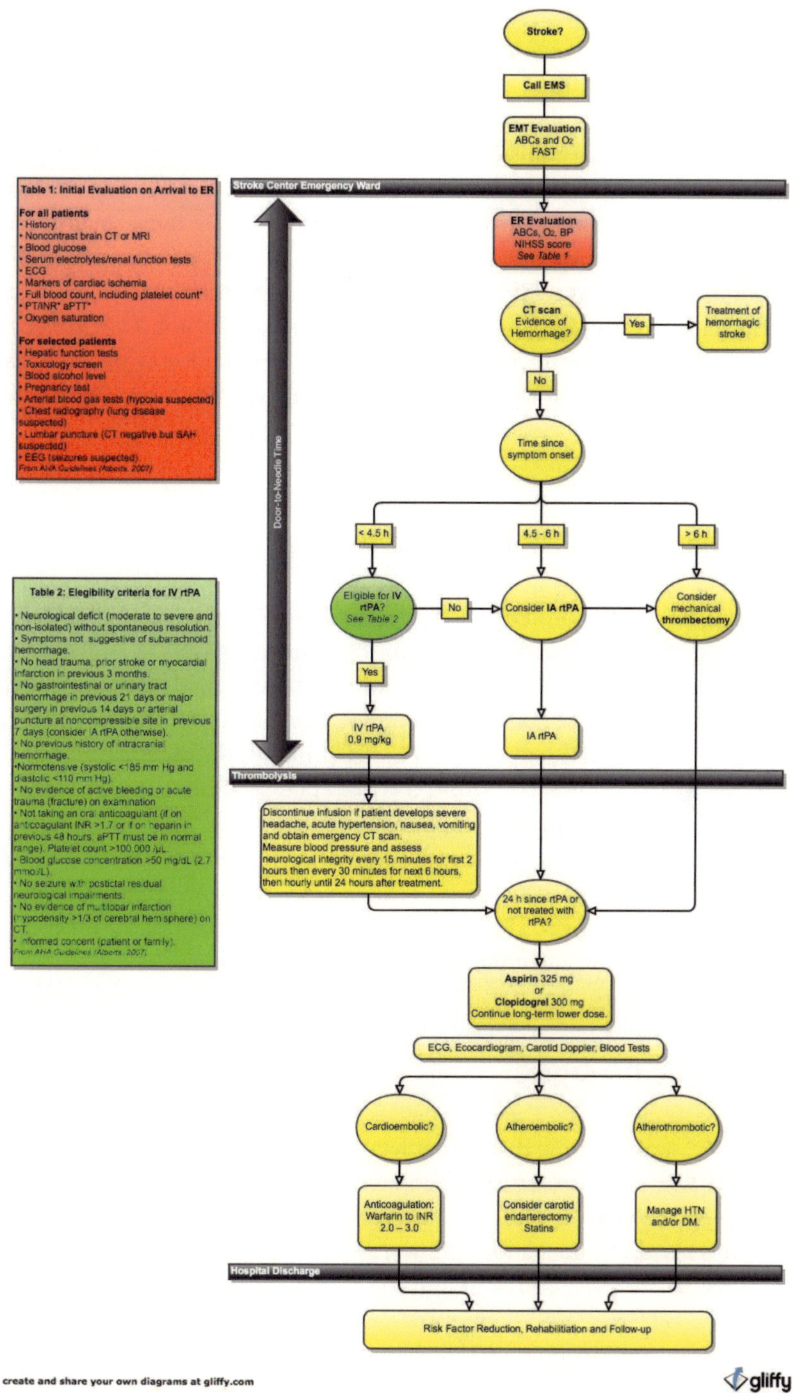

Figure 3. Treatment algorithm for AIS.

desmoteplase was associated with higher percentages of recanalization and neurological outcomes against a placebo. However, the therapeutic window being evaluated is 3-9 hours, highly similar to tPA [33]. Tenecteplase is a recombinant protein designed from the alteplase molecule, but it is modified at three sites. These modifications make it more fibrin-specific as opposed to tPA and targets the plasminogen within the thrombus allowing for more localized fibrinolysis. The clinical trials for this compound have been slow and mostly terminated, only arriving to phase II. Preliminary results did not yield convincing data compared to controls [34]. There are many limitations to thrombolytic therapy and these mainly reside in the hemorrhagic complications they may cause. The purpose of these is to reestablish CBF by means of arterial recanalization with the goal of saving the penumbra. An interesting alternative to this is mechanical thrombectomy but pharmacological thrombolytics should further be sought because they do not require a highly specialized team and may be administered in the emergency ward. These characteristics have made and continue making thrombolytics a promising area of research.

13. Combination therapies with thrombolytics

Thrombus formation depends on the function of several platelet surface proteins and blood-borne proteins (Figure 2B). A particularly important glycoprotein is IIb/IIIa, which aids in platelet aggregation. To optimize the function of fibrinolysis with tPA and further prevent thrombus formation, a combination scheme with GP IIb/IIIa inhibitors after administration of tPA was started. The Combined Approach to Lysis Utilizing Eptifibatide and rTPA (CLEAR) trial evaluated the use of eptifibatide within the therapeutic window of tPA. The preliminary data suggested that rtPA alone further improved the functional outcome as compared to the combination. The trial was restructured and is now in phase II, known as CLEAR-ER [35]. Other compounds that display synergistic effects with rtPA are matrix metalloproteinase inhibitors, free radical scavengers, NMDA receptor antagonists, AMPA receptor antagonists, antioxidants, anti-inflammatory agents, and antiplatelet drugs [93].

14. Antithrombotic therapies

Drugs that are aimed at preventing the further formation of thrombi are called antithrombotics. Ancrod is isolated from the venom of a pit viper [36]. This molecule degrades fibrinogen instead of fibrin as opposed to thrombolytics. Another example of a fibrinogen-depleting agent is an enzyme found also in snake venom known as batroxobin. Both of these agents have been taken to clinical trials with dismal results. In the preliminary results of ancrod in the Stroke Treatment with Ancrod Trial (STAT) it was suggested that there was a marked reduction in the frequency of symptomatic intracerebral hemorrhage in the group treated with ancrod. A revision of this trial was held by the European STAT database and they concluded that the study showed a lack of efficacy as it did not improve the outcome when administered 6 hours after symptom onset. Batroxobin trials concluded that it could effectively reduce the risk of recurrent stroke in patients with hyperfibrinogemia [37]. The true potential of fibrinogen-depleting agents has yet to be seen, but for now they are not considered a promising therapy.

15. Neuroprotection

15.1. Metal chelators

The prolyl hydroxylase inhibitor, deferoxamine mesylate is also an iron ion chelator. This molecule prevents the formation of hydroxyl radicals by neutralizing the reactive iron ions. It also upregulates and stabilizes the transcriptional activator hypoxia-inducible factor-1 (HIF-1) which is responsible for the transcription of several survival genes. The chelator is being studied in the Membrane-Activated Chelator Stroke Intervention (MACSI) trial and has had positive preliminary results [38]. Another metal chelator is DP-b99, which chelates zinc ions. Increased concentrations of zinc are known to be neurotoxic and it is also a cofactor in many degenerative processes. It is currently being studied alongside deferoxamine in the MACSI phase III trial with a intravenous administration route [39].

15.2. Growth factors

Erythropoyetin (EPO), a 30-kDa glycoprotein that is in charge of erythropoiesis by means of proliferation, maturation and survival of erythroid progenitor cells [40], was able to reduce infarct volumes and improve motor and memory functions, in rodent models of focal cerebral ischemia. A meta-analysis on the subject suggests that higher doses of EPO are linked to smaller infarct volumes and significant improvement of limb function; however, the effects are time-dependant, having almost no effect on infarct volume and limb function when administered 6 hours after stroke onset [41]. In addition, EPO was able to increase actively proliferating oligodendrocyte progenitor cells in the peripheral white matter zones and in the subventricular zone 7 days after stroke onset, but was unable to prevent the loss of myelinating oligodendrocytes. Nonetheless, a significant rise in myelinating oligodendrocytes and myelinated axons in the peripheral white matter area was observed 28 and 42 days after stroke onset and an improved recovery was also seen in a 6 week long time period, therefore increasing EPO's potential as a therapeutic agent in stroke [42]. On the other hand, Neuro-EPO, a nonerythropoietic variant of EPO, emerges as a potential therapeutic agent for stroke. Contrary to EPO, Neuro-EPO has the advantage of being available in an intranasal absorption route, has a short plasma half-life due to its low sialic acid content, and lacks erythropoietic activity [43]. Rodriguez-Cruz and colleagues, achieved a higher neuroprotective effect with intranasal Neuro-EPO, than the one obtained after intraperitoneal injection of EPO in gerbil models of stroke; this was evidenced by a better neurological state and functional cognitive improvement, as well as a protection of the temporal cortex, thalamus and the CA3 region of the hippocampus [44]. Immunoglobulin G-EPO (IgG-EPO) fusion protein is another re-engineered form of EPO that is fused to a heavy chain of a chimeric monoclonal antibody that is directed against the mouse transferring receptor. This form of EPO is able to easily penetrate the BBB when compared to original EPO and showed to reduce the hemispheric stroke volume 81% and the neural deficit 78% when administered in high doses (1.0 mg/kg) [45].

Granulocyte colony-stimulating factor was able to enhance not only leptomeningeal collateral growth in an ischemic stroke model, but also circulating blood monocytes and effectively reduced the infarct volume [46]. Granulocyte macrophage colony-stimulating factor (GM-CSF), has obtained similar results as the above when evaluated in adult mice models of cerebral ischemia [47]. A 6-week treatment with GM-CSF accomplished a complete recovery of cerebral blood flow and cerebrovascular capacity together with integrity of hippocampal hypoxia-vulnerable neurons in rat models of ischemia; a significantly higher number of arterioles in parenchymal and leptomeningeal regions were also observed [48].

15.3. Immunomodulators

Copolymer-1 (Cop-1) is a synthetic copolymer that suppresses encephalitogenic processes through an immunological cross-reactivity with myelin basic protein (MBP) [49]. Cop-1, also known as glatiramer acetate or its brand name Copaxone, has been FDA-approved for its use in multiple sclerosis and has shown neuroprotective effects in immune-based neurological pathologies [50] such as stroke. Cop-1 has been able to induce an environment with an adequate balance of Th1 and Th2 that tend to protect the brain tissue. The modulation of innate immunity, blockage of antigen presentation by MHC molecules and T cell receptor antagonism have also been proposed as probable neuroprotective mechanisms [51, 52]. Rina Aharoni and co-workers demonstrated infiltrating Th 2/3 cells' ability to induce an important expression of both neurotrophic factors, such as brain-derived neurotrophic factor (BDNF), and the potent anti-inflammatory cytokines, interleukin-10 (IL-10) and transforming growth factor β (TGFβ), by Cop-1-specific T cells *in situ*. All of these molecules play an important role on the protective and regenerative effects of Cop-1 [49]. Cop-1's action in cerebral ischemia was evaluated by our group in a transient MCAO model. Results showed a significant reduction in percentage of infarct volume, significant improvement on neurological recovery and higher tissue preservation when compared to control groups [53]. Cop-1's ability of acting on various mechanisms that present themselves after ischemic insult makes it a strong therapy to be used in stroke [54, 55]. The supporting evidence that has been obtained with the use of Cop-1 calls for more investigation in order to evaluate its overall potential. Poly-YE is a high molecular weight copolymer that has shown to have the ability of downregulating regulatory T cell activity and stimulating γδ T cells *in vitro* [56]. Poly-YE was used in an ischemic stroke model to enhance a spontaneous response of effector T cells recognizing antigens. In this study poly-YE not only generated a better clinical and behavioral outcome, but also induced neuroprotection and increased neurogenesis in the hippocampus and cerebral cortex. The beneficial effects in this study were observed even with administration of poly-YE up to 24 hours after ischemic stroke [57]. The long therapeutic window makes poly-YE a potential candidate for clinical use, however further research is needed. T cell-based therapeutic vaccination with MBP-derived peptides with attenuated pathogenic properties has also been proven effective in spinal cord injury in rats [58]. Recently; the neuroprotective effect of agents that stimulate toll-like receptor 9 (TLR9), such as K-type cytosine-guanine-rich DNA oligonucleotides was

http://dx.doi.org/10.5772/53774

Drug	Target	Phase	Name
Albumin	Hemodilution	III	Albumin in Acute Stroke (ALIAS)
Ancrod	Fibrinolytic	III	Stroke Treatment with Ancrod Trial (STAT)
Citicoline	Stabilizes membrane	III	ICTUS Study: International Citicoline Trial on Acute Stroke
Deferoxamine mesylate	Chelates iron molecules	II	-
Desmoteplase	Fibrinolytic	II	The Desmoteplase in Acute Ischemic Stroke Trial (DIAS)
DP-b99	Chelates metal ions	II	The Membrane-Activated Chelator Stroke Intervention (MACSI)
Ebselen	Free radical scavenger	III	-
Edaravone (MCI-186)	Free radical scavenger	III	-
Eptifibatide	Gp IIb/IIIa inhibitor	I/II	Study of the Combination Therapy of rt-PA and Eptifibatide to Treat Acute Ischemic Stroke (CLEAR-ER)
GM-CSF (Filgrastim)	Growth factor	II	AXIS 2: AX200 for the treatment of ischemic stroke
hCG (NTx-265)	Growth factor	II	-
Insulin	Glucose-lowering Hormone	III	-
Lovastatin	HMG CoA reductase inhibitor (statin)	II	Neuroprotection with Statin Therapy for Acute Recovery Trial (NeuSTART) I and II
Magnesium sulfate	NMDA cannel antagonist	III	The Field Administration of Stroke Therapy-Magnesium (FAST-MAG)
Minocycline	Antibiotic and antiapoptotic properties	III	Neuroprotection With Minocycline Therapy for Acute Stroke Recovery Trial (NeuMAST) and Minocycline to Improve Neurologic Outcome in Stroke (MINOS)
MLC601/901 (NeuroAiD™)	Nine herbal and five animal components	III	CHInese Medicine NeuroAid Efficacy on Stroke Recovery (CHIMES)
NXY-059 (Cerovive™)	Free radical scavenger	IIb/III	Stroke Acute Ischemic NXY-059 Treatment (SAINT) III.
Simvastatin	HMG CoA reductase inhibitor (statin)	III	-
Tenecteplase	Fibrinolytic	II	-

Table 1. Active Neuroprotection Clinical Trials

reported. These compounds induce tolerance (precondition) to ischemic brain injury. The beneficial effects of this therapy have been shown in both mice and nonhuman primate models of stroke [59]. Although further evaluation is needed, TLR9 agonists can be a possible strategy for stroke.

Tirilazad	Neurotrophins	Calpain inhibitors
Glutamate antagonists	Barbiturates	Gangliosides
Beta adrenergic receptor blockers	Aminophylline	Vasopressors
Anti-ICAM antibodies	Lubeluzole	Fosphenytoin
Basic Fibroblast Growth Factor	Enlimomab	Glycine antagonists
Naftidrofuryl	Nimodipine	Prostacyclins
Neutrophil inhibiting factor	Flunarizine	Opioid antagonists

Table 2. Neuroprotective drugs that have been clinically tested and have failed to improve AIS outcome

15.4. Free radical scavengers

Antioxidant nitrone-derived free radical trapping agents have lately received attention due to their therapeutic benefit [60]. The Stroke-Acute Ischemic NXY Treatment (SAINT-I) study, used NXY-059, in a phase 3 clinical trial and found this agent to reduce disability at 90 days when administered within 6 hours of stroke onset, but failed to markedly improve neurological functioning [61]. Nonetheless, the SAINT-II trial, a larger trial that sought to support SAINT-I trial results, concluded that NXY-059 is ineffective for acute ischemic stroke when administered 6 hours after onset [62]. Despite the stated, studies have shown that NXY-059, when administered 4 hours after stroke onset, was able to reduce BBB permeability, which is damaged by the ischemic insult. Reestablishing the BBB helps restore the brain endothelium and ameliorate endothelium-induced damage [63]. Moreover, NXY-059 was shown to be neuroprotective and safe in acute stroke patients at higher concentrations than the used in experimental models when administered 4 hours after insult [64]. NXY-059 is a potential stroke therapy agent but needs to go through further investigations that will help define its therapeutic window and dose regimens. NOX4 is a nicotinamide adenine dinucleotide phosphate (NADPH) oxidase type 4 that plays an important role in oxidative stress generation in cerebral ischemia; such action was supported when a significant improvement of long-term neurological outcome and reduced mortality was achieved when a NOX4 inhibitor, VAS2870, was applied several hours after ischemia induction. Effects were as protective as NOX4 deficient mice, further supporting their protective potential [65].

Agent	Mechanism of action	Reference
Glutamate oxaloacetate transaminase	Intravascular catabolic enzyme of glutamate	[66]
Prostaglandin E1	Antiapoptotic properties	[67]
Lithium	Antiapoptotic properties	[68]
Sigma-1 receptor agonists	Inhibition of inducible nitric oxide synthase	[69]
Fingolimod (FTY720)	Sphingosine-1-phosphate receptor agonist	[70, 71]
Opioid receptor agonists (Biphalin)	Inhibits postsynaptic potentials by lowering presynaptic Ca^{2+}	[72]
Cinnamophillin	Thromboxane A_2 receptor antagonist	[73]
Hawthorn extract	Antioxidant properties by incrementing glutathione levels	[74, 75]
Dichlorobenzamil	Sodium and/or calcium exchanger inhibitor	[76]
Cilostazol	Inhibitor of type III phosphodiesterase, antiplatelet agent	[77]
Magnesium sulfate	Inhibits the release of excitatory neurotransmitters	[78, 79]
Arundic acid (ONO-2506)	Astrocyte-modulating agent, inhibits S-100b protein synthesis	[80]
Repinotan	Serotonin or 5-Hydroxytryptophan (5-HT) 1A receptor agonist	[81]
Pioglitazone	Peroxisome proliferator-activated receptor (PPAR)-γ agonist	[82]
NADPH oxidase type 4 (NOX4) inhibitor	Inhibits enzyme that is major source of oxidative stress	[65]
C-Phycocyanin	Antioxidant	[83]
Ginsenoside Rd (*Panax ginseng*)	Antioxidant and anti-inflammatory	[84]
MFG-E8	Lactadherin glycoprotein that exerts tissue protection	[85]
YC-1	Hypoxia-inducible factor (HIF-1) inhibitor	[86]
Gelsolin	Actin- and calcium-binding protein	[87]

Table 3. Promising agents that are currently searching for clinical trial approval

16. Conclusion

16.1. Failure of clinical trials

Current science has very little to offer in the treatment of AIS. The guidelines available to the practicing clinician are limited and largely antiquated. The reason why these have not changed in the last 30 years is primarily because the field has made very little progress. This is not to say that the scientific community has stopped the search for an integral therapy for ischemic stroke, but there seems to be an error in translation. The main mistakes lie in the experimental model of stroke and the study design of both the preclinical and clinical phases of research.

16.2. Comorbidities

Adapting animal models to fit the human paradigm is an essential part of methodological design. However, these always seem to have limitations. Studies are designed to use young healthy animals from a homogenous population. However, in the clinical setting this is exactly the opposite. The population of individuals who suffer stroke are much older and almost all have comorbidities that either triggered the stroke (e.g. AF), or worsen the outcome (e.g. diabetes mellitus).

16.3. Stroke types

The research model of stroke that is most commonly used is middle cerebral artery occlusion (MCAo) with a filament; this model better represents ischemia-reperfusion after thrombolysis. The onset of stroke is carefully monitored and the duration of ischemia is also controlled. The reproducibility of a MCA ischemic stroke of the same duration across the study population provides for an incredibly standard sample size. The onset of AIS is highly variable with occlusion occurring in any vessel of both anterior and posterior circulation. Added to the variability in the type of stroke there are also differences in the anatomical conformation of the brain in rodents to humans. Humans have about 50% white matter and rodents have 10% [3, 88]. The majority of neuroprotective drugs are aimed at saving the neuronal soma, which constitutes the grey matter. In human studies many patients have a high frequency of sub-cortical damage and diffuse white matter ischemic lesions. This may suggest that grey matter-targeted neuroprotection benefits rodent brains more than it would a human. Attempt to neutralize this have been made by recent publications. The study used gyrencephalic non-human primates, which have the most similar cerebral structure to humans [89].

16.4. Reperfusion

As mentioned above, the model that is predominately used is MCAo. This model includes reperfusion after a time of ischemia; better emulating arterial recanalization after treatment with tPA. However, only about 2 to 5 % of patients with AIS receive this therapy [3]; and if patients do receive thrombolytics only a 30 % recanalization is observed after 6 hours of tPA infusion [90]. This model of reperfusion allows for better post-stroke CBF and allowing the adequate distribution of the drug. Also reperfusion injury causes BBB dysfunction allowing molecules that normally do not penetrate the BBB to enter into the brain.

16.5. Time window

The many syndromes seen secondary to vessel occlusion make the diagnosis of AIS difficult for the untrained eye. This heterogeneous presentation makes the arrival of emergency medical services volatile and the time that it takes for these patients to get to a stroke unit hospital is normally greater than 3 hours. In animal models, the administration of the agent is controlled and normally takes place immediately after the onset of stroke. The study of clinically unrealistic time windows for drugs is a major limitation when these are taken into human trials.

http://dx.doi.org/10.5772/53774

16.6. Neurological outcome measures

The criteria used to evaluate stroke varies greatly among basic and clinical research. In animal models the beneficial effect of an agent is measured by the change in size of the infarct zone through image analysis of histological slices. This morphohistological analysis of stroke is a very objective way of measuring a subjective parameter. The size of infarction can have a milieu of functional effects that varies greatly from subject to subject. In this case, the best way to evaluate stroke recovery is a functional outcome measure. This is the case for AIS in the clinic, the scales of the NIHSS, Barthel index, and Modified Rankin Scale all evaluate changes in the function, and not form, of the ischemic zone.

16.7. Study design

Most studies seen in the field are surrounded by heterogeneity and publication bias. Most preclinical studies do not perform randomized, double-blinded designs as opposed to clinical trials that do. In an attempt to standardize this, the Stroke Therapy Academic Industry Roundtable (STAIR) criterion drafted a set of recommendations [91]. The STAIR documents have the goal of smoothing the transition from the bench to the clinic and only the NXY-059 trial has rigorously adhered to them. The beneficial results observed in that trial suggest that the adherence to the STAIR criterion provide better translation into human studies.

17. Direction of future therapies

Increasingly many drugs are currently being tested as potential therapies in AIS. Most of these have demonstrated promising results in the preclinical phases of research and will probably never see the bedside. With every failed attempt at discovering an effective drug compound to treat stroke, the regulations to monitor which ones make it to the clinical setting will become stricter. A step in this direction is the STAIR criteria; these will unify the way in which science is conducted. The adherence to these recommendations allows for better drugs to reach patients but may also limit potentially beneficial drugs from ever passing the preclinical phase. Most neuroprotectants are designed to target one pathway of the multimechanistic pathophysiology of AIS. This reductionist approach to treatment yields modest results. A recent systematic review and meta-analysis by O'Collins and collaborators analyzed combination therapy in comparison to single treatments [92]. The study included 126 different treatments used in the management of animal models of AIS. Single treatments improved neurological score by 12 % in comparison to controls; when used in combination with a second therapy it improved that efficacy by an additional 25 %. In a separate analysis, combining thrombolysis with another compound extended the therapeutic window from 4.4 to 8 hours in animal models. This incredibly useful review suggests that the best approach to AIS therapy is in fact a combination scheme. A treatment strategy that will target most of the damaging mechanisms of stroke will perhaps allow the field to overcome the bench-to-bedside gap.

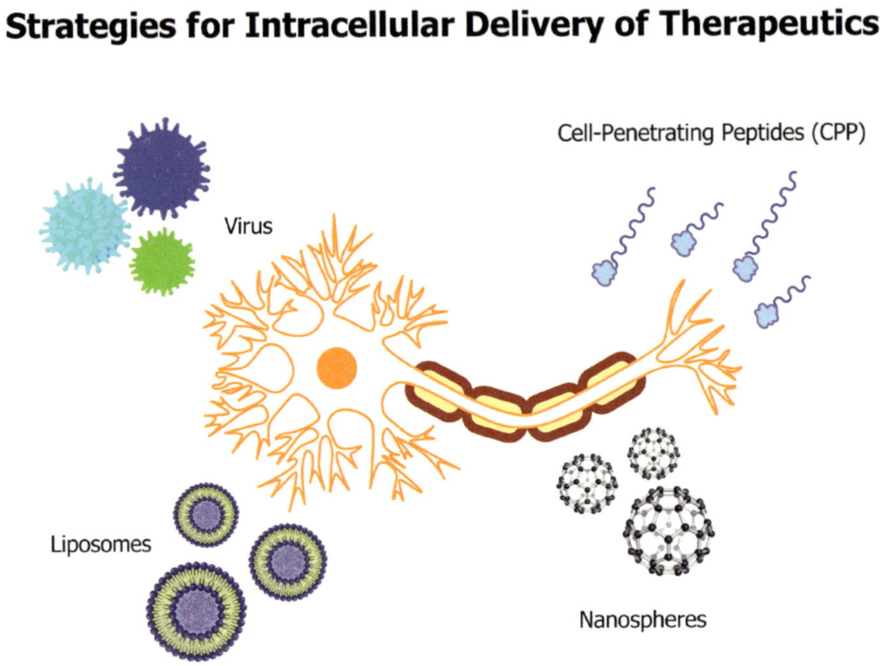

Figure 4. Neuron-specific strategies of drug delivery. Several molecules have been created or modified to be able to carry therapeutic compounds and home in on the target tissue. These strategies reduce secondary adverse side effects by decreasing the systemic concentration and increasing it at the site where it is needed.

One of the main problems of drug design in AIS is making the molecules small enough to diffuse across the BBB and reach the target tissue. In the case of NXY-059, the molecule disufenton sodium had very little BBB penetration and was limited to exerting its effect on the endothelium and neurovascular unit [93]. This particular limitation could be the culprit of why only modest beneficial effects were observed. In an attempt to increase the concentration of drugs that reach the target tissue, researchers have designed nanoparticles that will home in on the stressed neurons in the penumbra. These myriad molecules such as: virus, liposomes, nanospheres, and cell-penetrating peptides will target specific cell populations and spare secondary systemic effects. A very promising therapeutic strategy is cell-penetrating peptides (CPP). These use cell-specific homing proteins (cargo) such as viral surface proteins like trans-activator of transcription (Tat) and they are conjugated with proteins that will block intracellular protein-protein interactions (effector) (see Figure 5). Cook and collaborators recently published an example of this. They sidestepped several model limitations by using a gyrencephalic non-human primate that has a brain that shows genetic, anatomical and behavioral similarities to human brains [88]. In this study, they tested the neuroprotective effect of postsynaptic density protein-95 (PSD-95) inhibitors. These compounds uncouple PSD-95 from neurotoxic signaling pathways and results in increased neuroprotection. However, these inhibitors have limited transport into the cell, so in order to improve the effect they used a CPP. The following CPP was used: Tat-NR2B9c, comprising the nine carboxy-terminal amino acids of the N-methyl-D-aspartate receptor (NMDAR) NR2B subunit fused to the 11-mer HIV-1 Tat protein transduction domain. The results demonstrated that PSD-95 inhibitor CPP exert neuroprotection and improve the functional outcome seen after AIS. Another positive detail of this study is that it adhered completely to the STAIR criteria. The promising results seen with CPP suggest that they will soon be introduced into the clinical testing phase. Please refer to Figure 5 for more examples of CPPs that exert neuroprotective effects in AIS.

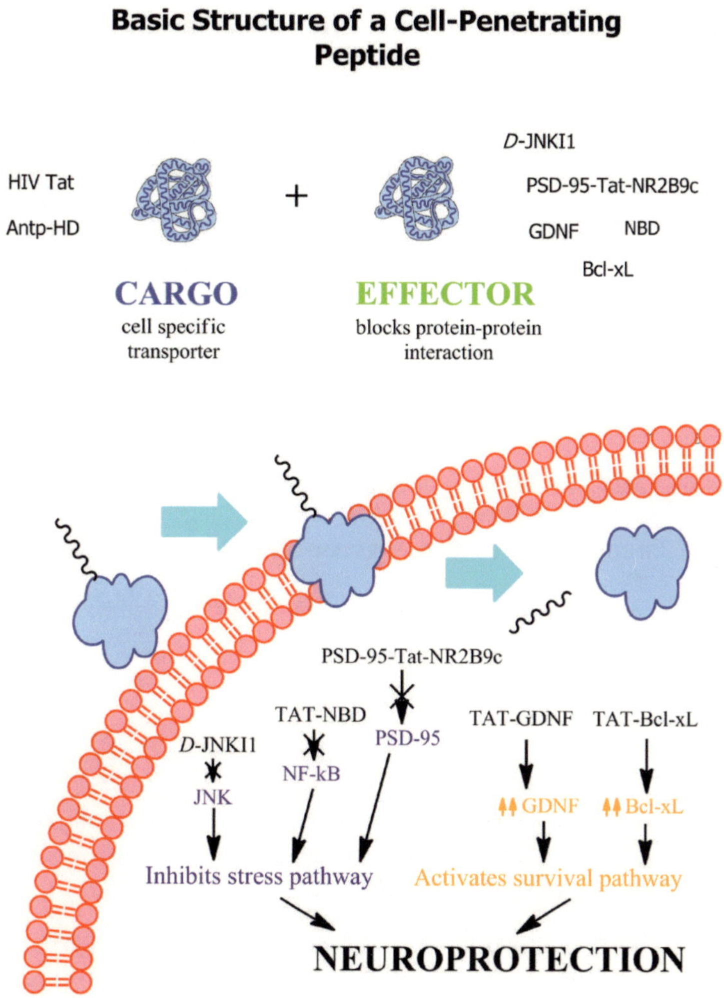

Figure 5. Cell-penetrating peptides and their role in AIS. The basic structure of a CPP includes a cell-specific targeting peptide coupled with an effector protein that once inside the cell will exert a protein-protein interaction. This interaction will either activate or inactivate certain metabolic processes and will confer neuroprotection to the ischemic penumbral neuron. Adapted from [94].

This review had the goal of jumpstarting drug discovery in AIS by providing a panorama of the field at present. Enormous strides have been made and shall continue to be made, but in order to focus our efforts and produce a revolutionary novel therapy in the foreseeable future several steps should be taken. This work urges the researchers of the field to become familiarized with the STAIR criteria and design all experiments in interventional stroke research around it. This will allow all publications to become more homogenous and if a truly promising compound or combination is discovered the distance from the bench-to-bedside will be shortened. The finality of this is to benefit as many people as possible in the shortest time available. The authors suggest that targeted molecules will result in better treatments by limiting adverse side effects at non-target sites. With the literature provided it should be considered that combination therapies hold greater promise than single therapies. The adherence to the STAIR criteria recommends that multiple types of stroke models be used and larger animals be sought. Also, strict analysis of pharmacodynamics and pharmacokinetic parameters shall be done on all experimental agents. The authors hope that with these steps being followed throughout the scientific community the cure for AIS is close at hand. However, until that moment comes the cornerstone of treatment is prevention. Possible therapies aimed at preventing the initial AIS will yield the highest benefits in neurological outcome; more research in this area is required.

Author details

Humberto Mestre[1], Yael Cohen-Minian[1], Daniel Zajarias-Fainsod[1,2] and Antonio Ibarra[1]

1 Faculty of Health Sciences, Universidad Anáhuac México Norte, Mexico

2 Institute of Biomedical Engineering, University of Oxford, UK

References

[1] Zhang, Y, Galloway, J. M, Welty, T. K, Wiebers, D. O, Whisnant, J. P, Devereux, R. B, et al. Incidence and risk factors for stroke in American Indians: the Strong Heart Study. Circulation. (2008). , 118(15), 1577-84.

[2] Roger, V. L, Go, A. S, Lloyd-jones, D. M, Benjamin, E. J, Berry, J. D, Borden, W. B, et al. Executive summary: heart disease and stroke statistics--2012 update: a report from the American Heart Association. Circulation. (2012). , 125(1), 188-97.

[3] Alberts, M. J. Cerebral hemorrhage, warfarin, and intravenous tPA: the real risk is not treating. JAMA. (2012). , 307(24), 2637-9.

[4] Kleindorfer, D, Lindsell, C. J, Brass, L, Koroshetz, W, & Broderick, J. P. National US estimates of recombinant tissue plasminogen activator use: ICD-9 codes substantially underestimate. Stroke. (2008). , 39(3), 924-8.

[5] Reeves, M. J, Arora, S, Broderick, J. P, Frankel, M, Heinrich, J. P, Hickenbottom, S, et al. Acute stroke care in the US: results from 4 pilot prototypes of the Paul Coverdell National Acute Stroke Registry. Stroke. (2005). , 36(6), 1232-40.

[6] Balami, J. S, Chen, R-L, Grunwald, I. Q, & Buchan, A. M. Neurological complications of acute ischaemic stroke. The Lancet Neurology. (2011). , 10(4), 357-71.

[7] Tiehuis, A. M, Visseren, F. L, Vincken, K. L, Biessels, G. J, et al. Diabetes increases atrophy and vascular lesions on brain MRI in patients with symptomatic arterial disease. Stroke. (2008).

[8] Quinn, T. J, & Dawson, J. Sugar and stroke: cerebrovascular disease and blood glucose control. (2011).

[9] Candelario-jalil, E. Injury and repair mechanisms in ischemic stroke: Considerations for the development of novel neurotherapeutics. Curr Opin Investig Drugs. (2009). , 10(7), 644-54.

[10] Dirnagl, U. U, & Iadecola, C. C. Moskowitz MAM. Pathobiology of ischaemic stroke: an integrated view. Trends Neurosci. (1999). , 22(9), 391-7.

[11] Xing, C, Arai, K, Lo, E. H, & Hommel, M. Pathophysiologic cascades in ischemic stroke. Int J Stroke. (2012). , 7(5), 378-85.

[12] Kostandy, B. B. The role of glutamate in neuronal ischemic injury: the role of spark in fire. Neurol. Sci. (2012). , 33(2), 223-37.

[13] Lipton, P. Ischemic cell death in brain neurons. Physiol Rev. (1999). , 79(4), 1431-568.

[14] Lo, E. H, Dalkara, T, & Moskowitz, M. A. Mechanisms, challenges and opportunities in stroke. Nat Rev Neurosci. (2003). , 4(5), 399-415.

[15] Ibarra, A, García, E, Flores, N, Martiñón, S, Reyes, R, Campos, M. G, et al. Immunization with neural-derived antigens inhibits lipid peroxidation after spinal cord injury. CORD Conference Proceedings. (2010). , 476(2), 62-5.

[16] Pallast, S, Arai, K, Wang, X, Lo, E. H, & Van Leyen, K. Lipoxygenase targets neuronal mitochondria under oxidative stress. J Neurochem. (2009). , 111(3), 882-9.

[17] Waldmeier PCPProspects for antiapoptotic drug therapy of neurodegenerative diseases. Prog Neuropsychopharmacol Biol Psychiatry. (2003). , 27(2), 303-21.

[18] Kuzhandaivel, A, Nistri, A, & Mladinic, M. Kainate-Mediated Excitotoxicity Induces Neuronal Death in the Rat Spinal Cord In Vitro via a PARP-1 Dependent Cell Death Pathway (Parthanatos). Cell Mol Neurobiol. (2010). , 30(7), 1001-12.

[19] Dreier, J. P. The role of spreading depression, spreading depolarization and spreading ischemia in neurological disease. Nature Medicine. (2011). , 17(4), 439-447.

[20] Strbian, D, Meretoja, A, Putaala, J, Kaste, M, et al. Cerebral edema in acute ischemic stroke patients treated with intravenous thrombolysis. Int J Stroke. (2012).

[21] Tissue plasminogen activator for acute ischemic strokeThe National Institute of Neurological Disorders and Stroke rt-PA Stroke Study Group. N. Engl. J. Med. (1995). , 333(24), 1581-7.

[22] Parise, P, Hauert, J, Iorio, A, et al. Streptokinase and rt-PA activate platelets by a different way: implications on the rethrombosis rate after their administration in myocardial infarction. J. Lab. Clin. Med. (1995). , 125(2), 212-21.

[23] Penny, W. F, & Ware, J. A. Platelet activation and subsequent inhibition by plasmin and recombinant tissue-type plasminogen activator. Blood. (1992). , 79(1), 91-98.

[24] Callahan, K. P, Malinin, A. I, et al. Platelet Function and Fibrinolytic Agents: Two Sides of a Coin? Cardiology. (2001).

[25] del Zoppo GJSaver JL, Jauch EC, Adams HP. Expansion of the Time Window for Treatment of Acute Ischemic Stroke With Intravenous Tissue Plasminogen Activator. Stroke. (2009).

[26] Adams, H. P. del Zoppo G, Alberts MJ, Bhatt DL, Brass L, Furlan A, et al. Guidelines for the Early Management of Adults With Ischemic Stroke. Circulation. (2007). ee534., 478.

[27] Lansberg, M. G, Donnell, O, Khatri, M. J, Lang, P, Nguyen-huynh, E. S, & Schwartz, M. N. NE, et al. Antithrombotic and Thrombolytic Therapy for Ischemic Stroke: Antithrombotic Therapy and Prevention of Thrombosis, 9th ed: American College of Chest Physicians Evidence-Based Clinical Practice Guidelines. Chest. (2012). suppl) e601S-e636S.

[28] Tijssen JGPLow-dose and high-dose acetylsalicyclic acid, with and without dipyridamole: A review of clinical trial results. Neurology. (1998). Suppl 3) SS16., 15.

[29] Broussalis, E, Killer, M, Mccoy, M, Harrer, A, Trinka, E, & Kraus, J. Current therapies in ischemic stroke. Part A. Recent developments in acute stroke treatment and in stroke prevention. Drug Discov. Today. (2012).

[30] Woodruff, R. S, Sullenger, B, & Becker, R. The many faces of the contact pathway and their role in thrombosis. J. Thromb. Thrombolysis. (2011). , 32(1), 9-20.

[31] Shahpouri, M, Mousavi, S, Khorvash, F, et al. Anticoagulant therapy for ischemic stroke: A review of literature. Journal of Research in Medical Sciences. (2012). , 17(6), 396-401.

[32] Miller, C. S, Grandi, S. M, Shimony, A, Filion, K. B, & Eisenberg, M. J. Meta-analysis of efficacy and safety of new oral anticoagulants (dabigatran, rivaroxaban, apixaban) versus warfarin in patients with atrial fibrillation. Am. J. Cardiol. (2012). , 110(3), 453-60.

[33] Hacke, W, Albers, G, Al-rawi, Y, Bogousslavsky, J, Davalos, A, Eliasziw, M, et al. The Desmoteplase in Acute Ischemic Stroke Trial (DIAS): a phase II MRI-based 9-hour

window acute stroke thrombolysis trial with intravenous desmoteplase. Stroke. (2005)., 36(1), 66-73.

[34] Haley EC JrThompson JL, Grotta JC, Lyden PD, et al. Phase IIB/III trial of tenecteplase in acute ischemic stroke: results of a prematurely terminated randomized clinical trial. Stroke. (2010)., 41(4), 707-711.

[35] Pancioli, A. M, Broderick, J, Brott, T, Tomsick, T, Khoury, J, Bean, J, et al. The combined approach to lysis utilizing eptifibatide and rt-PA in acute ischemic stroke: the CLEAR stroke trial. Stroke. (2008)., 39(12), 3268-76.

[36] Levy, D. E, Trammel, J, & Wasiewski, W. W. Ancrod Stroke Program (ASP) Study Team. Ancrod for acute ischemic stroke: a new dosing regimen derived from analysis of prior ancrod stroke studies. J Stroke Cerebrovasc Dis. (2009)., 18(1), 23-7.

[37] Xu, G, Liu, X, Zhu, W, Yin, Q, Zhang, R, & Fan, X. Feasibility of treating hyperfibrinogenemia with intermittently administered batroxobin in patients with ischemic stroke/transient ischemic attack for secondary prevention. Blood Coagul. Fibrinolysis. (2007)., 18(2), 193-7.

[38] Zhao, Y, & Rempe, D. A. Prophylactic neuroprotection against stroke: low-dose, prolonged treatment with deferoxamine or deferasirox establishes prolonged neuroprotection independent of HIF-1 function. J Cereb Blood Flow Metab. (2011). , 31(6), 1412-23.

[39] Rosenberg, G, Bornstein, N, Diener, H-C, Gorelick, P. B, Shuaib, A, Lees, K, et al. The Membrane-Activated Chelator Stroke Intervention (MACSI) Trial of DP-b99 in acute ischemic stroke: a randomized, double blind, placebo-controlled, multinational pivotal phase III study. Int J Stroke. (2011)., 6(4), 362-7.

[40] Fisher, J. W. Erythropoietin: physiology and pharmacology update. Exp. Biol. Med. (2003).

[41] Minnerup, J, Heidrich, J, Rogalewski, A, Schabitz, W. R, & Wellmann, J. The efficacy of erythropoietin and its analogues in animal stroke models: a meta-analysis. Stroke. (2009).

[42] Zhang, L, Chopp, M, Zhang, R. L, Wang, L, Zhang, J, Wang, Y, Toh, Y, Santra, M, Lu, M, & Zhang, Z. G. Erythropoietin amplifies stroke-induced oligodendrogenesis in the rat. PLoS One. (2010). e11016.

[43] Hermann, D. M. Nonhematopoietic variants of erythropoietin in ischemic stroke: need for step-wise proof-of-concept studies. Scientific World Journal. (2010).

[44] Rodriguez, C. Y, Mengana, T. Y, Munoz, C. A, Subiros, M. N, Gonzalez-quevedo, A, & Sosa, T. I. Garcia Rodriguez JC. Treatment with nasal neuro-EPO improves the neurological, cognitive, and histological state in a gerbil model of focal ischemia. Scientific World Journal. (2010).

[45] Fu, A, Hui, E. K, Lu, J. Z, Boado, R. J, & Pardridge, W. M. Neuroprotection in stroke in the mouse with intravenous erythropoietin-Trojan horse fusion protein. Brain Res. (2011).

[46] Sugiyama, Y, Yagita, Y, Oyama, N, Terasaki, Y, Omura-matsuoka, E, Sasaki, T, & Kitagawa, K. Granulocyte colony-stimulating factor enhances arteriogenesis and ameliorates cerebral damage in a mouse model of ischemic stroke. Stroke. (2011).

[47] Todo, K, Kitagawa, K, Sasaki, T, Omura-matsuoka, E, Terasaki, Y, Oyama, N, Yagita, Y, & Hori, M. Granulocyte-macrophage colony-stimulating factor enhances leptomeningeal collateral growth induced by common carotid artery occlusion. Stroke. (2008).

[48] Schneider, U. C, Schilling, L, Schroeck, H, Nebe, C. T, Vajkoczy, P, & Woitzik, J. Granulocyte-macrophage colony-stimulating factor-induced vessel growth restores cerebral blood supply after bilateral carotid artery occlusion. Stroke. (2007).

[49] Aharoni, R, Kayhan, B, Eilam, R, Sela, M, & Arnon, R. Glatiramer acetate-specific T cells in the brain express T helper 2/3 cytokines and brain-derived neurotrophic factor in situ. Proc. Natl. Acad. Sci. U. S. A. (2003).

[50] Angelov, D. N, Waibel, S, Guntinas-lichius, O, Lenzen, M, Neiss, W. F, Tomov, T. L, Yoles, E, Kipnis, J, Schori, H, Reuter, A, Ludolph, A, & Schwartz, M. Therapeutic vaccine for acute and chronic motor neuron diseases: implications for amyotrophic lateral sclerosis. Proc. Natl. Acad. Sci. U. S. A. (2003).

[51] Arnon, R, & Aharoni, R. Mechanism of action of glatiramer acetate in multiple sclerosis and its potential for the development of new applications. Proc. Natl. Acad. Sci. U. S. A. (2004). Suppl 2) 14593-14598.

[52] Gorantla, S, Liu, J, Sneller, H, Dou, H, Holguin, A, Smith, L, Ikezu, T, Volsky, D. J, Poluektova, L, & Gendelman, H. E. Copolymer-1 induces adaptive immune anti-inflammatory glial and neuroprotective responses in a murine model of HIV-1 encephalitis. J. Immunol. (2007).

[53] Ibarra, A, Avendano, H, & Cruz, Y. Copolymer-1 (Cop-1) improves neurological recovery after middle cerebral artery occlusion in rats. Neurosci. Lett. (2007).

[54] Aharoni, R, Arnon, R, & Eilam, R. Neurogenesis and neuroprotection induced by peripheral immunomodulatory treatment of experimental autoimmune encephalomyelitis. J. Neurosci. (2005).

[55] Yuan, T. F. BDNF signaling during olfactory bulb neurogenesis. J. Neurosci. (2008).

[56] Cady, C. T, Lahn, M, Vollmer, M, Tsuji, M, Seo, S. J, Reardon, C. L, Brien, O, & Born, R. L. WK. Response of murine gamma delta T cells to the synthetic polypeptide poly-Glu50Tyr50. J. Immunol. (2000).

[57] Ziv, Y, Finkelstein, A, Geffen, Y, Kipnis, J, Smirnov, I, Shpilman, S, Vertkin, I, Kimron, M, Lange, A, Hecht, T, Reyman, K. G, Marder, J. B, Schwartz, M, & Yoles, E. A

novel immune-based therapy for stroke induces neuroprotection and supports neurogenesis. Stroke. (2007).

[58] Schwartz, M, & Hauben, E. T cell-based therapeutic vaccination for spinal cord injury. Prog. Brain Res. (2002).

[59] Bahjat, F. R, Williams-karnesky, R. L, Kohama, S. G, West, G. A, Doyle, K. P, Spector, M. D, Hobbs, T. R, & Stenzel-poore, M. P. Proof of concept: pharmacological preconditioning with a Toll-like receptor agonist protects against cerebrovascular injury in a primate model of stroke. J. Cereb. Blood Flow Metab. (2011).

[60] Green, A. R, Ashwood, T, Odergren, T, & Jackson, D. M. Nitrones as neuroprotective agents in cerebral ischemia, with particular reference to NXY-059. Pharmacol. Ther. (2003). , 100, 195-214.

[61] Lees, K. R, Zivin, J. A, Ashwood, T, Davalos, A, Davis, S. M, Diener, H. C, Grotta, J, Lyden, P, Shuaib, A, Hardemark, H. G, & Wasiewski, W. W. NXY-059 for acute ischemic stroke. N. Engl. J. Med. (2006).

[62] Diener, H. C, Lees, K. R, Lyden, P, Grotta, J, Davalos, A, Davis, S. M, Shuaib, A, Ashwood, T, Wasiewski, W, Alderfer, V, Hardemark, H. G, & Rodichok, L. for the SAINT NXY-059 for the Treatment of Acute Stroke: Pooled Analysis of the SAINT I and II Trials. Stroke. (2008).

[63] Culot, M, Mysiorek, C, Renftel, M, Roussel, B. D, Hommet, Y, Vivien, D, Cecchelli, R, Fenart, L, Berezowski, V, Dehouck, M. P, & Lundquist, S. Cerebrovascular protection as a possible mechanism for the protective effects of NXY-059 in preclinical models: an in vitro study. Brain Res. (2009).

[64] Lees, K. R, Barer, D, Ford, G. A, Hacke, W, Kostulas, V, Sharma, A. K, & Odergren, T. Tolerability of NXY-059 at higher target concentrations in patients with acute stroke. Stroke, (2003).

[65] Kleinschnitz, C, Grund, H, Wingler, K, Armitage, M. E, Jones, E, Mittal, M, Barit, D, Schwarz, T, Geis, C, Kraft, P, Barthel, K, Schuhmann, M. K, Herrmann, A. M, Meuth, S. G, Stoll, G, Meurer, S, Schrewe, A, Becker, L, Gailus-durner, V, Fuchs, H, Klopstock, T, De Angelis, M. H, Jandeleit-dahm, K, Shah, A. M, Weissmann, N, & Schmidt, H. H. Post-stroke inhibition of induced NADPH oxidase type 4 prevents oxidative stress and neurodegeneration. PLoS Biol. (2010). e1000479.

[66] Campos, F, Sobrino, T, Ramos-cabrer, P, Argibay, B, Agulla, J, Pérez-mato, M, et al. Neuroprotection by glutamate oxaloacetate transaminase in ischemic stroke: an experimental study. J Cereb Blood Flow Metab. (2011). , 31(6), 1378-86.

[67] Kawamura, T, Horie, S, Maruyama, T, Akira, T, Imagawa, T, Nakamura, N, & Prostaglandin, E. transported into cells blocks the apoptotic signals induced by nerve growth factor deprivation. J Neurochem. (1999). , 72(5), 1907-14.

[68] Gold, A. B, Herrmann, N, & Lanctot, K. L. Lithium and its neuroprotective and neurotrophic effects: potential treatment for post-ischemic stroke sequelae. Curr. Drug Targets. (2011). , 12(2), 243-255.

[69] Vagnerova, K, Hurn, P. D, Bhardwaj, A, & Kirsch, J. R. Sigma 1 receptor agonists act as neuroprotective drugs through inhibition of inducible nitric oxide synthase. Anesth. Analg. (2006). , 103(2), 430-4.

[70] Wei, Y, Yemisci, M, Kim, H-H, Yung, L. M, Shin, H. K, Hwang, S-K, et al. Fingolimod provides long-term protection in rodent models of cerebral ischemia. Ann. Neurol. (2011). , 69(1), 119-29.

[71] Liesz, A, Sun, L, Zhou, W, Schwarting, S, Mracsko, E, Zorn, M, et al. FTY720 reduces post-ischemic brain lymphocyte influx but does not improve outcome in permanent murine cerebral ischemia. PLoS ONE. (2011). e21312.

[72] Zhang, Z, Chen, T-Y, & Kirsch, J. R. Toung TJK, Traystman RJ, Koehler RC, et al. Kappa-opioid receptor selectivity for ischemic neuroprotection with BRL 52537 in rats. Anesth. Analg. (2003). , 97(6), 1776-83.

[73] Chen, T-Y, Tai, S-H, Lee, E-J, Huang, C-C, Lee, A-C, Huang, S-Y, et al. Cinnamophilin offers prolonged neuroprotection against gray and white matter damage and improves functional and electrophysiological outcomes after transient focal cerebral ischemia. Crit. Care Med. (2011). , 39(5), 1130-7.

[74] Elango, C, & Jayachandaran, K. S. Niranjali Devaraj S. Hawthorn extract reduces infarct volume and improves neurological score by reducing oxidative stress in rat brain following middle cerebral artery occlusion. Int. J. Dev. Neurosci. (2009). , 27(8), 799-803.

[75] Elango, C, & Devaraj, S. N. Immunomodulatory effect of Hawthorn extract in an experimental stroke model. J Neuroinflammation. (2010).

[76] Kaur, H, Jaggi, A. S, & Singh, N. Modulation of neuroprotective effect of ischemic post-conditioning by dichlorobenzamil a Na (+)/Ca (2+) exchanger inhibitor in mice. Biol. Pharm. Bull. (2010). , 33(4), 585-91.

[77] Nonaka, Y, Tsuruma, K, Shimazawa, M, Yoshimura, S, Iwama, T, & Hara, H. Cilostazol protects against hemorrhagic transformation in mice transient focal cerebral ischemia-induced brain damage. Neuroscience Letters. (2009). , 452(2), 156-61.

[78] Saver, J. L. Target brain: neuroprotection and neurorestoration in ischemic stroke. Rev Neurol Dis. (2010). Suppl 1) S, 14-21.

[79] Saver, J. L, Kidwell, C, Eckstein, M, & Starkman, S. FAST-MAG Pilot Trial Investigators. Prehospital neuroprotective therapy for acute stroke: results of the Field Administration of Stroke Therapy-Magnesium (FAST-MAG) pilot trial. Stroke. (2004). e, 106-8.

[80] Pettigrew, L. C, Kasner, S. E, Albers, G. W, Gorman, M, Grotta, J. C, Sherman, D. G, et al. Safety and tolerability of arundic acid in acute ischemic stroke. J. Neurol. Sci. (2006).

[81] Green, A. R, & Shuaib, A. Therapeutic strategies for the treatment of stroke. Drug Discov. Today. (2006).

[82] Medhi, B, Aggarwal, R, & Chakrabarti, A. Neuroprotective effect of pioglitazone on acute phase changes induced by partial global cerebral ischemia in mice. Indian J. Exp. Biol. (2010). , 48(8), 793-9.

[83] Pentón-rol, G, Marín-prida, J, Pardo-andreu, G, Martínez-sánchez, G, Acosta-medina, E. F, Valdivia-acosta, A, et al. C-Phycocyanin is neuroprotective against global cerebral ischemia/reperfusion injury in gerbils. Brain Res. Bull. (2011).

[84] Ye, R, Kong, X, Yang, Q, Zhang, Y, Han, J, & Zhao, G. Ginsenoside Rd attenuates redox imbalance and improves stroke outcome after focal cerebral ischemia in aged mice. Neuropharmacology. (2011). , 61(4), 815-24.

[85] Cheyuo, C, Jacob, A, Wu, R, Zhou, M, Qi, L, Dong, W, et al. Recombinant human MFG-E8 attenuates cerebral ischemic injury: its role in anti-inflammation and anti-apoptosis. Neuropharmacology. (2012). , 62(2), 890-900.

[86] Yan, J, Zhou, B, Taheri, S, & Shi, H. Differential effects of HIF-1 inhibition by YC-1 on the overall outcome and blood-brain barrier damage in a rat model of ischemic stroke. PLoS ONE. (2011). e27798.

[87] Le, H. T, Hirko, A. C, Thinschmidt, J. S, Grant, M, Li, Z, Peris, J, et al. The protective effects of plasma gelsolin on stroke outcome in rats. Exp Transl Stroke Med. (2011).

[88] Broussalis, E, Trinka, E, Killer, M, Harrer, A, Mccoy, M, & Kraus, J. Current therapies in ischemic stroke. Part B. Future candidates in stroke therapy and experimental studies. Drug Discov. Today. (2012).

[89] Cook, D. J, Teves, L, & Tymianski, M. Treatment of stroke with a PSD-95 inhibitor in the gyrencephalic primate brain. Nature. (2012). , 483(7388), 213-7.

[90] Arakawa, S, Nilupul, P, & Doonan, G. Neuroprotection in Stroke. Advances in Clinical Neuroscience and Rehabilitation. (2005). , 5(5), 10-11.

[91] Fisher, M, Albers, G. W, Donnan, G. A, Furlan, A. J, Grotta, J. C, Kidwell, C. S, et al. Enhancing the development and approval of acute stroke therapies: Stroke Therapy Academic Industry roundtable. Stroke. (2005).

[92] Collins, O, Macleod, V. E, Donnan, M. R, & Howells, G. A. DW. Evaluation of combination therapy in animal models of cerebral ischemia. J Cerebr Blood F Met. (2012). , 32(4), 585-97.

[93] Sutherland, B. A, Sutherland, B. A, Minnerup, J, & Minnerup, J. MRCP JSB, Balami JS, et al. Neuroprotection for ischaemic stroke: Translation from the bench to the bedside. Int J Stroke. (2012). , 7(5), 407-18.

[94] Antoniou, X, & Borsello, T. Cell Permeable Peptides: A Promising Tool to Deliver Neuroprotective Agents in the Brain. Pharmaceuticals. Molecular Diversity Preservation International. (2010). , 3(2), 379-92.

Chapter 25

Cognitive Dysfunction Syndrome in Senior Dogs

Camilo Orozco Sanabria, Francisco Olea and
Manuel Rojas

Additional information is available at the end of the chapter

http://dx.doi.org/10.5772/54903

1. Introduction

Human history has been closely linked to some animal species, and very specifically to dog. This close relationship has endured, therefore the dog is considered the domestic specie closest to man, because for today plays socially important roles as a member of many families and / or as executor of activities that helps or facilitates human life. However, this closeness to man has promoted, either by love or not, that care provided to dogs is increasing, and therefore on the increase in life expectancy of these animals [1].

However, just as in humans, increased life expectancy of dogs, is often associated with behavioral disturbances and cognitive deficits related with clinical signs of disorientation, loss of social interaction, sleep disturbances, decreased general activity and progressive loss of acquired memories [2-3]. Initially, these behavioral changes have been assumed by some veterinarians, as evidence of senility [4]. It was recently proposed the term "Cognitive Dysfunction Syndrome of Geriatric Dogs" (CDS), to describe the cognitive deficits observed in some geriatric dogs [2,3,5,6], which seems being closely related with Alzheimer's disease (AD), therefore, it is likely that CDS can be known as Dog's Alzheimer's disease [7,8,9,10]

Cognition refers to mental processes such as perception, consciousness, learning, memory and making decisions, it allows obtaining information from the environment in order to interact normally with environment [11, 12, 13, 14]. Nevertheless, cognition alterations could be considered by some owners, as "normal" signs of aging, so these symptoms are always not informed to veterinarian. Other common modifications are inability to recognize the family members and to perform easy tasks such as eating and exercise, sleep-wake cycle changes are common too [15]. These behavioral modifications can cause limitation of social interaction of dogs; consequently can lead to rejection of certain owners to take care of these patients, so increasing the risk of some pets to be sacrificed.

To date it has been identified several similarities between CDS and AD, therefore it has been suggested that studies of geriatric canines that suffering CDS, could be a useful tool for recognizing clinicopathological aspects yet not clarified of AD, and thereby possibly give more effective management to disease [17-18]. However, despite the many similarities, there are also some important differences, such as the involvement factors that predispose to humans, but not dogs to diseases like EA. These factors including, gender [19] and background family [20].

Despite the large contribution that means owning a dog as the experimental model, which develops a disease with many similarities to that seen in humans [17], shall be taken into account that the results obtained from the use of this model is not always reflect a completely accurate information. Therefore, there are several voices that suggest that the results obtained in animals cannot always be extrapolated to humans because the techniques used to assess cognitive functions differ in their ability to describe functions such as perception, discrimination, storage and retrieval of cognitive flexibility [10]. However, after considering the possible similarities and differences in EA and SDC, this chapter is to describe in detail the clinical and patho-physiological characteristic of this canine dementia syndrome, likewise presents diagnostic and therapeutic tools that seek to stop the progression clinical signs of the disease, as well as discuss their clinic-pathologic similarities with the EA, and finally, discuss the facts that today are considered to CDS as a valid experimental model for human neurodegenerative diseases.

2. Clinical features

The behavioral abnormalities in geriatric dogs, are sometimes considered as traits of aging process, however, it is important to differentiate between those behavioral alterations that are related to serious damage of cognitive processes and slight decrease in psychomotor activity or "normal aging" [2,13,15,16]. The intensity which behavioral changes affect each animal, are characteristic of each patient and it is possible to identify a big variety of cognitive impairment, for example, some dogs are unable to distinguish to family's members, whereas others dogs, with lesser cognitive deficits, are able to remember instructions learned during training [17].

It is probably that altered urination habits, but not defecation habits, are the most frequent signs observed by owners in pets that suffering CSD [17], nevertheless, polyuria can occur without renal system diseases or without secondary environmental changes that prevent access to appropriate area of evacuation.

Other common signs reported are episodes of confusion and disorientation [18], in which pet gets lost in house or garden, going to wrong door or wrong side of the door. Clinical signs include reduced interaction with owners, slowness to obey orders, alterations in the sleep-wake cycle, excessive vocalization, exercise intolerance, difficulty climbing stairs, increased irritability and new fears or phobias. [17,18].

Besides in wide variety of behavioral alterations reported, some authors have suggested to use rating scales for diagnosing CDS in dogs, as proposed by Landsberg [3]. Landsberg's method sorts clinical signs in following topics: 1. Spatial disorientation and / or confusion, 2. Impaired learning abilities and memory (loss of home grooming habits, incompetence to obey certain orders or previously learned tasks), 3.Decreased activity or repetitive activities, 4.Alteration and reduction of social interactions, 5.Decreased perception and / or responsiveness, 6.Increased anxiety or restlessness, 7.Alteration of appetite associated with confusional states that could prevent to find their food, 8.Alteration of day-night cycles (sleep-wake) [19, 20].

3. Prevalence

The life expectancy of humans and dogs has increased steadily over the past decades, due to improved medical and health conditions available [21]. However, this increase in life expectancy has increased the prevalence of certain diseases related to aging, such as AD and CDS.

Therefore, after considering reports that suggest world presence of 52 million dogs around 7 years old [22], and taking into account that dogs over 7 years old could be considerate in geriatric condition, it is possible to suppose that these both conditions could generate a big population with great risk to suffer CDS [20. 23]. Some regional studies, have designed and implemented various observational questionnaires, for the geriatric canine pet owners, that try to identify behavioral changes in their pets and achieving determine CDS prevalence in animals evaluated. Recently, an Italian study that included 124 geriatric dogs, revealed prevalence about 50% of CDS, 75 dogs older than 7 years showed signs consistent with CDS [13]. Similarly, another study [1] conducted with 180 dogs between 11 and 16 years old, reported that 28% of dogs between 11 and 12 years showed some degree of cognitive impairment, while those individuals between 15 and 16 years had a probability close to 68% to develop CDS, these data suggests a close relationship between the aging process and likelihood of developing SDC.

However, although researches mentioned above are obviously important, it is worth noting that their impact is restricted to local areas where researches were develop and, therefore, data on the global prevalence of CDS have not yet been achieved, in part, due to tendency of pet owners to not report to veterinarian the possible behavioral changes in geriatric pets [13], which probably has limited accurate data to estimate the prevalence of CDS to worldwide.

4. Patho-physiological basis of CDS

To date have been identified several pathophysiological changes that matching for diseases such as AD and CDS. Neurodegeneration defines pathological neural death observed in several neurodegenerative diseases such as CDS, which is characterized morphologically by a decrease in the number of cholinergic neurons in hippocampus and cerebral cortex (areas especially related with changes in behavior and cognitive memory) [3.24]. Although the causes of neuronal death is unknown, some authors have suggested to oxidative stress and accumulation of beta-amilode peptide (βA) as possible causal factors of clinical signs observed in CDS [2].

βA peptide, which plays an important role in pathophysiology of canine dementia [2,8,25-26] and AD [2], generates its neurotoxic effects by intra-neuronal accumulation [6], hence, it induces degeneration of cholinergic neurons and it seems that quantity of accumulated βA is associated with severity of clinical signs [1,10, 23,25,27, 28]. Reactive oxygen species (ROS), which are recognized as inductors of oxidative stress, has been involved in presentation of CDS and other demential syndromes as AD. Oxidative stress induces its deleterious effects on neuronal cells and their effects are similar in dogs and older adults [2]. Mitochondria is the first organelle involved in production of ROS due to its aerobic metabolism [29], nevertheless, other sources could be also considerating as metabolic sources of ROS generation, such as peroxisomes and release of oxidants by neutrophils. Similarly, exogenous influence such as ionizing radiation, pollution and carcinogens, can contribute to production of free radicals in mammalian systems [30].

According to some authors, oxidative damage is a key mechanism for development of diseases associated with age that cause cognitive dysfunction [31]. Brain is highly predisposing to suffer lesions induced by oxidative stress because it is common accumulation of oxidants substances and because it is probably that protective mechanisms, such as superoxide dismutase and vitamin E, can be less efficient to prevent alterations induced by oxidative stress [32], and thus FR could potentially damage neuronal function causing cell death [2]. Neuronal death leads to uncontrolled release of excitatory neurotransmitters such as acetylcholine, involved in practically all cognitive functions especially in the memory, dopamine, which is associated with control of movement (motor); norepinephrine, associated with wakefulness, attention and serotonin, which is related to mood and sleep control [23,24,33,34]. In this sense, it is possible suggest that neurochemical changes which occurring in brain of aged patients, are the responsible of severity and clinical manifestation in patients with CDS.

5. Pathological lesions

Many morphological features which occur in brains of old dogs are similar to those observed in the brains of aged humans [34]. These changes, which are related to age, include cortical atrophy and increased ventricular spaces, morphological changes in meninges and choroid plexus, changes in cerebral and meningeal vasculature; it is also evident degraded protein accumulation and DNA damage [43 - 44.16]. Other lesions in dogs include inflammation of meninges, gliosis, amyloid deposits, degeneration of myelin in white matter and accumulation of oxidative stress products which have a close relationship with apoptotic processes. Apoptotic cell death has been described in brains from AD patients and in geriatric dogs affected with CDS. Neuronal death by apoptosis processes is related to amyloid accumulation, and according to various authors, may be the main responsible factor for age-related dementia [1]. These morphological changes are related to the characteristic signs of dementia in dogs [2,37, 41,42,45], therefore these has received much attention from researchers who have considered dog as a model for studying human neurodegenerative diseases [29].

http://dx.doi.org/10.5772/54903

In contrast, brains of patients with AD show neurofibrillary plaques and intra-neuronal formation of tau protein products. Tau protein normally is a essential constituent of cytoskeleton in neurons [46], however, in people with AD, protein is hyper-phosphorylated, then it starts a process which induces formation of paired helical filaments which saturate the cytoplasm and induce destruction of microtubules and neurodegeneracion [47-49]. Neurofibrillary plaques are rare in other species and their presence is a major difference between CDS and AD, especially because dogs not develop these structures, because tau's protein sequence is different in dogs and human beings, it could affect formation of neurofibrillary plaques. However, recent studies suggest presence of immature nascent plaques in brains of aged dogs [2,5].

6. Pathological lesions

Many morphological features which occur in brains of old dogs are similar to those observed in the brains of aged humans [25]. These changes, which are related to age, include cortical atrophy and increased ventricular spaces, morphological changes in meninges and choroid plexus, changes in cerebral and meningeal vasculature, it is also evident degraded protein accumulation and DNA damage [35, 36, 37]. Other lesions in dogs include inflammation of meninges, gliosis, amyloid deposits, degeneration of myelin in white matter and accumulation of oxidative stress products which have a close relationship with apoptotic processes. Apoptotic cell death has been described in brains from AD patients and in geriatric dogs affected with CDS. Neuronal death by apoptosis processes is related to amyloid accumulation, and according to various authors, may be the main responsible factor for age-related dementia [38]. These morphological changes are related to the characteristic signs of dementia in dogs [10,39,40,41,42], therefore these has received much attention from researchers who have considered dog as a model for studying human neurodegenerative diseases [2].

In contrast, brains of patients with AD show neurofibrillary plaques and intraneuronal formation of tau protein products. Tau protein normally is a essential constituent of cytoskeleton in neurons [43], however, in people with AD, protein is hyperphosphorylated, then it starts a process which induces formation of paired helical filaments which saturate the cytoplasm and induce destruction of microtubules and neurdegeneracion [44, 45]. Neurofibrillary plaques are rare in other species and their presence is a major difference between CDS and AD, especially because dogs not develop these structures, because tau's protein sequence is different in dogs and human beings, it could affect formation of neurofibrillary plaques. However, recent studies suggest presence of immature nascent plaques in brains of aged dogs [10, 23].

Neurochemical changes such as low levels of dopamine, norepinephrine, serotonin, acetylcholine, choline acetyl-transferase and decreased number of D2 receptors, are characteristics that are commonly observed in CDS and AD [34]. However, there are disease-specific changes as decrease of muscarinic receptor number [46] and increase of activity of enzyme acetylcholinesterase, which are factors present only in AD [47]. In contrast, in affected dogs have been detected increased MAO activity and increased sensitivity to glutamate neurotransmitter, which is capable of initiating processes neurotoxicity [23]. However, the most consistent alteration in brains of dogs and humans with AD is βA peptide accumulation in hippocampus and frontal cortex (areas especially related cognitive behavioral changes) [10, 48]. In neuron, βA is initially concentrated in microdomains of plasma membrane in neurons of the prefrontal cortex and subsequently affects other brain regions such as the parietal and entorhinal cortices [49].

7. Diagnosis

Veterinarians commonly faced with behavioral disturbances in older dogs, however, although it is true that CDS may be the main responsible for these changes, it is also true that behavioral disturbances could be induced by other multifactorial causes [6,10,28]. Therefore, considering the variety and inspecificity of clinical signs associated with CDS, it is important to use clinical history for obtain patient-specific data, which ensures that owners had provided a complete list of all medical and behavioral signs observed in their pets. This information could provide a solid support in finding potential medical problems that may be responsible for the development or exacerbation of clinical signs [3], furthermore this information along with clinical and neurological examination, which can be developed using assessment tests cognitive, may let to veterinarian obtain an early diagnosis [23].

However, we must emphasize difficulty for obtaining accurate information, because in many cases information obtained from pet owners could be little objective, possibly leading to false diagnosis. Thus, shortage of reliable diagnostic tests to ensure presence or absence of disease, gives to early identification of clinical signs a crucial role in establishment of effective treatment, capable of improvement the quality of life of affected patients. In this sense, and according to some authors, the most effective way to detect the condition is through the routinely establishment of behavioral questionnaires in geriatric dogs [2.10]. These questionnaires that ask to owners about your pet's behavior, which have been obtained from various researches [15.35], pretend classifying the behavior of affected patients. Within these cognitive evaluation questionnaires, neuropsychological tests are looking classify systematic cognitive impairment through methods such as modified apparatus of Wisconsin General Test (University of Toronto), in which the dogs are rewarded for each correct answer they obtain. Overall, in this test the dogs have access to a removable tray containing three food wells built in, which can be covered to test visual learning and memory [50, 51].

These neurophysiological tests allow assessment objective and quantitative of deficits in learning and memory, without relying on questionnaires applied to owners. These evaluation tests look for three specific objectives: 1. Identification of non-subjective cognitive changes that are characteristic of aging in dogs, 2. Characterization of the neurobiological basis of decline in cognitive abilities due to aging, and 3. Preparation of potential interventions in order to eliminate or minimize the adverse effects on quality of life [2, 50, 51].

Although learning and memory are quite susceptible to decline with aging, it is necessary evaluating too the spatial memory (the ability to remember the location of food, for example) and the object recognition memory (the ability to recall objects seen with 10-120 seconds ahead) [10], because it is well accepted that these both two memory types are affected in neurodegenerative processes, therefore several studies have developed scales that evaluate the spatial memory and the recognition abilities for indirect evaluation of dementia in dogs [52]. For example, it has been proposed a dementia evaluation index that discriminates between normal, pre-dementia and dementia states [17]. ARCAD scale (assessing cognitive and affective disorders associated with age), where dog's behavior is assessed indirectly through a questionnaire applied to owner, in order to assess the deficit by a scale evaluation of 1 to 5 [53].

Although various tests have shown be able to diagnose the cognitive dysfunction syndrome, we must consider that the results obtained with each test, can vary according to the test, it is possible that cognitive skills, may have a different meaning on the outcome of the test [11.13]. Moreover, besides the possibility to compare results obtained in each test, it is necessary to correlate the results of behavior modifications in dogs examined with paraclinical test results, such as electroencephalography. This relationship could establish whether the test results are able to correlate disturbances in learning, memory and cognitive with disorders of brain circuits that are involved in CDS. It is possible that paraclinical tests can predict dysfunctional brain diseases in dogs?

Finally, it is worth mentioning that several cognitive domains that are affected during the CDS (language, memory, visuospatial skills) and observation of a sign, is not sufficient for beginning a treatment. However, the onset of cognitive impairment in some specific domain could be related into a worsening of other existing signs, therefore it is important following up clinical evaluations routinely [10].

In conclusion, to determine if a dog shows signs of cognitive dysfunction, the veterinarian must rely on information provided by the owner in the medical record, however, the design and implementation of a questionnaire, and possibly paraclinical tests, are necessary to detected signs of CDS during the early stages of development, especially if it comes from animals that have previously had a high level of training [3].

8. Therapeutic alternatives for the treatment of CDS

Currently there are several therapeutic strategies that have been developed along different studies in geriatric dogs affected by CDS.

9. Behavioral type therapy

One consequence of age-associated diseases in dogs is loss of memories acquired during professional or home training, therefore dog may lose its ability to perform simple tasks or to answer previously learned commands. Faced with this kind of behavioral changes, which may be observed in patients with CDS, the establishment of behavioral therapy, in the early stages of the disease, has been suggested as appropriate, when it is accompanied with additional therapeutic tools like drug treatment. Re-training dogs with cognitive dysfunction requires patience and it is necessary to use simple commands with a clear reward and it is important that re-training begins as soon as possible to prevent the development of unwanted behaviors in the dog [2.6].

10. Pharmacological treatment alternatives

Drug therapy is aimed, on the one hand, restoring neurotransmitter concentrations and, on other hand, preventing too rapid advancement of neurodegenerative process [54, 55]. Most treatments used for people affected with AD, have not yet been tested in dogs, nevertheless it is necessary perform clinical studies which be able to clarify which treatments work and which do not. However, there are some options available as selegiline, this was the first therapeutic agent approved by the FDA in 1998 for use in dogs [5.56], this is a selective irreversible inhibitor of the enzyme monoamine oxidase B (MAO B) which increases the concentration of dopamine in brain and it seems to prevent oxidative stress, therefore it could decrease neuronal death. The therapeutical efficacy of selegiline has been shown by studies that verify a decrease in the progression of degenerative changes in AD patients and a significant improvement in dogs with CDS [1]. Therefore, regulating the concentration of neurotransmitters has been considered the main therapeutic alternative for treatment of CDS in dogs, nevertheless, it is possible that new studies could verify a major efficiency of other drugs, for example drugs with anticholinenterase activity or NMDA blockers drugs, which have been effective for treatment of AD, could be could be effective for dogs.

11. Nutritional therapies

After recognizing the role of ROS (reactive oxygen species) in neurodegenerative diseases, some researchers have recommended reduce the amount of free radicals formed from exogenous influences or include in habitual diet nutritional supplements capable to scavenge ROS, nowadays it is well accepted which these supplements can maximize the benefits of psychopharmacological therapy, improving quality of life promoting positive changes in behavior of canines that suffering CDS [5, 57].

Within the beneficial effects attributed to the antioxidant products, could be considered potentiating of mitochondrial function during aging, which resulting in decreased production of ROS [2-3,8,58]. As a result of these effects, some authors have suggested that dogs suffering CDS, and have received a supplement of antioxidants in diet, show an improvement in cognitive ability [59]. Besides, a variety of studies have shown that intake of fruits and vegetables may decrease the risk of cognitive declines associated with age in rodents, dogs, and even humans, attributing this property to its antioxidant and anti-inflammatory capabilities [3,5,58].

There are several compounds which have been described their antioxidant activity, among them we can mention the vitamins E and C, beta-carotene, selenium, L-carnitine and alpha lipoic acid, all them have shown to improve mitochondrial function and likely by some neuroprotective effect it is explains the improvement of memory. Similarly, some authors suggest that GingkoBiloba, besides possessing antioxidant effect, has a variety of properties such as anti-inflammatory, cerebral vasodilator, mitochondrial function enhancer and MAO enzyme inhibitor [3,13,60], therefore, it has been suggested that GingkoBiloba could reduce the severity of clinical symptoms observed in patients with CSD. Additionally, natural compounds of animal origin, such as propolis, which our research group studies its neuroprotective properties, currently are valued for their antioxidant and neuroprotective qualities [61], however, there are still no studies describing the positive effects of this compound on CDS.

Other group of compounds with ROS activity is composed of certain molecules classified as mitochondrial cofactors (acidolipoico, L-carnitine) which can potentiate the function of mitochondria, resulting in a lower production of ROS during aerobic respiration. Nutritional supplementation with these mitochondrial cofactors induces their cell acumulation where they restore mitochondrial efficiency and reduces oxidative damage to RNA [62]. It has also been suggested the use of mitochondrial cofactors along with antioxidants, in order to cause an improvement in learning processes and memory, through a synergistic action [19].

It is probably the best evidence of positive effect of dietary supplementation on cognitive impairment in dogs, was found after applying neuropsychological tests for a period exceeding two years. The study aimed to supplement diet of dogs with mitochondrial cofactors and antioxidants of broad spectrum to enhance antioxidant defenses and reduce ROS accumulation. Results indicated that these products slowed the age associated cognitive decline [3]. However, to develop a diet supplemented with antioxidants, it should be noted that the selection of components, the ranges of dosage and route of administration, vary considerably between species. Also, some antioxidants are absorbed more quickly than others, species-specific factors, metabolic differences due to inherent bioavailability: thus, different species may benefit from different types of antioxidants, but not all species may benefit from the same antioxidants [2].

Author details

Camilo Orozco Sanabria, Francisco Olea and Manuel Rojas

Departamento de Ciencias para la Salud Animal, Facultad de Medicina Veterinaria y de Zootecnia, Universidad Nacional de Colombia, Sede Bogota, Colombia

References

[1] Neilson J, Hart B, Cliff K, Ruehl W. Prevalence of behavioral changes associated with age-related cognitive impairment in dogs. JAVMA 2001; 218(11):1787-1791.

[2] Head E, Zicker S. Nutraceuticals, aging, and cognitive dysfunction. Vet Clin North Am Small Anim Pract 2004; (34):217-228.

[3] Landsberg G. Therapeutic agents for the treatment of cognitive dysfunction syndrome in senior dogs. Prog Neuropsychopharmacol Biol Psychiatry 2005; 29(3): 471-479.

[4] Ruehl WW, Bruyette DS, DePaoli A, Cotman CW, Head E, Milgram NW, Cummings BJ. Canine cognitive dysfunction as a model for human age-related cognitive decline, dementia and Alzheimer's disease: clinical presentation, cognitive testing, pathology and response to l-deprenyl therapy. Prog Brain Res 1995; (106):217-225.

[5] Zicker S. Cognitive and behavioral assessment in dogs and pet food market applications. Prog Neuropsycho Biol Psychiatry 2005; (29): 455-459.

[6] Koppang N. Canine ceroid lipofuscinososis-a model for human neuronal ceroid lipofuscinososis and aging. Mech Ageing Dev. 1973; 2:421-445.

[7] Ruehl WW, Bruyette DS, De Paoli A, Cotman CW, Head E, Milgran NW, et al. Canine cognitive dysfunction as a model for human age-related cognitive decline, dementia and Alzheimer's disease: clinical presentation, cognitive testing, pathology and response to l-deprenyl therapy. Prog Brain Res 1995; 106:217-225.

[8] Ruehl WW, Hart BL. Canine cognitive dysfunction. In: Dodman N, Shuster L, eds. Psychopharmacology of animal behavior disorders. Malden, Mass: Blackwell Scientific Publications, 1998; 283-304.

[9] Chan A, Nippak P, Murphey H, Ikeda-Douglas C, Muggenburg B, Head E, Cotman C, Milgram N. Visuospatial impairments in aged canines (Canis familairis): the role of cognitive behavioral therapy. Behav. Neurosci. 2002; 116: 443-454.

[10] Head E. Brian aging in dogs: Parallels with human brain aging and Alzheimer's disease. Vet Ther 2001; 2(3):247-260.

[11] Shettleworth SJ. Animal cognition and animal behaviour. Anim Behav 2001; 61(2): 277-286.

[12] Boutet I, Ryan M, Kulaga V, McShane C, Christie LA, Freedman M, Milgram NW. Age-associated cognitive deficits in humans and dogs: a comparative neuropsychological approach. Prog Neuropsychopharmacol Biol Psychiatry 2005; 29(3):433-441.

[13] Osella M, Re G, Odore R, Girardi C, Badino P, Barbero R, et.al. Canine cognitive dysfunction syndrome: Prevalence, clinical signs and treatment with a neuroprotective Natraceutical. Appl Anim Behav Sci 2007; (105):297-310.

[14] Frank D. Cognitive dysfunction in dog. In: Hill's European Symposia on Canine Brain Ageing (en línea) 2002. (fecha de acceso 27 de mayo de 2009). URL disponible en: http://www.ivis.org/proceedings/Hills/brain/frank.pdf?LA=1.

[15] Rofina JE, van der Meer I, Goossens M, Secrève M, Ederen van AM, Schilder M, et.al. Preliminary inquiry to assess behavior changes in aging pet dogs. En: Bely M, Apathy A editores. Amyloid and Amyloidosis IX; Budapest, Hungary: Apathy A editores; 2001.

[16] Peinado MA, del Moral ML, Esteban FJ, Martínez Lara E, Siles E, Jiménez A, et.al. Envejecimiento y neurodegeneración: bases moleculares y celulares. Rev Neurol 2000; 31(11):1054-1065.

[17] Frank D. Cognitive dysfunction in dog. In: Hill's European Symposia on Canine Brain Ageing (en línea) 2002. (fecha de acceso 27 de mayo de 2009). URL disponible en: http://www.ivis.org/proceedings/Hills/brain/frank.pdf?LA=1.

[18] Landsberg G, Ruehl W. Geriatric behavioral problems. Vet Clin North Am Small Anim Pract 1997; 27(6):1537-1559.

[19] Cummings BJ, Su JH, Cotman CW, White R, Russell M. b-Amyloid accumulation in aged canine brain. A model of early plaque formation in Alzheimer's disease. Neurobiol Aging 1993; (14):547-556.

[20] Gerosa R. Geriatría canina: trastornos y lesiones orgánicas en perros de edad avanzada. Buenos Aires: Ed Interamerica; 2007.

[21] Organización de las Naciones Unidas ONU. Follow-up to the 2nd World Assembly on ageing: Report of the secretary-general 2009; http://documents.un.org/mother.asp.

[22] Association AVM. US Pet Ownership & Demographics Sourcebook. Schaumburg, Illinois: American Veterinary Medical Association; 1997

[23] Pérez-guisado J. El Síndrome de disfunción cognitiva en el perro. Disponible en. RECVET (en línea) 2007 (fecha de acceso 05 de junio de 2009); 2(01-04). URL disponible en: http://www.veterinaria.org/revistas/recvet/n01a0407/01a040701.pdf.

[24] Pérez J. La descripción de los ovillos neurofibrilares en la enfermedad de Alzheimer. Rev Esp Patol 2007; (40)1:60-65.

[25] Cummings BJ, Satou T, Head E, Milgram NW, Cole GM, Savage MJ, et.al. Diffuse plaques contain C-terminal Ab 42 and not Ab 40: evidence from cats and dogs. Neurobiol Aging 1996; 17(4):653-659.

[26] Dimakopoulos A, Mayer R. Aspects of Neurodegeneration in the Canine Brain. J Nutr 2002; 132(Supl 1):1579-1582.

[27] Head E, Callahan H, Muggenburg BA, Cotman CW, Milgram NW. Visual-discriminación learning ability and beta-amyloid accumulation in the dog. Neurobiol Aging 1998; 19(5):415-425.

[28] Colle MA, Hauw JJ, Crespeau F, Uchiara T, Akiyama H, Checler F, et al. Vascular and parenchymal Ab deposition in the aging dog: correlation with behavior. Neurobiol Aging 2000; (21):695-704.

[29] Pageat P. Description, clinical and histological validation of the A.R.C.A.D. score (evaluation of age-related cognitive and affective disorders). En: Lynne Seibert DVM, MS editors. Newsletter of the American Veterinary Society of Animal Behavior. Third International Congress on Behavioural Medicine; Boston 7-8 de Agosto de 2001. Boston: Lynne Seibert DVM, MS editors; 2001.

[30] Dimakopoulos A, Mayer R. Aspects of Neurodegeneration in the Canine Brain. J Nutr 2002; 132(Supl 1):1579-1582.

[31] Cotman C, Head E, Muggenburg B, Zicker S, Milgram N. Brain aging in the canine: a diet enriched in antioxidants reduces cognitive dysfunction. Neurobiol Aging 2002; (23):809-818.

[32] Kiatipattanasakul W, Nakamura S, Kuroki K, Nakayama H, Doi K. Immunohistochemical detection of anti-oxidative stress enzymes in the dog brain. Neuropathology 1997; (17):307-12.

[33] Pugliese M, Gangitano C, Ceccariglia S, Carrasco J, Rodríguez M, Michetti F, et.al. Canine cognitive dysfunction and the cerebellum: Acetylcholinesterase reduction, neuronal and glial changes. Brain Res Rev 2007; (1139):85-94.

[34] Lieberman D, Mody I, Pike C, Cotman C. â-Amyloid (25-35) prolongs opening of NMDA channels through an intracellular pathway. Soc Neurosci 1994; (20):602.

[35] Cotman C, Head E, Muggenburg B, Zicker S, Milgram N. Brain aging in the canine: a diet enriched in antioxidants reduces cognitive dysfunction. Neurobiology of Aging. 2002; 23: 809-818.

[36] Dimakopoulos A, Mayer R. Aspects of Neurodegeneration in the Canine Brain. J. Nutr. 2002; 132: 1579S-1582.

[37] Pugliese M, Gangitano C, Ceccariglia S, Carrasco J, Rodríguez M, Michetti F, et al. Canine cognitive dysfunction and the cerebellum: Acetylcholinesterase reduction, neuronal and glial changes. B. Resear. 2007; 1139: 85-94. 45.

[38] Borrá D, Ferrer I, Pumarola. Age-related Changes in the Brain of the Dog. Vet Pathol. 1999; 36: 202-211.

[39] Galdzicki Z, Fukuyama R, Wadhwani K, Rapoport S, Ehrenstein G. b-Amyloid increases choline conductance of PC12 cells: Possible mechanism of toxicity in Alzheimer's disease. Brain Research 1994; 646: 332- 336.

[40] Kiatipattanasakul W, Nakamura S, Hossain M, Nakayama H, Uchino T, Shumiya S, et al. Apoptosis in the aged dog brain. Acta Neuropathol. 1996; 92: 242-248.

[41] Rofina JE, Singh K, Skoumalova-Vesela A, van Ederen AM, van Asten AJ, Wilhelm J, Gruys E. Histochemical accumulation of oxidative damage products is associated with Alzheimer-like pathology in the canine. Amyloid. 2004; 11: 90-100.

[42] Su JH, Anderson AJ, Cummings BJ, Cotman CW. Immunohistochemical evidence for apoptosis in Alzheimer's disease. Neuro Report. 1994; 5: 2529- 2533.

[43] Trojanowski JQ, Schmidt ML, Shin R-W, Bramblett GT, Goedert M, Lee VM-Y. PHFT (A68): From pathological marker to potential mediator of neuronal dysfunction and degeneration in Alzheimer's disease. Clin Neurosci. 1993; 1:184-191.

[44] Goedert M. Tau protein and the neurofibrillary pathology of Alzheimer's disease. Trends Neurosci. 1993; 16: 460-65.

[45] Pérez J. La descripción de los ovillos neurofibrilares en la enfermedad de Alzheimer. Rev Esp Patol. 2007; 40: 60-65.

[46] Ashford JW, Schmitt F, Kumar V. Diagnosis of Alzheimer's disease. In: Kumar V, Eisdorfer C, eds. Advances in the diagnosis and treatment of Alzheimer's disease. New York: Springer Publishing Co. 1998; 111-136.

[47] Rinne JO. Muscarinic and dopaminergic receptors in ageing human brain. Brain Res. 1987;404: 161-168.

[48] Neilson J, Hart B, Cliff K, Ruehl W. Prevalence of behavioral changes associated with age-related cognitive impairment in dogs. JAVMA. 2001; 218: 1787-1791.

[49] Studzinski C, Araujo J, Milgram N. The canine model of human Cognitive aging and dementia: Pharmacological validity of the model for assessment of human cognitive-enhancing drugs. Progr Neuro-Psychoph Biol Psych. 2005; 29: 489-498.

[50] Adams B, Chan A, Callahan H, Siwak C, Tapp D, Ikeda-Douglas C, et al. Spatial learning and memory in the dog as a model of cognitive aging. Behav Brain Res 2000; 108(1):47-56.

[51] Milgram NW, Head E, Weiner E, Thomas E. Cognitive functions and aging in the dog: acquisition of nonspatial visual tasks. Behav Neurosci 1994; (108):57-68.

[52] Uchino T, Kida M, Baba A, Ishii K, Okawa N, Hayashi Y, Shumiya S. Senile dementia in aged dogs and the diagnostic standards. Proceedings of the 17th Symposium of Japan Society for Biomedical Gerontology. Biomed Gerontol 1995; (19):24-31.

[53] Pageat P. Description, clinical and histological validation of the A.R.C.A.D. score (evaluation of age-related cognitive and affective disorders). En: Lynne Seibert DVM, MS editors. Newsletter of the American Veterinary Society of Animal Behavior. Third International Congress on Behavioural Medicine; Boston 7-8 de Agosto de 2001. Boston: Lynne Seibert DVM, MS editors; 2001.

[54] Orozco C, de Los Rios C, Arias E, León R, García AG, Marco JL, Villarroya M, López MG. ITH4012 (ethyl 5-amino-6,7,8,9-tetrahydro-2-methyl-4-phenylbenzol(1,8)naph-

thyridine-3-carboxylate), a novel acetylcholinesterase inhibitor with "calcium promotor" and neuroprotective properties. J Pharmacol Exp Ther. 2004 Sep;310(3):987-94

[55] Orozco C, García-de-Diego AM, Arias E, Hernández-Guijo JM, García AG, Villarroya M, López MG. Depolarization preconditioning produces cytoprotection against veratridine-induced chromaffin cell death. Eur J Pharmacol. 2006 Dec 28;553(1-3):28-38

[56] Campbell S, Trettien A, Kozan B. A non comparative open-label study evaluating the effect of selegiline hydrocloride in a clinical setting. Vet Ther 2001; (2):24-39.

[57] Head E. Oxidative Damage and Cognitive Dysfunction: Antioxidant Treatments to Promote Healthy Brain Aging. Neurochem Res 2009; (34): 670-678.

[58] Cotman C, Head E, Muggenburg B, Zicker S, Milgram N. Brain aging in the canine: a diet enriched in antioxidants reduces cognitive dysfunction. Neurobiol Aging 2002; (23):809-818.

[59] Head E, Liu J, Hagen T, Muggenburg B, Milgram N, Ames B, Cotman C. Oxidative damage increases with age in a canine model of human brain aging. J Neurochem 2002; (82): 375-381.

[60] Launer LJ, Andersen K, Dewey M, Lettenneur L, Ott A, Amaducci L. Rates and risk factors for dementia and Alzheimer's disease. Results from EURODEM pooled analyses. Neurology 1999; (52):78-74.

[61] Shimazawa M, Chikamatsu S, Morimoto N, Mishima S, Nagai H, Hara H. Neuroprotection by Brazilian Green Propolis against In vitro and In vivo Ischemic Neuronal Damage. Ecam 2005; 2(2):201-207.

[62] Liu J, Killilea DW, Ames BN. Age-associated mitochondrial oxidative decay: improvement of carnitine acetyltransferase substrate-binding affinity and activity in brain by feeding old rats acetyl-L-carnitine and/or R-alpha -lipoic acid. Proc Natl Acad Sci USA 2002; 99(4):1876-1881.